FAMILY HEALTH CARE NURSING

Theory, Practice and Research

4th Edition

FAMILY HEALTH CARE NURSING

Theory, Practice and Research

4th Edition

Joanna Rowe Kaakinen, PhD, RN
Professor, School of Nursing
University of Portland
Portland, Oregon

Vivian Gedaly-Duff, DNSc, RN
Associate Professor, School of Nursing
Oregon Health & Science University
Portland, Oregon

Deborah Padgett Coehlo, PhD, RN, PNP
Assistant Professor, Family Studies
Oregon State University
Bend, Oregon

Shirley May Harmon Hanson, PMHNP, PhD, RN, FAAN, CFLE, LMFT
Professor Emerita, School of Nursing
Oregon Health & Science University
Portland, Oregon

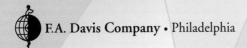

F.A. Davis Company • Philadelphia

F. A. Davis Company
1915 Arch Street
Philadelphia, PA 19103
www.fadavis.com

Printed in the United States of America

Last digit indicates print number: 10 9 8 7 6 5 4 3 2 1

Publisher, Nursing: Joanne Patzek DaCunha, RN, MSN
Director of Content Development: Darlene D. Pedersen
Senior Project Editor: Padraic J. Maroney
Design and Illustrations Manager: Carolyn O'Brien

As new scientific information becomes available through basic and clinical research, recommended treatments and drug therapies undergo changes. The author(s) and publisher have done everything possible to make this book accurate, up to date, and in accord with accepted standards at the time of publication. The author(s), editors, and publisher are not responsible for errors or omissions or for consequences from application of the book, and make no warranty, expressed or implied, in regard to the contents of the book. Any practice described in this book should be applied by the reader in accordance with professional standards of care used in regard to the unique circumstances that may apply in each situation. The reader is advised always to check product information (package inserts) for changes and new information regarding dose and contraindications before administering any drug. Caution is especially urged when using new or infrequently ordered drugs.

Library of Congress Cataloging-in-Publication Data

Family health care nursing : theory, practice, and research / [edited by] Joanna Rowe Kaakinen . . . [et at.]. — 4th ed.
        p. ; cm.
    Includes bibliographical references and indexes.
    ISBN 978-0-8036-2166-4
    1. Family nursing. 2. Families—Health and hygiene. I. Kaakinen, Joanna Rowe, 1951-
    [DNLM: 1. Family Nursing. 2. Family. WY 159.5 F1985 2010]
    RT120. F34F35 2010
    610.73—dc22

                                                                                    2009043352

I am blessed with loving, supportive, and compassionate family. Without my family, I would not be who I am today. My family gave me time to write, brought in take-out dinners, shared my home office (quietly most of the time), and always asked about "the book." I love my family and want to dedicate this book to my husband John, my son Thomas, my sister Vicki, my brother-in-law Peter, my nephew Scott and his wife Subin, and Christopher—my nephew who dedicated his short life to his children. Your love helps me be all that is possible. Blessings and Namaste.

Joanna Rowe Kaakinen

This is a special dedication to my parents, Hazel and Al Gedaly, and my husband, Robert W. Duff. By the time I was twenty years old, my family had lived in California, New York, Kentucky, Austria, Washington, Morocco, New Mexico, Spain, Germany, and England. Travel meant seeing in new ways. My parents' "being there" and sense of "adventure" provided stability and ignited my curiosity to learn. Whenever I lament, "I haven't gone anywhere," my husband laughs out loud, reminding me in his teasing, that I just returned from a conference 3000 miles away that included a Broadway theater show. In the tapestry of family life, families experience big things like travel that are the pictures. The laughter, the sharing of worries and hopes with family and friends are the threads that weave the pictures together. My parents, my husband, my family are my threads, knotted together into a colorful textured fabric. Upon the mind's eye, the colors shift, some images come into focus while others recede as the eye and heart move to different moments in family life. My thread, added to the others, strengthens the tapestry cloth, and as I follow my thread woven to the others, I have a "sense of place in the world."

Vivian Gedaly-Duff

This is a special dedication to my family, who has inspired my life long journey to learn about and help families grow together across the life span. My brother taught me to fight for what I believe in. My sisters taught me to cherish female friendships. My dad taught me to care for all, even the downtrodden. My mom taught me to use my brain with my heart, always. My husband taught me to love in the midst of all other emotions. And, my daughters—well, they taught me the most about loving and living and dedicating my work to their lives. Yes, family brings joy and pain, and it just does not get any better.

Deborah Padgett Coehlo

To dedicate a book is one way to acknowledge and pay tribute to those who played a significant role in one's personal and professional life. I am grateful to my *family of origin* including my deceased parents who gave me three loving and supportive sisters. My sisters continue to validate me as a person and professional. Thank you—Marjorie, Peggy, and Kathleen. In my *family of procreation*, I was blessed with two children, Derek and Gwen, who grew up to be more than I deserved and who presented me with three beautiful grandsons to love and cherish. I am also indebted to the children, couples, and families for whom I served as nurse practitioner and marriage/child/family therapist over many years. They all taught me the various meanings and ways of what is takes to be a "family." Finally, I dedicate this book to the many hundreds of nursing and child/family therapy students I was privileged to mentor over 49 years of professional life. These students now stand on my shoulders in service to families across the globe and serve as mentors to the next generation of clinicians and teachers of family nursing and family therapy. May their journey be as blessed as mine!

Shirley May Harmon Hanson

I am especially honored to write the foreword for this fourth edition of *Family Health Care Nursing: Theory, Practice and Research*. It seems odd to write the foreword for your own book, but as I near the end of my long nursing and academic career, it is a treasured time and opportunity to share my vision and commitment with my co-editors, the contributors of this edition, and future nurses.

Merriam-Webster defines *compendious* to mean "concise and comprehensive." *Family Health Care Nursing: Theory, Practice and Research* (editions 1-4) is an ever changing compendious textbook originally developed to reflect the state of the art and science of family nursing. This all-inclusive, far-reaching approach has continued throughout the history of this textbook. As the original title implied, the book represents an integration of theory, practice, and research pertaining to family nursing. With today's vernacular, we could easily rename this textbook "Theory-Guided Evidence-Based Nursing Practice With Families."

This is the **fourth** edition of this distinctive textbook, all of which were published by F. A. Davis Company. This book originated when I was teaching family nursing at Oregon Health and Science University (OHSU) School of Nursing in Portland, Oregon. At that time, no comprehensive or authoritative textbook on the nursing care of families was available that matched our program of study. This was the impetus I needed to write and edit the first edition of *Family Health Care Nursing: Theory, Practice and Research*. The first edition met a need of nursing educators in many other schools around the world. F. A. Davis asked me to revise and update the second edition, which was published in 2001 (Hanson, 2001). For the third edition (Hanson, Gedaly-Duff, & Kaakinen, 2005), I invited two trustworthy colleagues to help write and edit the book: Dr. Vivian Gedaly-Duff from OHSU and Dr. Joanna Rowe Kaakinen from the University of Portland (UP). The *Instructors' Manual*, a new

feature of the third edition, was developed by Dr. Deborah Coehlo from Oregon State University (OSU). The result of collaboration with additional nursing scholars elevated the integrity of the textbook. For this fourth edition, our professional collaboration has resulted in yet another cutting edge family nursing textbook. Our working team remained the same, but our roles for this edition shifted as I retired from active teaching and began to bring closure to my professional practice. Dr. Joanna Rowe Kaakinen (UP) is the lead editor for this fourth edition (Kaakinen, Gedaly-Duff, Coehlo, & Hanson, 2009), with the editorial team of Dr. Vivian Gedaly-Duff (OHSU), Dr. Deborah Padgett Coehlo (OSU), and myself, Professor Emerita (retired from OHSU). In addition, the *Instructors' Manual* was written by Dr. Deborah Coehlo with contributions by Diane Bauer, MS, RN, from Oregon Health & Science University and Kari Firestone, MSN, RN, from the University of Portland.

The first three editions were recognized as excellent family nursing texts. These editions received awards, including the *American Journal of Nursing* Book of the Year Award and the Nursing Outlook Brandon Selected Nursing Books Award. Every new edition has been well received around the world, and every edition has brought forth new converts to family nursing. The previous editions of the text have been translated into Japanese and Portuguese. More recently, the book was published in India, Pakistan, Bangladesh, Burma, Bhutan, and Nepal. I anticipate even more international interest in this fourth edition as the message of family nursing spreads across the world.

Contributors to this edition were selected from among distinguished practitioners, researchers, theorists, scholars, and teachers from nursing, as well as family social scientists across the United States, Canada, and England. Like many textbooks, some of the contributors have changed over time for a variety of reasons. As family nursing evolved over time, more authors were added to the writing team. For example, the third edition had 28 contributors, and the fourth edition has 37 contributors. In total there are 26 *new* contributors in this fourth edition. This textbook is a massive undertaking that involved many committed nurses and family scholars. The four book editors are grateful for this national and international dedication to family nursing. Together, we continue to increase nursing knowledge pertaining to the nursing care of families.

This fourth edition builds on the previous editions. The primary shift in the direction of the book for this edition is to make family nursing practice more meaningful and realistic for nursing students. The first unit of the fourth edition of this family nursing textbook sets the critical foundational knowledge pertaining to families and the nursing of families. The second unit concentrates on theory-guided, evidence-based practice of the nursing care of families across the life span and in a variety of specialties. Important new chapters have been added to this edition: Culturally Sensitive Nursing Care of Families, Canadian Context of Family Nursing, Families in Palliative and End-of-Life Care, Nursing Care of Families in Disaster and War, and Advancing Family Nursing. The chapters that were retained from the third edition have been rewritten to emphasize more fully the latest practice of family nursing. New features of this edition include:

- A strong emphasis on evidence-based practice in each chapter
- Five selected family nursing theories interwoven throughout the book
- Family case studies that demonstrate the practice of family nursing
- Content that addresses families and nursing in both Canada and the United States

Family nursing as an art and science has transformed in response to paradigm shifts in the profession and in society over time. As a nursing student in one of the earliest baccalaureate programs in the United States during the 1950s, the focus of care was on individuals and was centered in hospitals. As time passed and the profession matured, nursing education and practice expanded and shifted to more family-centered care and community-based nursing. My first master's degree was from the University of Washington in Community Health Nursing/Public Health. Ever since, I have felt like a "family nurse"

even though this paradigm of nursing practice was only recently called *family nursing*. The codified version of family nursing really emerged and peaked during the 1980s and 1990s in the United States and Canada, where the movement was headquartered. Even though this initial impetus for family nursing came from North America, the concept spread quickly worldwide. Asian countries, in particular, embraced these ideas and translated the English-language North American textbooks to their own languages. In actuality, many Asian and other worldwide countries already practiced family nursing, but they had not yet formally taught family nursing in their educational institutions. Nursing schools in other countries incorporated family nursing into their own educational curriculums. Now, family nursing textbooks and journals are being published in multiple languages as other countries conduct their own family nursing research and tailor family nursing to their unique countries and populations. Some other English-speaking countries continue to modify the North American versions of textbooks for their nursing programs. Today, it could be said that *family nursing is without borders,* and that no one country owns family nursing!

My final point about the historical development of modern family nursing is about the establishment of an international family nursing association. Internationally, family nursing theory, practice, and research has been heavily influenced by the startup of a series of nationwide workshops in the United States. This was then followed by international family nursing conferences consequently held in Canada, United States, Chile, Thailand, and Iceland. The next International Family Nursing Conference will be held in Japan in 2011. As a result of these international conferences, a group of family nurses from several countries has been charged with developing bylaws for a new, more structured format by creating an international family nursing organization that will ensure continuity of family nursing over time. This new professional body will presumably assume the leadership for keeping family nursing at the forefront of theory development, practice, research, education, and social policy.

Family nursing has become more than just a "buzzword," it is a reality. Family nursing is practiced internationally in many educational institutions, many health care settings, and by many nurses. Most everyone in the nursing profession agrees that a profound, reciprocal relationship exists among families, health, and nursing.

This book and this current edition recognize that nursing as a profession has a close alignment with families because nurses share many of the responsibilities that families have for the care and protection of their family members. Nurses have an obligation to help families promote and advance the care and growth of both individual family members and families as a unit. This textbook provides nursing students the knowledge base and the processes to become effective in their nursing care with families. In addition, families can benefit when already registered nurses use this knowledge to reorganize their nursing practice to be more family centered and to develop working partnerships with families to strengthen family systems. *Family Health Care Nursing: Theory, Practice and Research,* 4th edition, is written for nurses by nurses who practice and study the nursing of families. Students will learn how to tailor their assessment and interventions with families in health and illness, in physical and mental health, across the life span, and in the settings in which nurses and families interface. I firmly believe that this fourth edition of this textbook is at the cutting edge of this practice challenge for the next decade, and will help to marshal the nursing profession toward providing better nursing care of families here in North America and in other countries across the world.

Shirley May Harmon Hanson, PMHNP, PhD, RN, FAAN, CFLE, LMFT
Professor Emerita, Oregon Health and Science University School of Nursing

If you asked anyone to tell you of a time they were affected by something that happened to one of their family members, you would be overwhelmed with the intensity of the emotions and the exhaustive details. Everyone is influenced significantly by their families and the structure, function, and processes within their families. Even individuals who do not interact with their families have been shaped by their families. The importance and connection between individuals and their families have been studied expansively in a variety of disciplines, including nursing.

The importance of working in partnerships with families in the health care system seems so obvious, yet many health care providers view dealing with patients' families as an extra burden and way too demanding. Some nurses are baffled when a family acts or reacts in certain ways that are foreign to their own professional and personal family experiences. Some nurses avoid the tensions and anxiety that exist in families during a crisis situation. But it is in just such situations that families most need nurses' understanding, knowledge, and guidance. The purpose of this book is to provide nursing students, as well as practicing nurses, knowledge to practice family nursing. This fourth edition of the textbook focuses on theory-guided, evidence-based practice of the nursing care of families throughout the family life cycle and across a variety of clinical specialties.

Family Health Care Nursing: Theory, Practice and Research, 4th edition, is organized so that it can be used in its entirety for a course in family nursing. An alternative approach for the use of this text is for students to purchase the book at the beginning of their program of study so that specific chapters can be assigned for specialty courses throughout the curriculum. For example, Chapter 16, Family Mental Health Nursing, would be assigned when students took their mental health nursing course, and Chapter 13, Family Child Health Nursing,

would be studied during a pediatric rotation. Thus this textbook could be integrated throughout the undergraduate or graduate nursing curriculum.

Moreover, this fourth edition builds on successes of the past editions. In response to the needs of families and the changing dynamics of the health care system, the editors added new chapters, consolidated chapters and deleted some old chapters. The new chapters include Culturally Sensitive Nursing Care of Families (Chapter 6), Canadian Context of Family Nursing (Chapter 7), Families in Palliative and End-of-Life Care (Chapter 11), Nursing Care of Families in Disaster and War (Chapter 18), and Advancing Family Nursing (Chapter 19). The previous chapter on family social policy is expanded to the new Chapter 5, Family Social Policy and Health Disparities. New also to this edition is the inclusion of Canadian content. The chapters that most directly include Canadian information are Demography and Family Health (Chapter 2), Culturally Sensitive Nursing Care of Families (Chapter 6), Canadian Context of Family Nursing (Chapter 7), and Advancing Family Nursing (Chapter 19). The introductory chapter has been updated to help streamline the book and also combines content from two chapters contained in the third edition: Family Health Care Nursing: An Introduction and Family Structure, Function, and Process.

Each chapter begins with the critical concepts that are addressed within that chapter. The purpose of placing the critical concepts at the beginning of the chapter is to help focus the readers' thinking and learning. Another organizing framework for the book is initially presented in Chapter 3, Theoretical Foundations for the Nursing of Families. This chapter covers the importance of using theory to guide the nursing of families and presents five theoretical perspectives with a case study demonstrating how to apply these five theoretical approaches in practice. These five theories are then threaded throughout the book and are used for examples in many of the chapter case studies. Most chapters have a case study designed to demonstrate theory-guided, evidence-based nursing practice. All of the case studies contain family genograms and ecomaps.

The main body of the book is divided into four units: Unit 1: Foundations in Family Health Care Nursing, which includes Chapters 1 to 5; Unit 2: Families Across the Health Continuum, which includes Chapters 6 to 11; Unit 3: Nursing Care of Families in Clinical Areas, which includes Chapters 12 to 18; and Unit 4: Looking to the Future, which concludes the book with one chapter that addresses advancing family nursing. In addition to the text, the *Family Health Care Nursing Instructors' Manual* is an online faculty guide that provides assistance to faculty using/teaching family nursing or the nursing care of families in a variety of settings. The *Instructors' Manual* (IM) contains a summary of each chapter with study questions, discussion guides, exam questions, a case study, teaching strategies, and most importantly, a teacher's guide, including a PowerPoint presentation.

UNIT 1: FOUNDATIONS IN FAMILY HEALTH CARE NURSING

Chapter 1: Family Health Care Nursing: An Introduction provides foundational materials essential to understanding families and nursing. Three nursing scholars were involved in writing this chapter: Joanna Rowe Kaakinen, PhD, RN, Professor at the University of Portland School of Nursing; Shirley May Harmon Hanson, PMHNP, PhD, RN, FAAN, CFLE, LMFT, Professor Emerita, Oregon Health and Science University School of Nursing; and Sharon A. Denham, DSN, RN, Professor, School of Nursing, Ohio University.

The first half of the chapter discusses dimensions of family nursing and defines family, family health, and healthy families. Family health care nursing and the nature of interventions in the nursing care of families is explained, together with the four approaches to family nursing (context, client, system, and component of society). The chapter then presents the concepts or variables that influence family nursing, family nursing roles, obstacles to family nursing practice, and the history of family nursing.

The second half of the chapter elaborates on theoretical ideas involved with understanding family structure, family functions, and family processes. All three of these family concepts enable readers to comprehend changing dimensions inherent within families and family systems. This section of the chapter is explicated in detail, and is essential knowledge for students of family nursing and family social science.

Chapter 2: Demography and Family Health provides nurses with a basic contextual orientation to the demographics of families and health. Three sociologists joined to update and write this chapter: Lynne M. Casper, PhD, Professor of Sociology and Director of the South California Population Research Center, University of Southern California (USC); John G. Haaga, PhD, Deputy Director, Behavior and Social Research at the National Institute on Aging; and Radheeka R. Jayasundera, BS, graduate student/research assistant, Population Research Center at USC Department of Sociology. All three authors are experts in statistics and demographics of families. The purpose of this chapter is to present changing family demographics in the United States and Canada, as well as discuss trends of population health in both of these countries. This information includes: (1) changing economy and society, such as changing family norms, the aging society, immigration, and ethnic diversity; (2) living arrangements of the elderly, young adults, and unmarried couples; (3) parenting by unmarried couples living together, single mothers, single fathers, and grandparents; and (4) trends in population health. The last section of the chapter, pertaining to trends in population health, discusses overall trends in life expectancy/disability, obesity, adult behavioral risk factors, child health, and adolescent health. Each section concludes with relevant implications for nurses working with families.

Chapter 3: Theoretical Foundations for the Nursing of Families is coauthored by two of the editors of this textbook: Joanna Rowe Kaakinen, PhD, RN, Professor, University of Portland School of Nursing, and Shirley May Harmon Hanson, RN, PMHNP, PhD, FAAN, LMFT, CFLE, Professor Emerita, Oregon Health and Science University School of Nursing. This chapter lays the groundwork for the theoretical foundation needed to practice family nursing. The introduction builds a case for why nurses need to understand the interactive relationship among theory, practice, and research. It also makes the point that no single theory adequately describes the complex relationships of family structure, function, and processes. Theories, concepts, propositions, hypotheses, and conceptual models are defined and explained. Selected for this textbook, and explained in this chapter, are five theoretical/conceptual models: *Family Systems Theory, Developmental and Family Life Cycle Theory, Bioecological Theory, Family Cycle of Health and Illness Model,* and the *Family Assessment and Intervention Model.* Starting with a basic family case study, each of the five theories assists readers understanding of how each theoretical model could be used to assess and plan interventions for this exemplar family. This approach enables learners to see how different interventions are derived from different theoretical perspectives. Each theoretical approach provides a rich opportunity for learning the difficult subject of theories and their usefulness in planning care.

Chapter 4: Family Nursing Process: Family Nursing Assessment Models is authored by Joanna Rowe Kaakinen, PhD, RN, Professor, University of Portland School of Nursing. The purpose of this chapter is to present a systematic approach to thinking about and working with families to develop a plan of action for the family to address its most pressing needs. This author built on the traditional nursing process model as visualized by recent nursing scholars to create a "dynamic systematic family nursing process" approach. Assessment strategies are presented, including how to select assessment instruments, determine the need for interpreters, assess for health literacy, and learn how to diagram family genograms and ecomaps. The chapter also explores ways to involve families in shared decision making. Analysis is a critical step in the family nursing process that helps focus the nurse and the family on identification of the family's primary concern(s). Intervention strategies are discussed, including the family action plan. The chapter uses a family case study as an exemplar to demonstrate the family nursing process. The chapter concludes with a brief introduction to three family assessment and intervention models developed by nurses: *Family Assessment and Intervention Model and Family Systems Stressor-Strength Inventory (FS³I), Friedman's Family Assessment Model,* and *Calgary Family Assessment Model (CFAM) and Calgary Family Intervention Model (CFIM).*

Chapter 5: Family Social Policy and Health Disparities exposes nurses to social issues that affect the health of families and strongly challenges nurses to become more involved in the political aspects of health policy. This chapter is coauthored by two experienced nurses in the social policy arena: Lorraine B. Sanders, DNSc, CNM, FNP-BC,

PMHNP, RN, Associate Professor, Hunter Bellevue School of Nursing, and Kristine M. Gebbie, DrPH, RN, FAAN, Joan Grabe (Acting) Dean, School of Nursing at Hunter College. These authors discuss the practice of family nursing within the social and political structure of society. They encourage the readers to understand their own biases and how these contribute to health disparities. In this chapter, students learn about the complex components that contribute to health disparities. Nurses are called to become politically active, advocate for vulnerable families, and assist in the development of creative alternatives to social policies that limit access to quality care and resources. These authors present the difficulties families face in the current political climate as the legal definition of family is being challenged. Social policies, or lack of them, are discussed, specifically policies that affect education, socioeconomic status, and health insurance.

The chapter also explores determinants of health disparities, which include infant mortality rates, obesity, asthma, HIV/AIDS, aging, women's issues, and health literacy. The chapter concludes with a case study that demonstrates how quickly a family can become homeless and lose access to health care. The call to nurses to become politically active is clear throughout this chapter.

UNIT 2: FAMILIES ACROSS THE HEALTH CONTINUUM

Chapter 6: Culturally Sensitive Nursing Care of Families is coauthored by Deborah Padgett Coehlo, PhD, RN, PNP, Assistant Professor at Oregon State University, and Margaret M. Manoogian, PhD, Associate Professor in Child and Family Studies at Ohio University. This new chapter is built on the growing understanding of cultural diversity in the context of ethnicity, ability, age, family structure, socioeconomic status, and/or geographic location using family systems, development, and life span perspectives to view diversity from a family and community level. The purpose of this chapter is to present a culturally sensitive systematic approach to the nursing assessment and intervention of diverse families. Assessment strategies are presented, including how to assess families with chronic illnesses from diverse backgrounds, and how to assess cultural adaptation.

Chapter 7: Canadian Context of Family Nursing is a new chapter coauthored by Canadian nursing scholars Colleen Varcoe, PhD, RN, Associate Professor at the University of British Columbia, School of Nursing in Vancouver, British Columbia, Canada, and Gweneth Hartrick Doane, PhD, RN, Professor, School of Nursing, University of Victoria, British Columbia, Canada. The importance of attending to context in family nursing practice is the central tenet of this chapter. Specifically, these family scholars highlight the interface of sociopolitical, historical, geographic, and economic elements in shaping the health and illness experiences of families in Canada. The chapter begins by discussing why consideration of context is important to nursing. Then, some of the key characteristics of Canadian society are presented including how those characteristics shape health, families, health care, and family nursing. Finally, the authors propose how nurses might practice more responsively and effectively based on this understanding. Two family cases are presented in this chapter to show how attending to and working with families in context influences family health and the outcomes.

Chapter 8: Genomics and Family Nursing Across the Life Span is coauthored by two nurses with extensive knowledge in genomics and genetics: Janet K. Williams, PhD, RN, CGC, PNP, FAAN, who holds the Kelting Professor of Nursing at the University of Iowa, and Heather Skirton, PhD, MSc, RGN, Registered Genetic Counsellor, who is a Professor of Applied Health Genetics and the Deputy Head for Research of the School of Nursing and Community Studies at the University of Plymouth in the United Kingdom. The chapter begins with a brief introduction to genomics and genetics. The chapter, then, explains how families react to finding out they are at risk for genetic conditions, and decide how and with whom to disclose genetic information, and the critical aspect of confidentiality. The authors describe how some families decide to conceal genetic information and the processes parents undergo when deciding how to share genetic information with their children. The authors share what occurs when individuals have preselection beliefs and decide to undergo or not undergo predictive or presymptomatic testing. The components of conducting a genetic assessment and history are outlined. Interventions are offered that include education and resources. The authors use several specific case examples and a detailed case study to show the application of nurses working with families who have a genetic condition.

Chapter 9: Family Health Promotion is written by Yeoun Soo Kim-Godwin, PhD, MPH, RN, Associate Professor of Nursing, and Perri J. Bomar, PhD, RN, Professor Emeritus, who are both from the School of Nursing at the University of North Carolina, Wilmington. This chapter on family health promotion presents ways that nurses work with families to empower them to achieve healthier lives for each member and for the family as a whole. The purpose of this chapter is to introduce family health and family health models, and examine internal and external factors that influence family health promotion. External factors that influence family health promotion include health and family polices, environment, influence of the media, and science and technology. Internal factors are explained that influence family health including family type and developmental stage, lifestyle patterns, processes, personalities, role models, coping strategies, resilience, and culture. The chapter includes a case study of a family to discuss the applicable models for family assessment and interventions. In addition, this chapter discusses the role of nurses and intervention strategies in maintaining and regaining the highest level of family health. Specific interventions presented include family empowerment, anticipatory guidance, offering information, and encouraging family rituals, routines, and time together.

Chapter 10: Families with Chronic Illness is coauthored by Sharon A. Denham, DSN, RN, Professor of Nursing at Ohio University, and Wendy Sue Looman, PhD, RN, CPNP, Assistant Professor of Nursing at University of Minnesota. These authors conducted a current review of literature on the nursing care of families facing the challenge of chronic illness. The chapter reviews the life span perspective for working with families who experience chronic illness, including community and hospital care. Two case studies, one a child with diabetes and the other an adult with diabetes, are threaded throughout the chapter to demonstrate the concepts explained in the chapter. The authors emphasize the many factors that influence the outcome of care for chronic illness, including family culture, developmental stage, availability of resources, stages of illness, timing, and expected outcome. The chapter concludes with recommendations for nurses to build positive partnerships with families, as families remain the biggest resource for caring of members with chronic illness.

Chapter 11: Families in Palliative and End-of-Life Care is written by Rose Steele, PhD, RN, Professor, York University School of Nursing, Toronto, Ontario, Canada; Carole Robinson, PhD, RN, Associate Professor, University of British Columbia, Okanagan School of Nursing, British Columbia, Canada; Lissi Hansen, PhD, RN, Assistant Professor, Oregon Health and Science University School of Nursing; and Kimberly Widger, PhD(c), RN, Lawrence S. Bloomberg School of Nursing, University of Toronto, Canada. These authors conducted an extensive review of the literature to describe the concepts of palliative and end-of-life nursing care. Nurses are encouraged to explore personal assumptions about death and dying. These authors emphasize the importance of working with interdisciplinary teams to help manage death and dying. This new chapter focuses on family needs and barriers to providing compassionate nursing during palliative and end-of-life care. Nurses learn how to facilitate a positive end-of-life experience for families that includes connecting with families, relieving suffering, providing information, facilitating choices, managing negative feelings, and facilitating family conferences. Key issues are addressed for providing family-centered nursing care when a family member is dying. This section addresses care at the time of death and special situations such as the death of children, traumatic or sudden death, and dying at home. This chapter builds on the same family case study that was introduced in Chapter 3 as it demonstrates working with a family experiencing the death of a family member.

UNIT 3: NURSING CARE OF FAMILIES IN CLINICAL AREAS

Chapter 12: Family Nursing with Childbearing Families is written by Linda Veltri, MSN, RN, Instructor, University of Portland, School of Nursing. A review of literature provides current evidence about the processes families experience when deciding on and adapting to childbearing, including theory and clinical application of nursing care for families planning pregnancy, experiencing pregnancy, adopting and fostering children, struggling with infertility, and coping with illness during the early postpartum period. This chapter applies family nursing theories to specific clinical issues, including postpartum depression, attachment concerns, and postpartum illness, to help clinicians understand the benefit of considering the family as the client of care. Nursing interventions are integrated throughout this chapter to demonstrate how family nurses can help childbearing families prevent complications, increase coping strategies, and adapt to their expanded family structure, development, and function.

Chapter 13: Family Child Health Nursing, is written by Vivian Gedaly-Duff, DNSc, RN, Associate Professor; Ann Nielsen, MN, RN, Instructor; Marsha Heims, EdD, RN, Associate Professor; and Mary Frances D. Pate, DSN, RN, Assistant Professor. All four of these authors are faculty at the Oregon Health and Science University School of Nursing. This chapter addresses health care for families with children across the health care spectrum, including community, health promotion, hospitalization, and chronic illness. A major task of families is to nurture children to become healthy, responsible, and creative adults through their everyday parenting. The importance of family life for children's health and illness is often invisible, because families' everyday routines are commonplace and lie below the level of awareness. Families experience the stress of normative transitions with the addition of each child and situational transitions when children are ill. Knowledge of the family life cycle, child development, and illness trajectory provide a foundation to anticipatory guidance and coaching at stressful times. Family life influences the promotion of health and the experience of illness in children, and is influenced by their children's health and illness. This comprehensive chapter covers health promotion and prevention, care during chronic illness, and care during hospitalization. Nursing actions and interventions are woven throughout the chapter for caring for families with children in health and illness. A comprehensive case study addresses issues of cultural competence and health disparities, and demonstrates the application of theory for working with families who have children with health concerns.

Chapter 14: Nurses and Families in Adult Medical-Surgical Settings is written by a new team of scholars for this edition of this textbook. These four scholars are Anne M. Hirsch, DNS, ARNP, Senior Associate Dean from Washington State University Intercollegiate College of Nursing (WSU ICN) Spokane; Renee Hoeksel, PhD, RN, Professor of Nursing from WSU ICN Vancouver; Alice E. Dupler, JD, APRN-BC, Clinical Associate Professor from WSU ICN Spokane; and Joanna

Rowe Kaakinen, PhD, RN, Professor, University of Portland School of Nursing. This chapter describes family nursing with adult patients and families in medical-surgical units and critical care units. A review of literature summarizes major stressors that families experience during hospitalization of adult family members, the transfer of patients from one unit to another, visiting policies, family waiting rooms, home discharge, family presence during cardiopulmonary resuscitation, withdrawal or withholding of life-sustaining therapies, end-of-life family care in the hospital, and organ donation. Emphasis is placed on family needs during these critical events. This chapter also presents a family case study in a medical-surgical setting that demonstrates how the Family Assessment and Intervention Model and the FS^{3}I can be used as the framework to assess and intervene with this particular family. Finally, the chapter ends with implications for nursing education and health policy.

Chapter 15: Gerontological Family Nursing is coauthored by Diana L. White, PhD, Senior Research Associate in Human Development and Family Studies, Institute of Aging at Portland State University, and Jeannette O'Brien, PhD, RN Assistant Professor at Linfield College-Good Samaritan School of Nursing. The chapter presents a literature review on nursing care of older adults, including a review of the recent growth of assisted living choices for older adults with chronic illness. This chapter includes extensive information about caregiving for and by older adults, including spouses, adult children, and grandparents. The life course perspective, family systems models, and developmental theories are used throughout this chapter as the guiding organizational structure. A family case study that includes grandchildren, aging adult children, and old-old grandparents is used to illustrate the integrated generational challenges facing older adults today. Assessment recommendations and tools are provided to enhance understanding of many of the concepts introduced. The chapter concludes with a summary of recent changes that will continue to alter nursing care and settings for care of the elderly in the future.

Chapter 16: Family Mental Health Nursing is written by new contributors: Darcy Copeland, PhD, RN, Assistant Professor, University of Portland, School of Nursing, and Diane Vines, PhD, RN, Associate Professor, University of Portland, School of Nursing. Given the fact that such a large segment of the population is living with a disabling mental disorder, this chapter assists nurses in learning how to address their care and treatment not only from the perspective of preventing and treating these disorders at the individual level, but from a broader family perspective as well. This chapter provides the reader with a brief history of mental health policy in the United States. The literature review summarizes issues significant to families with members who have a mental illness; this includes the impact of mental illness on the family, obtaining social support, living with stigma, finding ways to cope, and obtaining assistance from the mental health professionals. Many individuals with mental illness have a dual diagnosis, and this chapter presents ways nurses can help families manage this situation. The chapter also offers practice strategies that nurses can implement in the provision of family mental health nursing both for the patient and for the family. These authors describe how nurses apply the family nursing process in working with families who have a member with mental illness. Family psychoeducation and case management are presented as intervention strategies. Nurses are called on to become politically active in lobbying for policy and care for the mentally ill and their families. This chapter concludes with a family case study using family systems theory that demonstrates the application of many of the concepts and strategies outlined in the chapter.

Chapter 17: Families and Community/Public Health Nursing is coauthored by a new writing team, Linda L. Eddy, PhD, RN, CPNP, Assistant Professor, and Dawn Doutrich, PhD, RN, CNS, Associate Professor. Both of these authors are faculty at Washington State University Intercollegiate College of Nursing Vancouver. The chapter begins by describing the importance of community/public health nurses understanding the reciprocal mutual relationship between families and communities. Community/public health nurses care for families in a variety of settings, such as in their homes, schools, clinics, adult day care or retirement centers, correctional facilities, under bridges, or in temporary housing during transitional or recovery programs. Regardless of the setting, these authors make the point that community health nursing is a mindset and not a place to provide nursing care. Throughout this chapter they stress how the community/public health nurse must understand the influences that affect the circumstances and choices of people/families living in the community. The authors analyze the definition of family and cultural competence in community/public health nursing practice. Various roles of the community/public health nurse are explored in the care of families. The chapter concludes with a family case study that demonstrates working with families in the community.

Chapter 18: Nursing Care of Families in Disaster and War is a new chapter in this book and is coauthored by Deborah C. Messecar, PhD, MPH, RN, Associate Professor, Oregon Health and Science University School of Nursing, and Lori Chorpenning, MS, RN, Instructor, University of Portland School of Nursing. Disasters and wars are challenging events in family life. Both are stressful for each individual in the family and the family as a whole, and are disruptive to family life. Certain families, and perhaps communities, are at greater risk for traumatization, family disorganization, and post-traumatic stress disorder (PTSD). This chapter examines the similarities and the particular challenges that families face in disaster and war situations, and then describes the nursing care of families experiencing these events. The chapter begins with a summary of the demographics of families affected by disasters and wartime, and the subsequent separation and reunion. A review of the evidenced-based literature is presented that identifies major common stressors families endure in these situations. Interventions are presented by the stage of disaster and interventions for two of the most common problems encountered in both war and disaster situations: PTSD and secondary traumatization of family members who have PTSD.

Two case studies using Family Systems Theory illustrate the many ways that family-focused nurses can expeditiously intervene and help the family cope.

UNIT 4: LOOKING TO THE FUTURE

Chapter 19: Advancing Family Nursing is a new chapter written by Joanna Rowe Kaakinen, PhD, RN, Professor, University of Portland, School of Nursing. The primary purpose of this chapter is to stimulate thoughtful debate, discussion, and ideas about the crucial future direction for family nursing. The author examines the health care reform debate in the United States and Canada, and outlines some of the challenges being faced. Nurses in Canada and the United States are encouraged to become more politically informed and active in health care issues and policy. To demonstrate the power of family nursing practice, the chapter describes three models of successful nurse-managed programs. Family nurse educators are challenged to keep family nursing a central thread in curriculums and programs of study. It is absolutely necessary that nursing education require competency in family nursing. This fourth edition of the *Family Health Care Nursing* text emphasizes theory and evidence-based practice. In this chapter, the author offers a critical review of the current state of the evidence used in family nursing practice. The chapter concludes with a call for an organized international family nursing association to give voice and to assure the continued vision and practice of family nursing.

Perri J. Bomar, PhD, RN
Professor Emeritus, School of Nursing
University of North Carolina at Wilmington
Wilmington, North Carolina

Lynne M. Casper, PhD
Professor of Sociology
University of Southern California
Los Angeles, California

Lori Chorpenning, MS, RN
Instructor, School of Nursing
University of Portland
Portland, Oregon

Deborah Padgett Coehlo, PhD, RN, PNP
Assistant Professor, Family Studies
Oregon State University
Bend, Oregon

Darcy Copeland, PhD, RN
Assistant Professor, School of Nursing
University of Portland
Portland, Oregon

Sharon A. Denham, DSN, RN
Professor, School of Nursing
Ohio University
Athens, Ohio

Gweneth Hartrick Doane, PhD, RN
Professor, School of Nursing
University of Victoria
Victoria, British Columbia, Canada

Dawn Doutrich, PhD, RN, CNS
Associate Professor, Intercollegiate College
of Nursing
Washington State University
Vancouver, Washington

Alice E. Dupler, JD, APRN-BC
Clinical Associate Professor, Intercollegiate
College of Nursing
Washington State University
Spokane, Washington

Linda L. Eddy, PhD, RN, CPNP
Assistant Professor, Intercollegiate College
of Nursing
Washington State University
Vancouver, Washington

Kristine M. Gebbie, DrPH, RN, FAAN
Joan Grabe (Acting) Dean, School of Nursing
Hunter College, City University of New York
New York, New York

Vivian Gedaly-Duff, DNSc, RN
Associate Professor, School of Nursing
Oregon Health & Science University
Portland, Oregon

John G. Haaga, PhD
Deputy Director, Behavioral and Social Research
National Institute on Aging
Bethesda, Maryland

Lissi Hansen, PhD, RN
Assistant Professor, School of Nursing
Oregon Health & Science University
Portland, Oregon

Shirley May Harman Hanson, PMHNP, PhD, RN, FAAN, CFLE, LMFT
Professor Emerita, School of Nursing
Oregon Health & Science University
Portland, Oregon

Marsha L. Heims, EdD, RN
Associate Professor, School of Nursing
Oregon Health & Science University
Portland, Oregon

Anne M. Hirsch, DNS, ARNP
Senior Associate Dean, Intercollegiate College
of Nursing
Washington State University
Spokane, Washington

Renee Hoeksel, PhD, RN
Professor, Intercollegiate College of Nursing
Washington State University
Vancouver, Washington

Radheeka R. Jayasundera, BS
Graduate Student, Population Research Center
University of Southern California
Los Angeles, California

Joanna Rowe Kaakinen, PhD, RN
Professor, School of Nursing
University of Portland
Portland, Oregon

Yeoun Soo Kim-Godwin, PhD, MPH, RN
Associate Professor, School of Nursing
University of North Carolina, Wilmington
Wilmington, North Carolina

Wendy Sue Looman, PhD, RN, CPNP
Assistant Professor, School of Nursing
University of Minnesota
Minneapolis, Minnesota

Margaret M. Manoogian, PhD
Associate Professor, Child and Family Studies
Ohio University
Athens, Ohio

Deborah C. Messecar, PhD, MPH, RN
Associate Professor, School of Nursing
Oregon Health & Science University
Portland, Oregon

Ann Nielsen, MN, RN
Instructor, School of Nursing
Oregon Health & Science University
Portland, Oregon

Jeannette O'Brien, PhD, RN
Assistant Professor, School of Nursing
Linfield College
Portland, Oregon

Mary Frances D. Pate, DSN, RN
Assistant Professor, School of Nursing
Oregon Health & Science University
Portland, Oregon

Carole Robinson, PhD, RN
Acting Associate Dean, Faculty of Health & Social
Development
Associate Professor, School of Nursing
University of British Columbia, Okanagan
Kelowna, British Columbia, Canada

**Lorraine B. Sanders, DNSc, CNM, FNP-BC,
PMHNP, RN**
Associate Professor
Hunter Bellevue School of Nursing
New York, New York

**Heather Skirton, PhD, MSc, RGN,
Registered Genetic Counsellor**
Professor of Applied Health Genetics and Deputy
Head for Research School of Nursing and
Community Studies
University of Plymouth
Taunton, United Kingdom

Rose Steele, PhD, RN
Professor, School of Nursing, Faculty of Health
York University
Toronto, Ontario, Canada

Colleen Varcoe, PhD, RN
Associate Professor, School of Nursing
University of British Columbia
Vancouver, British Columbia, Canada

Linda Veltri, MSN, RN
Instructor, School of Nursing
University of Portland
Portland, Oregon

Diane Vines, PhD, RN
Associate Professor, School of Nursing
University of Portland
Portland, Oregon

Diana L. White, PhD
Senior Research Associate, Institute on Aging
Portland State University
Portland, Oregon

Kimberley A. Widger, PhD(c), RN
PhD candidate, Lawrence S. Bloomberg Faculty
of Nursing
University of Toronto
Toronto, Ontario, Canada

Janet K. Williams, PhD, RN, CGC,
PNP, FAAN
Kelting Professor of Nursing
University of Iowa
Iowa City, Iowa

Ellen J. Argust, MS, RN
Lecturer
State University of New York
New Paltz, New York

Amanda J. Barton, DNP, FNP, RN
Assistant Professor of Nursing
Hope College
Holland, Michigan

Kathleen J. Bell, RN, MSN, CNM, RN
Instructor, School of Nursing
University of Portland
Portland, Oregon

Barbara S. Broome, PhD, RN
Associate Dean and Chair
University of South Alabama
Mobile, Alabama

Sharon L. Carlson, PhD, RN
Professor
Otterbein College
Westerville, Ohio

Michele D'Arcy-Evans, PhD, CNM
Professor
Lewis-Clark State College
Lewiston, Idaho

Margaret C. Delaney, MS, CPNP, RN
Faculty Instructor in the School of Nursing
Benedictine University
Lisle, Illinois

Sandra K. Eggenberger, PhD, RN
Professor, School of Nursing
Minnesota State University Mankato
Mankato, Minnesota

Brian Fonnesbeck, RN
Associate Professor of Nursing and Health Sciences
Lewis Clark State College
Lewiston, Idaho

Sheila Grossman, PhD, FNP-BC
Professor and FNP Specialty Track Director
Fairfield University
Fairfield, Connecticut

Anna Jajic, MN-NP, MSc, RPN, BSsN
Faculty, Nurse Practitioner
Douglas College
New West Minster, British Columbia, Canada

Molly Johnson, MSN, CPNP, RN
Nursing Instructor
Ohio University
Ironton, Ohio

Kathy Kollowa, MSN, RN
Nurse Educator
Platt College
Aurora, Colorado

Ken Kustiak, RN, RPN, BScN, MHS(C)
Nursing Instructor
Grant MacEwan College
Ponoka, Alberta, Canada

Maureen Leen, PhD, RN, CNE
Professor
Madonna University
Livonia, Michigan

Karen Elizabeth Leif, BA, RN, MA
Nurse Educator
Globe University/Minnesota School of Business
Richfield, Minnesota

Barbara McClaskey, PhD, MN, RNC, ARNP
Professor, Department of Nursing
Pittsburg State University
Pittsburg, Kansas

Vicki A. Moss, DNSc, RN
Associate Professor
University of Wisconsin Oshkosh
Oshkosh, Wisconsin

Verna C. Pangman, MEd, MN, RN
Senior Instructor
Faculty of Nursing
University of Manitoba
Winnipeg, Manitoba, Canada

Cindy Parsons, DNP, PMHNP, BC, RN
Assistant Professor of Nursing
University of Tampa
Tampa, Florida

Susan Perkins, MSN, RN
Lead Faculty/Instructor for Child and Family Health
Washington State University Intercollegiate College
of Nursing
Spokane, Washington

Cindy Peternelj-Taylor, RN, BScN, MSc, PhD(c)
Professor
University of Saskatchewan College of Nursing
Saskatoon, Saskatchewan, Canada

Thelma Phillips, MSN, RN, NRP
Instructor, McAuley School of Nursing
University of Detroit Mercy McAuley School
of Nursing
Detroit, Michigan

Nancy Ross, PhD, ARNP
Professor of Nursing
University of Tampa
Tampa, Florida

Jill Strawn, EdD, APRN
Associate Professor
Southern Connecticut State University
New Haven, Connecticut

Sara Sturgis, MSN, CRNP
Manager, Pediatric Clinical Research
Hershey Medical Center
Hershey, Pennsylvania

MaryAnn Troiano, MSN, RN, APN
Assistant Professor and Family Nurse Practitioner
Monmouth University
West Long Branch, New Jersey

Lois Tschetter, EdD, RN, IBCLC
Associate Professor
South Dakota State University
Brookings, South Dakota

Maria Wheelock, MSN, NP
Clinical Assistant Professor/Nurse Practitioner
State University of New York Upstate Medical
University
Syracuse, New York

ACKNOWLEDGMENTS

We are deeply grateful to the contributors for this fourth edition of *Family Health Care Nursing*. As the list of contributors became finalized, we were in awe of the wealth of expertise, dedication, and willingness to share their knowledge with nursing students. To write for a book is not an easy task. Thank you for your commitment to the nursing of families.

We thank our excellent editorial team at F. A. Davis. Joanne DaCunha, nursing acquisitions editor, who has walked this journey for all four editions. We are grateful to you for helping our vision of family nursing continue to be offered worldwide. We could not have pulled all the millions of details together without the constant direction from Padraic J. Maroney, our project editor. It takes this type of professional teamwork to publish a book. Thank you.

Joanna, Vivian, Debbie, and Shirley

Shirley Hanson is the consummate mentor. She is a trusted friend, a skilled counselor, and always a teacher. We were deeply moved and honored by the trust she placed in us when she asked us to join her writing team. Shirley wrote her first family nursing textbook because she saw a need for nurses to focus on more than the patient. Whereas the content of the book has changed as the practice and research has become more evidence-based, the vision that the nursing of families is crucial knowledge for nurses remains the central drive behind this book. Shirley, thank you for sharing your lifework of the nursing of families and guiding us on this journey.

Joanna, Vivian, and Debbie

In this fast paced dynamic world of nursing and health care, it is essential that we work in groups that share a common vision and spirit. Working with this team of dedicated nursing scholars has been an academic highlight for me. I am glad I shared this journey with Shirley, Vivian, and Debbie. This book is the result of many discussions, some tension, and the pooling, of our strengths as conceptual thinkers, problem-solvers, and caring people. A common ground of teaching is what pulled us together. Our zeal and commitment to sharing and advancing family nursing is what binds us as scholars. Our friendship is true and genuine. My deep gratitude and respect to my friends and colleagues, Dr. Shirley Hanson, Dr. Vivian Gedaly-Duff, and Dr. Debbie Coehlo. Thank you.

Joanna Rowe Kaakinen

CONTENTS

1

Foundations in Family Health Care Nursing

CHAPTER 1

Family Health Care Nursing: An Introduction

Joanna Rowe Kaakinen, PhD, RN

Shirley May Harmon Hanson, PMHNP, PhD, RN, FAAN, CFLE, LMFT

Sharon A. Denham, DSN, RN

CRITICAL CONCEPTS

✦ Family health care nursing is an art and a science that has evolved as a way of thinking about and working with families.

✦ Family nursing is a scientific discipline based in theory.

✦ Health and illness are family events.

✦ The term *family* is defined in many ways, but the most salient definition is, "the family is who the members say it is."

✦ An individual's health (on the wellness-to-illness continuum) affects the entire family's functioning, and in turn, the family's ability to function affects each individual member's health.

✦ Family health care nursing knowledge and skills are important for nurses who practice in generalized and in specialized settings.

✦ The structure, function, and processes of families have changed, but the family as a unit of analysis and service continues to survive over time.

✦ Nurses need to practice in ways that impact families' structure, function, and processes.

✦ Nurses should intervene in ways that promote health and wellness, as well as prevent illness risks, treat disease conditions, and manage rehabilitative care needs.

✦ Knowledge about each family's structure, function, and process informs the nurse in how to optimize nursing care in families and provide individualized nursing care, tailored to the uniqueness of every family system.

amily health care nursing is an art and a science that has evolved since the early 1980s as a way of thinking about, and working with, families when a member experiences a health problem (Hanson, 2005). Family nursing comprises a philosophy and a way of interacting with clients that affects how nurses collect information, intervene with patients, advocate for patients, and approach spiritual care with families. This philosophy and practice incorporates the following assumptions: health affects all members of families, health and illness are family events, and families influence the process and outcome of health care. All health care practices, attitudes, beliefs, behaviors, and decisions are made within the context of larger family and societal systems.

Families vary in structure, function, and processes. Families even vary within given cultures because every family has its own unique culture. People who come from the same family of origin create different families over time. Nurses need to be knowledgeable in the theory of families, as well as the structure, function, and processes of families to assist them in achieving or maintaining a state of health.

When families are considered the unit of care, nurses have much broader perspectives for approaching health care needs of both individual family members and the family unit as a whole (Hanson, 2005). The structure, function, and processes of the family influence and are influenced by individual family member's health status and the overall health status of the whole family. Understanding families enables nurses to assess the family health status, ascertain the affects of the family on individual family members' health status, predict the influence of alterations in health status of the family system, and work with members as they plan and implement action plans customized for improved health for each individual family and family member.

Recent advances in health care, such as changing health care policies and health care economics, ever-changing technology, shorter hospital stays, and health care moving from the hospital to the community/family home, are prompting changes from an individual person paradigm to the nursing care of families as a whole. This paradigm shift is affecting the development of family theory, practice, research, social policy, and education, and it is critical for nurses to be knowledgeable about and at the forefront of this shift. The centrality of family-centered care in health care delivery is emphasized by the American Nurses Association (ANA) in a recent publication, *Nursing's Social Policy Statement* (ANA, 2003a). In addition, ANA's *Nursing: Scope and Standards of Practice* mandates that nurses provide family care (ANA, 2003b).

The overall goal of this book is to enhance nurses' knowledge and skills in the theory, practice, research, and social policy surrounding nursing care of families. This chapter provides a broad overview of family health care nursing. It begins with an exploration of the definition of family, family health care nursing, and the concept of healthy families. This chapter goes on to describe four approaches to working with families: family as context, family as client, family as system, and family as a component of society. The chapter presents the varied, but ever-changing, family structures and explores *family functions* relative to reproduction, socialization, affective function, economic issues, and health care. Finally, the chapter discusses *family processes,* so that nurses know how their practice makes a difference when families experience stress because of the illness of individual family members.

DIMENSIONS OF FAMILY NURSING

Three foundational components of family nursing are: (1) determining how family is defined, (2) understanding the concepts of family health, and (3) knowing the current evidence about the elements of a healthy family.

What Is the Family?

No universally agreed-on definition of *family* exists. Now more than ever, the traditional definition of family is being challenged, with Canadian recognition of same-sex marriages and the push to legalize same-sex marriages in the United States. *Family* is a word that conjures up different images for each individual and group, and the word has evolved in its

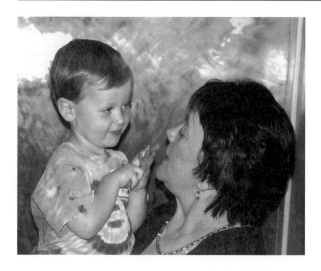

meaning over time. Definitions differ by discipline, for example:

- *Legal:* relationships through blood ties, adoption, guardianship, or marriage
- *Biological:* genetic biological networks among people
- *Sociological:* groups of people living together
- *Psychological:* groups with strong emotional ties

Early family social science theorists (Burgess & Locke, 1953, pp. 7–8) adopted the following traditional definition in their writing:

> *The family is a group of persons united by ties of marriage, blood, or adoption, constituting a single household; interacting and communicating with each other in their respective social roles of husband and wife, mother and father, son and daughter, brother and sister; and creating and maintaining a common culture.*

Currently, the U.S. Census Bureau defines *family* as two or more people living together who are related by birth, marriage, or adoption (Tillman & Nam, 2008). This traditional definition continues to be the basis for the implementation of many social programs and policies.

Nevertheless, this definition excludes many diverse groups who consider themselves to be families and who perform family functions, such as economic, reproductive, and affective functions, as well as child socialization. Depending on the social norms, all of the following examples could be viewed as "family": married couple with children, cohabitating same-sex couple, two sisters living together, and a grandmother raising two grandchildren without their parents.

The definition for *family* adopted by this textbook and that applies in the previous edition (Hanson, 2005) is as follows:

> *Family refers to two or more individuals who depend on one another for emotional, physical, and economical support. The members of the family are self-defined.*

Nurses who work with families should ask clients who they consider to be members of their family and should include those persons in health care planning with the patient's permission (Hanson, 2005). The family may range from traditional notions (Dad, Mom, child, grandparents, uncles, aunts, cousins), to such "postmodern" family structures as single-parent families, step families, and same-sex families.

What Is Family Health?

The World Health Organization (2008) defines *health* to include a person's characteristics, behaviors, and physical, social, and economic environment. This definition applies to individuals and to families. Anderson and Tomlinson (1992) suggest that the analysis of family health must include simultaneously health and illness, the individual and the collective. They underscore evidence that the stress of a family member's serious illness exerts a powerful influence on family function and health, and that familial behavioral patterns or reactions to illness influence the individual family members. The term *family health* is often used interchangeably with the terms *family functioning, healthy families,* or *familial health.* To some, family health is the composite of individual family members' physical health, because it is impossible to make a single statement about the family's physical health as a single entity.

The definition of *family health* adopted in this textbook and that applies in the previous edition (Hanson, 2005) is as follows:

> *Family health is a dynamic changing state of well-being, which includes the biological, psychological, spiritual, sociological, and culture factors of individual members and the whole family system.*

This definition and approach combines all aspects of life for individual members, as well as for the whole family. An individual's health (on the wellness-to-illness continuum) affects the entire family's functioning, and in turn, the family's ability to function affects each individual member's health. Assessment of family health involves simultaneous data collection on individual family members and the whole family system.

What Is a Healthy Family?

It is possible to define family health, but what about healthy family? Characteristics used to describe healthy families or family strengths have varied throughout time in the literature (Hanson, 2005). Otto (1963), the first scholar to develop psychosocial criteria for assessing family strengths, emphasizes the need to focus on positive family attributes instead of the pathologic approach that accentuates family problems and weaknesses. Pratt (1976) has introduced the idea of the "energized family" as one whose structure encourages and supports individuals to develop their capacities for full functioning and independent action, thus contributing to family health. Curran (1985) investigates not only family stressors but also traits of healthy families, incorporating moral and task focus into traditional family functioning. These traits are listed in Box 1-1.

For more than three decades, Driver, Tabares, Shapiro, Nahm, and Gottman (2005) have studied the interactional patterns of marital success or failure. The success of a marriage does not depend on the presence or the amount of conflict. Success of a marriage depends primarily on how the couple handles conflict. The presence of four characteristics of couple interaction has been found to predict divorce with 94% accuracy (Carrere, Buehlman, Coan, Gottman, & Ruckstuhl, 2000):

1. *Criticism:* These are personal attacks that consist of negative comments, to and about each other, that occur over time and that erode the relationship.
2. *Contempt:* This is the most corrosive of the four characteristics between the couple. Contempt includes comments that convey disgust and disrespect.
3. *Defensiveness:* Each partner blames the other in an attempt to deflect a verbal attack.
4. *Stonewalling:* One or both of the partners refuse to interact or engage in interaction, both verbally and nonverbally.

BOX 1-1
Traits of a Healthy Family

- Communicates and listens
- Fosters table time and conversation
- Affirms and supports each member
- Teaches respect for others
- Develops a sense of trust
- Has a sense of play and humor
- Has a balance of interaction among members
- Shares leisure time
- Exhibits a sense of shared responsibility
- Teaches a sense of right and wrong
- Abounds in rituals and traditions
- Shares a religious core
- Respects the privacy of each member
- Values service to others
- Admits to problems and seeks help

Source: From Hanson, S. M. H. (2005). Family heath care nursing: An introduction. In S. M. H. Hanson (Ed.), *Family health care nursing: Theory, practice & research* (3rd ed., p. 9). Philadelphia: F.A. Davis.

In contrast, conflict is addressed in three ways in positive, healthy marriages. *Validators* talk their problems out expressing emotions and opinions, and are skilled at reaching a compromise. *Volatiles* are two partners who view each other as equals, as they engage in loud, passionate, explosive interactions that are balanced by a caring, loving relationship. Their conflicts do not include the four negative characteristics identified earlier. The last type of couples is the *Avoiders.* Avoiders simply agree not to engage in conflicts, thus minimizing the corrosive effects of negative conflict resolution. The crucial point in all three styles of healthy conflict is that both partners engage in a similar style.

In happily married couples, the positive interactions occur far more often than the negative interactions. These couples find ways to work out their differences and problems, are willing to yield to each other during their arguments, and make purposeful attempts to repair their relationship.

Olson and Gorall (2005) have conducted longitudinal research on families, in which they merged the concepts of marital and family dynamics in the Circumplex Model of Marital and Family Systems. They found that the ability of the family to demonstrate flexibility is related to its ability to alter family leadership roles, relationships, and rules including control, discipline, and negotiation role sharing. Functional families have the ability to change the above factors in response to situations. Dysfunctional families have less ability to adapt and flex in response to changes (see Fig. 1-1 and Fig. 1-2, which depict the differences in families relative to these factors). Balanced families will function more adequately across the family life cycle. The family communication skills enable balance and help families to adjust and adapt to situations. Couples and families modify their levels of flexibility and cohesion to adapt to stressors (Olson & Gorall, 2005).

FAMILY HEALTH CARE NURSING

The specialty area of **family health care nursing** has been evolving since the early 1980s. For some, blurring of lines exists as to how family health care nursing is distinctive from other specialties that involve families, such as maternal-child health nursing, community health nursing, and mental health nursing. The definition for *family health care nursing* adopted

by this textbook and that applies in the previous edition (Hanson, 2005) is as follows:

> *The process of providing for the health care needs of families that are within the scope of nursing practice. This nursing care can be aimed toward the family as context, the family as a whole, the family as a system or the family as a component of society.*

Family nursing takes into consideration all four approaches to viewing families mentioned in Hanson's definition and discussed later. At the same time, it cuts across the individual, family, and community for the purpose of promoting, maintaining, and restoring the health of families. This framework illustrates the intersecting concepts of the individual, the family, nursing, and society (Fig. 1-3).

Another model for family nursing practice is where family nursing is seen conceptually as the confluence of theories and strategies from nursing, family therapy, and family social science as depicted in Figure 1-4. Over time, family nursing continues to incorporate ideas from family therapy and family social science into the practice of family nursing. See Chapter 3 for discussion about how theories

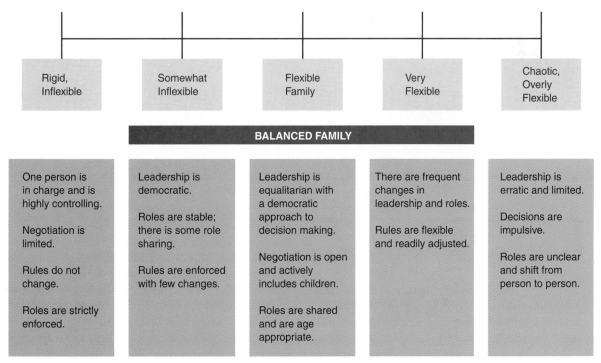

Rigid, Inflexible	Somewhat Inflexible	Flexible Family	Very Flexible	Chaotic, Overly Flexible

BALANCED FAMILY

One person is in charge and is highly controlling.	Leadership is democratic.	Leadership is equalitarian with a democratic approach to decision making.	There are frequent changes in leadership and roles.	Leadership is erratic and limited.
Negotiation is limited.	Roles are stable; there is some role sharing.	Negotiation is open and actively includes children.	Rules are flexible and readily adjusted.	Decisions are impulsive.
Rules do not change.	Rules are enforced with few changes.	Roles are shared and are age appropriate.		Roles are unclear and shift from person to person.
Roles are strictly enforced.				

FIGURE 1-1 Family flexibility continuum.

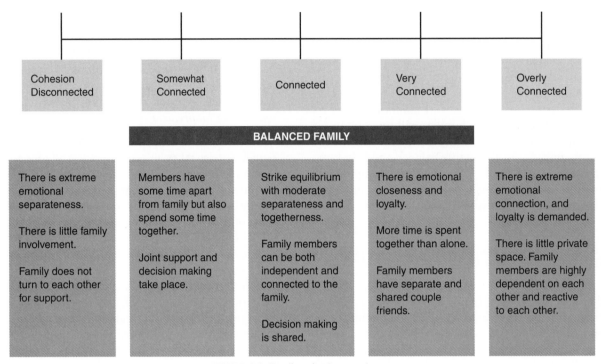

FIGURE 1-2 Family cohesion continuum.

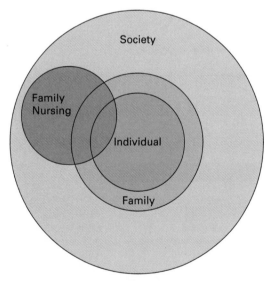

FIGURE 1-3 Family nursing conceptual framework.

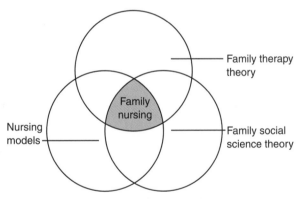

FIGURE 1-4 Family nursing practice.

from family social science, family therapy, and nursing converge to inform the nursing of families.

Several family scholars have written about levels of family health care nursing practice. For example, Wright and Leahey (2005) differentiate among several levels of knowledge and skills that family nurses need for a generalist versus specialist practice, and they define the role of higher education for the two different levels of practice. They propose that nurses receive a generalist or basic level of knowledge and skills in family nursing during their undergraduate work, and advanced specialization in family nursing or family therapy at the graduate level. They recognize that advanced specialists in family nursing have a narrower focus than generalists; they purport, however, that family assessment is an important skill for all nurses practicing with families. Bomar (2004) further delineates five levels of family health care nursing practice. Table 1-1 describes how the two levels of generalist and advanced practice have been delineated further with levels of education and types of clients, and relates them to Benner's paradigm of novice to expert (Benner, 2001).

NATURE OF INTERVENTIONS IN FAMILY NURSING

Ten distinctive interventions for family nurses emphasize the multivariate nature of the relationship between family health and the health of individual members (Gilliss, Roberts, Highley, & Martinson, 1989):

1. Family care is concerned with the experience of the family over time. It considers both the history and the future of the family group.

2. Family nursing considers the community and cultural context of the group. The family is encouraged to receive from, and give to, community resources.

3. Family nursing considers the relationships between and among family members, and recognizes that, in some instances, all individual members and the family group will not achieve maximum health simultaneously.

4. Family nursing is directed at families whose members are both healthy and ill. Family health is not indexed by the degree of individual health or illness.

5. Family nursing is often offered in settings where individuals have physiologic or psychological problems. Together with competency in treatment of individual health problems, family nurses must recognize the reciprocity between individual family members' health and collective health within the family.

6. The family system is influenced by any change in its members. Therefore, when caring for

TABLE 1-1

Levels of Family Nursing Practice

LEVEL OF PRACTICE	GENERALIST/SPECIALIST	EDUCATION	CLIENT
Expert	Advanced Specialist	Doctoral degree	All levels
			Family nursing theory development
			Family nursing research
Proficient	Advanced Specialist	Master's degree with added experience	All levels
			Beginning family nursing research
Competent	Beginning Specialist	Master's degree	Individual in the family context
			Interpersonal family nursing
			Family unit
			Family aggregates
Advanced Beginner	Generalist	Bachelor's degree with added experience	Individual in the family context
			Interpersonal family nursing (family systems nursing)
			Family unit
Novice	Generalist	Bachelor's degree	Individual in the family context

Source: Bomar, P. J. (Ed.) (2004). *Promoting health in families: Applying family research and theory to nursing practice* (pp.19). Philadelphia: Saunders/Elsevier.

individuals in health and illness, the nurse must elect whether to attend to the family. Individual health and collective health are intertwined and will be influenced by any nursing care given.

7. Family nursing requires the nurse to manipulate the environment to increase the likelihood of family interaction. The absence of family members does not preclude the nurse from offering family care, however.

8. The family nurse recognizes that the person in a family who is most symptomatic may change over time; this means that the focus of the nurse's attention will also change over time.

9. Family nursing focuses on the strengths of individual family members and the family group to promote their mutual support and growth.

10. Family nurses must define with the family which persons constitute the family and where they will place their therapeutic energies.

These are the distinctive intervention statements specific to family nursing that appear continuously in the care and study of families in nursing, regardless of the theoretical model in use.

APPROACHES TO FAMILY NURSING

Four different approaches to care are inherent in family nursing: (1) family as the context for individual development, (2) family as a client, (3) family as a system, and (4) family as a component of society (Hanson, 2005). Figure 1-5 illustrates these approaches to the nursing of families. Each approach derived its foundations from different nursing specialties: maternal-child nursing, primary care nursing, psychiatric/mental health nursing, and community health nursing, respectively. All four approaches have legitimate implications for nursing assessment and intervention. The approach that nurses use is determined by many factors, including the health care setting, family circumstances, and nurse resources. Figure 1-6 shows how a nurse can view all four approaches to families through just one set of eyes. It is important to keep all four perspectives in mind when working with any given family.

Family as Context

The first approach to family nursing care focuses on the assessment and care of an individual client in which the **family is the context**. This is the traditional nursing focus, in which the individual is foreground and the family is background. The family serves as context for the individual as either a resource or a stressor to their health and illness. Most existing nursing theories or models were originally conceptualized using the individual as a focus. Alternate labels for this approach are family centered or family focused. This approach is rooted in the specialty of maternal-child nursing and underlies the philosophy of many maternity and pediatric health care settings. A nurse using this focus might say to an individual client: "Who in your family will help you with your nightly medication?" "How will you provide for child care when you have your back surgery?" or "It is wonderful for you that your wife takes such an interest in your diabetes and has changed all the food preparation to fit your dietary needs."

Family as Client

The second approach to family nursing care centers on the assessment of all family members; the **family as client** is the focus of care. In this approach, all members of the family are in the foreground, and individuals are not mutually exclusive of the whole. The family is seen as the sum of individual family members, and the focus concentrates on each individual. Each person is assessed, and health care is provided for all family members. The family unit is not necessarily the primary consideration in providing care, however. Family care physicians provide the impetus for this approach to family care in community settings, but nurses and nurse practitioners (NPs) are also involved with this approach. This approach is typically seen in primary care clinics in the communities where primary care physicians (PCPs) or NPs provide care over time to all individuals in a given family. From this perspective, a nurse might ask a family member who has just become ill: "How has your diagnosis of juvenile diabetes affected the other individuals in your family?" "Will your nightly need for medication be a problem for other members of your family?" "Who in your family is having the most difficult time with your diagnosis?" or "How are the members of your family adjusting to your new medication regimen?"

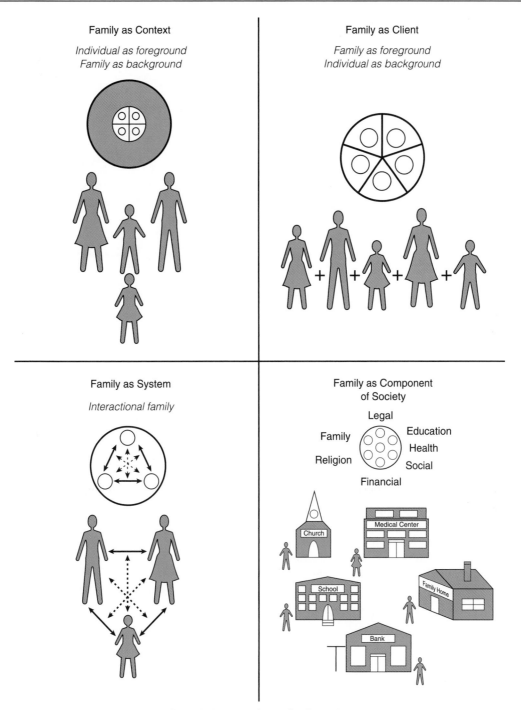

FIGURE 1-5 Approaches to family nursing.

Family as System

The third approach to care focuses on the **family as a system**. The focus is on the family as client, and the family is viewed as an interactional system in which the whole is more than the sum of its parts. In other words, the interactions between family members become the target for the nursing interventions, which flow from the assessment of the family as a whole. The family nursing system approach focuses on the

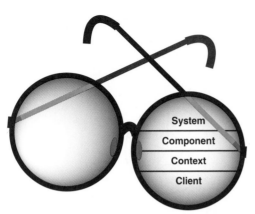

FIGURE 1-6 Four views of family through a lens.

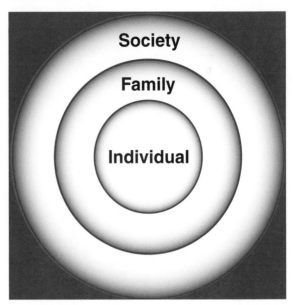

FIGURE 1-7 Family as primary group in society.

individual and family simultaneously. The emphasis is on the interactions between family members, for example, the direct interactions between the parental dyad or the indirect interaction between the parental dyad and the child. The more children there are in a family, the more complex these interactions become.

This interactional model had its start with the specialty of psychiatric and mental health nursing. The systems approach always implies that when something happens to one part of the system, the other parts of the system are affected. Therefore, if one family member becomes ill, it affects all other members of the family. Examples of questions that nurses may ask in a system approach are: "What has changed between you and your spouse since your child was diagnosed with juvenile diabetes?" or "How has the diagnosis of juvenile diabetes affected the ways in which your family is functioning and getting along with each other?"

Family as Component of Society

The fourth approach to care views the **family as a component of society**, in which the family is viewed as one of many institutions in society, similar to health, educational, religious, or economic institutions. The family is a basic or primary unit of society, and it is a part of the larger system of society (Fig. 1-7). The family as a whole interacts with other institutions to receive, exchange, or give communication and services. Family social scientists first used this approach in their study of families in society. Community health nursing has drawn many of its tenets from this perspective as it focuses on the interface between families and community agencies. Questions nurses may ask in this approach include: "What issues has the family been experiencing since you made the school aware of your son's diagnosis of HIV?" or "Have you considered joining a support group for families with mothers who have breast cancer? Other families have found this to be an excellent resource and a way to reduce stress."

VARIABLES THAT INFLUENCE FAMILY NURSING

The evolution of family health care nursing has been influenced by many variables that are derived from both historical and current events within society and the profession of nursing. Examples include changing nursing theory, practice, education, and research; new knowledge derived from family social sciences and the health sciences; national and state health care policies; changing health care behavior and attitudes; and national and international political events. Chapters 3 and 5 provide detailed discussions of these areas.

Figure 1-8 illustrates how many variables influence contemporary family health nursing, making

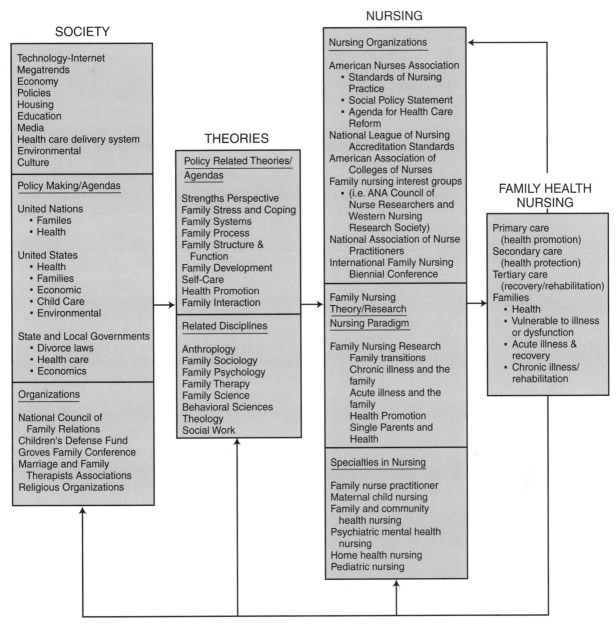

SOCIETY

Technology-Internet
Megatrends
Economy
Policies
Housing
Education
Media
Health care delivery system
Environmental
Culture

Policy Making/Agendas

United Nations
- Familes
- Health

United States
- Health
- Families
- Economic
- Child Care
- Environmental

State and Local Governments
- Divorce laws
- Health care
- Economics

Organizations

National Council of
  Family Relations
Children's Defense Fund
Groves Family Conference
Marriage and Family
  Therapists Associations
Religious Organizations

THEORIES

Policy Related Theories/
Agendas

Strengths Perspective
Family Stress and Coping
Family Systems
Family Process
Family Structure &
  Function
Family Development
Self-Care
Health Promotion
Family Interaction

Related Disciplines

Anthroplogy
Family Sociology
Family Psychology
Family Therapy
Family Science
Behavioral Sciences
Theology
Social Work

NURSING

Nursing Organizations

American Nurses Association
- Standards of Nursing
  Practice
- Social Policy Statement
- Agenda for Health Care
  Reform
National League of Nursing
  Accreditation Standards
American Association of
  Colleges of Nurses
Family nursing interest groups
- (i.e. ANA Council of
  Nurse Researchers and
  Western Nursing
  Research Society)
National Association of Nurse
  Practitioners
International Family Nursing
  Biennial Conference

Family Nursing
Theory/Research
Nursing Paradigm

Family Nursing Research
  Family transitions
  Chronic illness and the
  family
  Acute illness and the
  family
  Health Promotion
  Single Parents and
  Health

Specialties in Nursing

Family nurse practitioner
Maternal child nursing
Family and community
  health nursing
Psychiatric mental health
  nursing
Home health nursing
Pediatric nursing

**FAMILY HEALTH
NURSING**

Primary care
  (health promotion)
Secondary care
  (health protection)
Tertiary care
  (recovery/rehabilitation)
Families
- Health
- Vulnerable to illness
  or dysfunction
- Acute illness &
  recovery
- Chronic illness/
  rehabilitation

FIGURE 1-8 Variables that influence contemporary family health care.

the point that the status of family nursing is dependent on what is occurring in the wider society—family as community. A recent example of this point is that health practices and policy changes are under way because of the recognition that current costs of health care are escalating and, at the same time, greater numbers of people are underinsured or uninsured and have lost access to health care. The goal of this health care reform is to make access and treatment available for everyone at an affordable cost. That will require a major shift in priorities, funding, and services. A major movement toward health promotion and family care in the community will greatly affect the evolution of family nursing.

FAMILY NURSING ROLES

Nurses are challenged in their practice to guard against making assumptions based on personal history and beliefs, and to guard against consciously comparing the family they are working for with their own family. When nurses operate from a personal experience perspective, they are limited in their view of the family, and in ways to assist the family. Families are the basic unit of every society, but it is also true that families are complex, varied, dynamic, and adaptive, which is why it is crucial for all nurses to be knowledgeable about the scientific discipline of family nursing, and the variety of ways nurses may interact with families (Hanson, 2005).

The roles of family health care nurses are evolving along with the specialty. Figure 1-9 lists the many roles that nurses can assume with families as the focus. This figure was constructed from some of the first family nursing literature that appeared, and it is a composite of what various scholars believe to be some of the current roles of nurses (Bomar, 2004; Friedman, Bowden, & Jones, 2003; Hanson, 2005). The health care setting affects roles that nurses assume with families.

HEALTH TEACHER. The family nurse teaches about family wellness, illness, relations, and parenting, to name a few topics. The teacher-educator function is ongoing in all settings in both formal

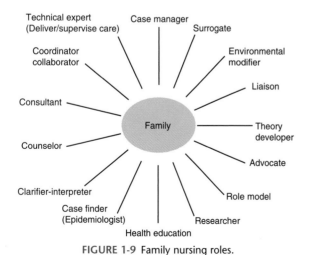

Family Nursing Roles

FIGURE 1-9 Family nursing roles.

and informal ways. Examples include teaching new parents how to care for their infant and giving instructions about diabetes to a newly diagnosed adolescent boy and his family members.

COORDINATOR, COLLABORATOR, AND LIAISON. The family nurse coordinates the care that families receive, collaborating with the family to plan care. For example, if a family member has been in a traumatic accident, the nurse would be a key person in helping families to access resources—from inpatient care, outpatient care, home health care, and social services to rehabilitation. The nurse may serve as the liaison among these services.

"DELIVERER" AND SUPERVISOR OF CARE AND TECHNICAL EXPERT. The family nurse either delivers or supervises the care that families receive in various settings. To do this, the nurse must be a technical expert both in terms of knowledge and skill. For example, the nurse may be the person going into the family home on a daily basis to consult with the family and help take care of a child on a respirator.

FAMILY ADVOCATE. The family nurse advocates for families with whom he or she works; the nurse empowers family members to speak with their own voice, or the nurse speaks out for the family. An example is the nurse who is advocating for family safety by supporting legislation that requires wearing seat belts in motor vehicles.

CONSULTANT. The family nurse serves as a consultant to families whenever asked or whenever necessary. In some instances, he or she consults with agencies to facilitate family-centered care. For example, a clinical nurse specialist in a hospital may be asked to assist the family in finding the appropriate long-term care setting for their sick grandmother. The nurse comes into the family system by request for a short period and for a specific purpose.

COUNSELOR. The family nurse plays a therapeutic role in helping individuals and families solve problems or change behavior. An example from the mental health arena is a family that requires help with coping with a long-term chronic condition, such as when a family member has been diagnosed with schizophrenia.

"CASE-FINDER" AND EPIDEMIOLOGIST. The family nurse gets involved in case-finding and becomes a tracker of disease. For example, consider the situation in which a family member has been recently diagnosed with a sexually transmitted disease. The nurse would engage in sleuthing out the sources of the transmission and in helping other sexual contacts to seek treatment. Screening of families and subsequent referral of the family members may be a part of this role.

ENVIRONMENTAL SPECIALIST. The family nurse consults with families and other health care professionals to modify the environment. For example, if a man with paraplegia is about to be discharged from the hospital to home, the nurse assists the family in modifying the home environment so that the patient can move around in a wheelchair and engage in self-care.

CLARIFY AND INTERPRET. The nurse clarifies and interprets data to families in all settings. For example, if a child in the family has a complex disease, such as leukemia, the nurse clarifies and interprets information pertaining to diagnosis, treatment, and prognosis of the condition to parents and extended family members.

SURROGATE. The family nurse serves as a surrogate by substituting for another person. For example, the nurse may stand in temporarily as a loving parent to an adolescent who is giving birth to a child by herself in the labor and delivery room.

RESEARCHER. The family nurse should identify practice problems and find the best solution for dealing with these problems through the process of scientific investigation. An example might be collaborating with a colleague to find a better intervention for helping families cope with incontinent elders living in the home.

ROLE MODEL. The family nurse is continually serving as a role model to other people. A school nurse who demonstrates the right kind of health in personal self-care serves as a role model to parents and children alike.

CASE MANAGER. Although case manager is a contemporary name for this role, it involves coordination and collaboration between a family and the health care system. The case manager has been formally empowered to be in charge of a case. For example, a family nurse working with seniors in the community may become assigned to be the case manager for a patient with Alzheimer's disease.

OBSTACLES TO FAMILY NURSING PRACTICE

Why has family nursing been practiced only in recent history? A number of reasons exist. First, a vast amount of literature is available about families, but there has been little taught about families in the nursing curricula until the past decade or two. Most practicing nurses have not had exposure to family concepts during their undergraduate education and continue to practice using the individualist medical paradigm.

Moreover, there has been a lack of valid and reliable comprehensive family assessment models, instruments, and strategies in nursing. More scholars are developing ideas and material in this arena (see Chapters 3 and 4).

Furthermore, some students and nurses may believe that the study of family and family nursing is "common sense," and therefore does not belong formally in nursing curricula, either in theory or practice. Nursing also has strong historical ties with the medical model, which has traditionally focused on the individual as client, rather than the family. At best, families have been viewed in context, and many times families were considered a nuisance in health care settings—an obstacle to overcome to provide care to the individual.

Another obstacle is the fact that the traditional charting system in health care has been oriented to the individual. For example, charting by exception focuses on the physical care of the individual and does not address the whole family or members of families. Likewise, the medical and nursing diagnostic systems used in health care are disease centered, and diseases are focused on individuals and have limited diagnostic codes that pertain to the family as a whole.

To complicate matters further, most insurance companies require that there be one identified patient, with a diagnostic code drawn from an individual disease perspective. Thus, even if health care providers are intervening with entire families, companies require providers to choose one person in the family group as the identified patient and to give that person a physical or mental diagnosis, even though the client is the whole family. A need exists for better family diagnostic codes that are accepted by vendors as legitimate reasons for reimbursement. See Chapter 4 for a detailed discussion on diagnostic codes.

The established hours during which health care systems provide services pose another obstacle to focusing on families. Traditionally, office hours take place during the day, when family members cannot accompany other family members. Recently, some urgent care centers and other outpatient settings have incorporated evening and weekend hours into their schedules, making it possible for family members to come in together. But many clinics and physician offices still operate on traditional Monday through Friday, 9:00 a.m. to 5:00 p.m. schedules. These obstacles to family-focused nursing practice are slowly changing; nurses should continue to lobby for changes that are more conducive to caring for the family as a whole.

HISTORY OF FAMILY NURSING

Family health nursing has roots in society from prehistoric times. The historical role of women has been inextricably interwoven with the family, for it was the responsibility of women to care for family members who fell ill, and to seek herbs or remedies to treat the illness. In addition, through "proper" housekeeping, women made efforts to provide clean and safe environments for the maintenance of health and wellness for their families (Bomar, 2004; Ham & Chamings, 1983; Whall, 1993).

During the Nightingale era, the development of families and nursing became more explicit. Florence Nightingale influenced both the establishment of district nursing of the sick and poor, and the work of "health missionaries" through "health-at-home" teaching. She believed that cleanliness in the home

could eradicate high infant mortality and morbidity rates. She encouraged family members of the fighting troops to come into the hospitals during the Crimean War to take care of their loved ones. Nightingale supported helping women and children achieve good health by promoting both nurse midwifery and home-based health services. In 1876, in a document entitled "Training Nurses for the Sick Poor," Nightingale encourages nurses to serve in nursing both sick and healthy families in the home environment. She appears to have given both home-health nurses and maternal-child nurses the mandate to carry out nursing practice with the whole family as the unit of service (Nightingale, 1979).

In colonial America, women continued the centuries-old traditions of nurturing and sustaining the wellness of their families and caring for the ill. During the Revolutionary War, women called *camp followers* provided nursing care. These untrained nurses performed many functions for the troops. During the Civil War (1861–1865), nursing of the wounded solders became more organized. Women formed Ladies Aid Societies, groups who met regularly to sew, prepare food and medicines, and gather other items needed by the soldiers. Dorothea Dix was named the Superintendent of Women Nurses of the U.S. Army. Hundreds of women received a month's training to prepare them for military nursing work.

During the industrial revolution of the late 18th century, family members began to work outside the home. Immigrants, in particular, were in need of income, so they went to work for the early hospitals. This was the real beginning of public health and school nursing. The nurses involved in the beginning of the labor movement were concerned with the health of workers, immigrants, and their families. Concepts of maternal child and family care were incorporated into basic curriculums of nursing schools.

Maternity nursing, nurse midwifery, and community nursing historically focused on the quality of family health. Margaret Sanger fought for family planning. Mary Breckenridge formed the famous Frontier Nursing Service (midwifery) to provide training for nurses to meet the health needs of mountain families.

A concerted expansion of public health nursing occurred during the Depression to work with families. However, before and during World War II, nursing became more focused on the individual, and care became centered in institutional and hospital settings, where it remained until recently.

Since the 1950s, at least 19 disciplines have studied the family and, through research, produced family assessment techniques, conceptual frameworks, theories, and other family material. Recently, this interdisciplinary work has become known as *family social science*. Family social science has greatly influenced family nursing in the United States largely because of the National Council of Family Relations and their large number of family publications. Many family nurses have become active in this organization. In addition, many nurses are now receiving advanced degrees in family social science departments around the country.

Nursing theorists started in the 1960s to systematize nursing practice. Scholars began to articulate the philosophy and goals of nursing care. Initially, theorists were concerned only with individuals, but gradually, individuals became viewed as part of a larger social system. See Chapter 3 for nursing theories that contribute to family nursing.

In the 1960s, the NP movement began espousing the family as a primary unit of care in their practice. In 1970, the grand theories of nursing focused primarily on the individual and not families.

During the 1980s, the refocusing on families as a unit of care was evident in America and Canada. Small numbers of people across these countries gathered together to discuss and share family nursing concepts. Family nurses started defining the scope of practice, family concepts, and how to teach this information to the next generation of nurses. Family

nursing has both old and new traditions and new definitions. Family nursing is now beyond youth, more like a young person, but still in a state of assuming itself. The Seventh International Family Nursing Conference was held in 2007 in Thailand, the Eighth International Family Nursing Conference took place in 2009 in Iceland, and the Ninth International Family Nursing Conference is scheduled for 2011 in Japan. See Table 1-2 for a composite representation of historical factors that contribute to the development of family health as a focus in nursing.

HISTORY OF FAMILIES

A brief macroanalytical history of families is important for understanding family nursing. The past helps to make the present realities of family life more understandable, because the influence of the past is evident in the present. This historical approach provides a means of conceptualizing family over time and within all of society. Finally, history helps to dispel preferences for family forms that are only personally familiar and broaden nurses' views of the world of families.

Prehistoric Family Life

Archaeologists and anthropologists have found evidence of prehistoric family life, existing before the time of written historical sources. These family forms varied from present-day forms, but the functions of

TABLE 1-2	
Historical Factors Contributing to the Development of Family Health as a Focus in Nursing	
TIME PERIOD	**EVENTS**
Pre-Nightingale era	Revolutionary War "camp followers" were an example of family health focus before Florence Nightingale's influence.
Mid-1800s	Nightingale influences district nurses and health missionaries to maintain clean environment for patient's homes and families.
	Family members provided for soldiers' needs during Civil War through Ladies Aid Societies and Women's Central Association for Relief.
Late 1800s	Industrial Revolution and immigration influence focus of public health nursing on prevention of illness, health education, and care of the sick for both families and communities.
	Lillian Wald establishes Henry Street Visiting Nurse Service (1893).
	Focus on Family during childbearing by maternal-child nurses and midwives.
	(Continued)

TABLE 1-2	
Historical Factors Contributing to the Development of Family Health as a Focus in Nursing—cont'd	
TIME PERIOD	**EVENTS**
Early 1900s	School nursing established in New York City (1903).
	First White House Conference on Children occurs (1909).
	Red Cross Town and Country Nursing Service was founded (1912).
	Margaret Sanger opens first birth control clinic (1916).
	Family planning and quality care become available for families.
	Mary Breckinridge forms Frontier Nursing Service (1925).
	Nurses are assigned to families.
	Red Cross Public Health Nursing Service meets rural health needs after stock market crash (1929).
	Federal Emergency Relief Act passed (1933).
	Social Security Act passed (1935).
	Psychiatry and mental health disciplines begin family therapy focus (late 1930s).
1960s	Concept of family as a unit of care is introduced into basic nursing curriculum.
	National League for Nursing (NLN) requires emphasis on families and communities in nursing curriculum.
	Family-centered approach in maternal-child nursing and midwifery programs is begun.
	Nurse-practitioner movement- programs to provide primary care to children are begun (1965).
	Shift from public health nursing to community health nursing occurs.
	Family studies and research produce family theories.
1970s	Changing health care system focuses on maintaining health and returning emphasis to family health.
	Development and refinement of nursing conceptual models that consider the family as a unit of analysis or care occur (e.g., King, Newman, Orem, Rogers, and Roy).
	Many specialties focus on the family (e.g., hospice, oncology, geriatrics, school health, psychiatry, mental health, occupational health, and home health).
	Master's and doctoral programs focus on the family (e.g., family health nursing, community health nursing, psychiatry, mental health and family counseling and therapy).
	ANA Standards of Nursing Practice are implemented (1973).
	Surgeon General's Report (1979).
1980s	ANA Social Policy Statement (1980).
	White House Conference on Families.
	Greater emphasis is put on health from very young to very old.
	Increasing emphasis is placed on obesity, stress, chemical dependency and parenting skills.
	Graduate level specialization is begun with emphasis on primary care outside of acute care settings, health teaching, and client self-care.
	Use of wellness and nursing models in providing care increases.
	Promoting Health/Preventing Disease: Objective for the Nation (1980) is released by U.S. Department of Health and Human Services.
	Family science develops as a discipline.
	Family nursing research increases.
	National Center for Nursing Research is founded, with a Health Promotion and Prevention Research section.
	First International Nursing Conference occurs in Calgary, Canada (1988).

TABLE 1-2

Historical Factors Contributing to the Development of Family Health as a Focus in Nursing—cont'd

TIME PERIOD	EVENTS
1990s	*Health People 2000: National Health Promotion and Disease Prevention Objective* (1990) is released by U.S. Department of Health and Human Services.
	Nursing's Agenda for Health Care Reform is developed (ANA, 1991).
	Family leave legislation is passes (1991).
	Journal of Family Nursing is created (1995).
2000s	*Nursing's Agenda for the Future* is written (ANA, 2002).
	Healthy People 2010 and 2020 are released from the U.S. Department of Health and Human Services.
	The quality and quantity of family nursing research continues to increase, especially in the international sector.
	Family related research is clearly a goal of the *National Institute of Nursing Research Themes for the Future* (NINR, 2003).
	World Health Organization document *Health for All in the 21st Century* calls for support of families.
	The National Council on Family Relations prepared the *NCFR Presidential Report 2001: Preparing Families for the Future.*
	International Family Nursing Conferences start meeting every two years instead of every three years.

Adapted from Bomar, P. J. (Ed.) (2004). *Promoting health in families: Applying family research and theory to nursing practice* (pp.12-13). Philadelphia: Saunders/Elsevier.

the family have remained somewhat constant over time. Families were then and are now a part of the larger community and constitute the basic unit of society.

Family structure, process, and function were a response to everyday needs. As communities grew, families and communities became more institutionalized and homogeneous as civilization progressed. Family culture was that aspect of life derived from membership in a particular group and shared by others. Family culture was composed of values and attitudes that allowed early families to behave in a predictable fashion.

The earliest human matings tended toward permanence and monogamy. Man and woman dyads are the oldest and most tenacious unit in history, which is perhaps why the "nuclear" family dominates modern experience. Biologically, human children need care and protection longer than other animals' offspring. This necessity led humans to marriage and permanent relationships—it did not dictate family structure, but it was essential for the activity of parenting.

Economic pairing was not always the same as reproductive pairing, but it was a by-product of reproductive pairing. A variety of skills were needed for living, and no single person possessed all skills; therefore, male and female role differentiation began to be more clearly defined. Early in history, children were part of the economic unit. In most societies, reproductive pairing merged also with the nurturing pair and the economic unit, as well as into respective gender role differentiation, and ultimately into socialization (education). As small groups of conjugal families formed communities, the complexity of the social order increased. This, in turn, changed the definition of the family.

European History

Many Americans are of European ancestry and come out of the family structure that was present there. Social organizations called *families* emphasized consanguineous (genetic) bonds. The tendency toward authority was concentrated in few individuals at the top of the hierarchical structure (kings, lords, fathers). The heads of families were men.

Property of family transferred through the male line. Women left home to join their husbands' families. Mothers did not establish strong bonds with their daughters because the daughters eventually left their home of origin to join their husband's family of origin.

Women and children were property to be transferred. Marriage was a contract between families, not individuals. Extended patriarchal family characteristics prevailed until the advent of industrialism.

Industrialization

Great stability existed within family systems until the Industrial Revolution. The revolution first appeared in England around 1750 and spread to Western Europe and North America. Some believe that the nuclear family idea started with the Industrial Revolution. Extended families had always been the norm until families left farms, moving into the cities, where men left home to work in the factories. This left women at home maintaining the home and caring for the children. Extended families were left behind. Some evidence has been reported that English families were nuclear from the 1600s, because family size has stayed constant at 4.75 people per family ever since.

Out of the religious Reformation came a strong movement for individuation, in which the Protestant ethic promoted the idea that the family unit was no longer paramount, but rather the individual within the family. This paradigm shift had a lot to do with the message of personal salvation of the Reformation and Protestantism.

When factories of the Industrial Revolution started to be built, people began moving about. The state had begun to provide services that families previously had performed for their members. Informal contractual arrangements between public and state power and nuclear families took place, in which the state gave fathers the power and authority over their families in exchange for male individuals giving the state their loyalty and service. This may be one of the ways in which families became controlled by patriarchy.

Women were not expected to love husbands but to obey them. Some feminists believe that the introduction of love into human consciousness was done as a purposeful and powerful force to limit female activity, and that it is hard to separate love and submission. This notion is controversial.

Society today is still living with bequests of patriarchal family life. Women are still struggling to get out from under the rules and expectations of the state and of men. The women's movement and the National Organization for Women (NOW) are two of the forces that have improved the level of equality of women in modern society. A lot more work needs to be done on the issues of equality for all Americans, including gender differences.

In recent years, men have also begun identifying the bondage they experience. They cannot meet all of the needs of families and feel inadequate for failing to do so. This is especially true of men who cannot access the resources of money, occupation, and occupational status through education. A men's movement is afoot that is promoting male causes, although this movement is not as dynamic as it may be in the future. One of the organizations supporting this work is the National Congress for Men.

American Families

American society and families were molded from the beginning by economic logic rather than consanguineous logic. America does not have the history of Europe's preindustrial age. English patriarchy was not transplanted in its pure form to America.

Women and men had to labor in the New World. This gave women new power. Also, the United States had an ethic of achieved status rather than inherited status through familial lines. Female suffrage was easier to obtain on the frontier, as is evidenced by Wyoming being one of the first states to give women the right to vote.

Children were also experiencing a changing status in American families. Originally, they were part of the economic unit and worked on farms. Then with the great immigration of the early 1900s, the expectation shifted to parents creating a better world for their children than they themselves had. To do this, children had to become more educated to deal with the developing society. Each generation of children obtained more education and income than their parents; they left the family farms and moved to distant cities. As a result of this change, parents lost assurance that their children would take care of them during their old age. This phenomenon is occurring in developing countries today. For example, the city of Seoul, Korea, has grown from 2 to 14 million people in one decade, largely because of young people coming into the cities for work and education.

In addition, the functions of families were changing greatly in earlier American society. The traditional roles that families played were being displaced by the growing numbers and kinds of social institutions. Families have been increasingly surrendering to public agencies many of the socialization functions they previously had performed.

Historically, adolescents worked on the family farms. With the burgeoning of cities in the industrialized world, adolescents lost their productive function on the farm. Teenagers could not be kept from jobs in the cities. The public school system was largely created to help keep adolescents off the streets. The concept of the generation gap occurred when the family economic and social functions no longer merged.

Families Today

Today, families cannot be separated from the larger system of which they are a part, nor can they be separated from their historical past. Some people argue that families are in terrible condition, like a rudderless ship in the dark. Other people hail the changes that continue to occur in families, and approve the diversity and options that address modern needs. Idealizing past family arrangements and decrying change has become commonplace in the media. Just as some families of both the past and present engage in behaviors that are destructive to individuals and other social institutions, there are families of the past and present that provide healthy environments. The structure, function, and processes of families have changed, but the family will continue to survive and thrive. It is, in fact, the most tenacious unit in society (Hanson, 2005).

FAMILY STRUCTURE, FUNCTION, AND PROCESS

Knowledge about family structure, function, and processes is essential for understanding the complex family interactions that affect health, illness, and well-being (Denham, 2005). Knowledge emerging from the study of family structure, function, and process suggest concepts and a framework that nurses can use to provide effective assessment and intervention with families. Many internal and external family variables affect individual family members and the family as a whole. Internal family variables include unique individual characteristics, communication, and interactions, whereas external family variables include location of family household, social policy, and economic trends. Family members generally have complicated responses to all of these factors. Although some external factors may not be easily modifiable, nurses can assist family members to manage change, conflict, and care needs. For instance, a sudden downturn in the economy could result in the family breadwinner becoming unemployed. Although nurses are unable to alter this situation directly, understanding the implications on the family situation provides a basis for planning more effective interventions. Nurses can assist members with coping skills, communication patterns, location of needed resources, effective use of information, or creation of family rituals or routines (Denham, 2005).

Nurses who understand the concepts of family structure, function, and process can use this knowledge to educate, counsel, and implement changes that enable families to cope with illness, family crisis, chronic health conditions, and mental illness. Nurses prepared to work with families can assist them with needed life transitions (Denham, 2005). For example, when a family member experiences a chronic condition such as diabetes, family roles, routines, and power hierarchies may be challenged. Nurses must be prepared to address the complex and holistic family problems resulting from illness, as well as to care for the individual's medical needs.

In today's postindustrial society, families are reconfiguring and reconstructing novel types of structures. Froma Walsh called today's families a "hodgepodge of multiple evolving family cultures and structures" (Walsh, 2005a, p. 11). The structure of these families is changing to meet the functions of the families as they respond to the current economic, social, demographic, and political pressures in society.

Despite all of the changes in society and families, a recent U.S. survey by the Pew Research Center (2006, p. 1) reported the following results:

- Family members are staying in ever more frequent touch
- Families remain the greatest source of satisfaction in people's lives

- Most parents and children live within an hour's drive of one another
- 73% of adults report almost daily contact with family members living elsewhere, and
- 24% say they have a daily meal with a relative

So families are not necessarily getting further apart, but are finding different ways to connect, despite the pressures around them to do otherwise.

Family Structure

Family **structure** is the ordered set of relationships within the family, and between the family and other social systems (Denham, 2005). The clearest change in American families during the past few decades has been in the structure. In determining the family structure, the nurse needs to identify:

- The individuals that comprise family
- The relationships between them
- The interactions between the family members
- The interactions with other social systems

Family patterns of organization tend to be relatively stable over time, but they are modified gradually throughout the family life cycle and often change radically when divorce, separation, or death occurs.

In today's information age and global society, several ideas about the "best family" coexist simultaneously. Different family types have their strengths and limitations, which directly or indirectly affect individuals and family health. Many families still adhere to more customary forms and patterns, but many of today's families fall into categories more clearly labeled nontraditional (Table 1-3). Nurses will confront families structured differently from their own families of origin and will encounter family types that conflict with personal value systems. For nurses to work effectively with families, they must maintain open and inquiring minds.

Discussions of family structure often begin with a focus on the decline of the nuclear family and the emergence of diverse family types in the American society during the late 20th century. The notion that the traditional nuclear family is the "gold standard" by which to evaluate family forms needs to change (Hanson, 2005). Nuclear families are defined as one with parents and children only. Extended families are the nuclear family plus other blood-related kin or relationships formed by a marriage tie. Contemporary families may take on several different forms, including single parent (biological, adoptive, step, foster), intact nuclear (biological, adoptive), intergenerational, extended without parent present headed

TABLE 1-3	
Variations of Family and Household Structures	
FAMILY TYPE	**COMPOSITION**
Nuclear dyad	Married couple, no children
Nuclear	Husband, wife, children (may or may not be legally married)
Binuclear	Two post-divorce families with children as members of both
Extended	Nuclear family plus blood relatives
Blended	Husband, wife, and children of previous relationships
Single Parent	One parent and child(ren)
Commune	Group of men, women, and children
Cohabitation (domestic partners)	Unmarried man and woman sharing a household
Homosexual	Same-gender couple
Single person (adult)	One person in a household

Source: Kaakinen, J. R., & Hanson, S. M. H. (2008). Family development and family nursing assessment. In M. Stanhope & J. Lancaster (Eds.). *Public Health Nursing* (7th ed.). St. Louis, MO: Mosby.

by grandparent (usually grandmother), same-sex, co-habitating or domestic partnerships, and institutions (foster care, group homes, residential or treatment centers). Regardless of the family structure, each type or configuration has strengths and weaknesses (Denham, 2005).

The nuclear family (parents and child) is becoming a demographic oddity as many cultures around the world redefine what family is. The structure and norms of families are in transition worldwide (Walsh, 2005b), and they are changing at a rapid rate (Hanson, 2005). Although it is not uncommon to hear people say that today's family is unstable and its future uncertain, evidence suggests that much of what has been viewed as truth about families is merely myth (Coontz, 1998). Many of the perceptions about families ignore the diversity that has always existed (Allen, Fine, & Demo, 2000).

Families in the past were more homogeneous than they are today. Whereas the past norm was a two-parent family (traditional nuclear family) living together with their biological children, many other family forms are acknowledged and recognized today. It is important to note that the average person born today will experience many family forms during his or her lifetime. Figure 1-10 depicts the many familial forms that the average person can live through today. It is clear that life is not as simple as it used to be, and that nurses are not only experiencing this proliferation of variation in their own personal lives but also with the patients with whom

they work in health care settings (Kaakinen & Birenbaum, 2008).

Understanding family structure enables nurses assisting families to identify effective coping strategies for daily life disturbances, health care crises, wellness promotion, and disease prevention (Denham, 2005). In addition, nurses are central in advocating and developing social policies relevant to family health cares needs. For example, taking political action to increase the availability of appropriate care for children could reduce the financial and emotional burden of many working and single-parent families when faced with providing care for sick children. Similarly, caregiving responsibilities and health care costs for acutely and chronically ill family members place increasing demands on family members. Nurses well informed about different family structures can identify specific needs of unique families, provide appropriate clinical care to enhance family resilience, and act as change agents to enact social policies that reduce family burdens.

Family Functions

A functional perspective has to do with the ways families serve their members. One way to describe the **functional aspect of family** is to see the unit as made up of intimate, interactive, and interdependent persons who share some values, goals, resources, responsibilities, decisions, and commitment over time

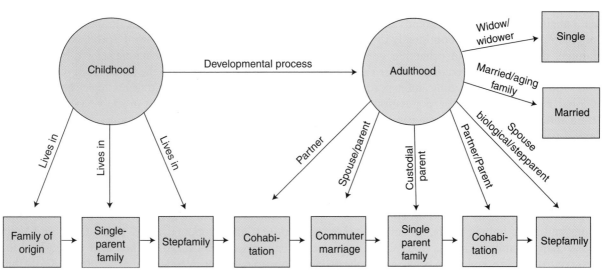

FIGURE 1-10 An individual's potential family life experiences.

(Steinmetz, Clavan, & Stein, 1990). **Family functioning** has been described as "the individual and cooperative processes used by developing persons as to dynamically engage one another and their diverse environments over the life course" (Denham, 2003a, p. 277). Specific functional aspects include the ways a family reproduces offspring, interacts to socialize its young, cooperates to meet economical needs, and relates to the larger society. Nurses should ask about specific characteristics that factor into achieving family or societal goals, or both. Families' functional processes such as socialization, reproduction, economics, and health care provision are areas nurses can readily address during health care encounters. Nursing interventions can enhance the family's protective health function when teaching and counseling is tailored to explicit learning needs. Family cultural context and individual health literacy needs are closely related to functional needs of families. Nurses become therapeutic agents as they assist families to identify social supports and locate community resources during times of family transitions and health crisis. Five family functions are described in this book: reproductive, socialization, affective, economic, and health care.

REPRODUCTIVE FUNCTIONS OF THE FAMILY

The survival of a society is linked to patterns of reproduction. Sexuality serves the purposes of pleasure and reproduction, but associated values differ from one society to another. Traditionally, the family has been organized around the biological function of reproduction. Reproduction was viewed as a major concern for thousands of years when populating the earth was continually threatened by famine, disease, war, and other life uncertainties. Norms about sexual intercourse affect the fertility rate. Birth control has long influenced families. Global concerns about overpopulation and environmental threats, as well as personal views of morality and financial well-being, have been reasons for limiting numbers of family births.

Since the 1980s, the reproductive function has become increasingly separated from the family (Robertson, 1991). Individuals tend to organize themselves into families based on cultural prescriptions and basic human needs. As cultural prescriptions change, families change. Today's families have less control over reproductive behaviors (Robertson, 1991). Abstinence, various forms of contraception, tubal ligation, vasectomy, family planning, artificial insemination, and abortion have various degrees of social acceptance as means to control reproduction. For centuries, the state, religion, and family have fought over rights to control reproduction. In 1973, in the *Roe v. Wade* decision, based on the privacy rights, the U.S. Supreme Court ruled that during the first trimester of pregnancy, states could not interfere with decisions about terminating pregnancy. The abortion issue continues to be debated with strong "pro-choice" and "pro-life" positions taken by some, with others giving assent to abortion in some situations but not others. In 2006, South Dakota became the first to ban access to abortion services, directly challenging *Roe v. Wade*. In South Dakota it is a felony for a health care provider to perform an abortion unless the mother's life is at risk.

The ethical dilemmas mirrored in the abortion controversy seem compounded by technologic advances that affect reproduction and problems of infertility. Reproductive technologies are guided by few legal, ethical, or moral guidelines. In fact, 47 states have a policy that allows health care practitioners to refuse to participate in the delivery of reproductive health services (Guttmacher Institute, 2005). Artificial insemination by husband or donor, in vitro fertilization, surrogate mothers, and artificial embryonation, in which a woman other than the woman who will give birth to and raise the child donates an egg for fertilization, create financial and moral dilemmas when pregnancy cannot occur through usual reproductive processes. Although assistive reproductive technologies can provide a biological link to the child, some families are choosing to adopt children. Many are wrangling over the issues implicit in cross-racial and cross-cultural adoptions. Reproductive technologies and adoption are being considered by all family types to add children to the family unit. Religious, legal, moral, economic, and technologic challenges will continue to cause debates in the years ahead about family control over reproduction.

SOCIALIZATION FUNCTIONS OF THE FAMILY

A major function for families is to raise and socialize their children to fit into society. Families have great variability in the ways they address physical, emotional, and economic needs of children, and these patterns are influenced by the larger society and the historical point in time (Coontz, 2000, 2006). Children are born into families without knowledge of the values, language, norms, or roles of the society where they will become members. A major function of the family continues to be to socialize them about family life, educate them for the labor market, and ground them in the societal identity of which they are a part.

Although the family is not the only institution of society that participates in children's socialization, it is generally viewed as having primary responsibility. When children fail to meet societal standards, it is common to blame this on family deficits and parental inadequacies.

Although Americans have traditionally viewed the nuclear family as the optimum type, other societies have spread the responsibility of child-rearing among other adults. Kin are very involved in child rearing, especially to provide after-school care (Hansen, 2005).

Today, patterns of socialization require appropriate developmental care that fosters dependence and leads to independence (Denham, 2005). Socialization is the primary way children acquire the social and psychological skills needed to take their place in the adult world. Parents combine social support and social control as they equip children to meet future life tasks. Parental figures interact in multiple roles such as friends, lovers, child-care providers, housekeepers, providers, recreation specialists, and counselors. Children growing up within families learn the values and norms of their parents and extended families.

Another role of families in the socialization process is to guide children through various rites of passage. Rites of passage are ceremonies that announce a change in status in the ways members are viewed. Examples include events such as a baptism, communion, circumcision, puberty ritual, graduation, wedding, and death. These occasions signal to others changes in role relationships and new expectations. Understandings about families' unique rites of passage can assist nurses working with diverse health care needs.

AFFECTIVE FUNCTIONS OF THE FAMILY

Affective function has to do with the ways family members relate to one another and those outside the immediate family boundaries. Families provide a sense of belonging and identity to their members. This identity often proves to be vitally important throughout the entire life cycle. Within the confines of families, members learn dependent roles that later serve to launch them into independent ones. Families serve as a place to learn about intimate relationships and establish the foundation for future personal interactions. Families provide the initial experience of self-awareness, which includes a sense of knowing one's own gender, ethnicity, race, religion, and personal characteristics. Families help members become acquainted with who they are and experience themselves in relationships with others. Families provide the substance for self-identity, as well as a foundation for other-identity. Within the confines of families, individual members learn about love, care, nurturance, dependence, and support of the dying.

Resilience implies an ability to rebound from stress and crisis, the capacity to be optimistic, solve problems, be resourceful, and develop caring support systems. Although unique traits alter potential for emotional and psychological health, individuals exposed to resilient family environments tend to have greater potential to achieve normative developmental patterns and positive sibling and parental relationships (Denham, 2005).

Research on parent-child interactions needs to consider the quantity and quality of time spent together, the kinds of activities engaged in, and patterns of interaction to understand member feelings toward each other. More needs to be known about relationships with nonresidential parents. Variables such as the quality of the couple's relationship, the ways family conflict is handled, whether abuse or violence has previously occurred in the household or member lives, frequency of children's contact with nonresidential parents, shared custody arrangements, and emotional relationships between parents and children seem important predictors of family affective functions. Affective functions can best be understood by gathering information from all of the various members involved within a household.

ECONOMIC FUNCTIONS OF THE FAMILY

During the 20th century, the most obvious change in family function is related to economics. In the early stages of American history, the household was the major source of commodity production (Hanson, 2005). In the past, families worked together under the leadership of a household head, usually a man, and family economics reflected these familial relationships. With the emergence of capitalism in the early 19th century, the family households and their patriarchal systems served as a source for workers. The heads of household who earned the wages for the family also contributed family members to work for the fledgling but growing industrial enterprises. Later in the 20th century, young and unmarried women constituted an important part of the labor pool in World War I (1914–1918). With the rise of capitalism in the late 19th and early 20th centuries, the division of labor between work and home increased, and became viewed as men's versus women's work, respectively.

After World War II, the majority of women returned home, but many elected to remain in the labor force. Over the years since then, the shift from an industrial to a service economy has meant an increased number of women in the labor force. Wage differences and familial desires for broader services have been reasons why dual-wage earners have become more common. Women continue to earn less than men even when they perform the same job (Walsh, 2005a). Young men, in particular, are experiencing a worsening of their economic position, and older men are leaving the labor force in record numbers. Many families today require dual earners to keep pace with costs.

Families have an important function in keeping the nation's economy viable. Economic conditions significantly affect families. When the economy is turbulent so is family structure, functions, and processes. People make decisions about when to enter the labor force, when to marry, when to have children, and when to retire or come of out of retirement based on economic factors (Bianchi, Casper, & King, 2005). For a detailed discussion on family and economics see Chapter 2.

Family income provides a substantial part of family economics, but an equally important aspect has to do with economic interactions and consumerism related to household consumption and finance. Money management, housing decisions, consumer spending, insurance choices, retirement planning, and savings are some of the issues that affect family capacity to care for the economic needs of its members. Financial vulnerability and bankruptcy have increased even for middle-class families as they have assumed greater debt, opted to use more credit cards, paid higher interest rates, and made increasingly larger credit payments. The ability of the family to earn a sufficient income and to manage its finances wisely is a critical factor related to economic well-being.

HEALTH CARE FUNCTIONS OF THE FAMILY

Family members often serve as the primary health care providers to their families. Individuals regularly seek services from a variety of health care professionals, but it is within the family that health instructions are followed or ignored. Family members tend to be the primary caregivers and sources of support for individuals during health and illness. Families influence well-being, prevention, illness care, maintenance care associated with chronic illness, and rehabilitative care. Family members often care for one another's health conditions from the cradle to the grave. Families can become particularly vulnerable when they encounter health threats, and family-focused nurses are in a position where they can provide education, counseling, and assist with locating resources. Family-focused care implies that when a single individual is the target of care, the entire family is still viewed as the unit of care (Denham, 2003a).

Health care functions of the family include many aspects of family life. Family members have different ideas about health and illness, and often these ideas are not discussed within families until problems arise. Availability and cost of health care insurance is a concern for many families, but many families lack clarity about what is and is not covered until they encounter a problem. Lifestyle behaviors, such as healthy diet, regular exercise, alcohol and tobacco use, are areas that family members may not associate with health and illness outcomes. Risk reduction, health maintenance, rehabilitation, and caregiving are areas where families often need information and assistance. Family members spend far more time taking care of health issues of family members than professionals do.

Family Processes

Family process is the ongoing interaction between family members through which they accomplish their instrumental and expressive tasks (Denham, 2005). In part, this is what makes every family unique within its own particular culture. Families with similar structures and functions may interact differently. Family process, at least in the short term, appears to have a greater effect on the family's health status than family structure and function, and in turn, processes within families are more affected by alterations in health status. Family process certainly appears to have the greatest implications for nursing actions. For example, for the chronically ill, an important determinant for successful rehabilitation is the ability to assume one's familial roles. For rehabilitation to occur, family members have to communicate effectively, make decisions about atypical situations, and use a variety of coping strategies. The usual familial power structure may be threatened or need to change to address unique individual needs. Ultimately, the success or failure of the adaptation processes will affect individual and family well-being.

Alterations in family processes most likely occur when the family faces a transition brought about by developmental changes (adding or subtracting family members), an illness or accident, or other potential crisis situations, such as natural disasters, wars, or personal crises. The family's current modes of operation may become ineffective, and members are confronted with learning new ways of coping with change. For example, when coping with the stress of a chronic illness, families experience alterations in role performance and in power. When individuals are unable to perform usual roles, other members are expected to assume them. A shift in family roles may result in the loss of individual power. During times of change, family nurses can assist family members to communicate, make decisions, identify ways to cope with multiple stressors, reduce role strain, and locate needed resources.

Family communication patterns, member interactions, and interaction with social networks are a few areas related to family processes that nurses need to assess systematically. Nursing interventions that promote resiliency in family processes vary with the degree of strain faced by the family. Families have complex needs related to adaptation, goal attainment, integration, pattern, and tension management. When family processes are ineffective or disrupted, the families and their members may be at risk for problems pertinent to health outcomes, and the family itself could be in danger of disintegrating.

Following is a discussion of a few family processes that nurses can influence through their relationships with families in caregiving situations. The family processes covered are family coping, family roles, family communication, family decision making, and family rituals and routines.

FAMILY COPING

Every family has their own repertoire of coping strategies, which may or may not be adequate in times of stress, such as when a family member experiences an altered health event. Coping consists of "constantly changing cognitive and behavioral efforts to manage specific external and/or internal demands that are appraised as taxing or exceeding the resources of the person" (Lazarus & Folkman, 1984, p. 141). Families with support can withstand and rebound from difficult stressors (Walsh, 2005b), which is called *family resilience.*

Not all families have the same ability to cope because of multiple reasons. Key processes in family resiliency include belief system, organizational patterns, and family communication (Walsh, 2005b). The family's belief system involves making meaning of adversity, maintaining a positive outlook, and being able to transcend adversity through a spiritual/faith system (Walsh, 2005b). The families' organization patterns, which speak to their flexibility, connectedness, and social and economic resources, help the family maintain resilience. Finally, families who communicate with clarity, allow open emotional expression, and have a collaborative problem-solving approach facilitate family resiliency (Walsh, 2005b).

Nurses have the ability to support families in times of stress and crisis through empowering processes that work well and are familiar to the family. Families need help in establishing priorities and responding to everyday needs. For example, when an unexpected death in the family occurs, family members are called on to make multiple decisions. At the same time, they may not remember phone numbers, cannot think of whom to call in what order, decide who should pick up the kids, determine which funeral home to use, or how or what to tell children or aging parents. Helping families work through steps and setting priorities during this situation is an important aspect of family nursing.

Even families who function at optimal levels may experience difficulties when stressful events pile up. Even when families cope well, they may still be stressed (Measley, Richardson, & Dimico, 1989). The outcomes of coping strategies are difficult to evaluate in the short term. The long-term impact of various coping strategies and styles is best understood over time. For example, an individual's grieving may appear adaptive during the first few weeks after the death of a family member, but the individual may go into deep depression and grieving weeks or months after the actual death. These initial reactions may send the wrong message to other family members who think the bereaved person is "taking it well."

Today's families encounter many challenges that leave them vulnerable to a myriad of stressors. Vulnerability can result from poverty, illness, abuse, and violence, and even the location of the family residence. Coping capacities are enhanced whenever families demonstrate resilience or the capacity to survive in the midst of struggle, adversity, and long-term conflict. Families who recover from crisis tend to be more cohesive, value unique member attributes, support one another without criticism, and focus on strengths.

FAMILY ROLES

Within the family, regardless of structure, each family position has a number of attached roles, and each role is accompanied by expectations. After a review of the family literature, Nye (1976) identified eight roles associated with the position of spouse/partner:

- Provider
- Housekeeper
- Child care
- Socialization
- Sexual
- Therapeutic
- Recreational
- Kinship

Additional roles that affect the family are those of family caregiver and the sick role the person takes on during illness. Traditionally, the provider role has been assigned to husbands, whereas wives assumed the housekeeper, child care, and other caregiving roles. With societal changes and variations in family structure, however, the traditional enactment of these roles is not viable for many families anymore. Families are organized by gender roles (Haddock, Zimmerman, & Lyness, 2005), generation, and location in the family, for example, middle child, mother, father, stepsister, niece, and grandfather. Attitudes have changed somewhat in regard to rigid gender role enactment (who does what), but the research shows that, in reality, little change has occurred, and most families remain gender based (Haddock et al., 2005). For example, 70% of all mothers work, and women continue to provide 80% of the child care and household obligations (Walsh, 2005a). Men are participating and doing more in the home and with child care in the family than ever before, but this responsibility still remains largely with women.

In every household, members have to decide the ways work and responsibilities will be divided and shared. Roles are negotiated, assigned, delegated, or assumed. Division of labor within the family household occurs as various members assume roles, and as families change over time and over the family life cycle. For example, family members may become unable to perform their roles, and the family needs to reconfigure role allocation after the birth or death of family members.

PROVIDER ROLE. The provider role has undergone significant change in the past few decades. Whereas American men were once viewed as the primary family breadwinner, this has changed significantly. In today's world, many families need more than one income to meet basic needs. Factors that contribute to the need for increased income are an increase in number of families with no wage earners, and an increased number of families being solely supported by someone other than a male householder (Walsh, 2005a). Work conditions have become increasingly stressful for men and women, and external work obligations increasingly impinge on members' abilities to meet familial role obligations.

HOUSEKEEPER AND CHILD CARE ROLES. Today, many women experience significant role strain in balancing provider and other familial roles. Women who work continue to be responsible for most housekeeping and child care responsibilities (Haddock et al., 2005). Women who work outside the home still perform 80% of the child care and household duties (Walsh, 2005a). Although husbands' roles in child care are increasing, their focus is often on playing with the children rather than meeting basic needs. Women still are primary in meeting health care needs of all family members, including children and men.

SOCIALIZATION ROLE. In relation to socialization of the children, the role expectations have become more egalitarian over the past few decades (Haddock et al., 2005). Socialization includes things such as the ways children learn to interact with others, care for themselves, create boundaries for relationships with extended family, peers, or others, and act as citizens of the larger society. Parents assume the major socialization roles through teaching, guiding, directing, disciplining, and counseling children. Although involvement of both parents promotes the healthy development of children, the father-child relationship is qualitatively different than the mother-child relationship. Mothers assume the larger share of the responsibility for children's socialization.

SICK ROLE. Individuals learn health and illness behaviors in their family of origin. Health behaviors are related to the primary prevention of disease, and include health promotion activities to reduce susceptibility to disease and actions to reduce the effects of chronic disease. Once a family member becomes ill, he or she demonstrates various illness behaviors or enacts the "sick role." Parsons (1951) defines the classic four characteristics of a person who is sick:

1. While sick, the person is temporarily exempt from carrying out normal social and family roles. The more severe the illness, the freer one is from role obligations.
2. In general, the sick person is not held responsible for being ill.
3. The sick person is expected to take actions to get well, and therefore has an obligation to "get well."
4. The sick person is expected to seek competent professional medical care and to comply with medical advice on how to "get well."

Voluminous research has been conducted on the theoretical concepts of the sick role. Some criticisms of the theory are: (1) some individuals reject the sick role; (2) some individuals are blamed for their illness, such as alcoholics or individuals with AIDS; and (3) sometimes independence is encouraged in persons who have a chronic illness as a way to "get well."

Regardless of the debates about the sick role, individuals in families experience acute and chronic illness. Each family, depending on its family processes, defines the sick role differently. Most "sick" people require some level of care; someone needs to assume the family caregiver role. The caregiving role may be as simple as a stop at the store on their way home to buy chicken soup or pick up medicines, or as involved as providing around-the-clock care for someone. The female individuals in our society still provide the majority of the care required when family members become sick or injured. The specific needs of families who experience health events are discussed in other chapters in this book.

ROLE STRAIN, CONFLICT, AND OVERLOAD

Family roles are affected, some more than others, when a family member becomes ill. Usually the women in the family add the role of family caregiver to their other roles. Nurses have a crucial role in helping families by discussing and exploring role strain, role conflict, and role overload. Nurses can facilitate family adaptation by helping to problem-solve role negotiations and helping families access outside resources.

ROLE STRAIN. Lack of competence in role performance may be a result of role strain. Some researchers have found that sources of role strain are cultural and interactional. Interactional sources of role strain are related to difficulties in the delineation and enactment of familial roles. Heiss (1981) identifies five sources of difficulties in the interaction process that place strain on a family system:

- Inability to define the situation
- Lack of role knowledge
- Lack of role consensus
- Role conflict
- Role overload

The *inability to define the situation* creates ambiguity about what one should do in a given scenario. Continual changes in family structures and gender roles means that members increasingly encounter situations in which guidelines for action are unclear. Single parents, stepparents, nonresident fathers, and cohabitating partners deal daily with situations for which there are no norms. What right does a stepparent have to discipline the new spouse's child? Is a nonresident father expected to teach his child about AIDS? What name or names go on the mailbox of cohabitating partners?

Regardless of whether the issues are substantive, they present daily challenges to the people involved. Some choose to withdraw from the situation, and others choose to redefine the situation when they are uncertain how to act. For instance, a blended family might want to operate in the same way as a traditional family but may experience conflict when thinking about who and who not to include in family decision making. When a solution cannot be found, family members suffer the consequences of role strain.

Role strain sometimes results when family members lack *role knowledge,* or they have no basis for choosing between several roles that might seem appropriate. In America, most people are not clearly taught how to be parents, and much leaning is observational and experiential. Socialization related to caregiving of a chronically ill family member is seldom done, and many individuals are unfamiliar with and unprepared to assume the roles necessary for providing care. When an individual is learning how to be a parent or a caregiver, role training may be required. Knowledge may be acquired by peer observation, trial and error, or explicit instruction. Parents may have limited opportunities to observe peers, and other family members may not have the knowledge necessary to help. Thus, the family may need to seek external resources or obtain needed information using other means such as child care classes, self-help groups, or instruction from health professionals. If individuals are unable to figure out their roles in a situation, problem-solving abilities are limited.

Family members may lack *role consensus,* or be unable to agree about the expectations attached to a role. One family role that is often the source of family disagreement is the housekeeping role, especially for dual-career couples. Men who have been socialized into more traditional male roles are less inclined to accept responsibility for household tasks readily and may limit the amount of time they are willing to spend on these activities. When active participation does not meet the wife's expectations, she tends to assume responsibility for the greater number of household tasks. If she has been socialized into thinking that women are accountable for traditional housekeeping roles, then she may feel guilty or neglectful if she asks for help. Lack of agreement about the role sometimes results in familial discord and taxes levels of satisfaction with the partner. Although persuasion, manipulation, and coercion may be used to reduce role strain, negotiation is usually required and is most likely to be effective in reaching consensus about things that can be done.

ROLE CONFLICT. Role conflict occurs when the expectations about familial roles are incompatible. For example, the therapeutic role might involve becoming a caregiver to an elderly parent, but expectations of this new role may be incompatible with that of provider, housekeeper, and child care provider. Does one go to the child's baseball game or to the doctor with the elderly parent? Role conflict may occur when roles present conflicting demands. Individuals and families often have to set priorities. Demands of caregiver and provider roles may be conflicting and may conflict with other therapeutic familial tasks. The caregiver may withdraw from activities that, in the short term, seem superfluous, but in the long term are sources of much needed energy. Family nurses are likely to encounter members facing many strains because of role conflict, and may need to assist by providing information and suggesting ways the family could negotiate roles, to discover meaningful solutions.

ROLE OVERLOAD. A source of role strain closely related to role conflict is role overload. In role overload, the individual lacks resources, time, and energy to meet role demands. As with role conflict, the first option usually considered is withdrawal from one of the roles. Maintaining a balance between energy-enhancing and energy-depleting roles reduces role strain. An alternative to withdrawing from a role might be to seek time away from some role responsibilities that are personally satisfying and energy producing. For example, a friend of the family member could relieve the primary caregiver for several hours. Nurses could arrange for a home-health aide to assist with personal care hygiene. The dependent family member can be temporarily cared for in a residential facility while the other family members go on a vacation.

It is the role of the nurse to help families who experience role strain, conflict, and overload. Using anticipatory guidance, nurses work closely with families to discuss and define the family flow of energy and resources when confronted with a family caregiving situation. See Chapter 4 for ways to work with families.

FAMILY COMMUNICATION

Communication is an ongoing, complex, changing activity and is the means through which people create, share, and regulate meaning in a transactional process to make sense of their world (Dance, 1967). In all families, communication is continuous in that it defines their present reality and constructs family relationships (Dance, 1967). "Rather than attempting to understand the family from one specific instance of communication or from one family member, the family should be understood as a whole" (Segrin & Flora, 2005, p. 1).

It is through communication that families find ways to adapt to changes as they seek family stability. Families that are highly adaptive change more easily in response to demands. Families with low adaptability have a fixed or more rigid style of interacting (Olson & Gorall, 2005). "Family adaptability is manifested in how assertive family members are with each other, the amount of control in the family, family discipline practices, negotiation, how rigid family roles are adhered to, and the nature and enforcement of rules in the family" (Segrin & Flora, 2005, p. 17).

Family communication affects family physical and mental health. Most programs and intervention strategies for improving family communication are beyond the role and experience of nurses with undergraduate education. The role of the nurse is to facilitate family communication at times when families are stressed by changes that occur with its members, such as birth of an infant, growth and development issues of children, when family members become ill, or the death of family members. It is the role of the nurse to assist family communication to achieve healthful outcomes.

FAMILY DECISION MAKING

Communication and power are family processes that influence decision making. Family decision making is not an individual effort but a joint one. Most health care decisions should be made from a family perspective. Each decision has at least five features: the person raising the issue, what is being said about the issue, supporting action to what is being said, the importance of what is being said, and the responses of the individuals (Friedman et al., 2003).

Decision making provides opportunity for various family members to make a contribution to the process, support one another, and jointly set and strive to achieve goals. Disagreements within a family are natural as members often have different points of view. It is important for members to share their various viewpoints with one another. Problem solving is part of the decision-making process, and frequently means that differences in opinion and emotions need to be considered.

Family communication processes influence decision-making outcomes. In the Pew Research Center 2006 report on family communication, 46% of the 3,014 subjects indicated that they turned to their families for help and advice when they have problems. In family conflicts, the expression of anger is not necessarily destructive, but contempt, belligerence, and defensiveness are counterproductive (Gottman, Coan, Carrere, Swanson, 1998). The expression of negative emotions tends to lead to conflict as an outcome of decision making. Using "I" messages rather than blaming or accusing the other person is helpful in talking through differences. Consensus or, at the least, continuation of negotiations is the preferred outcome when disagreements occur. Nurses working with families can facilitate family communication skills to help families find an effective way for resolving differences and making decisions.

Families want to be involved in varying degrees with health care decisions. Families are often asked to help make end-of-life decisions, to not resuscitate a loved one or to withdraw/withhold life-sustaining therapies. Decision making between families and health care professionals is addressed in more detail in Chapter 4.

FAMILY RITUALS AND ROUTINES

Rituals and routines have been identified in the literature as having health implications (Denham, 2003a). Rituals are associated with celebrations, traditions, religious observances, and symbolic events, whereas routines are behaviors closely linked with daily or regular activities. Families have unique rituals and routines that provide organization and give meaning to family life. The habitual behaviors associated with rituals and routines have potential for health and illness outcomes (Denham, 1995). Family culture, context, and function affect these rituals and routines. The importance and value of rituals in everyday life has been clearly explored in anthropologic and sociologic literature, but the significance of rituals is largely ignored by nurses (Denham, 2003b).

Family routines are continuous behaviors, and family members use them in their roles to define responsibilities, organize daily life, and identify family characteristics or traits (Bennett, Wolin, & McAvity, 1988; Steinglass, Bennett, Wolin, & Reiss, 1987). Examples of family routines include mealtimes, bedtime routines, leisure-time activities, greetings and good-byes, and treatment of guests.

Rituals and routines are family life processes with important consequences for individual and family health outcomes. Assessing rituals and routines related to specific health or illness needs provides a basis to envision distinct family interventions and to devise specific plans for health promotion and disease management, especially when adherence to medical regimens is critical or caregiving demands are burdensome to the families (Denham, 2003b). Nurses can help families maintain routines and rituals as a way to decrease stress, pull the family together, and help keep a focus on family strength.

SUMMARY

This chapter provides an introduction and broad overview to family health care nursing. The chapter explores definitions of family and family health, and presents characteristics of healthy families and couples based on longitudinal studies. The chapter also discusses the nature of interventions in family nursing, the four approaches to family nursing, and the variables that influence family nursing, together with the obstacles to family nursing practice and family nursing roles.

The second section of the chapter, Family Structure, Function, and Process, provides a broad view into the workings of families with specific focus on families who are experiencing a health event in one of its members. Nursing interventions offer nurses ideas about actions that support families. Family health care nursing is at the core of all nursing practice everywhere and at any time. Because health and illness are family events, nurses interface with families at these crossroads, and the informed nursing care of families makes a difference for all.

REFERENCES

Allen, K. R., Fine, M. A., & Demo, D. H. (2000). An overview of family diversity: Controversies, questions, and values. In D. Demo, K. Allen, & M. Fine (Eds.), *Handbook of family diversity* (pp. 1–14). New York: Oxford University Press.

American Nurses Association. (2003a). *Nursing's social policy statement* (2nd ed.). Washington, DC: American Nurses Association.

American Nurses Association. (2003b). *Nursing: Scope and standards of practice.* Washington, DC: American Nurses Association.

Anderson, K. H., & Tomlinson, P. S. (1992). The family health system as an emerging paradigmatic view for nursing. *Image: Journal of Nursing Scholarship, 24,* 57–63.

Benner, P. (2001). *Novice to expert: Excellence and power in clinical nursing practice.* Menlo Park, CA: Prentice Hall

Bennett, L. A., Wolin, S. J., & McAvity, K. J. (1988). Family identity, ritual, and myth: A cultural perspective on life cycle transitions. In C. J. Falicov (Ed.), *Family transitions: Continuity and change over the life cycle* (pp. 211–233). New York: The Guilford Press.

Bianchi, S. M., Casper, L. M., & King, R. B. (2005). *Work, family, health, & well-being.* Mahwah, NJ: Lawrence Erlbaum Associates.

Bomar, P. J. (Ed.). (2004). *Promoting health in families: Applying family research and theory to nursing practice* (3rd ed.). Philadelphia: Saunders/Elsevier.

Burgess, E. W., & Locke, H. J. (1953). *The family: From institution to companionship.* New York: American Book Company.

Carrere, S., Buehlman, K. T., Coan, J., Gottman, J. M., & Ruckstuhl, L. (2000). Predicting marital stability and divorce in newlywed couples. *Journal of Family Psychology, 14*(1), 42–58.

Coontz, S. (1998). *The way we really are: Coming to terms with America's changing families.* New York: Basic Books.

Coontz, S. (2000). Historical perspectives on family diversity. In D. Demo, K. Allen, & M. Fine (Eds.), *Handbook of Family Diversity* (pp. 15–31). New York: Oxford University Press.

Coontz, S. (2006). *Marriage, a history: How love conquered marriage.* New York: Peguin Press.

Curran, D. (1985). *Stress and the healthy family.* Minneapolis, MN: Winston Press (Harper and Row).

Dance, F. E. X. (1967). Toward a theory of human communication. In F. E. X. Dance (Ed.), *Human communication theory* (pp. 288–309). New York: Holt.

Denham, S. A. (1995). Family routines: A construct for considering family health. *Holistic Nursing Practice, 9*(4), 11–23.

Denham, S. A. (2003a). *Family health: A framework for nursing.* Philadelphia: F.A. Davis.

Denham, S. A. (2003b). Relationships between family rituals, family routines, and health. *Journal of Family Nursing, 9*(30), 305–330.

Denham, S. A. (2005). Family structure, function and process. In S. M. H. Hanson, V. Gedaly-Duff, & J. R. Kaakinen (Eds.), *Family health care nursing: Theory, practice and research* (3rd ed., pp. 119–157). Philadelphia: F.A. Davis.

Driver, H., Tabares, A., Shapiro, A., Nahm, E. Y., & Gottman, J. M. (2005). Interactional patterns in marital success and failure: Gottman laboratory studies. In F. Walsh (Ed.), *Normal family processes: Growing diversity and complexity* (3rd ed., pp. 493–514). New York: The Guilford Press.

Friedman, M. H., Bowden, V. R., & Jones, E. G. (2003). *Family nursing: Research, theory and practice* (5th ed.). Norwalk, CT: Appleton & Lange.

Gilliss, C. L., Roberts, B. M., Highley, B. L., & Martinson, I. M. (1989). What is family nursing? In C. L. Gilliss, B. L. Highley, B. M. Roberts, & I. M. Martinson (Eds.), *Toward a science of family nursing* (pp. 64–73). Menlo Park, CA: Addison-Wesley.

Gottman, J. M., Coan, J., Carrere, S., & Swanson, C. (1998). Predicting marital happiness and stability from newlywed interactions. *Journal of Marriage and the Family, 60,* 5–22.

Guttmacher Institute. (2005). *Striking a balance between a provider's right to refuse and a patient's right to receive care.* Retrieved July 9, 2008, from www.guttmacher.org/media/presskit/2005/04/index.html

Haddock, S. A., Zimmerman, T. S., & Lyness, K. P. (2005). Changing gender norms: Transitional dilemmas. In F. Walsh (Ed.), *Normal family processes: Growing diversity and complexity* (3rd ed., pp. 301–336). New York: The Guilford Press.

Ham, L. M., & Chamings, P. A. (1983). Family nursing: Historical perspectives. In I. Clements, & F. B. Roberts (Eds.), *Family health care: Vol. 1. A theoretical approach to nursing care* (pp. 88–109). San Francisco: McGraw-Hill.

Hansen, K. V. (2005). *Not-so-nuclear families: Class, gender, and networks of care.* New Brunswick, NJ: Rutgers University Press.

Hanson, S. M. H. (2005). Introduction to family health care nursing. In S. M. H. Hanson, V. Gedaly-Duff, & J. R. Kaakinen (Eds.), *Family health care nursing: Theory, practice and research* (3rd ed., pp. 3–38). Philadelphia: F.A. Davis.

Heiss, J. (1981). Family theory 20 years later. *Contemporary Sociology, 9*(2), 201–205.

Kaakinen, J. R., & Birenbaum, L. K. (2008). Family development and family nursing assessment. In M. Stanhope and J. Lancaster (Eds.), *Community and public health nursing* (7th ed., pp. 550–579). St. Louis, MO: Mosby.

Kaakinen, J. R., & Hanson, S. M. H. (2008). Family development and family nursing assessment. In M. Stanhope & J. Lancaster (Eds.). *Public Health Nursing* (7th ed.). St. Louis, MO: Mosby.

Lazarus, R. S., & Folkman, S. (1984). *Stress, appraisal, & coping.* New York: Springer.

Measley, A. R., Richardson, H., & Dimico, G. (1989). Family stress management. In P. J. Bomar (Ed.), *Nurses and family health promotion: Concepts, assessment, and interventions* (pp. 179–196). Baltimore, MD: Williams & Wilkins.

Nightingale, F. (1979). *Cassandra.* Westbury, NY: The Feminist Press.

Nye, F. I. (1976). *Role structure and analysis of the family.* Beverly Hills, CA: Sage.

Olson, D. H., & Gorall, D. N. (2005). Circumplex model of marital and family systems. In F. Walsh (Ed.), *Normal family processes: Growing diversity and complexity* (3rd ed., pp. 514–548). New York: The Guilford Press.

Otto, H. (1963). Criteria for assessing family strengths. *Family Process, 2,* 329–338.

Parsons. T. (1951). *The social system.* Glencoe, IL: The Free Press.

Pew Research Center. (2006). *Families drawn together by communication revolution: A social trends report.* Retrieved April 24, 2009, from http://pewresearch.org/assets/social/pdf/FamilyBonds.pdf

Pratt, L. (1976). *Family structure and effective health behavior: The energized family.* Boston: Houghton Mifflin.

Robertson, A. F. (1991). *Beyond the family: The social organization of human reproduction.* Berkeley: University of California Press.

Segrin, C., & Flora, J. (2005). Defining family communication and family functioning. In C. Segrin, & J. Flora (Eds.), *Family communication* (pp. 3–27). Mahwah, NJ: Lawrence Erlbaum Associates.

Steinglass, P., Bennett, L., Wolin, S., & Reiss, D. (1987). *The alcoholic family.* New York: Basic Books.

Steinmetz, S. K., Clavan, S., & Stein, K. F. (1990). *Marriage and family realities: Historical and contemporary perspectives.* New York: Harper & Roe.

Tillman, K. H., & Nam, C. G. (2008). Family structure outcomes of alternative family definitions. *Population Research and Policy Review, 27,* 367–384.

Walsh, F. (2005a). Changing families in a changing world: Reconstructing family normality. In F. Walsh (Ed.), *Normal family processes: Growing diversity and complexity* (3rd ed., pp. 3–27), New York: The Guilford Press.

Walsh, F. (2005b). Family resilience: Strengths forged through adversity. In F. Walsh (Ed.), *Normal family processes: Growing diversity and complexity* (3rd ed., pp. 399–423). New York: The Guilford Press.

Whall, A. L. (1993). The family as the unit of care in nursing: A historical review. In G. D. Wegner, & R. J. Alexander (Eds.), *Readings in family nursing* (pp. 3–12). Philadelphia: J. B. Lippincott.

World Health Organization. (2008). *The determinants of health.* Retrieved on July 9, 2008, from http://www.who.int/hia/evidence/doh/en/index.html

Wright, L. M., & Leahey, M. (2005). *Nurses and families: A guide to family assessment and intervention* (4th ed.). Philadelphia: F.A. Davis.

CHAPTER 2

Demography and Family Health

Lynne M. Casper, PhD

John G. Haaga, PhD

Radheeka R. Jayasundera, BS

CRITICAL CONCEPTS

✦ Economic and cultural changes have increased family diversity in North America. More families are maintained by single mothers, single fathers, cohabiting couples, and grandparents than in the past.

✦ Increases in women's labor force participation, especially among mothers, have reduced the amount of nonwork time that families have to attend to health care needs.

✦ Single-mother families are particularly vulnerable. They are more likely to be in poverty than are other families. These mothers are usually the sole wage earners and care providers in their families. Thus, these families are more likely than other families to be both monetarily poor and time poor.

✦ North Americans are more likely to live alone than they were a few decades ago. Thus, people are less likely to have family members living with them who can assist them when they become ill or injured.

✦ The aging of the population presents significant challenges for both informal caregivers and the health care system. An increased need will exist for nurses who specialize in caring for the elderly.

✦ More North Americans are immigrants than was the case a couple of decades ago. Family nurses provide care for an ethnically, culturally, and linguistically diverse population.

*I*f there is one "mantra" about family life in the last half century, it is that the family has undergone tremendous change. No other institution elicits as contentious debate as the North American family. Many argue that the movement away from marriage and traditional gender roles has seriously degraded family life. Others view family life as amazingly diverse, resilient, and adaptive to new circumstances (Popenoe, 1993; Stacey, 1993).

Any assessment of the general "health" of family life in North America, and the health and well-being of family members, especially children, requires a look at what we know about demographic and socioeconomic trends that affect families. A pragmatic approach to family nursing requires an understanding of the broader changes in family and health within the population. The latter half of the 20th century was characterized by tumultuous change in the economy, in civil rights, in sexual freedom, and by dramatic improvements in health and longevity. Marriage and family life felt the reverberations of these societal changes.

In the first decade of the 21st century, as we reassess where we have come from and where we are going, one thing stands out: Rhetoric about the dramatically changing family may be a step behind the reality. Recent trends suggest a quieting of changes in the family in Canada, as well as the United States, or at least of the pace of change. Little change occurred in the proportions of two-parent or single-mother families between the mid-1990s and the mid-2000s (U.S. Census Bureau, 2008a). The living arrangements of children stabilized, as did the living arrangements of young adults and the elderly. The divorce rate had been in decline for more than two decades. The rapid growth in cohabitation among unmarried adults has also slowed.

Yet, family life is still evolving. Young adults have often postponed marriage and children to complete college before attempting to enter labor markets that have become inhospitable to poorly educated workers. Accompanying this delay in marriage was the continued increase in births to unmarried women, though here, too, the pace of change slowed in the 1990s and the mid-2000s (Ventura et al., 1995). Within marriage or marriage-like relationships, the appropriate roles for each partner are shifting as North American societies accept and value more equal roles for men and women. The widening role of fathers has become a major agent of change in the family. More father-only families exist than in the past, and after divorce, fathers are more likely to share custody of children with the mother. Within two-parent families, fathers are also more likely to be involved in the children's care than in the past.

Whether the slowing, and in some cases, cessation, of change in family living arrangements is a temporary lull or part of a new, more sustained equilibrium will only be revealed in the coming decades of the 21st century. New norms may be emerging about the desirability of marriage, the optimal timing of children, and the involvement of fathers in child rearing and mothers in breadwinning. Understanding the evolution of North American families and the implications these changes have for family nursing requires taking the pulse of contemporary family life.

This chapter describes North American families and changes in the health and health behaviors of adults, children, and adolescents, so that we can understand what these changes portend for family health care nursing during the first half of this century. This chapter draws on information pertaining to family demography and population health from a variety of data sources (Box 2-1). The practice, research, education, and policy implications for nurses are discussed within each section of this chapter to ensure that readers understand the implications of these demographic patterns for practicing family nursing.

Where possible, statistics have been reported for both the United States and Canada. Comparable data for Canada were not always readily accessible for the topics covered in this chapter. Readers should note that data are not always collected in the same year, and that some family and health indicators are defined and measured differently across the two countries.

A CHANGING ECONOMY AND SOCIETY

Consider the life of a North American young woman reaching adulthood in the 1950s or early 1960s. Such a woman was likely to marry straight

---

BOX 2-1

Sources of Information on Demography and Public Health

Many of the statistics discussed in this chapter draw on information from the **Current Population Surveys** (CPS) collected by the U.S. Census Bureau. This is a continuous survey of about 60,000 households, selected at random to be representative of the national population. Each household is interviewed monthly for two 4-month periods. During February through April of each year, the CPS collects additional demographic and economic data, including data on health insurance coverage, from each household. This Annual Demographic Supplement is the most frequently used source of data on demographic and economic trends in the United States, and is the data source for the majority of statistics presented in this chapter regarding changes in the family.

For estimates for small areas or subgroups of the population, demographers often use data from the "long form" of the decennial **census**, which collects data from one-sixth of all households. The census collects a range of economic and demographic information, including incomes and occupations, housing, disability status, and grandparent responsibility for children. The census cannot match the detail found in more specialized surveys. For example, only four short questions measure disability for children; surveys designed for precise and complete estimates of disabilities will usually have dozens of such questions. Beginning in 2004, the **American Community Survey** replaced the sample data from the census and now provides a more continuous flow of estimates for states, cities, counties, and even towns and rural areas, for which estimates were made only once a decade.

Several large health-related surveys are conducted by the National Center for Health Statistics. The **National Health Interview Survey (NHIS)** is a large, continuous survey of about 43,000 households per year, covering the civilian, noninstitutionalized population of the United States. The NHIS is the major source of information on health status and disability, health-related behaviors, and health care utilization for all age groups. The **National Health and Nutrition Examination Survey (NHANES)** includes physical examinations, mental health questionnaires, dietary data, analyses of urine and blood, and immunization status from a random sample of Americans (about 10,000 in each 2-year cycle). NHANES also collects some basic demographic and income data. It is the major source of information on trends in obesity, cholesterol status, and a host of other conditions in the national population, and in particular age groups, racial and ethnic groups, and so on. The **National Survey of Family Growth (NSFG)** is the primary source of information on marriage and divorce trends, pregnancy, contraceptive use, and fertility behaviors, and the ways in which they vary among different groups and over time.

Birth and death certificates, sent by hospitals and funeral homes to state offices of vital events registration, provide the raw material for calculating fertility and mortality rates and life expectancy. The data are collected from the states and analyzed by the National Center for Health Statistics.

In Canada, the **National Population Health Survey** has interviewed a panel of respondents every 2 years since 1994 to 1995 to track changes in health-related behaviors, risk factors, and health outcomes.

---

out of high school or to take a clerical or retail sales job until she married. She would have moved out of her parents' home only after she married, to form a new household with her husband. This young woman was likely to marry by about age 20 in the United States (U.S. Census Bureau, 2008b) and age 22 in Canada, and begin a family soon after. If she were working when she became pregnant, she would probably have quit her job and stayed home to care for her children and husband while her husband had a steady job that paid enough to support the entire family. Thus, usually someone was at

home with the time to care for the health needs of family members, to schedule routine checkups with doctors and dentists, and to take family members to these appointments.

Fast-forward to the first decade of the 21st century. A young woman reaching adulthood in the first decade of the 21st century is not likely to marry before her 25th birthday. She will probably attend college and is likely to live by herself, with a boyfriend, or with roommates before marrying. She may move in and out of her parents' house several times before she gets married. Like her counterpart reaching adulthood in the 1950s, she is likely to marry and have at least one child, but the sequence of those events may well be reversed. She probably will not drop out of the labor force after she has children, although she may curtail the number of hours she is employed. She is much more likely to divorce and possibly even to remarry, compared with a young woman in the 1950s or 1960s. Because she is more likely to be a single mother and to be working outside of the home, she is also not as likely to have the time necessary to devote to caring for the health of family members.

A dramatic change in women's participation in market work (work for pay) occurred after 1970, as mothers with young children began entering the labor force in greater numbers. Historically, unmarried mothers (either never married or formerly married) of young children had higher labor force participation rates than married mothers. These women often were the only earners in their families. One notable change has been the increase in the combination of paid work and mothering among married mothers. In 1960, for example, in the United States, only 19% of married mothers with children younger than 6 were in the labor force. By 2005, the proportion increased to 60%. Another truly remarkable change has been the increase in the labor force participation of single mothers from 44% to 68% between 1980 and 2005 (U.S. Census Bureau, 2008c). What does this trend imply for family nursing? The majority of North American families with young children in the mid-20th century had mothers who were home full-time to care for the health needs of family members, whereas at the beginning of the 21st century, such families were in the minority.

Changes in the Economy

Economic conditions have an influence on young people's decisions about when to enter the labor force, when to marry, and when to have children (and how many children to have). After World War II, the United States and Canada enjoyed an economic boom characterized by rapid economic growth, full employment, rising productivity, higher wages, low inflation, and increasing earnings. A man with a high-school education in the 1950s and 1960s could secure a job that paid enough to allow him to purchase a house, support a family on one income, and join the swelling ranks of the middle class.

The economic realities of the 1970s and 1980s were quite different. The two decades after the oil crisis, which began in 1973, were decades of economic change and uncertainty marked by a shift away from manufacturing and toward services, stagnating or declining wages (especially for less-educated workers), high inflation, and a slowdown in productivity growth. The 1990s were just as remarkable for the turnaround: sustained prosperity, low unemployment, and economic growth that seems to have reached many in the poorest segments of society (Farley, 1996; Levy, 1998).

When the economy is on such a roller coaster, family life often takes a similar ride. Marriage occurred early and was nearly universal in the decades after World War II; mothers remained in the home to rear children, and the baby-boom generation was born and nurtured. When baby boomers hit working age in the 1970s, the economy was not as hospitable as it had been for their parents. They postponed marriage, delayed having children, and found it difficult to establish themselves in the labor market.

Many of the baby boomers' own children began reaching working ages in the 1990s and 2000s, when individuals' economic fortunes were increasingly dependent on their educational attainment. Those who attended college were much more likely to become self-sufficient and to live independently from their parents. High-school graduates who did not go to college discovered that jobs with high pay and benefits were in relatively short supply. In the United States, a high-school graduate in full-time work earned about 25% (allowing for inflation) less than a comparable new worker would have earned 20 years earlier (Farley, 1996). The increasing relative benefits of a college education probably encouraged more young men and women to delay marriage and attend college.

Partly because of these changes in the economy, both men and women are remaining single longer and are more likely to leave home to pursue a college education, to live with a partner, and to launch a career before taking on the responsibility of a family of their own. The traditional gender-based organization of home life (in which mothers have primary responsibility for care of the home and children, and fathers provide financial support) has not disappeared, but young women today can expect to be employed while raising children, and young men are more likely to share in some child-rearing and household tasks. Thus, in the first decade of this century, men are more likely to play a role in looking after the health of family members than they were in previous decades.

Before World War II, most men worked nearly to the end of their lives. Retirement was a privilege for the wealthy or the fortunate workers whose companies provided pensions. But since the passage of the Social Security Acts in 1936 and 1938 in the United States, and the institution of provincial (in the 1920s) and federal (since 1952) pensions in Canada, most workers can look forward to at least a modest guaranteed income for themselves, and their spouses and minor children. Social Security benefits constitute more than half the household income for two-thirds of Americans older than 65. The increased availability of public pensions made possible a growing period of retirement for most workers, a steady decrease in poverty rates for older people, and an increase in the proportion of older people maintaining their own households separately from their adult children.

Changing Family Norms

In 1950, in North America, there was one dominant and socially acceptable way for adults to live their lives. Those who deviated could expect to be censured and stigmatized. The "ideal" family was composed of a homemaker-wife, a breadwinner-father, and two or more children. Americans shared a common image of what a family should look like and how mothers, fathers, and children should behave. These shared values reinforced the importance of the family and the institution of marriage (McLanahan & Casper, 1995). This vision of family life showed amazing staying power, even as its economic underpinnings were eroding.

For this 1950s-style family to exist, North Americans had to support distinct gender roles, and the economy had to be vibrant enough for a man to support a family financially on his own.

Government policies and business practices perpetuated this family type by reserving the best jobs for men and discriminating against working women when they married or had a baby. Beginning in the 1960s, though, women and minorities gained legal protections in the workplace, and discriminatory practices began to recede.

A transformation in attitudes toward family behaviors also took place. People became more accepting of divorce, cohabitation, and sex outside marriage; less sure about the universality and permanence of marriage; and more tolerant of blurred gender roles and of mothers working outside the home (Cherlin, 1992; Thornton & Young-DeMarco, 2001). Society became more open-minded about a variety of living arrangements, family configurations, and lifestyles.

Although the transformation of many of these attitudes occurred throughout the 20th century, the pace of change accelerated in the 1960s and 1970s. These years brought many political, social, and medical upheavals affecting gender issues and views of the family. The women's liberation movement included a highly publicized, although unsuccessful attempt to pass the Equal Rights Amendment (ERA) to the Constitution of the United States. New and effective methods of contraception were introduced in the 1950s and 1960s. In 1973, the U.S. Supreme Court ruled that state laws banning abortion were unconstitutional. Popular literature and music heralded the sexual revolution and an era of "free love." In all industrialized countries, a new ideology was emerging during these years that stressed personal freedom, self-fulfillment, and individual choice in living arrangements and family commitments. People began to expect more out of marriage and to leave bad marriages that failed to fulfill their expectations. Certainly not all Americans approved of all these changes in beliefs and behaviors. The general North American culture changed, though, as divorce and single parenting became more widespread realities.

An Aging Society

For Americans born in 1900, the average life expectancy was less than 50 years. But the early decades of the 20th century brought such tremendous advances in the control of communicable diseases of childhood that life expectancy at birth increased to 70 years by 1960. Rapid declines in mortality from heart disease—the leading cause of death—significantly lengthened life expectancy for those aged 65 or older after 1960 (Treas & Torrecilha, 1995). By 2005, life expectancy at birth was nearly 77.9 years for Americans (National Center for Health Statistics, 2008) and 80.5 years for Canadians (World Health Organization, 2008). An American woman who reached age 65 in 2005 could expect to live an additional 15 years, on average, and a 65-year-old American man would live another 10 years. For Canadians, life expectancy at age 65 is even higher—17 years for women and 13 years for men. Women continue to outlive men in North America, though the gender gap in recent years has shrunk somewhat, primarily because of the delayed effects of smoking trends (men have always been more likely to smoke than women, but they have reduced smoking much more than women in recent decades). The gap in life expectancy between men and women means that women tend to outlive their husbands, and women predominate in the older age groups. Nearly two-thirds of Americans 75 years and older are women, and 56% of Canadians 75 and older are women (Statistics Canada, 2008a).

Partly because more North Americans are surviving until older ages, and partly because of a long-term decline in fertility rates, the proportion of the population aged 65 or older has grown. In 1900, only 1 of every 25 Americans was aged 65 or older. By 2000, the proportion was one in eight. By 2011, the first of some 78 million baby boomers will reach their 65th birthday, and the rate of increase of the elderly population will accelerate. By 2030, it is expected that one in five Americans will be aged 65 or older. The scenario for Canada is quite similar, although Canada has a slightly higher proportion of the population aged 65 and older; in 2006, 13.3% of Canada's population was 65 years and older compared with 12.5% of U.S. residents (U.S. Census Bureau, 2008d, Table 1300).

People do not suddenly become old on their 65th birthday, of course. Together with improvements in life expectancy have come improvements in the disability rates at older ages, so that North Americans are not only living longer than in the past but also enjoying more years of life without chronic illness or disabilities. In the United States, 65 is still a convenient marker for "old age" in health policy terms, because it is the age at which most Americans become eligible for medical and hospital insurance funded mainly by the federal government through Medicare. By 65, as well, most workers (both men and women) have left full-time work, though many continue to work part-time, or for part of the year, often at different jobs than those they pursued during most of their careers.

The aging of the population is often considered a major cause of increasing demand for medical services and of the growth in medical expenditures. Population aging is, indeed, one factor, because older people in every country consume more medical care than younger adults. The major causes of increased health expenditures in industrialized countries, however, have been changes in medical technology, including increased use of pharmaceuticals, rather than the simple growth of the elderly population (Reinhardt, 2003).

Increased life expectancy translates into extended years spent in family relationships. A couple who marries in their 20s could spend the next 50 years together, assuming they remain married. Couples in the past were much more likely to experience the death of one spouse earlier in their adult years. Longer lives (together with lower birth rates) also mean that people spend a smaller portion of their lives parenting young children. More parents live long enough to be part of their grandchildren's and even great-grandchildren's lives. Many adults are faced with caring for extremely elderly parents about the time they reach retirement age and begin to experience health limitations of older age themselves.

Immigration and Ethnic Diversity

In 1965, the U.S. Congress amended the Immigration and Naturalization Act to create a fundamental change in the nation's policy on immigration. Visas for legal immigrants were no longer to be based on quotas for each country of origin; instead, preference would be given to immigrants joining family members in the United States. The legislation also removed limitations on immigration from Latin America and Asia. The numbers of legal immigrants to the United States increased, to an average of 900,000 persons per year in the 1990s and to 1.1 million in 2007. Immigration has likewise increased in Canada from about 140,000 in 1980 to 252,000 in 2006. In 2007, 65% of legal immigrants were admitted because family members already living in the United States petitioned the government to grant them entry (U.S. Department of Homeland Security, 2008). For Canada, the corresponding figure is 40% (Citizenship and Immigration Canada, 2006). Immigrant visas were also granted for economic reasons, usually after employers petitioned the government for admission of persons with special skills, and for humanitarian reasons, including asylum granted to refugees because of well-founded fear of persecution in their home countries.

In addition to legal immigrants, an estimated 11 to 13 million illegal immigrants lived in the United States in 2006, either because they entered without detection or because they stayed longer than allowed by a temporary visa (Passel, 2007). In 2002, the U.S. Census Bureau estimated that there were 34.2 million U.S. residents born outside the country, about one-eighth of the total population (U.S. Census Bureau, 2008e). Because immigrants tend to arrive in the United States early in their working careers, they are younger, on average, than the total U.S. population and account for a larger share of young families. In 2002, for example, 23% of all births in the United States were to mothers born outside the country.

Estimates based on the 2000 U.S. Census show that 47 million people older than 5 speak a language other than English at home, the most common being Spanish (28 million) and Chinese (2 million). About a quarter of the adult (age, 25–44 years) Latino population of the United States reported that they could not speak English well (Saenz, 2004). Keep in mind, however, that the overwhelming majority of those who do not speak English well are recent immigrants. More than 97% of Latino adults born in the United States report that they can speak English well.

The majority of foreign-born U.S. residents live in states that are the traditional "gateways" to immigrant populations: California, New York, Florida, Texas, and Illinois. In recent decades, however, significant increases have occurred in the immigrant populations of most parts of the country, including the rural South and the Upper Midwest, which had seen few immigrants for most of the 20th century.

Implications for Health Care Providers

The aging and the growing diversity of the American and Canadian populations, combined with shifts in the economy and changing norms, values, and laws, alter the context for the nursing care of families. As the population ages, the demand will increase for nurses who specialize in caring for the elderly, and even those who do not choose a geriatric specialty will find that older people constitute an increasing

portion of the patient population. Improvements in health and physical functioning among those aged 60 to 70 reduce the need for care among this group. Yet rates of population growth are greatest for those aged 80 and older, implying an increased demand for care among the "oldest old," who are likely to suffer from poorer health and require substantial care. Because women continue to outlive men, on average, nurses are more likely to be dealing with the health care needs of older women than of men. Extended lives and delayed childbearing have increased the chances that adults will experience the double whammy of having to provide care and financial support for their children and their parents. Families in these situations can face considerable time and money pressures.

At the same time that changing gender roles point to more men in families taking on caregiving duties, more women are in the labor force and unavailable to care for family members, and it is doubtful that the increase in men's time in caregiving will fully compensate for the decrease in women's time. Societal changes also influence individuals' life-course trajectories. All these changes in individual lives and family relationships are transforming North American households and families, and in turn, changing the context in which health needs are defined, and both formal and informal health care are provided.

The growth of the immigrant population, and its spread throughout both the United States and Canada, has meant that patient populations in many regions are more diverse than in the past. Nurses in North America work with families whose cultural backgrounds, perceptions of sickness, and expectations of healers may be different from those with which they are familiar. Everyone providing health care can expect to face both the challenges and the professional rewards of adapting to a diverse patient population.

LIVING ARRANGEMENTS

The demographic changes for individuals discussed earlier in this chapter are reflected in changes in living arrangements, which have become more diverse over time. For most statistical purposes, a family is defined as two or more people living together who are related by blood, marriage, or adoption

(Casper & Bianchi, 2002). Most households (defined by the U.S. Census Bureau as one or more people who occupy a house, apartment, or other residential unit, as opposed to "group quarters" such as nursing homes or student dormitories) are maintained by families. Demographic trends, including late marriage, divorce, and single parenting, have resulted in a decrease in the "family share" of U.S. and Canadian households. In 1960, in the United States, 85% of households were family households; by 2006, just 68% were family households (authors' calculations from U.S. Census Bureau, 2008f). Two-parent family households with children constituted 44% of all households in 1960, but only 23% of all households in 2006 (authors' calculations from U.S. Census Bureau, 2008f, 2008g). Nonfamily households, which consist primarily of people who live alone or who share a residence with roommates or with a partner, have been on the rise. The fastest growth was among persons living alone. The proportion of households with just one person doubled from 13% to 26% between 1960 and 2006 (authors' calculations from U.S. Census Bureau, 2008h). Thus, fewer Americans live with family members who can help care for them when they are ill or injured.

In Canada, in 1981, two-thirds of households were married-couple households, but by 2001, the percentage declined to 59% (U.S. Census Bureau, 2008d, Table 1304). As in the United States, the percentage of households that contained two parents with children declined from 36% in 1981 to 26% in 2001. The proportion of Canadian households that contained one person grew from 20% in 1981 to 26% in 2001, as was the case in the United States. Single-person households are the fastest growing type of household.

Living Arrangements of the Elderly

Improvements in the health and financial status of older Americans helped generate a revolution in lifestyles and living arrangements among the elderly. Older North Americans now are more likely to spend their later years with their spouse or live alone, rather than with adult children as in the past. The options and choices differ between elderly women and elderly men, however, in large part because women live longer than men yet have fewer financial resources.

At the beginning of the 20th century, more than 70% of Americans aged 65 or older resided with kin (Ruggles, 1994). In part because of increased incomes of the elderly but also because of declining numbers of children and increased divorce rates, the proportion of elderly adults living alone has increased dramatically. Just 15% of widows aged 65 or older lived alone in 1900, whereas 67% lived alone in 2006 (Ruggles, 1996; U.S. Census Bureau, 2008i).

A woman is likely to spend more years living alone after a spouse dies than will a man because life expectancy is about 3 years longer for an elderly woman than for an elderly man, and because women usually marry men older than themselves. As a result, older American women are more than twice as likely as men to be living alone (38% vs. 19%) (U.S. Census Bureau, 2008i). This pattern is similar in Canada; for example, among Canadians aged 75 to 84, 43% of women lived alone compared with only 18% of men (Statistics Canada, 2002). Just less than half of all American women aged 75 and older live by themselves (Federal Interagency Forum on Aging-Related Statistics, 2008). Living alone can mean delays in getting attention for illness or injury, and can complicate arrangements for informal care or transportation to formal care when needed.

American women are also almost twice as likely as men to be living with nonrelatives (20% vs. 11%), in part because they tend to live longer and reach advanced ages when they are most likely to need the physical care and the financial help others can provide. Similarly in Canada, a larger proportion of women (35%) than men (23%) aged 85 and older lived in institutional settings in 2001. Elderly men who need help with activities of daily living (ADLs) such as eating, bathing, or getting around generally receive informal care from their wives, whereas elderly women with disabilities are more likely to rely on assistance from grown children, to live with other family members, or to enter a nursing home (Kramarow, 1995; Silverstein, 1995; Weinick, 1995).

To explain trends in living arrangements among the elderly, researchers have focused on a variety of constraints and preferences that shape people's living arrangement decisions (Goldscheider & Jones, 1989). The number and sex of children generally affect the likelihood that an elderly person will live with relatives. The greater the number of children, the greater the chances that there will be a son or daughter who can take care of an elderly parent. Daughters are more likely than sons to provide housing and care for an elderly parent, presumably as an extension of the traditional female caretaker role. Geographic distance from children is also a key factor; having children who live nearby promotes co-residence when living independently is no longer feasible for the elderly person (Crimmins & Ingegneri, 1990; Spitze & Logan, 1990).

Older Americans with higher income and better health are more likely to live independently (Woroby & Angel, 1990). In the United States, since 1940, growth in Social Security benefits accounted for half of the increase in independent living among the elderly (McGarry & Schoeni, 2000). By contrast, elderly Americans in financial need are more likely to live with relatives (Speare & Avery, 1993).

Social norms and personal preferences also determine the choice of living arrangements for the elderly (Wister & Burch, 1987). Many elderly individuals are willing to pay a substantial part of their incomes to maintain their own residence, which suggests strong personal preferences for privacy and independence. Social norms involving family obligations and ties may be especially important when examining racial and ethnic differences in the living arrangements of the elderly. Despite the trend toward independent living among older Americans, many of them are not able to live alone without assistance. Many families who have older kin in frail health provide extraordinary care. One study in New York City, for example, found that 40% of those who reported caring for an elderly relative devoted 20 or more hours per week to such informal care, and 80% of caregivers had been providing care for more than a year (Navaie-Walsier et al., 2001).

Despite the growth of home-health services and adult day-care centers, most long-term care consists of care provided informally, usually by spouses or younger relatives (Stone, 2000). Adult women, in particular, are likely to have primary responsibility for home care of the frail elderly, often including parents-in-law. Some evidence suggests that female caregivers experience greater levels of stress than do male caregivers (Yee & Schulz, 2000). Research has shown that even relatively low-cost interventions to support informal caregivers can greatly reduce the harmful effects of such stress on caregivers' health (Schulz et al., 2006).

Living Arrangements of Young Adults

The young-adult years (ages 18–30) have been described as "demographically dense" because these years involve many interrelated life-altering transitions (Rindfuss, 1991). Between these ages, young people usually finish their formal schooling, leave home, develop careers, marry, and begin families, but these events do not always occur in this order. Delayed marriage extends the period during which young adults can experiment with alternative living arrangements before they adopt family roles. Young adults may experience any number of independent living arrangements before they marry, as they change jobs, pursue education, and move into and out of intimate relationships. They may also return to their parents' homes for periods of time, if money becomes tight or at the end of a relationship.

In 1890, half of American women had married by age 22, and half of American men had married by age 26. The ages of entry into marriage dipped to an all-time low during the post–World War II baby-boom years, when the median age at first marriage reached 20 years for women and 23 years for men in 1956. Age at first marriage then began to increase and reached 25 years for women and 27 years for men by 2006 (U.S. Census Bureau, 2008b). In Canada, the average age at marriage increased from 25 years in 1971 (Wu, 1998) to 27 years in 2004 for men and from 22.6 years to 24 years for women (Statistics Canada, 2008b). In 1960, it was unusual for a woman to reach age 25 without marrying; only 10% of women aged 25 to 29 had never married (Casper & Bianchi, 2002). In 2000, two-fifths of women aged 25 to 29 and more than half of men in the same age group had never been married.

This delay in marriage has shifted the family behaviors in young adulthood in three important ways. First, later marriage coincides with a greater diversity and fluidity in living arrangements in young adulthood. Second, delaying marriage has accompanied an increased likelihood of entering a cohabiting union before marriage. Third, the trend to later marriage affects childbearing; it tends to delay entry into parenthood and, at the same time, increases the chances that a birth (sometimes planned but more often unintended) occurs before marriage (Bianchi & Casper, 2000).

Many demographic, social, and economic factors influence young adults' decisions about where and with whom to live (Casper & Bianchi, 2002). Family and work transitions are influenced greatly by fluctuations in the economy, as well as by changing ideas about appropriate family life and roles for men and women. Since the 1980s, the transition to adulthood has been hampered by recurring recessions, tight job markets, slow wage growth, and soaring housing costs, in addition to the confusion over roles and behavior sparked by the gender revolution (Goldscheider & Goldscheider, 1994). Even though young adults today may prefer to live independently, they may not be able to afford to do so. Many entry-level jobs today offer low wages, yet housing costs have soared, putting independent living out of reach for many young adults. Higher education, increasingly necessary in today's labor market, is expensive, and living at home may be a way for families to curb college expenses. Even when young adults attend school away from home, they still frequently depend on their parents for financial help and may return home after graduation if they cannot find a suitable job.

The percentage of young men living in their parents' homes was 54% in 2006, about the same as in 1970, whereas the percentage increased for young women from 39% to 47% (U.S. Census Bureau, 2008j). From 1981 to 2001, the proportion of young adults in Canada who resided with their parents increased dramatically from 28% to 41% (Statistics Canada, 2002).

Young adults who leave home to attend school, join the military, or take a job have always had, and continue to have, high rates of "returning to the nest." Those who leave home to get married have had the lowest likelihood of returning home, although returns to the nest have increased over time even in this group.

American parents routinely take in their children after they return from the military or school, or when they are between jobs. In the past, however, many American parents apparently were reluctant to take children in if they had left home simply to gain "independence." This is not true today. Demographers Frances Goldscheider and Calvin Goldscheider (1994) argue that, in the past, leaving home for simple independence was probably the result of friction within the family, whereas today, leaving and returning home seems to be a common part of a successful transition to adulthood. In the past, a young adult may have been reluctant to move back in with parents because a return home

implied failure; fewer stigmas are attached to returning home these days (Casper & Bianchi, 2002).

Changing demographic behaviors among young adults have implications for family health care nursing. In the United States, young adults often lack health insurance and, in many cases, are not financially independent, reducing the likelihood that they will receive routine checkups or seek medical care when the need arises (Casper & Haaga, 2005). These increasing numbers of people showing up in emergency rooms and urgent care settings put additional pressure on the health care providers, especially nurses. Also, the acuity level of the medical problems in these young adults is greater because earlier treatment was not sought.

Unmarried Couples

One of the most significant household changes in the second half of the 20th century in North America was the increase in men and women living together without marrying. The increase of cohabitation outside marriage appeared to counterbalance some of the delay of marriage among young adults and the overall increase in divorce. Unmarried-couple households made up less than 1% of U.S. households in 1960 and 1970 (Casper & Cohen, 2000). This share increased to 2.2% by 1980, and to nearly 5% by 2006, or 5.3 million households (U.S. Census Bureau, 2008k). Unmarried-couple households also are increasingly likely to include children. In 1978, 24% of unmarried-couple households included children younger than 15; by 2006, 34% included children.

Although the percentage of U.S. households consisting of an unmarried couple is small, many Americans have lived with a partner outside marriage at some point. More than half of the couples who married in the mid-1990s had lived together before marriage, up slightly from 49% in 1985 to 1986, and a big jump from just 8% of first marriages in the late 1960s (Bumpass & Lu, 2000).

The 2001 Canadian Census showed that an increasing proportion of families was maintained by common-law couples (cohabiters): from 5.6% in 1981 to 13.8% in 2001 (Statistics Canada, 2002). As in the United States, more Canadian children are living with common-law (cohabiting) parents. In 2001, about 733,000 children aged 0 to 14 (13% of the total) lived with common-law parents. In both countries, the pace of the increase in cohabitation has slowed somewhat since the rapid increase in the 1970s and 1980s.

Why has cohabitation increased so much? Researchers have offered several explanations, including increased uncertainty about the stability of marriage, the erosion of norms against cohabitation and sexual relations outside of marriage, the wider availability of reliable birth control, economic changes, and increased individualism and secularization. Youths reaching adulthood in the past two decades are much more likely to have witnessed their parents' divorce than any generation before them. Some have argued that cohabitation allows a couple to experience the benefits of an intimate relationship without committing to marriage. If a cohabiting relationship is not successful, one can simply move out; if a marriage is not successful, one suffers through a sometimes lengthy and difficult divorce.

Nevertheless, most adults in the United States eventually do marry. In 2006, 91% of women aged 50 to 54 had been married at least once (U.S. Census Bureau, 2008l). An estimated 88% of U.S. women born in the 1960s will eventually marry (Raley, 2000). The meaning and permanence of marriage may be changing, however. Marriage used to be the primary demographic event that marked the formation of new households, the beginning of sexual relations, and the birth of a child. Marriage also implied that an individual had one sexual partner, and it theoretically identified the two individuals who would parent any child born of the union. The increasing social acceptance of cohabitation outside marriage has meant that these linkages could no longer be assumed. Couples began to set up households that might include the couple's children, as well as children from previous marriages or other relationships. Similarly, what it meant to be single was no longer always clear, as the personal lives of unmarried couples began to resemble those of their married counterparts.

Cohabiting households can pose unique challenges for health care providers, especially in the United States. Because cohabiting relationships are not legally sanctioned in most states, partners may not have the right to make health care decisions on behalf of each other or of the other's children (Casper & Haaga, 2005). Cohabiting couples report poorer health and have lower incomes than do married couples, on average (Waite & Gallagher, 2000). Thus, although they are more likely to need

health care services, they may be less likely to have the financial ability to secure them.

PARENTING

Even with the increase in divorce and cohabitation, postponement of marriage, and decline in childbearing, most North American adults have children, and most children live with two parents. In 2006, 67% of families with children were two-parent families (U.S. Census Bureau, 2008a). In Canada, in 2001, the level was comparable: 65% of Canadian families with children were married two-parent families (authors' calculations from Statistics Canada, 2002). In 2006, 26.4% of American families were mother-only families and only 6% were father-only families. "Lone-parent families" in Canada increased from 9% of all families (including those with no children) in 1971 to about 16% in 2001 (data are not reported for single mothers and single fathers separately). But the changes in marriage, cohabitation, and nonmarital childbearing over the past few decades have had a profound effect on North American families with children and are changing our images of parenthood.

Unmarried Parents Living Together

In the United States, changes in marriage and cohabitation tend to blur the distinction between one-parent and two-parent families. The increasing acceptance of cohabitation as a substitute for marriage, for example, may reduce the chance that a premarital pregnancy will lead to marriage before the birth (Raley, 1999). Greater shares of children today are born to a mother who is not currently married than in previous decades. Some of those children are born to cohabiting parents and begin life in a household that includes both their biological parents. Data from the 2002 National Survey of Family Growth show that 40% of recent nonmarital births were to cohabiting women (National Center for Health Statistics, 2007a). Cohabitation increased for unmarried mothers in all race and ethnic groups, but especially among whites. Cohabiting couples account for up to 16% of the white mothers classified as unmarried mothers in 1998, compared with 8% of black mothers and 10% of

Hispanic mothers (Casper & Bianchi, 2002). (In Canada cohabiting couples are not distinguished in official statistics from married two-parent families.) Unmarried American fathers living with children are much more likely than unmarried mothers to be living with a partner: 33% of the 2.1 million "single" fathers lived with a partner in 1998, more than twice the percentage for single mothers. In 1998, about 1.4 million American men were raising their children on their own, without a wife or partner (Bianchi & Casper, 2000).

Single Mothers

How many single mothers are there? This turns out to be a more difficult question to answer from official statistics than it would first appear. Over time, it is easiest to calculate the number of single mothers who maintain their own residence. In the United States between 1950 and 2006, the number of such single-mother families increased from 1.3 million to 8.4 million (U.S. Census Bureau, 2008g). These estimates do not include single mothers living in other persons' households but do include single mothers who are cohabiting with a male partner. The most dramatic increase was during the 1970s, when the number of single-mother families was increasing at 8% per year. The average annual rate of increase slowed considerably during the 1980s and was near zero after 1994 (Casper & Bianchi, 2002). By 2006, single mothers who maintained their own households accounted for 23% of all families with children, up from 6% in 1950 (U.S. Census Bureau, 2008a). Almost 2 million more single mothers live in someone else's household—1.6 million with relatives and 370,000 with nonrelatives (cohabiting or with roommates)—bringing the total number of single mothers to nearly 10 million (Casper & Bianchi, 2002). (Tabulated data for lone-single parents in Canada are reported for lone parents regardless of the parent's sex; it is impossible to distinguish lone mothers from lone fathers.)

Single mothers with children at home face a multitude of challenges. They usually are the primary breadwinners, disciplinarians, playmates, and caregivers for their children. They must manage the financial and practical aspects of a household and plan for the family's future. Many mothers cope remarkably well, and many benefit from financial support and help from relatives and from their children's fathers.

Women earn less than men, on average, and because single mothers are usually younger and less educated than other women, they are often at the lower end of the income curve. Never-married single mothers are particularly disadvantaged; they are younger, less well educated, and less often employed than are divorced single mothers and married mothers. Single mothers often must curtail their work hours to care for the health and well-being of their children.

Despite the fact that the majority of American single mothers are not poor, they are much more likely to be poor than other parents. Single-parent families who are poor are considered to be under the poverty line, which for a single-mother with two children translates into an annual income of less than $13,874 in 2000. The family income of children who reside with a never-married single mother is less than one-fourth that of children in two-parent families (Bianchi & Casper, 2000). Almost three of every five children who live with a never-married mother are poor. Mothers who never married are much less likely to get child support from the father than are mothers who are divorced or separated. Whereas 60% of divorced mothers with custody of children younger than 21 received some child support from the children's father, fewer than 20% of never-married mothers reported receiving regular support from their child's father (Bianchi & Casper, 2000).

Children who live with a divorced mother tend to be much better off financially than are children of never-married mothers. Divorced mothers are substantially better educated and more often employed than are mothers who are separated or who never married. Even so, the average incomes of families headed by divorced mothers is less than half that of two-parent families.

Likewise, Canadian lone-parent families with children younger than 18 are much more likely to have low incomes: In 2000, 46% of lone parents were classified as low income compared with 11% of couple families with children younger than 18.

In the United States, single mothers with children in poverty are particularly affected by major welfare reform legislation, such as the Personal Responsibility and Work Opportunity Reconciliation Act (PRWORA) (Box 2-2).

President Clinton claimed in his 1993 State of the Union Address that the 1996 law would "end welfare as we know it," and the changes embodied in

---

BOX 2-2
Welfare Reform in the United States

Federal and state programs in the United States to aid low-income families have been transformed during the past decade. The 1996 PRWORA was the legislative milestone at the federal level.

- PRWORA replaced the Aid to Families with Dependent Children program, an entitlement for poor families, with a program of block grants to the states called *Temporary Assistance to Needy Families* (TANF).
- It required states to impose work requirements on at least 80% of TANF recipients.
- It forbade payments to single mothers younger than 18 unless they lived with an adult or in an adult-supervised situation.
- It set limits of 60 months on TANF for any individual recipient (and 22 states have used their option to impose shorter lifetime limits).
- It gave states more latitude to let TANF recipients earn money or get child support payments without reduction of benefits and to use block grants for child care.

Welfare-reform proponents often supported efforts to "make work pay," as well as to discourage long-term dependence on welfare. The Earned Income Tax Credit, for example, was expanded several times during the 1980s and 1990s, and now provides twice as much money to low-income families, whether single- or two-parent families, as does TANF. Funding for child care was also expanded during the decade, though child care remains a problem for low-income working families in most places.

PRWORA accelerated a decline in welfare caseloads throughout the country. Because of a concern that former welfare recipients entering the workforce would lose insurance coverage through Medicaid for their children, the 1997 Balanced Budget Act set up the new State Child Health Insurance Program (SCHIP), providing federal money to states in proportion to their low-income population and recent success in reducing the proportion of uninsured children.

Lack of health insurance remains an important concern for children in the United States, however. The Kaiser Commission on Medicaid and the Uninsured (2007) estimates that, in 2005, about one of every eight children in the United States was not covered by any health insurance (and one in five adults between ages 21 and 64 were uninsured).

PRWORA—time limits on welfare eligibility and mandatory job-training requirements, for example—seemed far-reaching (Besharov & Fowler, 1993). Some argued that this legislation would end crucial support for poor mothers and their children; several high-level government officials resigned because of the law. Others heralded PRWORA as the first step toward helping poor women gain control of their lives and making fathers take responsibility for their children. Many states had already begun to experiment with similar reforms (Cherlin, 2000). The success of this program is open to dispute because it has been and continues to be such a political issue.

Why have mother-child families increased in number and as a percentage of North American families? Explanations tend to focus on one of two trends. First is women's increased financial independence, either through their own wages as more women entered the labor force and women's incomes increased relative to those of men, or because of the expansion of welfare benefits for single mothers during the 1960s and 1970s. Women today are less dependent on a man's income to support themselves and their children, and many can afford to live independently rather than stay in an unsatisfactory relationship. Second, the job market for men has tightened, especially for less-educated men. As the North American economy experienced a restructuring in the 1970s and 1980s, the demand for professionals, managers, and other white-collar workers expanded, whereas wages for men in lower-skilled jobs have declined in real terms over the past two decades. Men still earn more than women, on average, but the income gap narrowed during the 1970s and 1980s as women's earnings increased and men's earnings remained flat or declined (Cotter, Hermsen, & Vannemen, 2004).

In the early years of the 20th century, higher mortality rates made it more common for children to live with only one parent (Uhlenberg, 1996). As declining death rates reduced the number of widowed single parents, a counterbalancing increase in single-parent families occurred because of divorce. For example, at the time of the 1960 Census, almost one-third of

American single mothers living with children younger than 18 were widows (Bianchi, 1995). As divorce rates increased precipitously in the 1960s and 1970s, most single-parent families were created through divorce or separation. Thus, at the end of the 1970s, only 11% of American single mothers were widowed and two-thirds were divorced or separated. In 1978, about one-fifth of single American mothers had never married but had a child and were raising that child on their own (Bianchi & Casper, 2000). By 2006, 45% of single mothers had never married (U.S. Census Bureau, 2008m).

The remarkable increase in the number of single-mother households with women who have never married was driven by a dramatic shift to childbearing outside marriage. The number of births to unmarried women grew from less than 90,000 per year in 1940 to nearly 1.5 million per year in 2002 (National Center for Health Statistics, 2007a). Less than 4% of all births in 1940 were to unmarried mothers compared with 37% in 2005. The rate of nonmarital births—the number of births per 1,000 unmarried women—increased from 7.1 in 1940 to 47.5 in 2005. The nonmarital birth rate peaked in 1994 at 46.2 and leveled out in the latter 1990s, but it has picked back up to a all-time high in 2005 (Bianchi & Casper, 2000; National Center for Health Statistics, 2007a). Births to unmarried women have increased in Canada as well, from 12.8% in 1980 to 28.3% of all births in 2000 (U.S. Census Bureau, 2008d, Table 1301).

The proportion of births that occur outside marriage is even higher in some European countries than in the United States and Canada. But unmarried parents in European countries and Canada are more likely to be living together with their biological children than are unmarried parents in the United States (Heuveline, Timberlake, & Furstenberg, 2003). In the United States, the tremendous variation in rates of unmarried childbearing among population groups suggests that there may be a constellation of factors that determine whether women have children when they are not married. In 2005, the nonmarital birth rate for Hispanic women was highest, at 100.3 per 1,000, followed by black women at 67.8, non-Hispanic white women at 30.1, and Asian/Pacific Islander women at 24.9. The percentage of mother-only family households is much higher for African American families (51%) than for Hispanic (24%) and white families (18%).

Single-mother families present challenges for family health care nurses providing care for this vulnerable group. Single mothers today are younger and less educated than they were a few decades ago. This presents problems because these mothers have less experience with the health care system and are likely to have more difficulty reading directions, filling out forms, communicating effectively with doctors and nurses, and understanding their care instructions. These mothers are also more likely to be poor and uninsured, making it less likely they will seek care and more likely they will not be able to pay for it. Consequently, when the need arises, these women are more likely to resort to emergency rooms for noncritical illnesses and injuries. Time is also in short supply for single mothers. With the advent of welfare reform in the United States, more of them are working, which conceivably reduces the time they used in the past to care for themselves and their children (Box 2-3). Moreover, although many of these mothers can rely on their families for help, they are apt to have tenuous ties with their children's fathers.

Fathering

A new view of fatherhood emerged out of the feminist movement of the late 1960s and early 1970s. The new ideal father was a co-parent who was responsible for and involved in all aspects of his children's care. The ideal has been widely accepted throughout North American society; people today, as opposed to those in earlier times, believe that fathers should be highly involved in caregiving (Pleck & Pleck, 1997). Fathers do spend more time with their children and are doing more housework than in earlier decades. In 1998, married fathers in the United States reported spending an average of 4 hours per day with their children, compared with 2.7 hours in 1965 (Bianchi, 2000).

At the same time, other trends increasingly remove fathers from their children's lives. When the mother and father are not married, for example, ties between fathers and their children often falter. Family demographer Frank Furstenberg (1998) uses the label "good dads, bad dads" to describe the parallel trends of increased commitment to children and child rearing on the part of some fathers at the same time that there seems to be less connection to and responsibility for children on the part of other fathers.

BOX 2-3

Research Brief—Unsupervised Children

SAMPLE AND SETTING

The data used in this study are from Wave 9 of the Survey of Income and Program Participation (SIPP), collected in the fall of 1995 by the U.S. Census Bureau. The sample consisted of 6,189 children aged 5 to 13 years from across the United States.

METHODOLOGY

The Wave 9 SIPP interviewed 17,583 households in 1995, representing a total sample loss of 27% since the panel began in 1993. Data were collected either in person or over the phone by Census Field Representatives. Respondents identified as the designated parent—the mother, if she is in the household—responded to a variety of questions for the four youngest children younger than 15 about the child care arrangements used during the mother's work and nonwork hours.

FINDINGS

Sixteen percent of children aged 5 to 13 are primarily in self-care during the time they are not at school. Percentages range from 7% for children aged 5 to 7 to 25% for those aged 11 to 13. One of the most

important factors associated with parents selecting self-care over some other primary supervised child care arrangement is full-time work. Parents who work more hours have to cover more hours with child care than do parents who work part-time or do not work, and this care can be expensive. Parents who work full-time may use self-care as a way to cut down on the high costs of child care. Children who are more responsible and mature, and those who live in neighborhoods with safe places to play outside are more likely to care for themselves than those who are less responsible and mature or who live in unsafe neighborhoods.

IMPLICATIONS

Nurses dealing with families with grade-school-aged children should be aware that some children care for themselves on a regular basis. Children in these situations do not have parental supervision all of the time. Thus, parents may not be home when a child gets hurt or when a sick child requires medication (Casper & Smith, 2004).

How many years do men spend as parents? Demographer Rosalind King (1999) has estimated the number of years that American men and women will spend as parents of biological children or stepchildren younger than 18 if the parenting patterns of the late 1980s and early 1990s continue throughout their lives. Almost two-thirds of the adult years will be "child-free" years in which the individual does not have biological children younger than 18 or responsibility for anyone else's children. Men will spend, on average, about 20% of their adulthood living with and raising their biological children, whereas women will spend more than 30% of their adult lives, on average, raising biological children. Whereas women, regardless of race, spend nearly all of their parenting years rearing their biological children, men are more likely to live with stepchildren or a combination of their own children and stepchildren. Among men, white men will spend about twice as much time living with their biological children as African American men.

One of the new aspects of the American family in the last 50 years has been an increase in the number of single fathers. Between 1950 and 2006, the

number of households with children that were maintained by an unmarried father increased from 229,000 to 2 million (U.S. Census Bureau, 2008f, 2008g). An additional 328,000 unmarried fathers lived with their children in someone else's household, bringing the total count of single fathers to about 2.5 million for 2006. During the 1980s and 1990s, the percentage of single-father households nearly tripled for white and Hispanic families and doubled for African American families.

Recent demographic trends in fathering have changed the context of family health care nursing. The growth in single fatherhood and joint custody, together with the increased tendency for fathers to perform household chores, means that family health care nurses are more likely today than in decades past to be interacting with the fathers of children.

Grandparents

One moderating factor in children's well-being in single-parent families can be the presence of grandparents in the home. Although the image of single-parent families is usually that of a mother living on her own, trying to meet the needs of her young child or children, many single mothers live with their parents. For example, in the United States in 1998, about 17% of single mothers lived in the homes of their parents, compared with 10% of single fathers (Casper & Bianchi, 2002). This is a snapshot at one point in time, however. A much higher percentage of single mothers (36%) live in their parents' home *at some point* before their children are grown. African American single mothers with children at home are more likely than are others to live with a parent at some time.

The involvement of grandparents in the lives of their children has even become an issue for court cases, as there have been several rulings in recent years on grandparents' visitation rights. The 2000 U.S. Census included a new set of questions on grandparents' support of grandchildren.

Children whose parents for one reason or another cannot take care of them also live with their grandparents. In 1970, 2.2 million, or 3.2% of all American children, lived in their grandparents' household. By 2006, this number had increased to 3.7 million, or 5.1% of all American children (U.S. Census Bureau, 2008n). Substantial increases occurred among all types of households maintained by grandparents, regardless of the presence or absence of the grandchildren's parents, but increases were greatest among children without any parent present in the household.

In Canada, 3.3% of children aged 0 to 14 resided with at least one grandparent. Of these children, 51% also had both parents in the household, 33% had a lone parent (mostly the mothers) in the households, and 12% resided with their grandparents without a parent (Milan & Hamm, 2003).

Emerging research shows that grandparents play an important role in multigenerational households, which is at odds with the traditional image of grandparents as family members who themselves require financial and personal support. Although early studies assumed that financial support flowed from adult children to their parents, more recent research suggests that the more common pattern is for parents to give financial support to their adult children (Eggebeen & Hogan, 1990).

In most multigenerational households, the grandparents bring their children and grandchildren into a household that the grandparents own or rent. In

2006, 60% of multigenerational households were of this type. In nearly 40% of the grandparent-maintained families, grandparents lived with their grandchildren without the children's parents (authors' calculations based on data from U.S. Census Bureau, 2008n). Grandparents who own or rent homes that include grandchildren and adult children are younger, healthier, and more likely to be in the labor force than are grandparents who live in a residence owned or rented by their adult children. Grandparents who maintain multigenerational households are also better educated (more likely to have at least a high-school education) than are grandparents who live in their children's homes (Casper & Bianchi, 2002).

Parents who support both dependent children and dependent parents have been referred to as the "sandwich" generation, because they provide economic and emotional support for both the older and younger generations. Although grandparents in parent-maintained households tend to be older, in poorer health, and not as likely to be employed, many are in good health and are, in fact, working (Bryson & Casper, 1999). These findings suggest that, at the very least, the burden of maintaining a co-residential "sandwich family" household may be somewhat overstated in the popular press. Many of the grandparents who are living in the houses of their adult children are capable of contributing to the family income and helping with the supervision of children.

Many grandparents step in to assist their children in times of crisis. Some provide financial assistance or child care, whereas others are the primary caregivers for their grandchildren. The recent increase in the numbers of grandparents raising their grandchildren is particularly salient to health care providers because both grandparents and grandchildren in this situation often suffer significant health problems (Casper & Bianchi, 2002). Researchers have documented high rates of asthma, weakened immune systems, poor eating and sleeping patterns, physical disabilities, and hyperactivity among grandchildren being raised by their grandparents (Dowdell, 1995; Minkler & Roe, 1996; Shore & Hayslip, 1994). Grandparents raising grandchildren are in poorer health than are their counterparts. They have higher rates of depression, poorer self-rated health, and more multiple chronic health problems (Dowdell, 1995; Minkler & Roe, 1993).

It is important to keep in mind that, although many of the grandparents who live in their adult children's homes are in good health, some of these grandparents require significant care. Nurses should also be aware that there are also adults who provide care for their parents who are not living with them. Adults who provide care for both generations are likely to face both time and money concerns.

TRENDS IN POPULATION HEALTH

This chapter has highlighted profound changes in families and households, and the ethnic diversity and age composition of the North American population, all setting the social context in which health care is provided and demands are made on providers. The next section reviews no less profound changes in demographic measures of health status and its determinants.

Overall Trends in Life Expectancy and Disability

The health status of the North American population has improved greatly during the last half century. This improvement can be measured most precisely by reviewing mortality indicators (Box 2-4). Since the mid-1950s, age-standardized mortality rates in the United States have improved nearly every year, at an average rate of about 1% per year (Fuchs & Garber, 2003). Disability is a less precisely definable outcome of ill health. Different definitions and measures of different aspects of physical health and functioning exist. But despite the difficulties of comparing over time and across data sources, the disability trends confirm this picture of improving health. Among Americans aged 65 and older, age-standardized disability rates have also been declining during the same decades at a rate of about 1% per year, with some variation among different data sources (Freedman, Martin, & Schoeni, 2002).

BOX 2-4
Age-Standardized Rates and Life Expectancy

Demographers and epidemiologists usually adjust for differences in the proportions of a population in different age groups when they compare mortality or morbidity rates at different times or across different countries. This is because the risk of mortality for any individual is strongly associated with age, increasing slowly from the lowest point at about age 10, and steeply at ages older than 60. Because the proportion of older people in North America has increased considerably over time, and because this proportion is different among countries, it could be misleading to compare "crude" rates, that is, the simple percentage of people who get a serious illness or die in a given year and infer that people are healthier in the population with the lower crude rate.

"Life expectancy" is a statistic commonly used to summarize information about age-specific mortality rates, to make comparisons over time or across populations without letting differences in age structure confuse the issue. Life expectancy is calculated as the average number of years that a person would live, if the age-specific mortality rates prevailing in a given year in the population were to stay constant

throughout the person's whole life. It is usually calculated as a number of years beginning at birth, but demographers also calculate life expectancy at later ages.

In 2005, for example, a woman in the United States would live, on average, to age 80.4 if mortality rates for American women stayed exactly the same at every age as in the year 2005. For an American woman who had already reached age 65, remaining life expectancy would be 20.0 years, if mortality rates at every age older than 65 stayed exactly the same as in 2005. (For American men in 2005, life expectancy at birth was 75.2 years, and at age 65, remaining life expectancy was 17.2 years. Male death rates are higher than female death rates at every age.) Most experts think that there will continue to be improvement in mortality rates—"life expectancy" is not a prediction of the future but a convenient way to summarize the situation in 2005. Mortality rates are lower in Canada than in the United States at every age; therefore, life expectancy is higher: 82.7 years for women in 2005 and 78.0 years for men.

The general picture of progress in health holds true for segments of the North American population defined by race and ethnicity, by levels of income and education, or by geography. But disturbing inequalities in health outcomes persist, posing a challenge for the health care system and society at large. African American men have a lower life expectancy at birth than white American men (69.6 vs. 75.7 years). African American women have a life expectancy at birth about 4 years less than do white American women (76.5 vs. 80.8 years) (National Center for Health Statistics, 2008).

Latinos and Asian Americans, by contrast, have lower age-adjusted mortality rates than do non-Hispanic whites in the United States (National Center for Health Statistics, 2008, Table 28). In large part, this advantage is associated with "immigrant selectivity." Leaving one's native country to move to a new one has always required a certain degree of good health and optimism. Evidence also suggests that many immigrant families maintain healthy diets, social and family connections, and other behaviors that promote health and well-being. These advantages appear to dissipate as subsequent generations assimilate to the larger culture and patterns of behavior (Hernandez, 1999).

The Americans with Disabilities Act of 1990 (ADA) defines "disability" as a substantial limitation in a major life activity (Box 2-5). In 2002, 51.2 million people (18% of the population) had some level of disability, and 32.5 million (11.5% of the population) had a severe disability, according to Census Bureau estimates (Steinmetz, 2006). For all ages, the prevalence of severe disability was 7% for Asians and Pacific Islanders, 9% for Hispanics, 12% for non-Hispanic whites, and 14% for African Americans. Some of the overall differences among the different race/ethnic groups reflect differences in the age distributions of the populations. For individuals 65 years and older, non-Hispanic whites fared considerably better than the other racial or ethnic groups in the United States: 35% of non-Hispanic whites were severely disabled compared with 37% of Asians and Pacific Islanders, 43% of Hispanics, and 50% of African Americans.

About 8.1 million individuals (3.6% of the population) had difficulty with one or more ADLs. ADLs include difficulty getting around inside the

---

BOX 2-5

Definitions of Disability Status, Severe Disability, Functional Limitations, Activities of Daily Living, and Instrumental Activities of Daily Living

Demographers and epidemiologists use various ways to measure disability within the population. In recent U.S. Census Bureau studies using data from the SIPP, individuals 15 years old and older are typically identified as having a disability if they meet any of the following criteria (McNeil, 2001):

1. Use a wheelchair, a cane, crutches, or a walker
2. Have difficulty performing one or more **functional activities** (seeing, hearing, speaking, lifting/carrying, using stairs, walking, or grasping small objects)
3. Have difficulty with one or more **activities of daily living** (the **ADLs** include getting around inside the home, getting into or out of bed or a chair, bathing, dressing, eating, and toileting)
4. Have difficulty with one or more **instrumental activities of daily living** (the **IADLs** include going outside the home, keeping track of money and bills, preparing meals, doing light housework, taking prescription medicines in the right amount at the right time, and using the telephone)
5. Have one or more specified conditions (a learning disability, mental retardation or another developmental disability, Alzheimer's disease, or some other type of mental or emotional condition)
6. Have any other mental or emotional condition that seriously interfere with everyday activities (frequently depressed or anxious, trouble getting along with others, trouble concentrating, or trouble coping with day-to-day stress)
7. Have a condition that limits the ability to work around the house
8. If aged 16 to 67, have a condition that makes it difficult to work at a job or business
9. Receive federal benefits based on an inability to work

Individuals are considered to have a **severe disability** if they meet criteria 1, 6, or 9; if they have Alzheimer's disease, mental retardation, or another developmental disability; or if they are unable to perform or need help to perform one or more of the activities in criteria 2, 3, 4, 7, or 8.

home, getting into or out of bed or a chair, bathing, dressing, eating, and getting to or using the toilet. Instrumental activities of daily living (IADLs) include difficulty going outside the home, keeping track of money and bills, preparing meals, doing light housework, taking prescription medicines in the right amount at the right time, and using the telephone (Steinmetz, 2006). About 13.2 million people reported difficulty with at least one IADL. In the U.S. population aged 15 years and older, 2.7 million used a wheelchair (1% of the population). Another 4%, or 9.1 million, used some other ambulatory aid such as a cane, crutches, or a walker. About 7.8 million individuals 15 years old and older had difficulty seeing the words and letters in ordinary newspaper print; of them, 1.8 million were unable to see at all.

The ability to work is one of the major activities affected by the chronic conditions of the disabled. Individuals with a severe disability had an employment rate of 43% and median earnings of $12,781, compared with 82.0% and $21,980 for those with a nonsevere disability and 88% and $25,046 for those with no disability. Many people with disabilities live in poverty. The poverty rate among the population 25 to 64 years old with no disability was 8%; it was 26% for those with a severe disability (Steinmetz, 2006).

Obesity

In North America, one of the most disturbing trends in health over the past decade has been the increase in the proportion of the population that is overweight or obese (Box 2-6). Overweight and obese people are more likely than are those of normal weight to suffer from heart disease, diabetes, and some types of cancer. Hypertension, musculoskeletal problems, and arthritis tend to be more severe in obese and overweight people. Obesity increased little in the U.S. population between the early 1960s and 1980. Since 1980, however, obesity has increased dramatically in the United States. Fifteen percent of American adults were obese in the mid-to-late 1970s; the prevalence of obesity doubled in two decades to reach 31% by 1999 to 2000. In 2005 to 2006, more than one-third of U.S. adults were obese. The proportions of overweight individuals in the United States also increased dramatically over this period, from 47% in the mid-1970s to 65% by 1999 to 2000. Women (35.3%)

BOX 2-6
Definitions of Underweight, Overweight, and Obesity

The U.S. Centers for Disease Control define weight categories for adults using body mass index (BMI), calculated as an individual's height in meters (squared) divided by weight in kilograms.

BMI < 18.5 = underweight
BMI = 18.5 to 24.9 = healthy weight
BMI = 25.0 to 29.9 = overweight
BMI ≥ 30.0 = obese

Definitions for children are different, in part because boys and girls differ somewhat in the timing of growth and fat deposition before and after puberty.

BMI is a valuable indicator but is not a complete assessment of risk. The Centers for Disease Control and Prevention also recommends use of additional indicators such as measures of abdominal fat (not simply overall weight), physical inactivity, high blood pressure, among other indicators, for a more precise assessment of health risks for individuals.

Many Web sites will calculate BMI (doing the conversions from feet and inches to meters and pounds to kilograms, for those not accustomed to the metric system). A good site, with a significant amount of health information, is maintained by the National Heart Lung and Blood Institute: http://www.nhlbisupport.com/bmi/.

---

are more likely than are men (33.3%) to be obese (National Center for Health Statistics, 2007b).

Obesity rates are lower in Canada than in the United States, but Canadian rates have also increased rapidly in recent years. Twenty-three percent of Canadian adults were obese and 36% were overweight in 2005 (Tjepkema, 2005). In Canada, men are more likely to be obese than women, in contrast with the United States.

Adults: Behavioral Risk Factors

In 1990, at the urging of the Surgeon General of the United States, the U.S. Federal Government published a national agenda for health promotion, entitled *Healthy People 2000,* which identified 319 objectives for health promotion and set measurable goals for achieving them. (See National Center for Health Statistics [2001] for a complete list of objectives and an assessment of progress toward their achievement). Many of the objectives for the decade dealt with health behaviors such as physical activity and exercise; tobacco, alcohol, and drug use; violent and abusive behaviors; safer sexual practices; and behaviors designed to prevent or mitigate injuries. The effort was never meant to be just the responsibility of the health care, or even the public health, sectors alone. Rather, these objectives were set as national goals to be realized through a combination of public sector, private-sector, community, and individual efforts. The outcomes to date appear to be mixed, with considerable success in some areas, including increases in moderate physical activity; moderate improvements in some others, including decreases in binge drinking and increases in safer sexual practices; and little progress or worsening in some other behavioral objectives, including marijuana use and tobacco use during pregnancy (National Center for Health Statistics, 2001). A new set of objectives and measurable goals, *Healthy People 2010,* was adopted for the first decade of this century. The relevant *Healthy People* goals provide a good way to assess changes in behaviors that affect susceptibility to illness and injury. Numerous tables in the statistical yearbooks published by the National Center for Health Statistics form a "scorecard" for this national effort. Among the behaviors with the greatest negative impact on public health are tobacco use, use of alcohol and other drugs, lack of physical activity, and unsafe sexual practices.

Smoking has declined steadily among adults in the United States. In 1965, more than half of adult men smoked, as did a third of adult women. The prevalence has declined more rapidly for men than for women, and the gap between sexes has narrowed. By 2007, approximately 23.9% of adult men and 18% of adult women were current smokers. Prevalence of cigarette smoking is highest among American Indians/Alaska Natives (32.4%), followed by African Americans (23.0%), whites (21.9%), Hispanics (15.2%), and Asians (excluding Native Hawaiians and other Pacific Islanders) (10.4%) (U.S. Department of Health and Human Services, 2007, November).

In Canada, the proportion of daily smokers decreased from 24% to 17% between 1995 and 2005. In 2005, another 5% of Canadians reported being occasional smokers. As in the United States, more men

(23%) were smokers than women (20%) (Human Resources and Social Development Canada, 2008).

Use of alcohol is a risk factor for a wide range of poor physical and mental health outcomes. Alcohol use is legal for adults, though drunk driving and, to a lesser extent, public drunkenness are banned. Alcohol use is illegal for minors, though widely tolerated in the United States and Canada. In 2005, 64% of American adult men (aged 21 or older) and 49% of American adult women reported that they currently drank alcohol. Almost one-third of men and 15% of women reported "binge drinking" (defined as five or more drinks on one occasion) during the preceding month. In the United States, non-Hispanic whites were more likely than other race groups to be current drinkers, whereas Native Americans were more likely than other race groups to be binge drinkers (U.S. Department of Health and Human Services, 2005a). In 2002, about 35% of the adult population of Canada had engaged in binge drinking. Close to half (48%) of binge drinkers reported binge drinking on a monthly basis (Tjepkema, 2004).

The prevalence of illegal drug use, the particular drugs used, and the methods in which they are taken vary considerably over time, among racial and ethnic groups, across social and economic classes, and among regions of the country or even neighborhoods. In 2005, nearly 8% of Americans aged 18 and older who were interviewed in confidential household surveys reported that they had used one or more illicit drugs during the preceding 30 days (U.S. Department of Health and Human Services, 2005b). In 2002, 13% of the Canadian population aged 15 or older reported that they had used illicit drugs during the past year. Almost half of those who used drugs had done so at least monthly, and 9% acknowledged daily use (Tjepkema, 2004).

Children's Health

In many ways, the physical health of North American children has never been better. When American parents are asked to assess the overall health of their children, most (82% in 2004) rate their children's physical health as very good or excellent (Federal Interagency Forum on Child and Family Statistics, 2006). But fewer poor parents (67%) than nonpoor parents (88%) rate their children's overall health as being good or excellent. Fewer African American

(74%) and Hispanic (73%) children are reported to be in very good or excellent health when compared with white children (87%). Younger children are generally reported to be in better health than older children. The overall health of children was reported to be better in 2004 than in 1990 for children in each age, economic, and race/ethnic group except for Hispanic children (73% vs. 75%).

Living conditions for children have improved in many ways, especially in the poorest households (Mayer & Jencks, 1989). Poor children are increasingly better housed over time. The percentage of low-income children living in homes without a complete bathroom or with leaky roofs, holes in the floor, no central heat, no electric outlets, or no sewer or septic system has declined substantially.

Another indicator of the general health of North American children is activity limitations that result from chronic conditions. Few children who suffer from chronic health conditions have activity limitations that require help from adult persons, for their personal care needs, such as eating, bathing, toileting, dressing, getting around inside the home, or walking. In 2004, only 8.4% of American children aged 5 to 17 had limitation of activities associated with physical, mental, or psychological chronic conditions (Federal Interagency Forum on Child and Family Statistics, 2006). Almost twice as many boys as girls are reported to have limitations in their activities. This difference exists mainly because more boys experience limitations associated with the need for special education. White and African American children are more likely to have activity limitations than are Hispanic children. Poor children are more likely than nonpoor children to experience limitations.

About 4% of Canadian children aged 5 to 14 had activity limitations in 2001. Of these children, 57% experienced mild-to-moderate disabilities and 43% experienced severe-to-very-severe disabilities. Nearly one in four Canadian children with disabilities receives help for daily activities. More than one in four Canadian children aged 5 to 14 with disabilities received some form of special education during the 2005–2006 school year. Most of these children required special education because of their learning disabilities, and like in the United States, these disabilities were more common among boys (Canadian Council on Social Development, 2006).

Among the most important indictors demographers use to assess child health are the infant and child mortality rates. The infant mortality rate is a good indicator of societal development because, as the standard of living in a country goes up, the health of babies improves earlier and faster than the health of older people. The highest probability of death for children occurs within the first year of life. The infant mortality rate is measured by the number of deaths of children younger than 1 year for every 1,000 live births that occurred during the year. The simple number of infant deaths in a country does not provide a good comparison across countries because larger countries will have more deaths just because they have a greater number of babies at risk of dying. The denominator, per 1,000 live births, takes into account the size of the population, making the figure easier to compare across countries.

In Canada, infant mortality rates have declined significantly. In 1975, the infant mortality rate stood at 13.6 deaths per 1000 births. By 2005, it stood at 5.4. Although the U.S. infant mortality rate remains higher than in many other industrialized countries including Canada, both infant and child mortality rates have declined significantly since 1960. In the United States, the infant mortality rate stood at 6.9 deaths per 1,000 births in 2000 (Table 2-1).

Many serious illnesses, such as diphtheria and polio, have been entirely or nearly eradicated. Most children may not enter school unless they have been vaccinated against several major childhood diseases. A significant increase in the likelihood that children receive all immunizations occurred in the latter part of the 1990s, although minority children are still less likely than are white children to receive these vaccines (Fig. 2-1). Poor children (78%) are less likely to be immunized than are higher-income children (85%) (Federal Interagency Forum on Child and Family Statistics, 2006).

Infant mortality continues to decline, whereas the percentage of low weight births has been stable or slightly increasing (see Table 2-1). This trend is true in Canada as well. These two trends may be intertwined, as more premature babies are kept alive by improvements in technology than in the past. The most striking finding is that the prevalence of low birth weight for African American infants is about twice as high as the rates for infants of other races. The infant mortality rate for African Americans is twice as high as the rate for white, Hispanic, and Asian/Pacific Islander infants and substantially higher than the Native American/Alaska Native rate. The source of this difference is poorly understood. The

TABLE 2-1			
Low Birth Weight (<2,500 g) and Infant Mortality by Race, United States 1980 to 2000			
CHARACTERISTICS	1980	1990	2000
Percentage low birth weight			
Total	6.8	7.0	7.7
White	5.7	5.6	6.8
Black	12.7	13.3	13.1
Hispanic	6.1	6.1	6.5
Asian/Pacific Islander	6.7	6.5	7.3
American Indian/Alaska Native	6.4	6.1	6.8
Infant mortality rate (per 1,000)*			
Total	10.9	8.9	6.9
White	9.2	7.2	5.7
Black	19.1	16.9	13.6
Hispanic	9.5	7.5	5.6
Asian/Pacific Islander	8.3	6.6	4.9
American Indian/Alaska Native	15.2	13.1	8.3

*Infant mortality rates are for 1983 rather than 1980.

Source: Federal Interagency Forum on Child and Family Statistics, (2008a). HEALTH1 Low birth weight: Percentage of infants born with low birth weight by detailed mother's race and Hispanic origin, 1980–2006. *America's Children in Brief: Key National Indicators of Well-Being, 2008.* Retrieved online on April 13, 2008, from

http://www.childstats.gov/americaschildren/tables/health1.asp?popup=true

African American population, on average, is more likely to be poor and less educated than the white population. If poverty and low education were the root cause, however, one would expect that the mortality rates of Hispanics and Native Americans would be higher as well, because they are also more likely to be in poverty and have low education. In addition, African American infant mortality rates are higher than white rates within each socioeconomic group. Factors that affect infant mortality are complex and may include access to good prenatal care. An additional reason for the increase in low-birth-weight infants is that the number of multiple births has also been increasing, and multiple births such as twins, triplets, and so forth are much more likely to be of low birth weight (Federal Interagency Forum on Child and Family Statistics, 2006).

Adolescents

Once children survive the first year of life, their risk of death decreases dramatically. It increases again in the teen years as youths, especially male and minority youths, are subject to heightened risk of fatal motor vehicle accidents and homicides. In the United States, African American teenage men are more often victims of a homicide than teens in other racial and ethnic groups (Federal Interagency Forum on Child and Family Statistics, 2006). For young Americans aged 15 to 24, the most common causes of death are unintentional injuries, homicide, suicide, cancers, and heart disease, in that order (these five causes account for more than four-fifths of deaths to young people), and the risk of dying during these ages is more than twice as high for boys as for girls. Hispanic teenage girls have the lowest mortality rates, and African American teenage boys have the highest rates. Car accidents account for more deaths among white male and female adolescents than among minority adolescents.

As is the case with the older population, the percentage of teenagers who are overweight has been increasing dramatically. In the mid-1980s in the United States, only 5% of children were overweight (Federal Interagency Forum on Child and Family Statistics, 2006). Overweight is defined as body mass index (BMI) at or above the 95th percentile of

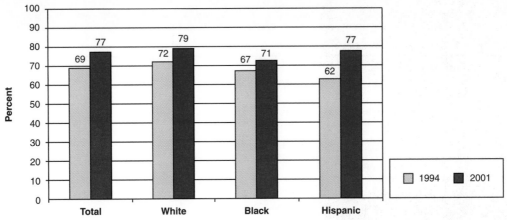

FIGURE 2-1 Percentage of children aged 19 to 35 months with complete immunization/vaccination, 1994 and 2001.

the 2000 Centers for Disease Control and Prevention BMI-for-age growth charts. BMI is calculated as weight in kilograms divided by the square of height in meters. By 2004, the percentage of teenagers who were overweight had increased to 18%. Boys and girls are about equal in their likelihood to be overweight. Non-Hispanic African American teenagers are more likely to be overweight than are non-Hispanic white and Mexican American teenagers. By 2004, the percentage of overweight Mexican American teenagers decreased from 25% to 16%.

By comparison, in 2005, 34% of 12- to 17-year-old Canadian boys were overweight compared with about 23% of girls (Human Resources and Social Development Canada, 2008). Over the past quarter century, the percentage of Canadian adolescents aged 12 to 17 who are overweight has more than doubled, and the percentage of those who are obese tripled. Canadian children who eat fruits and vegetables frequently are less likely to be overweight. By contrast, those who watch TV, play video games, or spend time on the computer are more likely to be overweight.

The teen years become the time of heightened experimentation with behaviors that engender health consequences. In the United States, from 1991 to 2005, adolescent smoking and alcohol consumption remained relatively stable, and the use of illicit drugs increased substantially in the mid-1990s but decreased in the mid-2000s (Table 2-2). A worrisome increase occurred in regular cigarette use among high-school seniors, however, from 19% in 1990 to 25% in 1997, but this rate declined to 14% by 2005 (Federal Interagency Forum on Child and Family Statistics, 2006). Interestingly, the risky behaviors of smoking, alcohol use, and drug use are all much more likely among white than among minority youths (Casper & Bianchi, 2002). African Americans were the least likely to report engaging in any of these behaviors. Research with large data sets that follow representative samples of young people over time, such as the National Study of Adolescent Health, is just beginning to untangle the effects of peer influences, family factors, school climate, and neighborhood contexts on youth risk-taking behavior (Duncan, Harris, & Boisjoly, 2001; Harris, Duncan, & Boisjoly, 2002).

Trends in alcohol use for Canadian adolescents have remained relatively stable since the late 1990s, hovering at just more than 70% for both boys and girls aged 15 to 19. By contrast, fewer Canadian adolescents smoke today than was the case a decade ago. In 2002, slightly more than 1 in 5 adolescents aged 15 to 19 smoked daily or occasionally compared with slightly less than 3 in 10 in 1994 (Canadian Council on Social Development, 2006).

Implications for Health Care Providers

What implications do these health trends have for nursing and the health care of families? Lower mortality means that more people will require nursing care at older ages. But declines in disability mean that seniors in their 60s and 70s are less likely to require intensive, around-the-clock care, at least in their 60s and 70s. Fewer adults smoke, so the incidence of diseases stemming from tobacco use such

TABLE 2-2		
Selected Risky Behaviors of Adolescents in the United States, 1991 and 2001		
CHARACTERISTICS	1991	2001
Adolescent birth rate (per 1,000)		
Age, yr		
15–17	38.7	24.7
18–19	94.4	76.1
Percentage smoking daily in past 30 days		
8th graders	7.2	5.5
10th graders	12.6	12.2
12th graders	18.5	19
Percentage consuming 5+ drinks in a row in past 2 weeks		
8th graders	12.9	13.2
10th graders	22.9	24.9
12th graders	29.8	28.6
Percentage using illicit drugs in past 30 days		
8th graders	5.7	11.7
10th graders	11.6	22.7
12th graders	16.4	25.7

Source: Federal Interagency Forum on Child and Family Statistics. (2008b). *America's Children in Brief: Key National Indicators of Well-Being, 2008.* Retrieved online on April 13, 2008, from http://www.childstats.gov/americaschildren/tables.asp

as lung cancer and emphysema may decline. Obesity is on the rise, however, increasing the need for counseling on diet, nutrition, and physical activities.

In popular discussions, and sometimes among professionals, health-related behaviors are treated as resulting solely from conscious choice by individuals, who are to blame if their risky behavior leads to poor health outcomes. Many health activists, by contrast, seek to place blame on commercial interests that profit from these behaviors or on government policies that protect them. Research on the causes of risky behaviors is much less developed than is research on their consequences, but even so, it is clear that behaviors are the results of multiple causes and can be influenced by health policy in multiple ways (Berkman & Mullen, 1997; Singer & Ryff, 2001). Obesity, for example, has a genetic component, as well as dietary, environmental, and economic correlates. Health promotion is concerned with generating improvements through whatever works. This orientation leads to combined approaches of research, public education, changes in the physical and social environment, regulation of disease- and injury-promoting activities

or behaviors, and improved access to high-quality health care.

SUMMARY

Families change in response to economic conditions, cultural change, and shifting demographics such as the aging of the population and immigration. North America has gone through a particularly tumultuous period in the last few decades, resulting in rapid changes in family structure, function, and process. Families have emerged more diversified. More single-mother families, single-father families, and families with both parents in the labor force exist than did in the past. This translates into less time for parents to take care of the health needs of the family. Single mothers may find it particularly challenging to meet the health care needs of their families because they tend to have the least time and money to do so. More fathers are taking responsibility for being primary parents of their children and will be increasingly likely to be the parent with whom the nurse interacts. More grandparents are raising their grandchildren, and these grandchildren may suffer from more health problems compared with other children. Many families maintained by grandparents are in poverty, and many of the grandparents in these families suffer from poor health themselves. Nurses increasingly may be likely to provide care to grandparent families, and they should be aware of the unique health and financial challenges these families face.

As mortality rates at the older ages continue to improve and baby boomers move into their retirement years, increasing proportions of the population will be elderly. This demographic shift will increase the need for nurses who specialize in caring for the elderly. More adults will have children and parents for whom they must care—caring in both directions of the younger and older. Working with the health care needs of both generations of the family system will be a challenge for health care professionals, especially nurses who are on the front line in most health care systems that take care of individuals and families.

Today, more North Americans come from other countries than was true in the past. Many of these Americans speak a language other than English. Health care providers will be serving a more ethnically and culturally diverse population.

Demographic health data indicate that mortality rates, disability, and smoking have been declining in the adult population. Obesity is on the rise, increasing the need for promotion of healthy diets and physical activity. The general health of children has improved since the late 1990s, but racial and economic disparities still exist, with minority and poor children faring the worst. Increasing proportions of teenagers are overweight, and more of them are using illicit drugs.

Poor American children today are more likely to receive medical attention than in the past. The percentage of children who did not visit a doctor in the previous year declined, especially during the 1970s. Poor children are more likely to be immunized than in the past. By contrast, obesity and illicit drug use are increasing among teenagers. Nurses should be aware of these negative trends, but more importantly, they should note that poor and minority children are likely to fare worse on nearly all of these measures.

Economics and family relationships remain intertwined. Issues growing in importance include balancing paid work with child rearing, income inequality between men and women, fathers' parenting roles, the expected increase in the number of frail elderly, and family relationship changes because of the increase in life expectancy. Families have been amazingly adaptive and resilient in the past; one would expect them to be so in the future.

REFERENCES

Berkman, L. F., & Mullen, J. M. (1997). How health behaviors and social environment contribute to health differences between black and white older Americans. In L. G. Martin & B. J. Soldo (Eds.), *Racial and ethnic differences in the health of older Americans* (pp. 163–182). Washington, DC: National Academy Press.

Besharov D. J., & Fowler, A. (1993). The end of welfare as we know it? *The Public Interest, 111,* 95–108.

Bianchi, S. M. (1995). The changing demographic and socioeconomic characteristics of single-parent families. *Marriage and Family Review, 20,* 71–97.

Bianchi, S. M. (2000). Maternal employment and time with children: Dramatic change or surprising continuity? *Demography, 37*(4), 401–414.

Bianchi, S. M., & Casper, L. M. (2000). *American families* (Population Bulletin, Vol. 55, No. 4, pp. 1–44). Washington, DC: Population Reference Bureau.

Bryson, K., & Casper, L. M. (1999). *Coresident grandparents and grandchildren* (Current Population Reports, P23–198). Washington, DC: U.S. Census Bureau.

Bumpass, L. L., & Lu, H. (2000). Trends in cohabitation and implications for children's family contexts in the United States. *Population Studies, 54*(1), 29–41.

Canadian Council on Social Development. (2006). *The progress of Canada's children and youth.* Ottawa, Ontario, Canada: Canadian Council on Social Development.

Casper, L. M., & Bianchi, S. M. (2002). *Continuity and change in the American family.* Thousand Oaks, CA: Sage.

Casper, L. M., & Cohen, P. (2000). How does POSSLQ measure up? Historical estimates of cohabitation. *Demography 37*(2), 237–245.

Casper, L. M., & Haaga, J. G. (2005). Family and health demographics. In Hanson, S. M. H., Gedaly-Duff, V., & Kaakinen, J. R. (Eds.), *Family health care nursing: Theory, practice and research* (3rd ed., pp. 39–68). Philadelphia: F.A. Davis.

Casper, L. M., & Smith K. E. (2004). Self care: Why do parents leave their children unsupervised? *Demography 41*(2), 285–301.

Cherlin, A. J. (1992). *Marriage, divorce, remarriage.* Cambridge, MA: Harvard University Press.

Cherlin, A. J. (2000). How is the 1996 welfare reform law affecting poor families? In A. J. Cherlin (Ed.), *Public and private families: A reader* (2nd ed.). New York: McGraw-Hill.

Citizenship and Immigration Canada. (2006). *Canada: Permanent residents by category, 1980 to 2006.* Retrieved April 13th, 2008, from http://www.cic.gc.ca/english/resources/statistics/facts2006/permanent/01.asp

Cotter, D. A., Hermsen, J. M., & Vannemen, R. (2004). In R. Farley, & J. Haaga (Eds.), *The American people.* New York: Russell Sage Foundation.

Crimmins, E. M., & Ingegneri, D. G. (1990). Interaction and living arrangements of older parents and their children. *Research on Aging, 12*(1), 3–35.

Dowdell, E. B. (1995). Caregiver burden: Grandparents raising their high-risk children. *Journal of Psychosocial Nursing, 33*(3), 27–30.

Duncan, G. J., Harris, K. M., & Boisjoly, J. (2001). Sibling, peer, neighbor and schoolmate Correlations as indicators of the importance of context for adolescent development. *Demography, 38*(3), 437–447.

Eggebeen, D. J., & Hogan, D. P. (1990). Giving between generations in American families. *Human Nature 1*(3), 211–232.

Farley, R. (1996). *The new American reality: Who we are, how we got here, where we are going.* New York: Russell Sage Foundation.

Federal Interagency Forum on Aging-Related Statistics. (2008). *Older Americans 2008: Key indicators of well-being.* Washington, DC: U.S. Government Printing Office.

Federal Interagency Forum on Child and Family Statistics. (2006). *America's children: Key national indicators of well-being, 2006.* Washington, DC: U.S. Government Printing Office.

Federal Interagency Forum on Child and Family Statistics. (2008a). HEALTH1 Low birth weight: Percentage of infants born with low birth weight by detailed mother's race and Hispanic origin, 1980–2006. *America's Children in Brief: Key National Indicators of Well-Being, 2008.* Retrieved April 13, 2008, from http://www.childstats.gov/americaschildren/tables/health1.asp?popup=true.

Federal Interagency Forum on Child and Family Statistics. (2008). *America's Children in Brief: Key National Indicators of Well-Being, 2008.* Federal Interagency Forum on Child and Family Statistics, Washington DC: U.S. Government Printing Office.

Freedman, V., Martin, L., & Schoeni, R. (2002). Recent trends in disability and functioning among older adults in the United States: A systematic review. *Journal of the American Medical Association, 288*(24), 3137–3146.

Fuchs, V. R., & Garber, A. M. (2003). Health and medical care. In H. J. Aaron, J. M. Lindsay, & P. S. Nivola (Eds.), *Agenda for the nation* (pp. 145–182). Washington, DC: Brookings Institution Press.

Furstenberg, F., Jr. (1998). Good dads–bad dads: Two faces of fatherhood. In A. J. Cherlin (Ed.), *The changing American family and public policy* (pp. 193–218). Washington, DC: The Urban Institute.

Goldscheider, C., & Goldscheider, F. K. (1994). *Leaving and returning home in 20th century America* (Population Bulletin, Vol. 48, No. 4). Washington, DC: Population Reference Bureau.

Goldscheider, C., & Jones, M. B. (1989). Living arrangements among the older population. In F. K. Goldscheider & C. Goldscheider (Eds.), *Ethnicity and the new family economy* (pp. 75–91). Boulder, CO: Westview Press.

Harris, K. M., Duncan, G. J., & Boisjoly, J. (2002). Evaluating the role of 'nothing to lose' attitudes on risky behavior in adolescence. *Social Forces, 80*(3), 1005–1039.

Hernandez, D. J. (Ed.). (1999). *Children of immigrants: Health, adjustment, and public assistance.* Washington, DC: National Academy Press.

Heuveline, P., Timberlake, J. M., & Furstenberg, F. F., Jr. (2003). Shifting child rearing to single mothers: Results from 17 Western nations. *Population and Development Review, 29*(1), 47–71.

Human Resources and Social Development Canada. (2008). *Indicators of well-being in Canada: Health.* Retrieved May 20, 2008, from http://www4.hrsdc.gc.ca/domain.jsp?lang=en&domainid=1

Kaiser Commission on Medicaid and the Uninsured (2007, May). Health insurance coverage and access to care for low-income non-citizen children. Retrieved October 6, 2009, from www.kff.org/medicaid/upload/7643.pdf

King, R. B. (1999). Time spent in parenthood status among adults in the United States. *Demography 36*(3), 377–385.

Kramarow, E. (1995). Living alone among the elderly in the United States: Historical perspectives on household change. *Demography 32*(2), 335–352.

Levy, F. (1998). *The new dollars and dreams.* New York: Russell Sage Foundation.

Mayer, S. E., & Jencks, C. (1989). Growing up in poor neighborhoods: How much does it matter? *Science 243*, 1441–1446.

McGarry, K., & Schoeni, R. F. (2000). Social security, economic growth, and the rise in elderly widows' independence in the twentieth century. *Demography 37*(2), 221–236.

McLanahan, S., & Casper, L. (1995). Growing diversity and inequality in the American family. In R. Farley (Ed.), *State of the union: America in the 1990s* (pp. 1–46). New York: Russell Sage Foundation.

McNeil, J. (2001). *Americans with disabilities 1997* (Current Population Reports, P70–73). Washington, DC: U.S. Census Bureau.

Milan, A., & Hamm, B. (2003). Across generations: Grandparents and grandchildren. *Canadian Social Trends, 71*, 1–7.

Minkler, M., & Roe, K. M. (1993). *Grandmothers as caregivers: Raising children of the crack cocaine epidemic.* Newbury Park, CA: Sage.

Minkler, M., & Roe, K. M. (1996). Grandparents as surrogate parents. *Generations 20*, 34–38.

National Center for Health Statistics. (2001). *Healthy people 2000 final review.* Hyattsville, MD: Public Health Service.

National Center for Health Statistics. (2007a). Births: Final data for 2005. *National Vital Statistics Reports 56*(6), 1–104.

National Center for Health Statistics. (2007b). *Obesity among adults in the United States.* Retrieved April 29, 2008, from http://www.cdc.gov/nchs/data/databriefs/db01.pdf

National Center for Health Statistics. (2008). Births, marriages, divorces, and deaths: Provisional data for February 2007 (Table A, p. 1). *National Vital Statistics Reports 56*(21).

Navaie-Walsier, M., Feldman, P. H., Gould, D. A., Levine, C., Kuerbis, A. N., & Donelan, K. (2001). The experiences and challenges of informal caregivers: Common themes and differences among whites, blacks, and Hispanics. *Gerontologist 41*(6), 733–741.

Passel, J. S. (2007). *The size and characteristics of the unauthorized migrant population in the United States.* Washington, DC: Pew Hispanic Center.

Pleck, E. H., & Pleck, J. H. (1997). Fatherhood ideals in the United States: Historical dimensions. In M. E. Lamb (Ed.), *The Role of the father in child development* (3rd ed., pp. 33–48). New York: John Wiley & Sons.

Popenoe, D. (1993). American family decline, 1960–1990: A review and appraisal. *Journal of Marriage and the Family 55*(3), 527–555.

Raley, R. K. (1999). Then comes marriage? Recent changes in women's response to a non-marital pregnancy. Presented at the annual meeting of the Population Association of America, New York.

Raley, R. K. (2000). Recent trends and differentials in marriage and cohabitation. In L. Waite (Ed.), *Ties that bind: Perspectives on marriage and cohabitation* (pp. 19–39). New York: Aldine de Gruyter.

Reinhardt, U. E. (2003). Does the aging of the population really drive the demand for health care? *Health Affairs 22*(6), 27–39.

Rindfuss, R. R. (1991). The young adult years: Diversity, structural change, and fertility. *Demography 28*(4), 493–512.

Ruggles, S. (1994). The transformation of American family structure. *American Historical Review 99*(1), 103–127.

Ruggles, S. (1996). Living arrangements of the elderly in America: 1880–1990. In T. Harevan (Ed.), *Aging and generational relations: Historical and cross-cultural perspectives* (pp. 254–263). New York: Aldine de Gruyter.

Saenz, R. (2004). *Latinos and the changing face of America.* Washington, DC: Population Reference Bureau.

Schulz, R., & REACH II investigators. (2006). Enhancing the quality of life of dementia caregivers from different ethnic or racial groups. *Archives of Internal Medicine, 145*(10), 727–738.

Shore, R. J., & Hayslip, B., Jr. (1994). Custodial grandparenting: Implications for children's development. In A. E. Gottfried & A. W. Gottfried (Eds.), *Redefining families: Implications for children's development* (pp. 171–218). New York: Plenum.

Silverstein, M. (1995). Stability and change in temporal distance between the elderly and their children. *Demography 32*(1), 29–46.

Singer, B. H., & Ryff, C. D. (Eds.). (2001). *New horizons in health: An integrative approach/committee on future directions for behavioral and social sciences research at the National Institutes of Health, Institute of Medicine.* Washington, DC: National Academy Press.

Speare, A., Jr., & Avery, R. (1993). Who helps whom in older parent-child families? *Journal of Gerontology: Social Sciences, 48*(2), S64–S73.

Spitze, G., & Logan, J. R. (1990). Sons, daughters, and intergenerational social support. *Journal of Marriage and the Family, 52*(2), 420–430.

Stacey, J. (1993). Good riddance to 'The Family': A response to David Popenoe. *Journal of Marriage and the Family, 55*(3), 545–547.

Statistics Canada. (2002). Profile of Canadian families and households: Diversification continues [electronic version]. *2001 census analysis series.* Statistics Canada: Ottawa, Ontario, Canada. Retrieved April 13th 2008, from http://www.statcan.gc.ca/bsolc/olc-cel/olc-cel?catno=96F0030XIE2001003&lang=eng

Statistics Canada. (2008a). *Projected population by age group and sex according to a medium growth scenario for 2006, 2011, 2016, 2021, 2026 and 2031, at July 1 (2006, 2011).* Retrieved April 13, 2008, from http://www40.statcan.ca/l01/cst01/demo23a.htm?sdi=age%20population

Statistics Canada. (2008b). *Mean age and median age at divorce and at marriage, by sex, Canada, Provinces and Territories, annual (years)* (Table 101-6502). Retrieved April 11, 2008, from http://cansim2.statcan.ca/cgi-win/CNSMCGI.PGM

Steinmetz, E. (2006). *Americans with disabilities: 2002* (Current Population Reports, P70–107). Washington, DC: U.S. Census Bureau.

Stone, R. I. (2000). *Long-term care for the elderly with disabilities: Current policy, emerging trends, and implications for the twenty-first century.* New York: Milbank Memorial Fund.

Thornton, A., & Young-DeMarco, L. (2001). Four decades of trends in attitudes toward family issues in the United States: The 1960s through the 1990s. *Journal of Marriage and the Family, 63*(4), 1009–1037.

Tjepkema, M. (2004). Alcohol and illicit drug dependence. *Supplement to Health Report, 15.* Ottawa, Ontario, Canada: Statistics Canada.

Tjepkema, M. (2005). *Adult obesity in Canada: Measured height and weight. Nutrition: findings from the Canadian community health survey, no. 1.* Ottawa, Ontario, Canada: Statistics Canada/Statistique Canada.

Treas, J., & Torrecilha, R. (1995). The older population. In R. Farley (Ed.), *State of the union: America in the 1990s* (pp. 47–92). New York: Russell Sage Foundation.

Uhlenberg, P. (1996). Mortality decline in the twentieth century and supply of kin over the life course. *Gerontologist, 36,* 681–685.

U.S. Census Bureau. (2008a). *All parent/child situations, by type, race, and Hispanic origin of householder or reference person: 1970 to present* (Table FM-2). Retrieved April 3, 2008, from http://www.census.gov/population/www/socdemo/hh-fam.html

U.S. Census Bureau. (2008b). *Estimated median age at first marriage, by sex: 1890 to the present* (Table MS-2). Retrieved April 3, 2008, from http://www.census.gov/population/www/socdemo/hh-fam.html

U.S. Census Bureau. (2008c). *Employment status of women, by marital status and presence and age of children: 1960 to 2005* (Table 580). Retrieved July 31, 2008, from http://www.census.gov/compendia/statab/cats/labor_force_employment_earnings/laborf orce_status.html

U.S. Census Bureau. (2008d). *Statistical abstract of the United States 2003.* Washington, DC: U.S. Government Printing Office.

U.S. Census Bureau. (2008e). *Foreign-born population by sex, age, and year of entry: 2004* (Table 2.1). Retrieved April 13, 2008, from http://www.census.gov/population/socdemo/foreign/ppl-176/tab02-1.pdf

U.S. Census Bureau. (2008f). *Households, by type: 1940 to present* (Table HH-1). Retrieved April 13, 2008, from http://www.census.gov/population/www/socdemo/hh-fam.html#ht

U.S. Census Bureau. (2008g). *Families by presence of own children under 18: 1950 to present* (Table FM-1). Retrieved April 3, 2008, from http://www.census.gov/population/www/schdemo/hh-fam.html

U.S. Census Bureau. (2008h). *Households by size: 1960 to present* (Table HH-4). Retrieved April 13, 2008, from http://www.census.gov/population/www/socdemo/hh-fam.html#ht

U.S. Census Bureau. (2008i). *Family status and household relationship of people 15 years and over, by marital status, age, sex, race, and Hispanic origin/1: 2006* (Table A2). Retrieved April 13, 2008, from http://www.census.gov/population/www/socdemo/hh-fam/cps2006.html

U.S. Census Bureau. (2008j). *Young adults living at home: 1960-present* (Table AD-1). Retrieved April 13, 2008, from http://www.census.gov/population/www/socdemo/hh-fam/cps2006.html

U.S. Census Bureau. (2008k). *Unmarried-couple households, by presence of children: 1960 to present* (Table UC-1). Retrieved April 13, 2008, from http://www.census.gov/population/www/socdemo/hh-fam.html#history

U.S. Census Bureau. (2008l). *Marital status of people 15 years and over, by age, sex, personal earnings, race, and Hispanic origin/1, 2006* (Table A-1). Retrieved April 13, 2008, from http://www.census.gov/population/www/socdemo/hh-fam/cps2006.html

U.S. Census Bureau. (2008m). *One-parent family groups with own children under 18, by marital status, and race and hispanic origin/1 of the reference person: 2006* (Table FG-6). Retrieved April 15, 2008, from http://www.census.gov/population/www/socdemo/hh-fam/cps2006.html

U.S. Census Bureau. (2008n). *Grandchildren living in the home of their grandparents: 1970 to present* (Table CH-7). Retrieved April 3, 2008, from http://www.census.gov/population/www/socdemo/hh-fam.html

U.S. Department of Health and Human Services. (2005a). *National survey on drug use & health: Detailed tables: Table 2.106B Alcohol use, binge alcohol use, and heavy alcohol use in the past month among persons aged 21 or older, by demographic characteristics: Percentages, 2004 and 2005*. Retrieved April 30, 2008, from http://www.cdc.gov/tobacco/data_statistics/Factsheets/adult_cig_smoking.html

U.S. Department of Health and Human Services. (2005b). *National survey on drug use & health: Detailed tables: Table 1.12B Types of illicit drug use in lifetime, past year, and past month among persons aged 18 or older: Percentages, 2004 and 2005*. Retrieved April 30, 2008, from http://www.oas.samhsa.gov/NSDUH/2k5nsduh/tabs/Sect1peTabs1to66.htm#Tab1.12A

U.S. Department of Health and Human Services. (2007, November). *Fact sheet: Adult cigarette smoking in the United States: Current estimates*. Retrieved April 29, 2008, from http://www.cdc.gov/tobacco/data_statistics/Factsheets/adult_cig_smoking.htm

U.S. Department of Homeland Security. (2008). *Annual flow report. U.S. legal permanent residents: 2007*. Washington, DC: Office of Immigration Statistics.

Ventura, S. J., Bachrach, C. A., Hill, L., Kaye, K., Holcomb, P., & Koff, E. (1995). The demography of out-of-wedlock childbearing. In National Center for Health Statistics (Ed.), *Report to congress on out-of-wedlock childbearing* (pp. 1–133). Washington, DC: U.S. Department of Health and Human Services.

Waite, L. J., & Gallagher, M. (2000). *The case for marriage: Why married people are happier, healthier and better off financially*. Garden City, NY: Doubleday.

Weinick, R. M. (1995). Sharing a home: The experiences of American women and their parents over the twentieth century. *Demography 32*(2), 281–297.

Wister, A. V., & Burch, T. K. (1987). Values, perceptions, and choice in living arrangements of the elderly. In E. F. Borgatte & R. J. V. Montgomery (Eds.), *Critical issues in aging policy* (pp. 180–198). Newbury Park, CA: Sage.

World Health Organization. (2008). Life tables for WHO member states 2005. Retrieved April 13, 2008, from http://www.who.int/whosis/database/life_tables/life_tables_process.cfm?path=whosis,life_tables&language=english

Woroby, J. L., & Angel, R. J. (1990). Functional capacity and living arrangements of unmarried elderly persons. *Journal of Gerontology: Social Sciences 45*(3), S95–S101.

Wu, Z. (1998, September). Recent trends in marriage patterns in Canada. *Policy options*, 3–6.

Yee, J. L., & Schulz, R. (2000). Gender differences in psychiatric morbidity among family caregivers: A review and analysis. *Gerontologist 40*(2), 147–164.

SUGGESTED READINGS

Bianchi, S. M., & Casper, L. M. (2000). *American families* (Population Bulletin, Vol. 55, No. 4, pp. 1–44). Washington, DC: Population Reference Bureau.

Bumpass, L. L. (1990). What's happening to the family? Interactions between demographic and institutional change. *Demography, 27*(4), 483–493.

Casper, L. M., & Bianchi, S. M. (2002). *Continuity and change in the American family*. Thousand Oaks, CA: Sage.

Cherlin, A. J. (1992). *Marriage, divorce, remarriage*. Cambridge, MA: Harvard University Press.

Decade in review: Understanding families into the new millennium. (2000). Special Issue, *Journal of Marriage and the Family, 62*(4).

Farley, R., & Haaga, J. (Eds.). (2004). *The American people*. New York: Russell Sage Foundation.

Federal Interagency Forum on Aging-Related Statistics. (2008). *Older Americans 2008: Key national indicators of well-being*. Washington, DC: U.S. Government Printing Office.

Federal Interagency Forum on Child and Family Statistics. (2008). *America's children key national indicators of well-being, 2008*. Washington, DC: U.S. Government Printing Office.

Fields, J., & Casper, L. M. (2001). *America's families and living arrangements, 2000* (Current population reports, P20-537). Washington, DC: U.S. Census Bureau.

Levy, F. (1998). *The new dollars and dreams*. New York: Russell Sage Foundation.

Mayer, S. E. (1997). *What money can't buy: Family income and children's life chances*. Cambridge, MA: Harvard University Press.

McLanahan, S., & Casper, L. (1995). Growing diversity and inequality in the American family. In R. Farley (Ed.), *State of the union: America in the 1990s* (pp. 1–46). New York: Russell Sage Foundation.

McLanahan, S., & Sandefur, G. (1994). *Growing up with a single parent: What helps, what hurts?* Cambridge, MA: Harvard University Press.

National Center for Health Statistics. (2001). *Healthy people 2000 final review*. Hyattsville, MD: Public Health Service.

National Center for Health Statistics. (2008). *Health, United States 2008, with chartbook on trends in the health of Americans*. Hyattsville, MD: Public Health Service.

Nock, S.L. (1998). *Marriage in men's lives*. New York: Oxford University Press.

Ruggles, S. (1994). The transformation of American family structure. *American Historical Review 99*(1), 103–127.

Spain, D., & Bianchi, S. M. (1996). *Balancing act: Motherhood, marriage, and employment among American women*. New York: Russell Sage Foundation.

Waite, L. J., Bachrach, C. A., Hinden, M., Thomson, E., & Thornton, A. T. (2000). *The ties that bind: Perspectives on marriage and cohabitation*. New York: Aldine de Gruyter.

CONTACTS

- *Child Trends:* www.childtrends.org
- *Federal Interagency Forum on Aging-Related Statistics:* www.agingstats.gov
- *Federal Interagency Forum on Child and Family Statistics:* www.childstats.gov
- *Kaiser Commission on Medicaid and the Uninsured:* www.kff.org
- *Kids Count: The Annie E. Casey Foundation:* www.aecf.org/kidscount
- *National Center for Health Statistics, U.S. Department of Health and Human Services, Centers for Disease Control and Prevention:* www.cdc.gov/nchs
- *National Institute on Aging, National Institutes of Health:* www.nia.nih.gov
- *National Institute of Child Health and Human Development, National Institutes of Health:* www.nichd.nih.gov
- *Population Reference Bureau:* www.prb.org
- *Statistics Canada/ Statistique Canada:* www.statcan.gc.ca
- *U.S. Census Bureau:* www.census.gov

CHAPTER 3

Theoretical Foundations for the Nursing of Families

Joanna Rowe Kaakinen, PhD, RN

Shirley May Harmon Hanson, PMHNP, PhD, RN, FAAN, CFLE, LMFT

CRITICAL CONCEPTS

✦ The relationship between theory, practice, and research is that through this knowledge nurses can consider options and interventions to support families. By understanding theories and models, nurses are prepared to think more creatively and critically about how health events affect family clients. Theories and models provide different ways of comprehending issues that may be affecting families. Simply put, theories offer choices for action.

✦ No single theory, model, or conceptual framework adequately describes the complex relationships of health events on family structure, function, and process.

✦ The major purpose of theory in family nursing is to provide knowledge and understanding that improves the quality of nursing care of families.

✦ The theoretical/conceptual frameworks and models that provide the foundations for nursing of families have evolved from three major traditions and disciplines: family social science, family therapy, and nursing.

✦ Nurses who use a singular theoretical approach to working with families limit the possibilities for families they serve. By integrating several theories, nurses acquire different ways to conceptualize problems, thus enhancing thinking about interventions. Nurses who use an integrated theoretical approach build on the strengths of families in creative ways.

✦ Theories inform the practice of nursing. Practice informs theory and research. Theory, practice, and research are interactive, and all three are critical to the profession of nursing and family care.

*B*y understanding theories and models, nurses are prepared to think creatively and critically about how health events affect the family client. The reciprocal or interactive relationship between theory, practice, and research is that each aspect informs the other, thereby expanding knowledge and nursing interventions to support families. Theories and models expand thinking to higher levels of understanding problems and circumstances that may be affecting families, and thereby offer more choice and options for nursing interventions.

Currently, no single theory, model, or conceptual framework adequately describes the complex relationships of family structure, function, and process, nor does one theoretical perspective give nurses a sufficiently broad base of knowledge and understanding to guide assessment and interventions with families. No one theoretical perspective is better, more comprehensive, or more correct than another (Doane & Varcoe, 2005; Hanson & Kaakinen, 2005). The goal for nurses is to have a deep understanding of the stresses that families experience when their family members have a health event, and to support and implement family interventions based on theoretical perspective(s) that best match the need(s) identified by the family.

Many theoretical approaches to understanding family exist. The purpose of this chapter is to demonstrate how the phenomena of a family with a member who experiences a health event is conceptualized differently depending on the theoretical perspective. In this chapter, nurses seek different data depending on which theory is being used to understand the family experience to determine the interventions offered to the family to help bring them back to a state of stability. This chapter begins with a brief review of the components of a theory and how these contribute to the nursing of families. The chapter then presents five theoretical approaches for working with families, ranging from a broader to a more specific perspective: Family Systems Theory, Developmental and Family Life Cycle Theory, Bioecological Theory, the Family Cycle of Health and Illness Model, and the Family Assessment and Intervention Model. Demonstrating the five different theoretical approaches to nursing care, the chapter presents a case study of a family with a member who is experiencing progressive multiple sclerosis (MS).

RELATIONSHIP BETWEEN THEORY, PRACTICE, AND RESEARCH

In nursing, the relationship of theory to practice constitutes a dynamic feedback loop rather than a static linear progression. Theory, practice, and research are mutually interdependent. Theory grows out of observations made in practice and is tested by research; then tested theory informs practice, and practice, in turn, facilitates the further refinement and development of theory. Figure 3-1 depicts the dynamic relationship between theory, practice, and research.

Theories do not emerge all at once but build slowly over time, as data are gathered through observation and analysis of evidence. Relating the various concepts together that emerge from observation and evidence occurs through a purposeful thoughtful reasoning process. *Inductive reasoning* is a process that moves from specific pieces of information toward a general idea; it is thinking about how the parts create the whole. *Deductive reasoning* goes in the opposite direction of inductive reasoning. Deductive reasoning is where the general ideas of a given theory generate more specific questions about what filters back into the cycle, and helps refine understanding of the theory and how to apply the theory to practice (White, 2005; White & Klein, 2008).

Theory

Theories are designed to make sense of the world, to show how one thing is related to another and how together they make a pattern that can predict

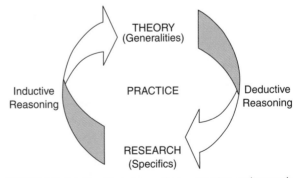

FIGURE 3-1 Relationship between theory, practice, and research. (Adapted from Smith, S. R., Hamon, R. R., Ingoldsby, B. B., & Miller, J. E. (2008). *Exploring family theories* (2nd ed.). New York: Oxford University Press, by permission.)

the consequences of certain clusters of characteristics or events. Theories are abstract, general ideas that are subject to rules of organization. All scientific theories use the same building blocks: concepts, relationships, and proposition. We live in a time when tremendous amounts of information are readily available and accessible quickly in multiple forms. Therefore, theories provide ways to transform this huge volume of information into knowledge and to integrate/organize the information to help us make better sense of our world (White, 2005, p. 6). Ideally, nursing theories represent logical and intelligible patterns that make sense of the observations nurses make in practice and enable nurses to predict what is likely to happen to clients (Polit & Beck, 2008). Theories can be used as a level of evidence on which to base nursing practice (Fawcett & Garity, 2008). The major function of theory in family nursing is to provide knowledge and understanding that improves nursing services to families.

Theories help nurses accumulate and organize evidence into meaningful patterns to develop and test hypotheses or predictions of what the world will look like; hence, theories allow us to see information in a particular way and to integrate it in such a way that it helps make sense of our world (White, 2005). Theories are systematic sets of ideas that make it possible to articulate ideas more clearly and specifically than what may be possible in everyday language. Theories demonstrate how ideas are connected to each other. Most importantly, theories explain what is happening; they provide answers to "how" and "why" questions, help to interpret and make sense of phenomena, and predict or point to what could happen in the future.

Concepts, the building blocks of theory, are words that create mental images or abstract representations of phenomena of study. Concepts, or the major ideas expressed by a theory, may exist on a continuum from empirical (concrete) to abstract (Powers & Knapp, 2005). The more concrete the concept, the easier it is to figure out when it applies or does not apply (White & Klein, 2008, p. 8). For example, one concept in Family Systems Theory is that families have boundaries. A highly abstract aspect of this concept is that the boundary reflects the energy between the environment and the system. A more concrete understanding of family boundaries is that families open and/or close their boundaries in times of stress.

Propositions are statements about the relationship between two or more concepts (Powers & Knapp, 2005). A proposition might be a statement such as: Families as a whole influence the health of individual family members. The word *influence* links the two concepts of "families as a whole" and "health of individual family members." Propositions denote a relationship between the subject and the object. Propositions may lead to hypotheses. Theories are generally made up of several propositions.

A **hypothesis** is a way of stating an expected relationship between concepts or an expected proposition (Powers & Knapp, 2005). The concepts and propositions in the hypothesis are derived and being driven by the original theory. For example, using the concepts of family and health, one could hypothesize that there is an interactive relationship between how a family is coping and the eventual health outcome of family members. In other words, the family's ability to cope with stress affects the health of individual family members, and in turn, the health of this individual family member influences the family's ability to cope. This hypothesis may be tested by a research study that measures family coping strategies and family members' health over time, and uses statistical procedures to look at the relationships between the two concepts.

A **conceptual model** is a set of general propositions that integrate concepts into meaningful configurations or patterns (Fawcett, 2005). Conceptual models in nursing are based on the observations, insights, and deductions that combine ideas from several fields of inquiry. Conceptual models provide a frame of reference and a coherent way of thinking about nursing phenomena. A conceptual model is more abstract and more comprehensive than a theory. Like a conceptual model, a conceptual framework is a way of integrating concepts into a meaningful pattern, but conceptual frameworks are often less definitive than models. They provide useful conceptual approaches or ways in which to look at a problem or situation, rather than a definite set of propositions.

In this chapter, the terms *conceptual model or framework* and *theory or theoretical framework* are often used interchangeably. In part, that is because no single theoretical base exists for the nursing of families. Rather, nurses draw from many theoretical conceptual foundations using a more pluralistic and eclectic approach. The interchangeable use of these various terms reflects the fact that there is considerable overlap among ideas in the various theoretical perspectives and conceptual models/frameworks, and many "streams of influence" are important for family nurses to incorporate into practice. As might be expected, a substantial amount of cross-fertilization among disciplines has occurred, such as social science and nursing, and concepts originating in one theory or discipline have been translated into similar concepts for use in another discipline. Currently, no single theory or conceptual framework adequately describes the complex relationships of family structure, function, and process, nor does one theoretical perspective give nurses a sufficiently broad base of knowledge and understanding to guide assessment and interventions with families.

THEORETICAL AND CONCEPTUAL FOUNDATIONS FOR THE NURSING OF FAMILIES

Nursing is a scientific discipline; thus, nurses are concerned about the relationships between ideas and data. Nurse scholars explain empirical observations by creating theories, which can be used as evidence in evidence-based-practice (Fawcett & Garity, 2008). Nurse researchers investigate and test the models and relationships. Nurses in practice use theories, models, and conceptual frameworks to help clients achieve the best outcomes (Hanson & Kaakinen, 2005). In nursing, evidence, in the form of theory, is used to explain and guide practice (Fawcett & Garity, 2008). The theoretical foundations, theories,

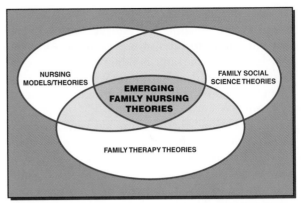

FIGURE 3-2 Theoretical frameworks that influence the nursing of families.

and conceptual models that inform the nursing of families are presented in the following section.

The theoretical/conceptual frameworks, models, and approaches that provide the foundation for the nursing of families have evolved from three major traditions and disciplines: family social science theories, family therapy theories, and nursing models and theories. Figure 3-2 shows the theoretical frameworks that influence the nursing of families.

Of these sources of theory, **family social science theories** are the best developed and informative about family phenomena; examples include family function, the environment-family interchange, interactions and dynamics within the family, changes in the family over time, and the family's reaction to health and illness. Box 3-1 summarizes the basic family social science theories and some major writers

---

BOX 3-1
Family Social Science Theories Used in Family Nursing Practice

Family Social Science Theory	Summary
STRUCTURAL FUNCTIONAL THEORY	
▪ Artinian (1994) ▪ Friedman, Bowden, & Jones (2003) ▪ Nye & Berado (1981)	The focus is on families as an institution and how they function to maintain family and social network.
SYMBOLIC INTERACTION THEORY	
▪ Hill and Hansen (1960) ▪ Rose (1962) ▪ Turner (1970) ▪ Nye (1976)	The focus is on the interactions within families and the symbolic communication.

Family Social Science Theories Used in Family Nursing Practice—cont'd

Family Social Science Theory	Summary
DEVELOPMENTAL THEORY AND FAMILY LIFE CYCLE THEORY	
▪ Duvall (1977) ▪ Duvall & Miller (1985) ▪ Carter & McGoldrick (2005)	The focus is on the life cycle of families and representing normative stages of family development.
FAMILY SYSTEMS THEORY	
▪ von Bertalanffy (1950, 1968)	The focus is on the circular interactions among members of family systems, which result in functional or dysfunctional outcomes.
FAMILY STRESS THEORY	
▪ Hill (1949, 1965) ▪ McCubbin & Paterson (1983) ▪ McCubbin & McCubbin (1993)	The focus is on the analysis of how families experience and cope with stressful life events.
CHANGE THEORY	
▪ Maturana (1978) ▪ Maturana & Varela (1992) ▪ Watzlawick, Weakland, & Fisch (1974) ▪ Wright & Watson (1988) ▪ Wright & Leahey (2005)	The focus is on how families remain stable or change when there is change within the family structure or from outside influences.
TRANSITION THEORY	
▪ White & Klein (2002) ▪ White (2005)	The focus on understanding and predicting the transitions families experience over time by combining Role Theory, Family Development Theory, and Life Course Theory.

who discuss these theories. It is somewhat challenging to use the purist form of family social science theories as a basis for nursing assessment and intervention because of their abstract nature. Despite this, in recent years, nursing scholars have made strides in extrapolating and morphing these theories for use in family nursing practice (Hanson & Kaakinen, 2005).

As discussed in Chapter 1, family structure is the ordered set of relationships among family members. Family function has to do with the purposes that the family serves in relation to the individual, the family, other social systems, and society, and between the family and other social systems. Family process represents the ongoing interactions between family members through which they accomplish their instrumental and expressive tasks.

Family therapy theories are newer than and not as well developed as family social science theories. Box 3-2 lists these theories and some of the people who expound them. These theories emanate from a practice discipline of family therapy, rather than an academic discipline of family social science. Family therapy theories were developed to work with troubled families and, therefore, focus primarily on family pathology. Nevertheless, these conceptual models describe family dynamics and patterns that are found, to some extent, in all families. Because these models are concerned with what can be done to facilitate change in "dysfunctional" families, they are both descriptive and prescriptive. That is, they not only describe and explain observations made in practice but suggest treatment or intervention strategies.

BOX 3-2
Family Therapy Theories Used in Family Nursing Practice

Family Therapy Theories	Summary
STRUCTURAL FAMILY THERAPY THEORY	
■ Minuchin (1974) ■ Minuchin, Rosman, & Baker (1978) ■ Minuchin & Fishman (1981) ■ Nichols (2004)	This systems-oriented approach views the family as an open sociocultural system that is continually faced with demands for change, both from within and from outside the family. The focus is on the whole family system, its subsystems, boundaries, and coalitions, as well as family transactional patterns and covert rules.
INTERNATIONAL FAMILY THERAPY THEORY	
■ Jackson (1965) ■ Watzlawick, Beavin, & Jackson (1967) ■ Satir (1982)	This approach views the family as a system of interactive or interlocking behaviors or communication processing. Emphasis is on the here and now rather than on the past. Key interventions focus on establishing clear, congruent communication, and clarifying and changing family rules.
FAMILY SYSTEMS THERAPY THEORY	
■ Toman (1961) ■ Kerr & Bowen (1988) ■ Freeman (1992)	This approach focuses on promoting differentiation of self from family and promoting differentiation of intellect from emotion. Family members are encouraged to examine their processes to gain insight and understanding into their past and present. This therapy requires a long-term commitment.

Finally, of the three types of theories, **nursing conceptual frameworks** are the least developed "theories" in relation to the nursing of families. Box 3-3 lists only a few of the theories and theorists from within the nursing profession. During the 1960s and 1970s, nurses placed great emphasis on the development of nursing models. Other than the Neuman Systems Model (Neuman, 2001) and the Behavioral Systems Model for Nursing (Johnson, 1980), both of which were based on family social science theories, the majority of the classic nursing theorists from the 1970s were originally focused on individual patients and on families as a unit. The nursing models, in large part, represent a deductive approach to the development of nursing science (general to specific). Although they embody an important part of our nursing heritage, these nursing conceptual frameworks and their deductive approach are viewed more critically today. More inductive approaches to nursing theory development (specific to the general) are now being advocated. Collectively, today more focus is on making qualitative and quantitative empirical observations to develop concepts and propositions to formulate new theory. In addition, nursing intervention studies need to be conducted to test and provide evidence that these approaches to working with families are best practice and evidence based. It is imperative that family nurses build a body of knowledge that stems from theory, is founded on best practice, and is evidence based.

Table 3-1 shows the differences between family social science theories, family therapy theories, and nursing models/theories as they inform the practice of nursing with families. The following case study is used to demonstrate five different theoretical approaches that may inform a nurse's work with one particular family.

BOX 3-3

Nursing Theories and Models Used in Family Nursing Practice

Nursing Theories and Models	Summary
NIGHTINGALE (1859)	
	Family is described as having both positive and negative influences on the outcome of family members. The family is seen as a supportive institution throughout the life span for its individual family members.
KING'S GOAL ATTAINMENT THEORY	
■ King (1981, 1983, 1987)	The family is seen as the vehicle for transmitting values and norms of behavior across the life span, which includes the role of a sick family member and transmitting health care function of the family. Family is seen as both an interpersonal and a social system. The key component is the interaction between the nurse and the family as client.
ROY'S ADAPTATION MODEL	
■ Roy (1976) ■ Roy & Roberts (1981)	The family is seen as an adaptive system that has inputs, internal control, and feedback processes and output. The strength of this model is understanding how families adapt to health issues.
NEUMAN'S SYSTEMS MODEL	
■ Neuman (1983, 1995)	The family is viewed as a system. The family's primary goal is to maintain its stability by preserving the integrity of its structure by opening and closing its boundaries. It is a fluid model that depicts the family in motion and not a static view of family from one perspective.
OREM'S SELF-CARE DEFICIT THEORY	
■ Orem (1983a, 1983b, 1985) ■ Gray (1996)	The family is seen as the basic conditioning unit in which the individual learns culture, roles, and responsibilities. Specifically, family members learn how to act when one is ill. The family's self-care behavior evolves through interpersonal relationships, communication, and culture that is unique to each family.
RODGER'S THEORY OF UNITARY HUMAN BEINGS	
■ Rodgers (1970, 1986, 1990) ■ Casey (1996)	The family is viewed as a constant open system energy field that is ever changing in its interactions with the environment.
FRIEDEMANN'S FRAMEWORK OF SYSTEMIC ORGANIZATION	
■ Friedemann (1995)	The family is described as a social system that has the expressed goal of transmitting culture to its members. The elements central to this theory are family stability, family growth, family control, and family spirituality.

Continued

BOX 3-3

Nursing Theories and Models Used in Family Nursing Practice—cont'd

Nursing Theories and Models	Summary
JOHNSON'S BEHAVIORAL SYSTEMS MODEL FOR NURSING	
▪ Johnson (1980)	The family is viewed as a behavioral system composed of a set of organized interactive interdependent and integrated subsystems that adjust and adapt with internal and external forces to maintain stability.
PARSE'S HUMAN BECOMING THEORY	
▪ Parse (1992, 1998)	The concept of family and who makes up the family is viewed as continually becoming and evolving. The role of the nurse is to use therapeutic communication to invite family members to uncover their meaning of the experience, to learn what the meaning of the experience is for each other, and to discuss the meaning of the experience for the family as a whole.
DENHAM'S FAMILY HEALTH MODEL	
▪ Denham (2003)	Family health is viewed as a process over time of family member interactions and health-related behaviors. Family health is described in relation to contextual, functional, and structural domains. Dynamic family health routines are behavioral patterns that reflect self-care, safety and prevention, mental health behaviors, family care, illness care, and family caregiving.

TABLE 3-1

Family Social Science Theory, Family Therapy Theories, and Nursing Models/Theories

CRITERIA	FAMILY SOCIAL SCIENCE THEORIES	FAMILY THERAPY THEORIES	NURSING THEORIES
Purpose of theory	Descriptive and explanatory (academic models); to explain family functioning and dynamics	Descriptive and prescriptive (practice models); to explain family dysfunction and guide therapeutic actions	Descriptive and prescriptive (practice models); to guide nursing assessment and intervention efforts
Discipline focus	Interdisciplinary (although primarily sociologic)	Marriage and family therapy; family mental health; new approaches focus on family strengths	Nursing focus
Target population	Primarily "normal" families (normality-oriented)	Primarily "troubled" families (pathology-oriented)	Primarily families with health and illness problems

Source: Adapted from Jones, S. L., & Dimond, S. L. (1982). Family theory and family therapy models: Comparative review with implications for nursing practice. *Journal of Psychiatric Nursing and Mental Health Services, 20*(10), 12–19.

Family Case Study

SETTING: Inpatient acute-care hospital

NURSING GOAL: Work with the family to assist them in preparation for discharge that is planned to occur in the next 2 days

FAMILY MEMBERS:
The Jones family is a nuclear family. The Jones family genogram is shown is Figure 3-3 and the Jones family ecomap is drawn in Figure 3-4.

+ Robert: 48 years old; father, software engineer, full-time employed
+ Linda: 43 years old; mother, stay-at-home home-maker, has progressive multiple sclerosis, which recently has worsened significantly
+ Amy: 19 years old; oldest child, daughter, fresh-man at university in town 180 miles away
+ Katie: 13 years old: middle child, daughter, sixth grade, usually a good student
+ Travis: 4 years old: youngest child, son, just started attending an all-day preschool because of his mother's illness

JONES FAMILY STORY

Linda was diagnosed with multiple sclerosis (MS) at age 30 when Katie was 3 months old. Pregnacy often masks the symptoms of multiple sclerosis (MS); therefore a pregnant woman who develops MS during pregnancy will show symptoms after the birth of the child. After she was diagnosed with MS Linda had a well controlled slow progression of her illness. Travis was a surprise pregnancy for Linda at age 39, but he is described as "a blessing." Linda and Robert are devout Baptists, but they did discuss abortion given that Linda's illness might progress significantly after the birth of Travis. Their faith and personal beliefs did not support abortion. They made the decision to continue with Linda's pregnancy knowing the risks, that it might exacerbate and speed up her MS. Linda had an un-complicated pregnancy with Travis. She felt well until 3 months postpartum with Travis when she noted a significant relapse of her MS.

Over the last 4 years, Linda has experienced develop-ment of progressive relapsing MS, which is a progressive disease from onset with clear acute relapses without full recovery after each relapse. The periods between her re-lapses are characterized by continuing progression of the disease. Because of her increased weakness, Robert and Linda are having sexual issues with decreased libido and painful intercourse for Linda. Both are experiencing stress in their marital roles and relationship.

Currently, Linda has had a serious relapse of her MS. She is hospitalized for secondary pneumonia from aspiration. She has weakness in all limbs, left foot drag, and increasing ataxia. Linda will be discharged with a

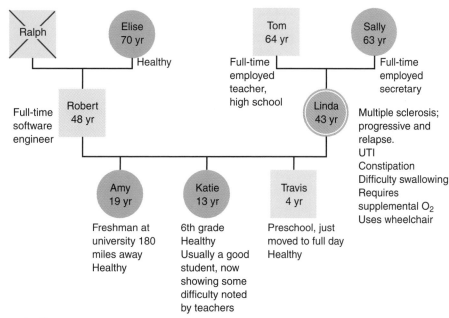

FIGURE 3-3 Jones family geogram.

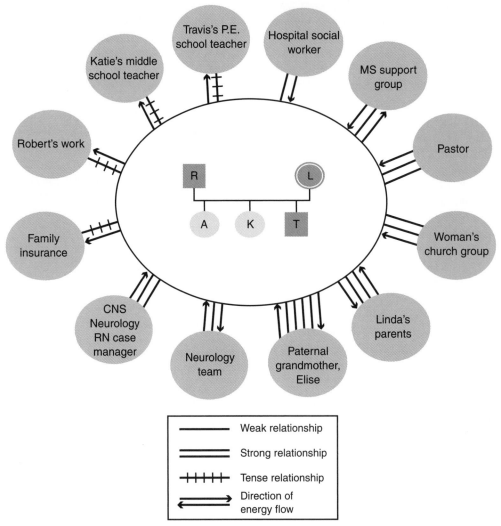

FIGURE 3-4 Jones family ecomap.

wheelchair (this is new as she has used a cane up until this admission). She has weakness of her neck muscle and cannot hold her head up steady for long periods. She has difficulty swallowing, which probably was the cause of her aspiration. She has numbness and tingling of her legs and feet. She has severe pain with flexion of her neck. Her vision is blurred. She experiences vertigo at times and has periodic tinnitus. Constipation is a constant problem together with urinary retention that causes periodic urinary tract infections.

HEALTH INSURANCE

Robert receives health insurance through his work that covers the whole family. Hospitalizations are covered 80/20, so they have to pay 20% of their bills out of pocket. Although Robert is employed full time, this adds heavily to the financial burden of the family. Robert has shared with the nurses that he does not know whether he should take his last week of vacation when his wife comes home, or whether he should save it for a time when her condition worsens. Robert works for a company that offers family leave, but he would have to take family leave without pay.

FAMILY MEMBERS

Robert reports being continuously tired with caring for his wife and children, as well as working full time. He asked the doctor for medication to help him sleep and decrease his anxiety. He said he is afraid that he may not hear Linda in the night when she needs help.

He is open to his mother moving in to help care for Linda and the children. He began counseling sessions with the pastor in their church.

Amy is a freshman at a university that is 180 miles away in a different town. Her mother is proud of Amy going to college on a full scholarship. Amy does well in her coursework but travels home weekends to help the family and her mother. Amy is considering giving up her scholarship to transfer home to attend the local community college. She has not told her parents about this idea yet.

Katie is in the sixth grade. She is typically a good student, but her latest report card showed that she dropped a letter grade in most of her classes. Katie is quiet. She stopped having friends over to her home about 6 months ago when her mother began to have more ataxia and slurring of speech. Linda used to be very involved in Katie's school but is no longer

involved because of her illness. Katie has been involved in Girl Scouts and the youth group at church.

Travis just started going to preschool 2 months ago for half days because of his mother's illness. This transition to preschool has been difficult for Travis because he has been home full time with Linda until her disease got worse. He is healthy and developmentally on target for his age.

Linda's parents live in the same town. Her parents, Tom and Sally, both work full time and are not able to help. Robert's widowed mother, Elise, lives by herself in her own home about 30 minutes out of town and has offered to move into the Jones home to help with the care of Linda and the family.

DISCHARGE PLANS: Linda will be discharged home in 2 days.

THEORETICAL PERSPECTIVES AND APPLICATION TO FAMILIES

This case of the Jones family is used throughout the rest of this chapter to demonstrate how different assessments, interventions, and options for care vary based on the particular theoretical perspective chosen by nurses caring for this family.

Family Systems Theory

Family Systems Theory has been the most influential of all the family social science frameworks (Hanson & Kaakinen, 2005; Wright & Leahey, 2005). Much of the understanding of how a family is a system derives from physics and biology perspectives that organisms are complex, organized, and interactive systems (von Bertalanffy, 1950, 1968; Bowen, 1978). Nursing theorists who have expanded the concept of systems theory include Johnson (1980), Neuman (1995, 2001), Neuman and Fawcett (2001), Hanson (2001), Walker (2005), Parker (2005), and Wilkerson and Loveland-Cherry (2005).

The Family Systems Theory is an approach that allows nurses to understand and assess families as an organized whole and/or as individuals within family units who form an interactive and interdependent system (Hanson & Kaakinen, 2005). Family Systems Theory is constructed of concepts and propositions that provide a framework for thinking about the family as a system. Typically, in family nursing, we look at a three-generation family system (Goldenberg & Goldenberg, 2007).

One of the major assumptions of Family Systems Theory is that family systems features are designed to maintain stability, although these features may be adaptive or maladaptive. At the same time, families change constantly in response to stresses and strains from both the internal and external environments. Family systems increase in complexity over time, and as a system, families increase their ability to adapt and to change (White & Klein, 2008). The family system theoretical perspective encourages nurses to see individual clients as participating members of a larger family system. Figure 3-5 depicts a mobile showing how family systems work. Any change in one member of the family affects all members of the family. As it applies to the Jones family, the nurses who are using this perspective would assess the impact of Linda's illness on the entire family, as well as the effects of family functioning on Linda. The goal of nurses is to help maintain or restore the stability of the family, to help them achieve the highest level of functioning that they can give. Therefore, emphasis should be on the whole, rather than on any given individual. Some of

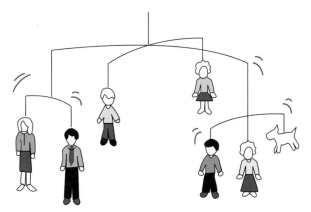

FIGURE 3-5 Mobile depicting family system.

the concepts of systems theory that helps nurses working with families are explained in the following sections.

CONCEPT 1: ALL PARTS OF THE SYSTEM ARE INTERCONNECTED.

What influences one part of the system influences all the parts of the system. When an individual in a family experiences a health event, all members are affected because they are connected. The effect on each family member varies in intensity and quality. In the Jones case study, all members of the Jones family were touched when the mother's health condition changed, requiring her to be hospitalized. Linda takes on the role of a sick person and must give up some of her typical at-home mother roles; she is physically ill in the hospital. She feels guilty about not being at home for her family. Robert was affected because he had to assume the care of Katie and Travis. This required getting them ready for school, transporting them to school and other events, and making lunches. Katie gave up some after-school activities to help Travis when he gets home from preschool. Travis misses the food his mother prepared for him, his afternoon alone time with his mother when they read a story, and being tucked into bed at night with songs and a back rub. Amy, who is a freshman in college, finds it difficult to concentrate while reading and studying for her college classes. The formal and informal roles of all these family members are affected by Linda's hospitalization. What affects Linda affects all the members of the Jones family in multiple ways.

CONCEPT 2: THE WHOLE IS MORE THAN THE SUM OF ITS PARTS.

The family is a whole is composed of more than the individual lives of family members. It goes beyond parents and children as separated entities. Families are not just relationships between the parent-child, but are all relationships seen together. As we look at the Jones family, it is a nuclear family—mother, father, and three children. They are a family system that is experiencing the stress of a chronically ill mother who is deteriorating over time; each of them is individually affected, but so is the family as a whole affected by this unexpected (non-normative) family health event. The individuals in this family may, at times, wonder what will happen to them as a family (whole) when Linda dies.

One way of visualizing the family as a whole is to think of how each family member acts during a family ritual or routine. For example, Linda always decorates the house and bakes several special dishes for the major holidays. This year, however, Linda has been too ill to decorate for Easter. Family traditions contribute to how the Jones family sees itself as a family unit. When Linda is so ill she cannot do the special Jones family decorating or baking, the family as a whole feels stressed by the loss of routine and ritual.

CONCEPT 3: ALL SYSTEMS HAVE SOME FORM OF BOUNDARIES OR BORDERS BETWEEN THE SYSTEM AND ITS ENVIRONMENT.

Families control the in-flow of information and people coming into its family system to protect individual family members or the family as a whole. Boundaries are conceptualized as a continuum ranging from closed to open or any variation in-between. Boundaries are physical or abstract imaginary lines that families use as barriers or filters to control the impact on the family system (White & Klein, 2008). Family boundaries include levels of permeability in that they can be closed, flexible, or too open to information, people, or other forms of resources. Some families have *closed boundaries* that can be exemplified by a family myth such as, "We as a family pull together and don't need help from others," or "We take care of our own." For example, if the Jones family was to have a *closed boundary,* they would not want to meet with the social worker, or if they did, they would reject the idea of a home-health aide and respite care. Some families have *flexible boundaries,* which they control and selectively open or close to gain balance or adapt to the situation. For example, the Jones family welcomes a visit from their pastor but turn down visits from some of the women in Linda's Bible study group. Some families have *too open boundaries* in which they are not discriminating about who knows their family situation or the number of people from whom they seek help. One of the concerns of people with open boundaries is that they could invite chaos if they are not selective in the quantity or quality of resources, thus contributing to a steady state of chaos and unbalance. If the Jones family were to have truly *open boundaries,* they may reach out to the larger community for resources and have different church members come stay with the children every evening. Boundaries are on a continuum and vary from family to family.

CONCEPT 4: SYSTEMS CAN BE FURTHER ORGANIZED INTO SUBSYSTEMS.
Rather than conceptualizing the family as a whole, nurses can think about the subsystems of the family, which may include parent to child, mother to child, father to child, child to child, grandparents to parents, grandparents to grandchildren, and so forth. These subsystems take into account three dimensions of families: structure, function (including roles), and processes (interconnection and dynamics). By understanding these three dimensions, family nurses can streamline interventions to achieve specific family outcomes. For example, the Jones family has the following subsystems: parents, siblings, parent-child, a daughter subsystem, in-law subsystem, and grandparent subsystem. The nurse may work to decrease family stress by focusing on the marital spouse subsystem to help Linda and Robert continue couple time, or the nurse may focus on the sibling subsystem of Katie and Travis and their after-school activities.

APPLICATION OF FAMILY SYSTEMS THEORY WITH THE JONES FAMILY

The focus of the nurses' practice from this perspective is family as the client. Nurses work to help families maintain and regain stability. Assessment questions of family members are focused on the family as a whole. Using the Jones family case study, a nurse would ask the following questions to explore with Linda or with Linda and Robert while they are planning discharge scheduled in the next couple of days:

- Who are members of your family? (see Concept 1)
- How do you see your family being involved in your care once you go home? (see Concept 1)
- Who in your family will experience the most difficulty coping with the changes, especially that you will be using a wheelchair? (see Concept 1)
- How are the members of your family meeting their personal needs at this time? (see Concept 1)
- The last time your condition worsened, what helped your family the most? (see Concept 2)
- The last time your condition worsened, what was the least help to your family? (see Concept 2)
- Who outside of your immediate family do you see as being a potential person to help your family during the next week when you go home? (see Concept 3)
- How do you feel your family would react to having a home-health aide come to help you twice a week? (see Concept 3)
- Are there some friends, church members, or neighbors who might be able to help with some of the everyday management issues, such as carpooling to school, providing some after-school care for Travis so Katie could go to her after-school activities? (see Concepts 3 and 4)
- What are your thoughts about how the children will react to having Grandma Elise here to help the family? (see Concept 4)

Interventions by family nurses must address individuals, subsystems within the family, and the whole family all at the same time. One strategy would be to assess the family process and functioning, and offer intervention strategies to assist families in their everyday functioning. Nurses could ask families the following types of questions about their functioning, which would help provide stability with the changes:

- Linda and Robert, from what you have told me, it appears that your oldest daughter, Amy, has been able to help take on some of the parental jobs in the family by being the errand runner, chauffeur, and grocery shopper. Now that Amy is off to college, which of your family roles will need to be covered by someone else for a while when you and Linda first come home: cooking, laundry, chauffeur, cleaning the house?

- Because you both shared with me that your family likes to go bowling on family night out, how do you envision how Linda being in a wheelchair might affect family night out?
- Robert and Linda, have the two of you discussed legal Durable Power of Attorney if you are unable to act on behalf of yourself?
- Linda, who would you prefer to make health care decisions for you, should you not be able to do so? Let us discuss what those health care decisions might involve.
- Tell me about your personal/sexual relationship that you, Linda, are experiencing now that you are more disabled.

The goal of using a family systems perspective is to help the family reach stability by building on their strengths as a family, using knowledge of the family as a social system, and understanding how the family is an interconnected whole that is adapting to the changes brought about by the health event of a given family member.

STRENGTHS AND WEAKNESSES

The strengths of the general systems framework is that this theory covers a large array of phenomena, and views the family and its subsystems within the context of its suprasystems (the larger community in which it is embedded). Moreover, this is an interactional and holistic theory that looks at processes within the family, rather than at the content and relationships between the members. The family is viewed as a whole, not as merely a sum of its parts. Another strength of this approach is that it is an excellent data-gathering method and assessment strategy.

Unfortunately, the strengths of the theory are also its limitations. Because this theoretical orientation is broad and general, it may not be specific enough for beginners, to define family nursing interventions. It is important for family nurses to be able to understand conceptually how important the family as a whole is to the practice of family nursing.

Developmental and Family Life Cycle Theory

Developmental Theory provides a framework for nurses to understand normal family changes and experiences over the members' lifetimes; the theory assesses and evaluates both individuals and families as a whole. Developmental stages for individuals have been elaborated by psychologists and sociologists, such as Erikson, Piaget, and Bandura. Family developmental theory is similar to individual developmental theories because the concept of normative development is systematic, and patterned changes can be applied to the family as a group. The family developmental theories are specifically geared to understanding families and not individuals (White & Klein, 2008, p. 122). Early in the intellectual exploration of family science it was believed that families, like individuals, are in constant movement and changing throughout time—the **Family Life Cycle** (White & Klein, 2008, p. 125). Family developmental theorists that inform the nursing of families include Duvall (1977), Duvall and Miller (1985), and Carter and McGoldrick (2005).

The original work of Duvall (1977), and later Duvall and Miller (1985), examined how families were affected or changed when all members experienced developmental changes cognitively, socially, emotionally, spiritually, and physically. The relationships among family members are affected by changes in individuals, and changes in the family as a whole affect the individuals within the family. These theorists recognized that families are stressed at common and predictable stages of change and transition, and need to undergo adjustment to regain family stability. This early theoretical work was primarily based on the experiences of White Anglo middle-class nuclear families, with a married couple, children, and extended family (Carter & McGoldrick, 2005, p. xiii).

Carter and McGoldrick (2005) expanded on the original Developmental and Family Life Cycle Theory because they recognized the dramatically changing landscape of family structure, functions, and processes, making it increasingly difficult to determine normal predictable patterns of change in families. They replace the concept of "nuclear family" with "immediate family," which takes into consideration all family structures, such as stepfamilies, gay families, and divorced families. Instead of addressing the legal aspects of being a married couple, they viewed the concept of couple relationships and commitment as a focal point for family bonds. Families are seen as a system in that what happens at one level has powerful ramifications at other levels of the system. Families are seen as the basic social unit of society and as the optimal level of intervention.

CONCEPT 1: FAMILIES DEVELOP AND CHANGE OVER TIME

According to Family Developmental Theory, family interactions among family members change over time in relation to structure, function (roles), and processes. The stresses created by these changes in family systems are somewhat predictable for different stages of family development.

The first way to view family development is to look at predictable stresses and changes as they relate to the age of the family members and the social norms the individuals experience throughout their development. The classic traditional work of Duvall (1977) and Duvall and Miller (1985) identify overall family tasks that need to be accomplished for each stage of family development that is related to the developmental trajectory of the individual family members. It starts with couples getting married and ends with one member of the couple dying. Refer to Table 3-2 for the complete list of the traditional family life cycle stages and developmental tasks. Carter and McGoldrick (2005) expanded the traditional developmental and family life cycle theory to address changes in the family that undergoes a divorce. Table 3-3 outlines the emotional process of a family undergoing a divorce and describes the developmental tasks the family deals with at different stages.

According to this theory, families have a predictable natural history. The first stage involves the simple husband-wife pairing, and the family group

TABLE 3-2	
Traditional Family Life Cycle Stages and Developmental Tasks	
STAGES OF FAMILY LIFE CYCLE	**FAMILY DEVELOPMENTAL TASKS**
Married couple	Establishing relationship as a married couple
	Blending of individual needs, developing conflict-and-resolution approaches, communication patterns, and intimacy patterns
Childbearing families with infants	Adjusting to pregnancy and then infant
	Adjusting to new roles, mother and father
	Maintaining couple bond and intimacy
Families with preschool children	Understanding normal growth and development
	If more than one child in family, adjusting to different temperaments and styles of children
	Coping with energy depletion
	Maintaining couple bond and intimacy
Families with school-age children	Working out authority and socialization roles with school
	Supporting child in outside interests and needs
	Determining disciplinary actions and family rules and roles
Families with adolescents	Allowing adolescents to establish their own identities but still be part of family
	Thinking about the future, education, jobs, working
	Increasing roles of adolescents in family, cooking, repairs, and power base
Families with young adults: launching	After member moves out, reallocating roles, space, power, and communication
	Maintaining supportive home base
	Maintaining parental couple intimacy and relationship
Middle-aged parents	Refocusing on marriage relationship
	Ensuring security after retirement
	Maintaining kinship ties
Aging families	Adjusting to retirement, grandparent roles, death of spouse, and living alone

TABLE 3-3
Family Life Cycle for Divorcing Families

PHASE	EMOTIONAL PROCESS OF TRANSITION: PREREQUISITE ATTITUDE	DEVELOPMENTAL ISSUES
Divorce		
The decision to divorce	Acceptance of inability to resolve marital tensions sufficiently to continue relationship	Acceptance of one's own part in the failure of the marriage
Planning the breakup of the system	Supporting viable arrangements for all parts of the system	a. Working cooperatively on problems of custody, visitation, and finances
		b. Dealing with extended family about the divorce
Separation	a. Willingness to continue cooperative co-parental relationship and joint financial support of children	a. Mourning loss of intact family
		b. Restructuring marital and parent-child relationships and finances; adaptation to living apart
	b. Work on resolution of attachment to spouse	c. Realignment of relationships with extended family; staying connected with spouse's extended family
The divorce	More work on emotional divorce: overcoming hurt, anger, guilt, among other emotions	a. Mourning loss of intact family
		b. Retrieval of hopes, dreams, expectations from the marriage
		c. Staying connected with extended families
Postdivorce Family		
Single parent (custodial household or primary residence)	Willingness to maintain financial responsibilities, continue parental contact with ex-spouse, and support contact of children with ex-spouse and his or her family	a. Making flexible visitation arrangements with ex-spouse and family
		b. Rebuilding own financial resources
		c. Rebuilding own social network
Single parent (noncustodial)	Willingness to maintain financial responsibilities and parental contact with ex-spouse, and to support custodial parent's relationship with children	a. Finding ways to continue effective parenting
		b. Maintaining financial responsibilities to ex-spouse and children
		c. Rebuilding own social network

Carter, B., & McGoldrick, M. (2005). The divorce cycle: A major variation in the American Family Life Cycle. In B. Carter & M. McGoldrick (Eds.). *The expanded family life cycle: Individual, family, and social perspectives* (3rd ed., pp. 373–380). New York: Allyn & Bacon.

becomes more complex over time with the addition of new members. When the younger generation leaves home to take jobs or marry, the original family group becomes less complex again. The original group ends with the death of one member of the couple. According to this theoretical approach, the Jones family would be considered *Families with Young Adults: Launching Phase,* because daughter Amy just left the family of origin for college.

The second way to view family development is to assess the predictable stresses and changes in families based on the stage of family development and how long the family is in that stage. For example, suppose each of the following couples have made a choice to be childless: a newly married couple, a couple who has been married for 3 years, and a couple who has been married for 15 years (White & Klein, 2008). The stresses each couple experiences from this decision are different.

A third way to view family development would be how a chronic illness in a given family member affects family stages over time. Rolland (1984, 1987,

2005) developed the Family Systems-Illness Model as a framework to understand the impact that chronic illnesses have on family development and function. Rolland outlined three types of chronic illness: progressive, constant, and relapsing/episodic.

PROGRESSIVE. When individual family members have a progressive chronic illness, the disability occurs in a stepwise fashion that requires families to make gradual changes in their roles to continually adapt to the losses. Families usually experience exhaustion, because they have few periods of relief from the demands of the illness. As the disease progresses, new family roles develop, and family caregiving tasks evolve over time.

CONSTANT. Chronic illness is considered constant when, after the initial chaos and stress caused by the acute illness, it evolves into a semipermanent change in condition that is stable and predictable over a time. The potential for family stress and exhaustion are present, but to a lesser degree than a progressive chronic illness.

RELAPSING/EPISODIC. With a relapsing/episodic chronic illness, families alternate between stable low symptomology periods with periods of exacerbation and flare-up. Families are strained by both the frequency of the transition between stable and unstable crisis modes of functioning, and the ongoing uncertainty of when the remission and exacerbation will occur.

To assess the Jones family relative to development and change over time, the nurse would take into consideration the formidable impact Linda's chronic illness had, moving from a relapsing/episodic chronic stage to a chronic progressive illness. The family is constantly adjusting and adapting to the course of Linda's illness and increasing incapacitation. The family is exhausted with the uncertainty of the future.

Two propositions are relevant to this concept that all families develop systematically and change over time:

Proposition 1: The family does not chronologically advance through the predictable normative stages of family development. Overlaps of the stages complicate and increase conflict within the family and for the family. The stages can be interrupted, for example, by the premature death of a spouse or the death of a child, a divorce, and a remarriage.

Proposition 2: Family development is regulated by societal timing and sequencing norms. Culture affects the concept of sequencing. For example, in Peru, a couple has a child and lives together traditionally for many years before they marry; cohabitation is the early family norm. The timing of becoming a young adult in an African culture may be much younger than the North American norm of the young adult. Cultures differ based on the importance of certain rights of passage or rituals. Cultures differ in the meaning of "family" (Hines, Preto, McGoldrick, Almeida, & Weltman, 2005).

CONCEPT 2: FAMILIES EXPERIENCE TRANSITIONS FROM ONE STAGE TO ANOTHER

Disequilibrium occurs in the family during the transitional periods from one stage of development to the next stage. When transitions occur, families experience changes in kinship structures, family roles, social roles, and interaction. Family stress is considered to be greatest at the transition points as families adapt to achieve stability, redefine their concept of family in light of the changes, and realign relationships as a result of the changes (Carter & McGoldrick, 2005). For example, marriage changes the status of all family members, creates new relationships for family members, and joins two different complex family systems (McGoldrick, 2005).

Family developmental theorists explore whether families make these transitions "on time" or "off time" according to cultural and social expectations (White & Klein, 2008, p. 131). For example, it is off time for a couple in their 40s to have their first child. It is still considered "on time" in North America to have a couple married before the birth of a child, but that norm may be changing according to the increased birth of babies to couples who are not married but cohabitate.

Even though some family developmental needs and tasks must be performed at each stage of the family life cycle, developmental tasks are general goals, rather than specific jobs that must be completed at that time. Achievement of family developmental tasks enables individuals within families to realize their own individual tasks. According to family developmental theory, every family is unique in its composition and in the complexity of its expectations of members at different ages and in different roles. Families, like individuals, are influenced by their history and traditions, and by the social context in which they live. Furthermore, families change and develop in different ways because their internal/external demands and situations differ. Families may also arrive at similar developmental levels using different processes. Despite their differences, however, families have enough in common to make it possible to chart family development over the life span in a way that applies to most, if not all, families (Friedman, Bowden, & Jones, 2003). Families experience stress when they transition from one stage to the next. The predictable changes experienced by the family based on these developmental steps is called a *normative* change. When changes occur in families out of sequence, "off time," or are caused by a different family event, such as illness, it is called *non-normative*.

In contrast with the Duvall (1977) and later Duvall and Miller's (1985) traditional developmental approach, Carter and McGoldrick (1989, 2005) build on this work by approaching family development from the perspective of family life cycle stages (Carter & McGoldrick, 2005). They explore what happens within families when family members enter or exit their family group; they focus on specific family experiences, such as disruption in family relationships, roles, processes, and family structure. Examples of a family member leaving would be divorce, illness, a miscarriage, or death of a family member. Examples of family members entering would include birth, adoption, marriage, or other formal union.

Today, the developmental framework and family life cycle theory remains useful as long as it is viewed generally for use with families, despite all the current variations of families. Carter and McGoldrick (2005) expand the Family Life Cycle to incorporate the changing family patterns, and broaden the view of both development and the family.

APPLICATION OF DEVELOPMENTAL AND FAMILY LIFE CYCLE THEORY TO THE JONES FAMILY

In conducting family assessments using the developmental model, nurses begin by determining the family structure and where this family lies on the continuum of family life cycle stages. Using the developmental tasks outlined in the developmental model, the nurse has a ready guide to anticipate stresses the family may be experiencing or to assess the developmental tasks that are not being accomplished. Family assessment would also entail determining whether the family is experiencing a "normative" or "non-normative" event in the family life cycle.

According to Duvall and Miller (1985), the Jones family is in the *Families with Young Adults: Launching Phase* because Amy left home and is now a freshman at a college. She is living away from home for the first time. Regardless of the fact that the Jones family is experiencing a non-normative event (unexpected, developmental stressor) because Linda, the mother, is now in the hospital, the family is also experiencing the normative or expected challenges for a family when the oldest child leaves home. This is a good example of where major individual and whole family events coincide and present challenges for families. Questions to explore with the family might include:

1. How has the family addressed the reallocation of family household physical space since Amy left for school? (For example, the allocation of bedrooms or the arrangement of space within the bedroom if Katie and Amy shared the bedroom).
2. How has Amy developed as an indirect caregiver (such as calling home to chat with dad and see how he is doing, talking with the siblings and teasing or supporting their efforts, or sharing with parents her school life to reduce their worry about her adjustment)?
3. How have family roles changed since Amy left for school? What roles did Amy perform for the family that someone else needs to pick up now? For example, who will perform such roles as chauffeur, grocery shopper, errand runner, and baby-sitter since Linda is not able and Amy is gone?
4. How has the power structure of the family shifted now that Katie is more responsible for the care of Travis?
5. How has the parents' couple time changed since Amy went off to college?

With the developmental approach, nursing interventions may include helping the family to understand individual and family developmental tasks. Interventions could also include helping the family understand the normalcy of disequilibrium during these transitional periods. Another intervention is to help the family punctuate these transitions through capitalizing family rituals. Family rituals serve to decrease the anxiety of changes in that they help link the family to other family members and to the larger community (Imber-Black, 2005).

Family nurses must recognize that every family must accomplish both individual and family developmental tasks for every stage of the Developmental and Family Life Cycle. Events at one stage of the cycle have powerful effects at other stages. Helping families adjust and adapt to these transitions is an important role for family nurses. It is important for nurses to keep in mind the needs and requirements of both the family as a whole and the individuals who make up the family.

STRENGTHS AND WEAKNESSES

A major strength of the developmental approach is that it provides a systematic framework for predicting what a family may be experiencing at any stage in the family life cycle. Family nurses can assess a family's stage of development, the extent to which the family has achieved the tasks associated with that stage of family development, and problems that may or may not exist. It is a superb theoretical approach for assisting nurses who are working with families on health promotion. Family strengths and available resources are easier to identify because they are based on assisting families to achieve developmental milestones.

A major weakness of the developmental framework is that it originated when the "traditional nuclear family" was considered the norm. Today, families vary widely in their makeup and in their roles. The traditional view of families moving in a linear direction from getting married, tracking children from preschool to launching, middle-aged parents, and aging families is no longer so clearcut and applicable. Carter and McGoldrick (1989, 2005; Carter, 2005) expanded the family developmental model to include stresses in the remarried family. As family structures continue to change in response to the culture and ecologic system, trajectories of families likely will not fit within the traditional developmental framework (White & Klein, 2008).

Bioecological Systems Theory

Urie Bronfenbrenner was one of the world's leading scholars in the field of developmental psychology (Bronfenbrenner, 1972a, 1972b, 1979, 1981, 1986, 1997; Bronfenbrenner & Morris, 1998). He created the Ecological Systems Theory, which he renamed the **Bioecological Systems** Theory (Bronfenbrenner & Lerner, 2004). The Bioecological System is the combination of a children's biological disposition and environmental forces coming together to shape the development of human beings. This theory seems to combine both Developmental Theory and Systems Theory to understanding individual and family growth.

Before Bronfenbrenner, child psychologists studied children, sociologists examined families, anthropologists the society, economists the economic framework of the times, and political scientists the political structure. Through Bronfenbrenner's groundbreaking work in "human ecology," environments from the family to larger economic/political structures have come to be viewed as part of the life course from childhood through adulthood. This "bioecological" approach to human development crosses over barriers among the social sciences and builds bridges among the disciplines, allowing for better understanding to emerge about key elements in the larger social structure that are vital for optimal human development (both individual and family) (Boemmel & Briscoe, 2001; Wikipedia, 2008).

The human ecology framework brings together other diverse influences. From evolutionary theory and genetics comes the view that humans develop as individual biological organisms with capacities limited by genetic endowment (*ontogenetic development*) leading to hereditary familial characteristics. From population genetics comes the perspective that populations change by means of natural selection. For the individual, this means that individuals/families demonstrate their fitness by adapting to ever changing environments (adaptation). From ecologic theories come the notion that human and family development is "contextualized" and "interactional" (White & Klein, 2008, p. 247). All of this leads to the never-ending debate related to the dual nature of humans as constructions of both biology and culture, hence the argument *nature* versus *nurture*. Although this debate has never been resolved, scientists have moved beyond this debate to realize that the development of most human traits depends on a nature/nurture interaction rather than on one versus the other (White & Klein, 2008 p. 248). Thus, Bronfenbrenner moves his own theory and ideas from the concept and terminology of ecology (environment) to bioecology (both genetics and society) to embrace two developmental origins for this theory. His Bioecological Systems Theory emphasizes the interaction of both the biological/genetics (ontologic/nature) and the social context (society)

characteristics of development (White & Klein, 2008, p. 260).

The human bioecological perspective consists of a framework of four locational/spatial contexts and one time-related context (Bengtson, Acock, Allen, Dilworth-Anderson, & Klein, 2005). A primary feature of this theory is the premise that individual and family development is contextual over time. According to Bronfenbrenner, individual development is

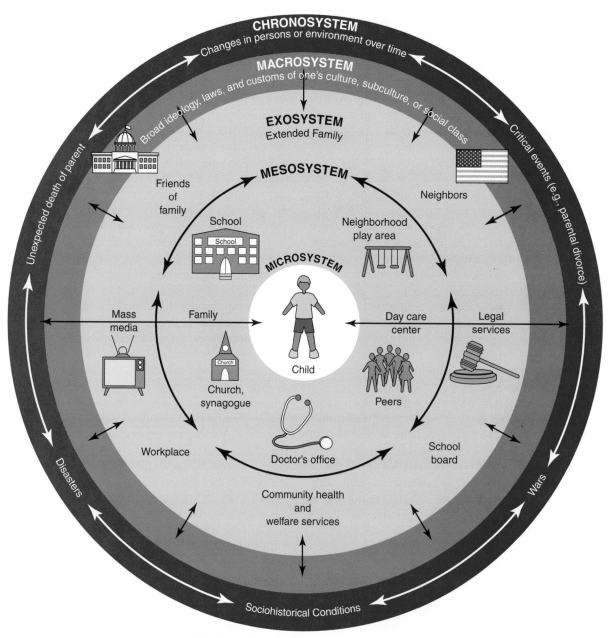

FIGURE 3-6 Bioecological systems theory model.

effected by five types or levels of environmental systems (Fig. 3-6) (Emory University, 2008). Family Bioecological Theory describes the interactions and influences on the family from systems at different levels of engagement.

Microsystems are the settings in which individuals/families experience and create day-to-day reality. They are the places people inhabit, the people with whom they live, and the things they do together. In this level, people fulfill their roles in families, with peers, in schools, and in neighborhoods where they are in the most direct interaction with agents around them.

Mesosystems are the relationships among major microsystems in which persons or families actively participate, such as families and schools, families and religion, and families to peers. For example, how does the interaction between families and school affect families? Can the relationship between families and their religious/spiritual communities be used to help families?

Exosystems are external environments that influence individuals and families indirectly. The person may not be an active participant within these systems, but the system has an effect on the persons/families. For example, a parent's job experience affects family life, which, in turn, affects the children (parent's job's travel requirements, job stress, salary). Furthermore, governmental funding to other microsystems environments—schools, libraries, parks, health care, and daycare—affect the experiences of children and families.

Macrosystems are the broad cultural attitudes, ideologies, or belief systems that influence institutional environments within a particular culture/subculture in which individuals/families live. Examples include the Judeo-Christian ethic, democracy, ethnicity, or societal values. Mesosystems and exosystems are set within macrosystems, and together they are the "blueprints" for the ecology of human and family development.

Chronosystems refers to time-related contexts where changes occur over time and have an effect on the other four levels/systems of development mentioned earlier. This includes the patterning of environmental events and transitions over the life course of individuals/families. These effects are created by time or critical periods in development and are influenced by sociohistorical conditions, such as parental divorce, unexpected death of a parent, or a

war. It is the evolution of external systems over time over which individuals/families have no control.

Within each one of these nested levels are roles, norms, and rules that shape the environment. Bronfenbrenner's model of human/family development acknowledges that people do not develop in isolation, but rather in relation to their larger environment: families, home, schools, communities, and society. Each of these interactive, ever changing, and multilevel environments over time are key to understanding human/family development.

Bronfenbrenner uses the term *bidirectional* to describe the influential interactions that take place between children and their relationships with parents, teachers, and society. All relationships among humans/families and their environment are bidirectional or interactional. The environment influences us as individuals or families, but in turn, individuals/families influence what happens in their own environments. This kind of interaction is also basic to family systems theory.

In the bioecological framework, what happens outside family units is as important as what happens inside individual members and family units. Developing families are on center stage as an active force shaping their social experiences for themselves. The ecologic perspective views children/families and their environments as mutually shaping systems, each changing and adapting over time (again, a systems perspective). The bioecological approach addresses both opportunities and risks. Opportunities mean that the environment offers families material, emotional, and social encouragement compatible with their needs and capacities. Risks to family development are composed of direct threats or the absence of opportunities.

APPLICATION OF THE BIOECOLOGICAL SYSTEMS THEORY WITH THE JONES FAMILY

Assessment consists of looking at all levels of the system when interviewing the family in a health care setting. Assessment of the *microsystem* shows that the Jones family consists of five members: two parents and three children. They live in a two-story home with four bedrooms in an older suburban section of the town. Mother Linda had been a full-time homemaker before experiencing health problems related to her diagnosis of MS. The *mesosystem* assessment for the family consists of identifying the schools the children attend, neighborhood/friends, extended family, and their religious affiliation. The oldest daughter is a college student who travels home on weekends to help the family. The second daughter is in a local middle school, and can walk back and forth to her school. The youngest child, a boy, attends an all-day preschool and is transported by his parents or other parents from the preschool. The family has attended a Protestant church in the neighborhood. The family lives in a house in an older established neighborhood, and they have made friends through the schools, church, and neighborhood contacts. Part of the extended family (grandparents) live nearby, and all of the family members get together for the holidays; neither parent has siblings who live nearby. The *exosystem* assessment shows that father Robert works 40 hours a week for an industrial plant at the edge of town, and he drives back and forth daily. He has some job stress, because the father is in a middle-management position. His salary is average for middle-class families in the United States. State and county funding to the area schools, libraries, and recreational facilities are always a struggle in this community. The town has physicians/clinics of all specialties and has one community hospital. An assessment of the *macrosystem* shows that this community is largely white, with only 10% of residents from ethnic backgrounds. Most people in the community embrace a Christian ethic.

The value system includes a family focus and a strong work ethic. Many of the people prefer the Democratic Party. In terms of the time-related contexts of the *chronosystem,* few things are notable. These time-related events put more stress on the family than usual non-normative events. Linda's disease process with MS has exacerbated in recent times, placing additional strain on the family system. Robert's own dad passed away in the past year, leaving him extra responsibility for his widowed mother, in addition to his responsibility for his own children and now ill wife. The economy in the country and region is going through a recession, leading people to feel some fear about their economic futures. Robert had hoped that his wife could go to work part time when the youngest child went to school, but that no longer seems to be a possibility. The family assessment would include how the family at each of the earlier-mentioned levels is influenced by the changes brought about by Linda's progressing debilitative disease and recent hospitalization. The family is experiencing disturbance at many of these levels.

Interventions include the following possibilities. In general, nurses can also look for additional systems with which the family could interact, to help support family functioning during this family illness event. Nurses could make home visits to assess the living arrangements of the family and to determine how the home could be changed to accommodate a wheelchair/walker. The nurses should talk with the parents about their relationship to the schools, church, and extended family support systems. The parents are advised to inform the school(s), church, workplace, and grandparents of what is happening to their family. The nurses could make suggestions relative to Travis's current behavior with having to go to all-day preschool. The nurses also could explore with the family the larger external environment, including community resources (i.e., MS Society, visiting nurse service, counseling services). The nurses should contact the medical doctor(s) and discharge planning nurse at the hospital to obtain information to interpret the diagnosis, prognosis, and treatment of MS to the family. The nurses might talk to the family about how their faith can be of help during these tough times, and what their primary concerns are as a family. The nurses should get in touch with the social workers at the hospital to coordinate care and social well-being strategies for the posthospitalization period, as well as in the future. This may involve application to social security for the disabled. A family care planning meeting is set up to involve as many caretakers and stakeholders as possible.

Evaluation of the interventions consists of follow-up with the family through periodic home visits and telephone contact. The nurses would be interested in how the family is adapting to its situation, how the father is dealing with the extra responsibility, how the children are coping, and the physical and mental health of the mother. Because MS is a chronic progressive relapsing disorder, a plan is put into place for periodic evaluations that might involve changing the plan of care.

STRENGTHS AND WEAKNESSES

The strength of the bioecological perspective is that it represents a comprehensive and holistic view of human/family development—a bio/psycho/socio/cultural/spiritual approach to the understanding of how humans and families develop and adapt to the larger society. It includes both the *nature* (biological) and *nurture* (environmental contexts) aspects of growth and development for both individuals and families. It directs our attention to factors that occur within, as well as to the layered influences of factors that occur outside individuals and families. The bioecological perspective provides a valuable complement to other theories that may offer greater insight into how each aspect of the holistic approach affects individuals and families over time.

The weakness of this approach is that the bio/psycho/socio/cultural/religious aspects of human/family growth and development are not detailed enough to define how individuals/families can accomplish or adapt to these contextual changes over time, given their biological imperative. Aspects to the theory require further delineation and testing, that is, influence of biological and cognitive processes, and how they interact with the environment.

The Family Cycle of Health and Illness Model

Families, as a whole, experience health events. When family members become ill, it triggers a stress response in the family to adapt to the needs of the individual and the family itself. The Family Cycle of Health and Illness Model (Danielson, Hamel-Bissell, & Winstead-Fry, 1993) describes common family stressors, reactions, and adaptations that families experience when members become ill. Their model is based on the Family Health and Illness Cycle (Doherty & McCubbin, 1985) and Stages of the Family Illness Experience (Coe, 1983, cited in Dery, 1983). Figure 3-7 depicts the family health and illness cycle, illustrating the eight phases of family reactions and potential stresses that can lead to family crisis as they experience a health event of one of their members. The model is circular to represent the continuum of family through the illness experience, even when a family must reorganize after the death of a family member.

Because this is a conceptual model and not a theory per se, each phase of the cycle represents several fields of inquiry around which the model has been built and data organized. It provides a more coherent way of thinking about families when members become ill. The areas of inquiry that inform this model include family health promotion and risk reduction, family vulnerability and illness onset, family illness appraisal, family acute response, family adaptation to illness, and family

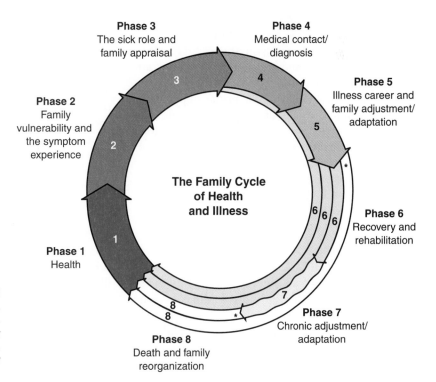

FIGURE 3-7 Family cycle of health and illness model. (From Danielson, C., Hamel-Bissell, B., & Winstead-Fry, P. (1993). *Families, health and illness: Perspectives on coping and intervention.* (p. 72). St. Louis, MO: Mosby, by permission.)

and health care system. The stresses families experience in each of the following eight phases and specific coping tasks of the family are outlined in the next section. More often the nature of the illness and the family's reaction to the situation determine the order of the phases (Danielson et al., 1993, p. 73). For example, the family could move immediately from phase 1, focused on family health, to phase 8, death and reorganization, when a phone call is received that a family member was seriously injured in a car accident and is in the intensive care unit and not expected to live through the night.

PHASES OF THE MODEL

PHASE 1: FAMILY AND THE FAMILY MEMBER HEALTH. The focus in phase 1 of the Family Cycle of Health and Illness is health promotion and risk-reduction needs of family members. Family health promotion is discussed in detail in Chapter 9. Families are stressed, to varying degrees, when family members change a behavior in an attempt to improve their state of health. Families find it difficult to change from established patterns as family members are required to reorganize, form new behaviors, and sustain the changes over time. Nurses need to capitalize on opportunities to work with families on health promotion and risk reduction. Well-child checks and health physicals for sports are excellent times for nurses to be asking questions and teaching families about sleep and rest, stress and overcommitment, nutrition, and relationships. When nurses work with adolescents, it is a prime opportunity to discuss and teach about recreational drug use, sexual behaviors, and nutrition. School nurses could aim health teaching at families by having exercises that have students gathering information or teaching their families about health principles. Nurses can teach during flu immunization clinics and other screening clinics.

PHASE 2: FAMILY VULNERABILITY AND THE SYMPTOM EXPERIENCE. When family members exhibit symptoms of an illness, other family members become aware that an individual has become ill. The family or someone in the family decides the seriousness of the illness based on person's ability to carry out normal activities, previous experience with similar symptoms, and medical knowledge

(Danielson et al., 1993, p. 75). The family may seek opinions from other family members or friends in helping to determine how to treat the symptoms, the seriousness of the illness, or whether they should see a physician.

The second aspect of this phase is the application of folk medicine or self-medicine. During an earlier phase of the illness, family and friends are a source of medical information and treatment suggestions. Given the plethora of health media messages available, families have numerous home remedies to offer. Offering advice is the family's way of showing support and caring for ill family members. It is critical for nurses to realize that the majority of patients and families already seek alternative and complementary therapies in addition to traditional allopathic medical treatments from physicians. Nurses should gather information about alternative therapies as a routine part of data collection and assessment.

Depending on the level of illness, and which family member is ill, the disruptions caused by the illness vary in their effects on family functioning. If the family is dealing with multiple stresses when individuals become ill, the family is more vulnerable or feels the stress of the illness more than if the family were in a stable state when the illness started.

PHASE 3: THE SICK ROLE AND FAMILY APPRAISAL. The family coping tasks are to accept, adjust, and adapt to the sick role, and to respond to the situation. When the family determines that a member is sick, it often excuses that individual from normal family responsibilities. The identified sick person is expected to comply with the behaviors and advice to get better, and is expected to assume previous roles as soon as possible. The family begins to experience the illness of the individual within the family. The family adapts or accommodates to the changes during the illness. How well the family adapts to the changes brought about by the illness varies. If the family member recovers and returns to previous roles, the family returns to its previous state of health. If the family member remains ill, becomes more ill, or determines the illness is more serious, the family moves to the next phase of seeking medical advice.

In addition to the sick role in phase 3, family appraisal considers the family's beliefs about illness and family decisions about health care. An example of a strategy that nurses may use to help families cope with a situation before the situation becomes more acute is identifying depressed teens who are at high risk for suicide. Then nurses can encourage families to place their adolescents into some form of mental health treatment as soon as possible.

PHASE 4: MEDICAL CONTACT AND DIAGNOSIS.

The family tasks in phase 4 are as follows: (1) establish a positive working relationship with health care providers, (2) gather information about the diagnosis, and (3) accept the diagnosis. At some point, families decide to seek medical advice and diagnosis. Families may already know a known health care provider, which typically generates less stress than if they need to seek out and establish a relationship with a new health care provider. The longer it takes to receive a diagnosis, the more stress that is generated for families. Once a diagnosis is given, families gather information about the diagnosis and are challenged to accept the diagnosis. Families vary in ability to seek resources, information, and understand the ramifications of the diagnosis. Nurses have a central role in providing information to families with new diagnoses and helping them navigate the health care system. Family education is critical to the health outcomes, specifically integrating the medical treatment plan into family life and family roles.

All diagnoses have the potential to create stress. The diagnostic process creates stress and uncertainty in families. Families may or may not accept the diagnosis. Some families may deny the diagnosis, and others will question the diagnosis and seek other opinions. Once a medical diagnosis is given to families, the diagnosis becomes public knowledge, which means that everyone who knows the diagnosis has a reaction and response. Families may choose to keep the information within their family unit and are discriminating in whom they tell.

PHASE 5: ILLNESS CAREER AND FAMILY ADJUSTMENT/ADAPTATION.

The family tasks of phase 5 are as follows: (1) accept the treatment plan, (2) reorganize family roles, and (3) maintain a positive relationship with health care providers. Once families accept the diagnosis, they move into what is called the "illness career," which is a way that families adapt and adjust to the illness on a day-by-day basis. The patients and families are expected to comply with treatment plans. The American medical model of patient autonomy, which is individual in focus, runs counter to the notion of involving families in the treatment plans. During this phase, families are constantly adjusting to the situation caused by the illness. Families vary in ability to adjust to the illness situation—the more problems adjusting, the more stress families experience. Depending on the length of the illness career, the short-term family adjustments put in place in phase 3 may create stress for the family when the illness is prolonged. Family role stress, role strain, and role overload can occur when the family deals with illness over a long period.

The family relationship with the health care provider(s) is a critical component of this phase. Families expect that they will be active members of the treatment team; when this expectation is not met to satisfaction, stress results.

PHASE 6: RECOVERY AND REHABILITATION.

The major task for families is to relinquish the sick role and to adjust to a new definition of "normal" or re-establish the original family system as they re-enter phase 1 of health. Recovery can occur after phase 3 without seeing a health care provider or after phase 5. The stress comes from families moving back into old familial patterns, roles, and responsibilities practiced before the onset of the illness. Families can recover fully and have complete confidence in the recovery. They may partially recover so that they worry that the illness may return or that the ill person is doing too much too fast. Families feel vulnerable during this time. They may not recover to their previous state of health because of a permanent disability of the sick member. The effects of the illness may require families to adjust to new roles, new relationships, or a new concept of normalcy and health.

PHASE 7: CHRONIC ADJUSTMENT/ADAPTATION.

Family tasks are to redefine normal, adjust to social stigma or altered relationships caused by the disability, continue to maintain a positive relationship with the health care team, and successfully grieve the loss incurred from the disability or chronic condition. The family must adjust continually to the remission and exacerbations of the illness during this phase of the cycle. One of the major tasks is to balance the needs of the family and the needs of ill family members.

Families must adapt to the demands of the chronic condition; thus, a whole body of information has evolved around family coping and family adaptation with medical regimens. How do families promote the recovery of ill members while preserving their energy to nurture other family members and perform other family functions? An example of an appropriate intervention would be to help families find respite care for family caregivers so that caregivers do not "burn out."

PHASE 8: DEATH AND FAMILY REORGANIZATION. The family tasks in phase 8 consist of working through the grieving process and integrating the loss into the family and family life. Each family member will respond differently to the loss, and the family will be forever changed by the loss. The loss requires the family to adjust and adapt to the finality of the loss and to develop or generate a different sense of identity of family without the person (see Chapter 11).

Nurses work with family stress responses related to relapses or exacerbations of chronic disorders (i.e., diabetes, MS, or schizophrenia). The development of support groups would be one nursing strategy for dealing with family members who have chronic illness.

APPLICATION OF THE FAMILY CYCLE OF HEALTH AND ILLNESS MODEL WITH THE JONES FAMILY The Jones family is in phase 7, Chronic Adjustment/Adaptation. Each family member, including Linda, and the family as a whole must continually adapt to the progression of Linda's MS, thus the chronic illness has become an assault on family stability and health (Danielson et al., 1993, p. 85). At the same time each member struggles with the changes brought about by Linda's progressive disease, the family as a whole has the ability to develop renewed growth and closeness as the family nurse helps them put in place interventions, such as the grandmother coming to live with the family. The role of the family nurse is to help the family maintain stability. Depending on the speed of decline of Linda's health, the Jones family may likely be in phase 7 for a long time, perhaps years, until the family moves into phase 8, Death and Reorganization.

STRENGTHS AND WEAKNESSES

This model depicts the cyclical nature of families as they respond and adjust to changes that illnesses bring to individual family systems. The strength of this model is that it shows how the family as a whole may move through the health and illness phases. It outlines the specific coping tasks that cause families stress during each of the phases. Nurses who are not intimately knowledgeable of these stressors can use this model to help them focus their health and illness care with the family. The weakness of this model is that nurses must have a broad depth of understanding of the current family literature in each of the phases.

Family Assessment and Intervention Model

The **Family Assessment and Intervention Model** was originally developed by Berkey and Hanson (1991). Figure 3-8 depicts the Family Assessment and Intervention Model, which is based on Neuman's Health Care Systems Model (Hanson, 2001; Hanson & Kaakinen, 2005; Hanson and Mischke, 1996). Neuman's model and theoretical constructs are based on systems theory, and were extended and modified to focus on the family rather than on the individual.

According to the Family Assessment and Intervention Model, families are viewed as a dynamic, open system in interaction with their environment. One of the roles for families is to help buffer its members or protect the family as a whole, as well from perceived threats to the family system. The core of the family system comprises basic family structure, function, processes, and energy/strength resources. This basic family structure must be protected at all costs, or the family ceases to exist. The family develops normal lines of defense as an adaptational mechanism and abstract flexible protective lines of defense when the system is threatened by significant stressors. Family systems are vulnerable to tensions produced when stressors in the form of problems or concerns penetrate the family's lines of defenses. Families also have lines of resistance to help prevent penetration into the basic family core. The lines of defense and resistance depicted in the model (see Fig. 3-8) demonstrate how unexpected/unwanted health status changes can affect the basic family unit or core.

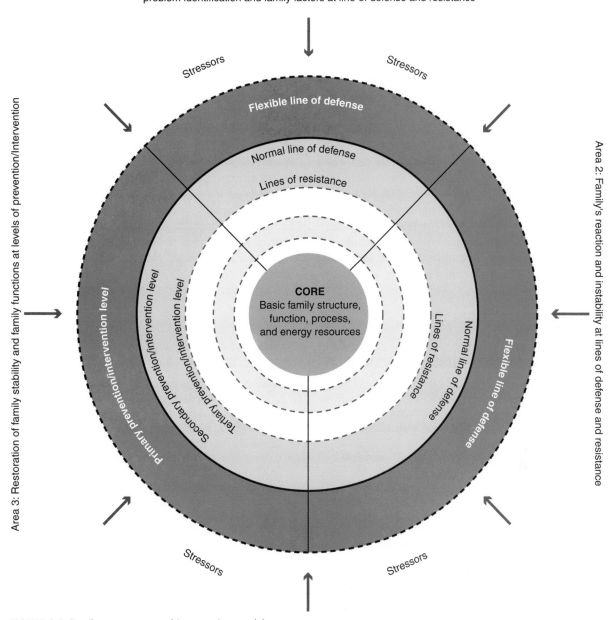

FIGURE 3-8 Family assessment and intervention model.

Families are subject to imbalance from normal homeostasis when stressors (i.e., physical or mental health problems) penetrate families' flexible and normal lines of defense. Furthermore, the stressors can challenge the families' lines of resistance, which have been put in place to keep stability and penetrate the basic family defense system. In other words, health events cause families to react to stressors created by changes in the health status of one of its members. Families vary in their response to the stressors and in their ability to cope based on how deeply the stressors penetrate the basic family unit, and how capable or experienced the family is in adapting to maintain its stability.

Reconstitution or adaptation is the work the family undertakes to preserve or restore family stability after stressors penetrate the family lines of defense and resistance. This process alters the whole of the family. The model addresses three areas: (1) wellness-health promotion activities—problem identification and family factors at lines of defense and resistance; (2) family reaction and instability at lines of defense and resistance; and (3) restoration of family stability and family functioning at levels of prevention and intervention. The basic assumptions of this family-focused model are listed in Box 3-4.

The Family Assessment and Intervention Model focuses specifically on what causes family stress and how families react to this stress. One critical concept is to build on the family's strengths by helping them identify its problem-solving strategies.

Berkey and Hanson (1991) developed an assessment, intervention, and measurement tool, Family Systems Stressor-Strength Inventory (FS³I), to help guide nurses working with families who are undergoing stressful health events and to build on the strengths of the family. The FS³I is divided into three sections: (1) family systems stressor—general; (2) family stressors—specific; and (3) family system strengths. Family stability is assessed by gathering information on family stressors and strengths. The assessment of general, overall stressors is followed by an assessment of specific issues or problems, such as birth of first child, automobile accident, or family divorce. Family strengths are identified to help determine potential or actual problem-solving abilities of the family system. Examples of family strengths could include supportive extended family, health insurance, and availability of family counseling. An updated blank copy of the instrument, with instructions for administration and a scoring guide, can be found in Appendix A. A summary of a completed instrument applied to the case study follows.

The FS³I is intended for use with multiple family members. Individual members of the family can

---

BOX 3-4
Basic Assumptions for Family Assessment and Intervention Model

- Although each family has a unique family system, all families have a common basic structure that is composite of common, known factors or innate characteristics within a normal given range of response.
- Family wellness is on a continuum of available energy to support the family system in its optimal state.
- The family, in both a state of wellness or illness, is a dynamic composite of inter-relationships of variables (physiological, psychological, sociocultural, developmental, and spiritual).
- A myriad of environmental stressors can impact the family. Each stressor differs in its potential for disturbing the family's stability level, or normal line of defense. The specific family interrelationships (physiological, psychological, sociocultural, developmental, and spiritual) affect the degree to which a family is protected by its flexible lines of defense against possible reactions to the stressors.
- Families evolve a normal range of response to the environment, which is called a *normal line of defense*, or its usual wellness or state of stability. The normal line of defense is flexible or accordion-like as it moves to protect the family.
- When the flexible line of defense is no longer capable of protecting the family or family system

against the environmental stressor, the stressor is said to break through the normal line of defense.
- Families have in internal resistance factor called *line of resistance* that functions to stabilize and return the family to its usual wellness state (normal line of defense), or possibly to a higher level of stability after an environmental stressor reaction.
- Primary prevention is general knowledge that is applied in family assessment and intervention for identification and mitigation of risk factors associated with environmental stressor to prevent possible reaction.
- Secondary prevention is symptomatology after reaction to stressors, appropriate ranking of intervention priorities, and treatment to reduce their noxious effects.
- Tertiary prevention is the adjustive processes that take place as reconstitution begins and maintenance factors move the client back in the circular manner toward primary prevention.
- The family is in dynamic, constant energy exchange with the environment.

Source: Adapted from Berkey, K. M. & Hanson, S. M. (1991). *Pocket guide to family assessment and intervention* (pp. 23–24), St. Louis, MO: Mosby Year Book, by permission.

complete the FS³I, or the entire family can sit together and complete the assessment. The nurse meets with family members and interviews them to clarify their perceived general stressors, specific stressors, and family strengths as identified by the family members.

After the interview, the nurse completes the quantitative summary and enters each respondent's score on the graph. Recording individual scores on the graph allows for a comparison of the family responses and visually shows the variability among family members' perceptions of general and specific health stressors. On a separate graph, one can see how individuals and nurses perceive the strengths of the family for prevention and intervention purposes. The nurse synthesizes the interview information gleaned from all the family participants on the qualitative summary. Together, the nurse and family develop a family care plan with intervention strategies tailored to the individual family needs and built on the strengths of the family.

A major benefit of using the FS³I for family assessment and intervention planning is that both quantitative and qualitative data are used to determine the level of prevention and intervention needed: primary, secondary, or tertiary (Pender, Murdaugh, & Parsons, 2006). Primary prevention focuses on moving the individual and family toward a state of improved health or toward health-promotion activities. *Primary interventions* include providing families with information about their strengths, supporting their coping and functioning capabilities, and encouraging movement toward health through family education. *Secondary interventions* attain system stability after stressors or problems have invaded the family core. Secondary interventions include helping the family to handle its problems, helping family members to find and use appropriate treatment, and intervening in crises. *Tertiary prevention* is designed to maintain system stability through intervention strategies that are initiated after treatment has been completed. Coordination of care after discharge from the hospital or rehabilitation services is an example of tertiary prevention.

In summary, the *Family Assessment and Intervention Model* focuses on the family as client. The *Family Systems Stressor-Strength Inventory (FS³I)* was developed to provide a concrete, focused assessment and intervention instrument that helps families identify current family stressors and strengths, and assists nurses and families in planning interventions to meet family needs. The model and inventory represent a nursing model made for nursing care of families.

APPLICATION OF THE FAMILY ASSESSMENT AND INTERVENTION MODEL WITH THE JONES FAMILY

The FS³I was used to assess stressors (problems) and the strengths (resources) that the Jones family had to cope with in their situation. The adult parents, Robert and Linda, were interviewed together by the nurse, but each person completed a separate FS³I. Scores were tallied using the scoring guide for the FS³I. Amy was away attending college, and Katie (13 years old) and Travis (4 years old) were too young to complete the assessment instrument (FS³I).

The general stressors were viewed similarly by both Robert and Linda, and these stressors were assessed as more serious by the nurse than by the couple. Robert, Linda, and the nurse concurred that the general stress level was high, which was consistent with their experience. The specific stressors were perceived slightly differently by Robert and Linda. The following figures summarize information gained from the Jones family: Figure 3-9, which applies the FS³I to the Jones Family; Figure 3-10, which presents an FS³I quantitative summary of family system stressors, general and specific, for the Jones family; Figure 3-11, which lists FS³I family and clinician perception scores of the Jones family; Figure 3-12, which is an FS³I qualitative summary, family and clinician, of the Jones family; and Figure 3-13, which provides an FS³I family care plan for the Jones family.

The *Qualitative Summary,* family and clinician form in Figure 3-12 serves as the groundwork for the Family Care Plan. This form synthesizes information pertaining to general stressors, specific stressors, family strengths, and the overall functioning and physical and mental health of the family members. The nurse completed this form using her assessment skills with information obtained from the verbal exchange and the written data obtained from the FS³I.

The family members and the nurse perceived that the chronic and debilitating diagnosis of MS was the major general stressor. Linda's specific stressors included her growing disability to function as a wife and mother; her physical problems such as growing physical weakness, swallowing, pain, vision impairment,

INSTRUCTIONS FOR ADMINISTRATION

The Family Systems Stressor-Strength Inventory (FS3I) is an assessment and measurement instrument intended for use with families (see Chapter 8). It focuses on identifying stressful situations occurring in families and the strengths families use to maintain healthy family functioning. Each family member is asked to complete the instrument on an individual form before an interview with the clinician. Questions can be read to members unable to read.

After completion of the instrument, the clinician evaluates the family on each of the stressful situations (general and specific) and the strengths they possess. This evaluation is recorded on the family member form.

The clinician records the individual family member's score and the clinician perception score on the Quantitative Summary. A different color code is used for each family member. The clinician also completes the Qualitative Summary, synthesizing the information gleaned from all participants. Clinicians can use the Family Care Plan to prioritize diagnoses, set goals, develop prevention and intervention activities, and evaluate outcomes.

Family Name _Jones_   **Date** _April 18, 2009_

Family Member(s) Completing Assessment _Robert and Linda_

Ethnic Background(s) _"American all mixed up"_

Religious Background(s) _Protestant_

Referral Source _Neurologist For Linda_

Interviewer _Meredith Rowe, RN_

Family Members	Relationship in Family	Age	Marital Status	Education (highest degree)	Occupation
1. _Robert_	_Father_	_48 yr_	_Married_	_MS_	_Software engineer_
2. _Linda_	_Mother_	_43 yr_	_Married_		_Home maker_
3. _Amy_	_Daughter_	_19 yr_	_Single_		
4. _Katie_	_Daughter_	_13 yr_	_Single_		
5. _Travis_	_Son_	_4 yr_	_Single_		
6.					

Family's current reasons for seeking assistance:

Linda MS is progressing family feels stressed.

Source: Hanson, S. M. H. (2001). *Family health care nursing: Theory, practice, and research* (2nd ed.), pp. 425-437. Philadelphia: F. A. Davis.

FIGURE 3-9 Family System Stressor-Strength Inventory: Jones family.

vertigo/tinnitus, constipation, urinary infections; and her mental health issues, such as guilt, anxiety, and depression. Specific stressors for Robert included his worry about Linda's health, loss of his life's partner in taking care of the family, household maintenance and raising children, fear of the unknown future and health outcomes, loss of sexual expression with his wife, and financial worries. The strengths of the family were seen as communication between the couple, religious faith, the social support network of extended family, and the availability of good health providers. The overall family functioning was considered to be as good as could be expected under the circumstances. Where the mother's physical health was compromised, the father's physical health was good. Both Linda and Robert expressed mental health concerns; see the *Qualitative Summary Family Form: Jones Family* (see Fig. 3-12), which includes frustration,

QUANTITATIVE SUMMARY OF FAMILY SYSTEMS STRESSORS: GENERAL AND SPECIFIC FAMILY AND CLINICIAN PERCEPTION SCORES

DIRECTIONS: Graph the scores from each family member inventory by placing an "X" at the appropriate location. (Use first name initial for each different entry and different color code for each family member.)

SCORES FOR WELLNESS AND STABILITY	FAMILY SYSTEMS STRESSORS (GENERAL)		SCORES FOR WELLNESS AND STABILITY	FAMILY SYSTEMS STRESSORS (SPECIFIC)	
	FAMILY MEMBER PERCEPTION SCORE	CLINICIAN PERCEPTION SCORE		FAMILY MEMBER PERCEPTION SCORE	CLINICIAN PERCEPTION SCORE
5.0			5.0		
4.8			4.8	X√1	
4.6			4.6		
		X			X
4.4			4.4		
	X√1			X√2	
4.2			4.2		
4.0	X√2		4.0		
3.8			3.8		
3.6			3.6		
3.4			3.4		
3.2			3.2		
3.0			3.0		
2.8			2.8		
2.6			2.6		
2.4			2.4		
2.2			2.2		
2.0			2.0		
1.8			1.8		
1.6			1.6		
1.4			1.4		
1.2			1.2		
1.0			1.0		

*PRIMARY Prevention/Intervention Mode: Flexible Line   1.0-2.3   √1 = Robert
*SECONDARY Prevention/Intervention Mode: Normal Line   2.4-3.6
*TERTIARY Prevention/Intervention Mode: Resistance Lines   3.7-5.0   √2 = Linda
*Breakdowns of numerical scores for stressor penetration are suggested values.

FIGURE 3-10 Quantitative summary of family systems stressors, general and specific: Jones family.

FAMILY SYSTEMS STRENGTHS FAMILY AND CLINICIAN PERCEPTION SCORES

DIRECTIONS: Graph the scores from the inventory by placing an "X" at the appropriate location and connect with a line. (Use first name initial for each different entry and different color code for each family member.)

SUM OF STRENGTHS AVAILABLE FOR PREVENTION/ INTERVENTION MODE	FAMILY SYSTEMS STRENGTHS	
	FAMILY MEMBER PERCEPTION SCORE	CLINICIAN PERCEPTION SCORE
5.0		
4.8		
4.6		
4.4		X
4.2		
	√2	
4.0		
3.8		
3.6		
3.4	√1	
3.2		
3.0		
2.8		
2.6		
2.4		
2.2		
2.0		
1.8		
1.6		
1.4		
1.2		
1.0		

*PRIMARY Prevention/Intervention Mode: Flexible Line   1.0-2.3   √1 = Robert
*SECONDARY Prevention/Intervention Mode: Normal Line   2.4-3.6
*TERTIARY Prevention/Intervention Mode: Resistance Lines   3.7-5.0   √2 = Linda
*Breakdowns of numerical scores for stressor penetration are suggested values.

FIGURE 3-11 Family and clinician perception scores: Jones family.

QUALITATIVE SUMMARY FAMILY AND CLINICIAN REMARKS
PART I: FAMILY SYSTEMS STRESSORS (GENERAL)

Summarize general stressors and remarks of family and clinician. Prioritize stressors according to importance to family members.

The major general stressor of the family as is the DX of MS and the impact of the progressive disabling illness on the entire family.

PART II: FAMILY SYSTEMS STRESSORS (SPECIFIC)

A. Summarize specific stressors and remarks of family and clinician.

> Linda's specific stressors: growing disability to function as wife/mother, physical signs of impairment and guilt, anxiety, and depression. Robert's specific stressors: loss of fully functional wife, fear of unknown; loss of sexual expression and finances.

B. Summarize differences (if discrepancies exist) between how family members and clinicians view effects of stressful situation on family.

> Each family member has some different stressors, but share in common the fears, anxiety, helplessness, sadness over their losses due to Linda's condition. Nurse views general and specific stressors higher than family.

C. Summarize overall family functioning.

> Functioning as best as can be expected. Physical health in question. Mental health standing up so far. Family addressing issues one by one.

D. Summarize overall significant physical health status for family members.

> Mother's physical health compromised. Father's physical health is okay.

E. Summarize overall significant mental health status for family members.

> Mother is frustrated and anxious. Expressed guilt, which makes her depressed. Father is also frustrated and worried about Linda, the children, and finances.

PART III: FAMILY SYSTEMS STRENGTHS

Summarize family systems strengths and family and clinician remarks that facilitate family health and stability.

> Couple communication, religious faith, social support of extended family and believe they have competent caring health care providers.

FIGURE 3-12 Qualitative summary, family and clinician: Jones family.

Diagnosis: General and Specific Family System Stressors	Family Systems Strengths Supporting Family Care Plan	Goals for Family and Clinician	Prevention/Intervention Mode		Outcomes Evaluation and Replanning
			Primary, Secondary, or Tertiary	Prevention/Intervention Activities	
Dx of MS weakness of swallowing, pain, vision impairment, vertigo/tinnitus, constipation, urinary infections, guilt/anxiety, depression, sexual dysfunction, over-load for caregiver father.	Couple communication, religious faith, social support of extended family, good medical care.	Restoration of stability and homeostasis at each level of progressive chronic illness.	Support of family changes, connect family with MS family support group, locate part-time family helper for home, coordinate with other medical groups involved, set up rehabilitation, and physical therapy.	Couple receives counseling, pain and symptom management; involve social worker to look at community agencies to offer assistance.	Evaluation to be done once plan implemented.

FIGURE 3-13 Family Care Plan: Jones family.

anxiousness, fear of unknown, worry, guilt, and depression. Overall, the family members had similar perceptions of their stressors and strengths, and the nurse concurred with their perceptions, although the nurse rated both stressors and strengths higher than the family members. The nurse perceived that this family had the strengths they needed to deal with both the general and specific stressors. After completing a genogram and ecomap of this family unit, the nurse concluded that the family was being supported by community/family resources. These social support systems are important factors in coping with stress, and the nurse concluded that this family could use assistance in utilizing these resources.

Figure 3-13, *Family Care Plan: Jones family*, was developed by the nurse in concert with the family members who completed the FS³I. The Family Care Plan addresses the diagnosis of general and specific family systems stressors and family systems strengths that support the Family Care Plan and the goals of the family and the clinician(s): interventions/prevention activities—primary/secondary/tertiary, and outcome/evaluation/replanning proposed for this family. The goal of this Family Care Plan was to achieve a restoration of optimum health that could provide homeostasis and stability for this family, and more positive health outcomes than the family could reach at the beginning of their health challenges. The outcome/evaluation/replanning section of the Family

Care Plan remains blank for now because it is dependent on feedback from the interventions proposed for the family, as well as the physical and mental health status of the entire family.

STRENGTHS AND WEAKNESSES

The strength of the FS³I approach is that both quantitative and qualitative data are used to determine the level of prevention and intervention needed: primary, secondary, or tertiary. The instrument is brief, easy to administer, and yields data to compare one family member with another member and one family with another family. The weakness of this model and instrument is that they focus only on family strengths and stressors. This model and instrument hold much promise for nursing assessment of families, but more work needs to be done on this approach.

SUMMARY

By understanding theories and models, nurses are prepared to think creatively and critically about how health events affect the family. This chapter introduces nurses to the concept of theory-guided, evidence-based family nursing practice. It presents the relationship between theory, practice, and research, and explains crucial aspects of theory. The chapter then explores five theories and models of working with families: Family Systems Theory, Developmental and Family Life Cycle Theory, Family Health and Illness Cycle Model, Bioecological Theory, and the Family Assessment and Intervention Model. The authors demonstrate how nurses can practice family nursing differently with the Jones family depending on different theoretical perspectives. Box 3-5 summarizes how the primary focus of the Jones family differs depending on which of the five theories/models were adopted. The following points highlight critical concepts that are addressed in this chapter:

- No single theory, model, or conceptual framework adequately describes the complex relationships of family.
- No one theoretical perspective gives nurses a sufficiently broad base of knowledge and understanding to guide assessment and interventions with all families.
- No one theoretical perspective is better than another.

- No one theoretical perspective is more comprehensive or more correct than another.
- Nurses who draw from multiple theories are more effective in tailoring their nursing practice and family interventions. Using multiple theories substantially increases the likelihood that the family will be able to achieve stability and health as a family unit.
- Theories that inform the nursing of families should be the "gold standard" of nursing practice (Segaric & Hall, 2005); hence, family nursing is a theory-guided evidence-based nursing practice.

In conclusion, regardless of the underlying model or theory, the authors of this chapter present ways of providing excellence of family health care nursing that is theory driven and evidenced based. Of significance is that by using different lenses to view family care problems, different solutions and options for care and interventions are more available. No one theoretical perspective stands out as representing the best and only way of nursing care for families. What is crucial is that nurses use multiple

---

BOX 3-5

Comparison of Theories as They May Apply to the Jones Family

FAMILY SYSTEMS THEORY

Conceptual

Family is viewed as a whole. What happens to the family as a whole affects each individual family member, and what happens to individuals impacts the totality of the family unit. Focus is on the circular interactions among members of family system resulting in functional or dysfunctional outcomes. This theory evolved out of general systems theory and was applied to families by family social scientists.

Assessment

The family may be assessed together or individually. Assessment questions relate to the *interaction* between the individual and the family, and the *interaction* between the family and the community in which they live.

Intervention Examples

- Complete a family genogram to understand patterns and relationships over several generations over time.

- Complete family ecomap to see how individuals/ family relate to the community around them.
- Collect data about the family as a whole and individual family members.
- Conduct care planning sessions that include family members.

Strengths

Focus is on family as a whole or its subsystems, or both. It is a generally understood and accepted theory in society.

Weaknesses

Theory is broad and general. It does not give definitive prescriptions for interventions.

Application to Jones Family

All members of Jones family are affected by the mother's progressive chronic health condition and changes. Family structure, functions, and processes of the family are impacted, changing family roles and dynamics. Everyone in the family has their own

Continued

concerns and needs attention by health care professionals.

FAMILY DEVELOPMENTAL AND LIFE CYCLE THEORY

Conceptual
Family is viewed as a whole over time. All families go through similar developmental processes starting with the birth of first child to death of the parents. Focus is on life cycle of families and represents normative stages of family development. Theory evolved out of individual growth and developmental theory, and elaborated by family social scientists.

Assessment
The family may be assessed together or individually. Assessment questions relate to the normative predictable events that occur in family life over time. It also includes non-normative, unexpected events including how the family is adapting to somewhat predictable developmental tasks.

Intervention Examples
- Conduct family interview to determine where family is in terms of cognitive, social, emotional, spiritual, and physical development.
- A family genogram and ecomap should be completed.
- Determine the normative and non-normative events that have occurred to the family as a whole or to individuals within the family.
- Analyze how an individual's growth and developmental milestones may impact the family developmental trajectory.

Strengths
Focus is on family as a whole. Theory provides a framework for predicting what a family will experience at given stage in the family life cycle. Anticipatory guidance can be given.

Weaknesses
The traditional linear family life cycle is no longer the norm. Modern families vary widely in their structure and roles. Divorce, remarriage, gay parents, and never-married parents have changed the traditional trajectory of growth and developmental milestones. The theory does not focus on how the family adapts to the transitions from one stage to the other, but it does predict what transitions will occur.

Application to Jones Family
The Jones family is in the "stage of families with adolescents" and "launching young adults." The

non-normative health condition of the mother is changing the predictable normative course of development for the individuals and the family as a whole. These health events will change the cognitive, social, emotional, spiritual, and physical development as the family shifts to integrate new roles into their lives as family members.

BIOECOLOGICAL SYSTEMS THEORY

Conceptual
Bioecological systems theory combines children's biological disposition and environmental forces that come together to shape the development of human beings. This theory has basis in both developmental theory and systems theory to understand individual and family growth. It combines the influence of both genetics and environment from the individual and family to the larger economic/political structure over time. Basic premise is that individual and family development is contextual over time. Theory evolved out of normal growth and development theory, but was further developed and contextualized ecologically by a developmental psychologist.

Assessment
Assess all levels of the larger ecological system when interviewing the family. Determine the microsystem, mesosystem, exosystem, macrosystem, and chrono-system of the individual and family as a whole.

Intervention Examples
- Conduct family interview to determine where family is in relationship to four locational/spatial contexts and one time-related context.
- A family genogram and ecomap should be completed.
- Determine how individuals are doing in relationship to their entire environment, which includes immediate family, extended family, home, school and community.
- Analyze family in its smaller and larger contextual aspects.

Strengths
Focus is on a holistic approach to human/family development. A bio/psycho/socio/cultural/spiritual approach to understanding how individuals and families develop and change/adapt over time in our society.

Weaknesses
This holistic approach is not specific enough to define contextual changes over time, given

individual biological imperatives. Nor can the larger context in which individuals/families are embedded be predicted or controlled.

Application to Jones Family

- Microsystem. Jones family consists of school aged children living at home. The parental roles have been traditional until recent health events.
- Mesosystem. Family has much interaction between the family and schools, church and extended family.
- Exosystem. Family influenced by father's work at the factory and other institutions in the community.
- Macrosystem. Family consistent with community culture, attitudes and beliefs. Their community is largely Caucasian, middle class and Christian.
- Chronosystem. At this time in history, but with mother's illness, the family is changing and is in crisis.

FAMILY CYCLE OF HEALTH AND ILLNESS MODEL
Conceptual

As this is a conceptual model and not a theory, each phase of the cycle represents several fields of inquiry area around which the model has been built and data organized to provide a coherent way of thinking about families when a member becomes ill, rather than a definite set of propositions. The areas of inquiry that inform this model are family health promotion and risk reduction, family vulnerability and illness onset, family illness appraisal, family acute response, family adaptation to illness, and family and health care system.

Assessment

The family as a whole is assessed to determine whether they are managing known stressors and meeting coping tasks in each phase of the family cycle of health and illness. Analyze how individual members of the family as a whole are coping with the predicted stressors associated with that phase of the family cycle of health and illness.

Intervention Examples

- Complete a family genogram and ecomap.
- Implement a plan of care to help facilitate family adaptation and coping strategies.
- Work with families to adjust family roles to help the family with managing the stressors identified.

Strengths

Focus is on family coping through identified predictable stressors that families experience who are in that stage of the health illness cycle. Anticipatory guidance can be provided. The model represents a continuum from health to death and presents how the family integrates death as it moves back into a healthy phase.

Weaknesses

The model is not specific enough to identify precise ways families cope; rather, it is more of a guideline of typical stressors and coping tasks. The model does not address transitional stress, but rather additional stress placed on the family from the illness.

Application to Jones Family

The Jones family is struggling to adapt during the rocky chronic illness phase. As the mother's illness has changed from being episodic to progressive in nature, the family is stressed with adapting to the mother losing ambulation and needing more physical support than in the past. The family is in a constant state of stress as it adjusts to the new patterns, regimens, and roles. The family is grieving as Linda becomes more disabled.

FAMILY ASSESSMENT AND INTERVENTION MODEL
Conceptual

Families are viewed as dynamic, open systems in interaction with their environment. A major role of family is to help protect themselves from events such as illness that may threaten the family's inner core. The inner core of the family consists of family structure, function, process, and energy/strength resources, and must be protected or the family ceases to exist. Adaptation is the work the family undertakes to preserve/restore family stability. This model evolved out of nursing and builds on general systems theory, stress theory, and change theory.

Assessment

Family may be assessed together, but all individuals are asked to complete the measurement instrument. The Family Systems Stressor-Strength inventory (FS^{3}I) is administered to determine general family stressors, specific family stressors, and family system strengths. The stressors that affect the balance of the family strengths are analyzed to assist the family to achieve stability.

Intervention Examples

- The FS^{3}I is completed by all adult individuals in the family. Scores are derived from the measurement scales and then analyzed. Health care providers

Continued

meet with families to go over results and provide different intervention strategies based on the specific stressors, how the family is coping, and what strengths are brought to the situation.
■ A family genogram and ecomap should be completed.

Strengths
The model and instrument provide a structure approach to family assessment and intervention based on both quantitative and qualitative data. These data help determine the primary, secondary, and tertiary levels of prevention and intervention. The focus on family strengths is unique to this model and approach.

Weaknesses
This model is used specifically when families enter the health care system. It is applicable when health problems have come up that cause stressors. Although the model per se is applicable to all families in terms of life stressors, the administration of the FS³I is specific to health events.

Application to Jones Family
The adults in this family were interviewed together with each person completing the FS³I. General stressors and specific stressors were rated similarly by each member of the couple. The nurse also rated her perceptions of the family stressors and strengths. Overall, family physical and mental functioning were also rated. The nurse concluded that this family had the strengths they needed to deal with both the general and specific stressors.

theoretical perspectives to guide their practice with the nursing care of families. Clearly, not one theoretical perspective gives all nurses in all settings a sufficiently broad base of knowledge on which to assess and intervene with the complex health events experienced by families.

REFERENCES

Artinian, N. T. (1994). Selecting model to guide family assessment. *Dimensions of Critical Care Nursing, 14*(1), 4–16.

Bengtson, V. L., Acock, A. C., Allen, K. R., Dilworth-Anderson, P., & Klein, D. M. (Eds.). (2005). *Sourcebook of family theory & research.* Thousand Oaks, CA: Sage.

Berkey, K. M., & Hanson, S. M. H. (1991). *Pocket guide to family assessment and intervention.* St. Louis, MO: CV Mosby.

Boemmel, J., & Briscoe, J. (2001). Web Quest Project Theory Fact Sheet of Urie Bronfenbrenner. Retrieved February 9, 2008, from http://pt3.nl.edu/boemmelbriscoewebquest

Bowen, M. (1978). *Family therapy in clinical practice.* New York: Jason Aronson.

Bronfenbrenner, U. (1972a). *Two worlds of childhood.* New York: Simon & Schuster.

Bronfenbrenner, U. (1972b). *Influences on human development.* Hinsdale, Il: Dryden Press.

Bronfenbrenner, U. (1979). *The ecology of human development.* Cambridge, MA: Harvard University Press.

Bronfenbrenner, U. (1981). *On making human beings human.* Thousand Oaks, CA: Sage.

Bronfenbrenner, U. (1986). Ecology of the family as a context for human development: Research perspectives. *Developmental Psychology, 22,* 723–742.

Bronfenbrenner, U. (1997). Ecology of the family as a context for human development: Research perspectives. In J. L. Paul, M. Churton, H. Rosselli-Kostoryz, W. C. Morse, K. Marfo, C. Lavely, et al. (Eds.), *Foundations of special education* (pp. 49–83). Pacific Grove, CA: Brooks/Cole.

Bronfenbrenner, U. & Lerner, R. M. (Eds.) (2004). *Making human beings human: Bioecological perspectives on human development.* Thousand Oaks, CA: Sage Publications.

Bronfenbrenner, U., & Morris, P.A. (1998). The ecology of developmental processes. In W. Damon (Series Ed.), & R. M. Lerner (Vol. Ed.), *Handbook of child psychology: Vol. 1. Theoretical models of human development* (pp. 993–1028). New York: John Wiley & Sons.

Carter, B., (2005). Becoming parents: The family with young children. In B. Carter, & M. McGoldrick (Eds.), *The expanded family life cycle: Individual, family and social perspectives* (3rd ed., pp. 249–273). New York: Allyn & Bacon.

Carter, B., & McGoldrick, M. (1989). *The changing family life cycle: A framework for family therapy.* New York: Gardner Press.

Carter, B., & McGoldrick, M. (2005). The divorce cycle: A major variation in the American Family Life Cycle. In B. Carter & M. McGoldrick (Eds.). *The expanded family life cycle: Individual, family, and social perspectives* (3rd ed., pp. 373–380). New York: Allyn & Bacon.

Carter, B., & McGoldrick, M. (Eds.). (2005). *The expanded family life cycle: Individual, family and social perspectives* (3rd ed.). New York: Allyn & Bacon.

Casey, B. (1996). The family as a system. In C. Bomar (Ed.), *Nurses and family health promotion: Concepts, assessment, and interventions* (2nd ed.). Philadelphia: Saunders.

Danielson, C. B., Hamel-Bissell, B., & Winstead-Fry, P. (1993). *Families, health & illness: Perspectives on coping and intervention.* St. Louis, Mo: CV Mosby.

Denham, S. (2003). *Family health: A framework for nursing.* Philadelphia: F.A. Davis.

Dery, G. K. (1983). Concepts of health and illness. In W. J. Phipps, B. C. Long, & N. F. Woods (Eds.), *Medical-surgical nursing: Concepts and clinical practice* (2nd ed., pp. 5–17). St. Louis, MO: Mosby-Year Book.

Doane, G. H., & Varcoe, C. (2005). *Family nursing as relational inquiry: Developing health-promoting practice.* Philadelphia: Lippincott Williams & Wilkins.

Doherty, W., & McCubbin, H. I. (1985). Families and health care: An emerging arena of theory, research, and clinical intervention. In W. Doherty, & H. I. McCubin (Eds.), *Family relations* (pp. 5–10). Minneapolis, MN: National Council of Family Relations.

Duvall, E. M. (1977). *Marriage and family development* (5th ed.). Philadelphia: Lippincott.

Duvall, E. M., & Miller, B. (1985). *Marriage and family development* (6th ed.). Philadelphia: J.B. Lippincott.

Emery University. (2008). *Urie Bronfenbrenner.* Retrieved February 9, 2008, from http://www.des.emory.edu/mfp/302/302bron.PDF

Fawcett, J. (2005). *Contemporary nursing knowledge: Analysis and evaluation of nursing models and theories* (2nd ed.). Philadelphia: F.A. Davis.

Fawcett, J., & Garity, J. (2008). *Evaluating research for evidenced-based nursing practice.* Philadelphia: F.A. Davis.

Freeman, D. S. (1992). *Multigenerational family therapy.* New York: The Haworth Press.

Friedman, M. M., Bowden, V. R., & Jones, E. G. (2003). *Family nursing: Research, theory and practice* (5th ed., pp. 103–150). Upper Saddle River, NJ: Prentice Hall.

Friedemann, M. L. (1995). *The framework of systemic organization: A conceptual approach to families and nursing.* Thousand Oaks, CA: Sage.

Goldenberg, H., & Goldenberg, I. (2007). *Family therapy: An overview* (7th ed.). Belmont, CA: Wadsworth.

Gray, V. (1996). Family self-care. In C. Bomar (Ed.), *Nurses and family health promotion: Concepts, assessment, and interventions* (2nd ed.). Philadelphia: Saunders.

Hanson, S. M. H. (2001). *Family health care nursing: Theory, practice and research* (2nd ed.). Philadelphia: F.A. Davis.

Hanson, S. M. H., & Kaakinen, J. R. (2005). Theoretical foundations for nursing of families. In S. M. H. Hanson, V. Gedaly-Duff, & J. R. Kaakinen (Eds.), *Family health care nursing: Theory, practice and research* (3rd ed., pp. 69–96). Philadelphia: F.A. Davis.

Hanson, S. M. H., & Mischke, K. M. (1996). Family health assessment and intervention. In P. J. Bomar (Ed.), *Nurses and family health promotion: Concepts, assessment and intervention* (2nd ed). Philadelphia: W.B. Saunders.

Hill, R. (1949). *Families under stress.* New York: Harper and Brothers.

Hill, R. (1965). *Challenges and resources for family development: Family mobility in our dynamic society.* Ames: Iowa State University.

Hill, R., & Hansen, D. (1960). The identification of conceptual frameworks utilized in family study. *Marriage and Family Living, 22*(4), 299–311.

Hines, P. M., Preto, N. G., McGoldrick, M., Almeida, R., & Weltman, S. (2005). Culture and the family life cycle. In B. Carter, & M. McGoldrick (Eds.), *The expanded family life cycle: Individual, family and social perspectives* (3rd ed., pp. 69–87). New York: Allyn & Bacon, Pearson Education Company.

Imber-Black, E. (2005). Creating meaningful rituals for new life cycle transitions. In B. Carter, & M. McGoldrick (Eds.), *The expanded family life cycle: Individual, family and social perspectives* (3rd ed., pp. 202–214). New York: Allyn & Bacon, Pearson Education Company.

Jackson, D. D. (1965). Family rules: Marital quid quo. *Archives of General Psychiatry, 12,* 589–594.

Johnson, D. (1980). The behavioral system model for nursing. In J. P. Riehl, & C. Roy (Eds.), *Conceptual models for nursing practice* (2nd ed., pp. 207–216). New York: Appleton-Century-Crofts.

Jones, S. L., & Dimond, S. L., (1982). Family theory and family therapy models: Comparative review with implications for nursing practice. *Journal of Psychiatric Nursing and Mental Health Services, 20*(10), 12–19.

Kerr, M., & Bowen, M. (1988). *Family evaluation: An approach based on Bowen's theory.* New York: Norton.

King, I. (1981). *Family therapy: A comparison of approaches.* Bowie, MD: Brady.

King, I. (1983). King's theory of nursing. In I. W. Clements, & J. B. Roberts (Eds.), *Family health: A theoretical approach to nursing* (pp. 177–187). New York: John Wiley & Sons.

King, I. (1987, May). *King's theory* (Cassette Recording). Recording presented at Nursing Theories Conference, Pittsburgh, PA.

Maturana, H. (1978). Biology of language: The epistemology of reality. In G. Millar, & E. Lenneberg (Eds.), *Psychology and biology of language and thought* (pp. 27–63). New York: Academic Press.

Maturana, H. R., & Varela, F. J. (1992). *The tree of knowledge: The biological roots of human understanding.* Boston: Shambhala (Random House).

McCubbin, H. I., & Patterson, J. M. (1983). The family stress process: The double ABCX model of adjustment and adaptation (pp. 7–27). In H. I. McCubbin, M. B. Sussman, & J. M. Patterson (Eds.), *Social stress and the family: Advances in Developments in Family Stress Theory and Research.* New York: Haworth.

McCubbin, M. A., & McCubbin, H. I. (1993). Family coping with illness: The Resiliency Model of Family Stress, Adjustment, and Adaptation. In C. Danielson, B. Hamel-Bissell, & P. Winstead-Fry (Eds.), *Families, health and illness: Perspectives on coping and intervention.* St. Louis, MO: CV Mosby.

McGoldrick, M. (2005). Becoming a couple. In B. Carter, & M. McGoldrick (Eds.), *The expanded family life cycle: Individual, family and social perspectives* (3rd ed., pp. 231–248). New York: Allyn & Bacon, Pearson Education Company.

Minuchin, S. (1974). *Families and family therapy.* Cambridge, MA: Harvard University Press.

Minuchin, S., & Fishman, H.G. (1981). *Family therapy techniques.* Cambridge, MA: Harvard University Press.

Minuchin, S., Rosman, B. L., & Baker, L. (1978). *Psychosomatic families: Anorexia nervosa in context.* Cambridge, MA: Harvard University Press.

Neuman, B. (1983). Family intervention using the Betty Neuman health care systems model. In I. W. Clements, & F. B. Roberts (Eds.), *Family health: A theoretical approach to nursing care.* New York: John Wiley.

Neuman. B. (1995). *The Neuman systems model* (3rd ed.). Stanford, CT: Appleton & Lange.

Neuman, B. (2001). The Neuman systems model. In B. Neuman, & J. Fawcett (Eds.), *The Neuman systems model* (4th ed.). Upper Saddle River, NJ: Prentice Hall.

Neuman, B, & Fawcett, J. (2001). *The Neuman systems model* (4th ed.). Upper Saddle River, NJ: Prentice Hall.

Nichols, M. P. (2004). *Family therapy: Concepts and methods* (6th ed.). Boston: Pearson/Allyn & Bacon.

Nightingale, F. (1859). *Notes on Nursing: What it is, and what it is not.* London: Harrison. Reprinted 1980. Edinburgh, NY: Churchill Livingstone.

Nye, F. I. (1976). *Role structure and analysis of the family, Vol. 24.* Beverly Hills, CA: Sage.

Nye, F. I., & Berardo, F. (Eds.). (1981). *Emerging conceptual frameworks in family analysis.* New York: Praeger.

Orem, D. (1983a). The family coping with a medical illness: Analysis and application of Orem's theory. In I. Clements, & F. Roberts (Eds.), *Family health: A theoretical approach to nursing care.* New York: John Wiley.

Orem, D. (1983b). The family experiencing emotional crisis: Analysis and application of Orem's self-care deficit theory. In I. Clements, & F. Roberts (Eds.), *Family health: A theoretical approach to nursing care.* New York: John Wiley.

Orem, D. (1985). *Nursing: Concepts of practice* (3rd ed.). New York: McGraw-Hill.

Parker, M. (2005). *Nursing theories and nursing practice.* Philadelphia: F.A. Davis.

Parse, R. R. (1992). Human becoming: Parse's theory of nursing. *Nursing Science Quarterly, 5,* 35–42.

Parse, R. R. (1998). *The human becoming school of thought: A perspective for nurses and other health professionals.* Thousand Oaks, CA: Sage.

Pender, N. J., Murdaugh, C. L., & Parsons, M. A. (2006). *Health promotion in nursing practice* (5th ed.). Upper Saddle River, NJ: Prentice Hall.

Polit, D., & Beck, C. (2008). *Nursing research: Generating and assessing evidence for nursing practice* (8th ed.). Philadelphia: Lippincott Williams & Wilkins.

Powers, B., & Knapp, T. (2005). *A dictionary of nursing theory and research* (3rd ed.). New York: Spring Publishing Company, Incorporated.

Rogers, M. (1970). *Introduction to the theoretical basis of nursing.* Philadelphia: F.A. Davis.

Rogers, M. (1986). Science of unitary human beings. In V. Malinski (Ed.), *Explorations on Martha Rogers' science of unitary human beings* (pp. 3–8). Norwalk, CT: Appleton-Century-Crofts.

Rogers, M. (1990). Nursing: Science of unitary, irreducible, human being: Update, 1990. In E. Barret (Ed.), *Visions of Rogers' science-based nursing* (pp. 5–11). New York: National League for Nursing.

Rolland, J. S. (1984). Toward a psychosocial typology of chronic and life-threatening illness. *Family Systems Medicine, 2,* 245–263.

Rolland, J. S. (1987). Chronic illness and the life cycle: A conceptual framework. *Family Process, 26*(2), 203–221.

Rolland, J. S. (2005). Chronic illness and the family life cycle. In B. Carter, & M. McGoldrick (Eds.), *The expanded family life cycle: Individual, family and social perspectives* (3rd ed., pp. 492–511). New York: Allyn & Bacon, Pearson Education Company.

Rose, A. M. (1962). *Human behavior and social processes.* Boston: Houghton Mifflin.

Roy, C. (1976). *Introduction to nursing: An adaptation model.* Englewood Cliffs, NJ: Prentice-Hall.

Roy, C., & Roberts, S. (1981). *Theory construction in nursing: An adaptation model.* Englewood Cliffs, NJ: Prentice-Hall.

Satir, V. (1982). The therapist and family therapy: Process model. In A. M., Horne & M. M. Ohlsen (Eds.), *Family counseling and therapy* (pp. 12–42). Itasca, IL: F.E. Peacock.

Segaric, C., & Hall, W. (2005). The family theory-practice gap: A matter of clarity? *Nursing Inquiry, 12*(3), 210–218.

Smith, S. R., Hamon, R. R., Ingoldsby, B. B., & Miller, J. E. (2008). *Exploring family theories* (2nd ed). New York: Oxford University Press.

Toman, W. (1961). *Family constellation: Its effects on personality and science behavior.* New York: Springer.

Turner, R. H. (1970). *Family interaction.* New York: John Wiley & Sons.

von Bertalanffy, L. V. (1950). The theory of open systems in physics and biology. *Science, 111,* 23–29.

von Bertalanffy, L. W. (1968). *General systems theory: Foundations, development, and applications.* New York: George Braziller.

Walker, P. H. (2005). Neumann's systems model. In J. J. Fitzpatrick, & A. L. Whall (Eds.), *Conceptual models of nursing: Analysis and application* (4th ed., pp. 194–224). Upper Saddle River, NJ: Pearson Prentice Hall.

Watzlawick, P., Beavin, J., & Jackson, D. (1967). *Pragmatics of human communication.* New York: W.W. Norton.

Watzlawick, P., Weakland, J., & Fisch, R. (1974). *Change: Principles of problem formulation and problem resolution.* New York: W.W. Norton.

White, J. M. (2005). *Advancing family theories.* Thousand Oaks, CA: Sage.

White, J. M., & Klein, D. M. (2002). *Family theories* (2nd ed.). Thousand Oaks, CA: Sage.

White, J. M., & Klein, D. M. (2008). *Family theories* (3rd ed.). Los Angles, CA: Sage.

Wikipedia. (2008). *Urie Bronfenbrenner.* Retrieved February 9, 2008, from http://en.wikipedia.org/wiki/Urie_Bronfenbrenner

Wilkerson, S., & Loveland-Cherry, C. (2005). Johnson's behavioral systems model. In J. J. Fitzpatrick, & A. L. Whall (Eds.), *Conceptual models of nursing: Analysis and application* (4th ed., pp. 83–103). Upper Saddle River, NJ: Pearson Prentice Hall.

Wright, L., & Leahey, M. (2005). *Nurses and families, A guide to family assessment and intervention* (4th ed.). Philadelphia: F.A. Davis.

Wright, L. M., & Watson, W. L. (1988). Systemic family therapy and family development. In C. J. Falicox (Ed.), *Family transitions: Continuity and change over the life cycle* (pp. 407–430). New York: Guilford Press.

CHAPTER 4

Family Nursing Process: Family Nursing Assessment Models

Joanna Rowe Kaakinen, PhD, RN

CRITICAL CONCEPTS

✦ Families are complex social systems, so the use of a logical systematic Family Nursing Process approach is important.

✦ In the context of family nursing, the creative nurse thinker must be aware of possibilities, be able to recognize the new and the unusual, be able to decipher unique and complex situations, and be inventive in designing an approach to family care.

✦ Nurses determine through which theoretical and practice lens the family event will be analyzed.

✦ Nurses begin family assessment from the moment of referral.

✦ Conducting family interviews requires knowledge of family assessment and intervention models, as well as skilled organizational communication techniques so that the interaction will be effective and efficient for all parties.

✦ The family genogram and ecomap are both assessment data-gathering instruments. The therapeutic interaction that occurs with the family while diagramming a genogram or ecomap is a powerful intervention in and of itself.

✦ Nurses need to approach assessment of family health literacy with sensitivity and understanding, because it is a crucial element to successful outcomes.

✦ One of the most critical aspects of family nursing is to encourage and seek family involvement in the decision-making process to plan family care.

✦ Nurses need to tailor their work with families based on the level of involvement preferred by the family, and the health literacy needs of the family.

(continued)

- ✦ Nurses and families who work together and build on family strengths are in the best positions to determine and prioritize the family needs, develop realistic outcomes, and design a plan of action that has a high probability of being implemented by the family.
- ✦ What the families perceive as important is critical to successful planning and implementation.
- ✦ The more specific the family interventions are, the more positive the outcomes.
- ✦ Nurses work with families to evaluate the ongoing family care plan and modify the course of action as needed.
- ✦ The final step in the Family Nursing Process should always be for nurses to engage in critical, creative, and concurrent reflection about the family, their work with the family, and professional self-reflection of their practice.

Families are complex social systems. Therefore, the use of logical, systematic approaches to family clients is essential for several reasons: (1) to assure that the needs of the family are met, (2) to uncover any gaps in the family plan of action, and (3) to offer multiple supports and resources to the family. Nurses use a variety of assessment models to collect information about families. In concert with the family, this information is used to develop the interventions families use to manage their current health event. Some assessment and intervention instruments are based on theoretical models, and some are developed using a psychometric approach to instrument development. Built on the traditional nursing process as visualized by Doegnes, Moorhouse, and Murr (2008) (Fig. 4-1) and combined with the Outcome Present State Testing Model (Pesut & Herman, 1999), this chapter presents a dynamic systematic Family Nursing Process (Fig. 4-2) approach and applies it to a case study. The chapter explores assessment strategies, including how to select assessment instruments, determine the need for interpreters, assess for health literacy, diagram family genograms, and develop family ecomaps. Intervention strategies follow assessment strategies to assist nurses and families in shared decision making. The chapter concludes

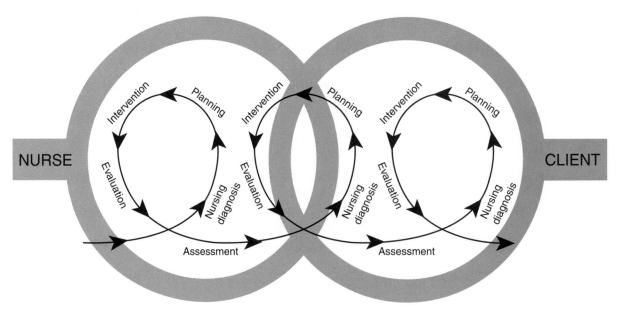

FIGURE 4-1 Nursing process model.

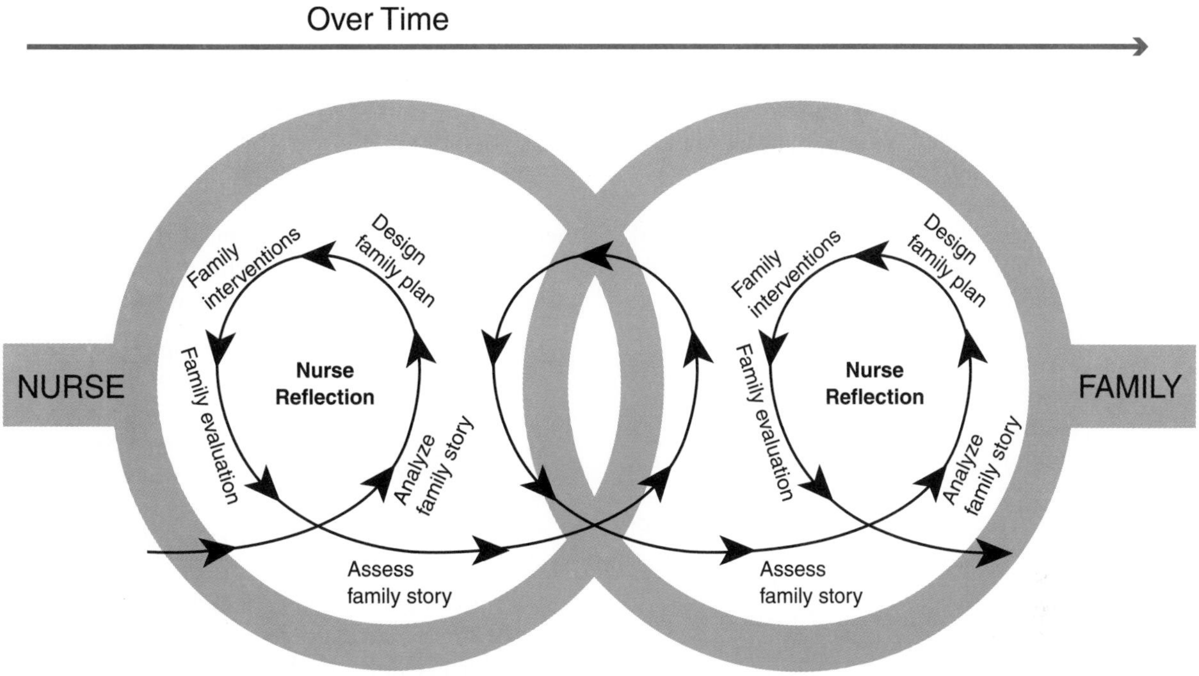

Over Time

FIGURE 4-2 Family nursing process model.

with a brief introduction to three family assessment and intervention models that were developed by nurses.

FAMILY NURSING PROCESS

Central to the delivery of safe and effective family nursing care is the nurse's ability to make accurate assessments, identify health problems, and tailor plans of care. Each step of working with families, whether applied to individuals within the family or the family as a whole, requires a thoughtful, deliberate reasoning process. Nurses decide what data to collect and how, when, and where that data are collected. Nurses determine the relevance of each new piece of information and how it fits into the emerging family story. Before moving forward, nurses decide whether they have obtained sufficient information on problem and strength identification, or whether gaps exist that require additional data gathering. Each family situation evolves as it is analyzed, and each item of new information must be evaluated for accuracy, clarity, and relevance.

Nurses must always be aware that "common" interpretations of data may not be the "correct"

interpretation in any given situation, and that commonly expected signs and symptoms may not appear in every case or in the same data pattern presentation. The ability of nurses to be open to the unexpected and to be alert to unusual or different responses is critical to determining the primary needs confronting the family. Nurses should be able to see that which is not obvious and to understand how this family story is similar or different from other family stories.

The steps of the Family Nursing Process include:

- Assessment of the family story: The nurse gathers data from a variety of sources to see the whole picture of the family experience.
- Analysis of family story: The nurse clusters the data into meaningful patterns to see how the family is managing the health event. The family needs are prioritized using a Family Reasoning Web.
- Design of a family plan of care: Together, the nurse and family determine the best plan of care for the family to manage the situation.
- Family intervention: Together, the nurse and family implement the plan of care incorporating the most family-focused, cost-effective, and efficient interventions that assist the family to achieve the best possible outcomes.

- Family evaluation: Together, the nurse and family determine whether the outcomes are being reached, partially reached, or need to be redesigned. Is the care plan working well, does a new care plan need to be put into place, or does the nurse/family relationship need to end?
- Nurse reflection: Nurses engage in critical, creative, and concurrent reflection about the family and their work with the family.

Assessment of the Family Story

Nurses encounter families in diverse health care settings for many different kinds of problems and circumstances. Every family has a story about how the potential or actual health event influences its individual members, family functioning, and management of the health event. Nurses filter data gathered in the story through different views or approaches, which affects how they think about the family as a whole and each individual family member. For example, a family who is faced with a new diagnosis of a chronic illness would have different needs than a family who is faced with a member dying of an end-stage chronic illness. Nurses might use different strategies if the patient is in the acute hospital setting, is in an assisted living center, or is living at home. Another example of how nurses would use a different approach to work with a family is when the family member who has been diagnosed with a serious illness is the mother, usually the primary caregiver of the child(ren). In this scenario, the other members of the family are more significantly affected by the illness than they would be if the family member who is ill were the grandfather, who is less central to family functioning because of his age.

The underlying family theoretical approach used by the nurses working with families influences how they ask questions and collect family data. For example, if the family is worried about how their 2-year-old child will react to the new baby, such as in the Bono family case study presented later in this chapter, the nurse may elect to base the assessment and interventions on a family systems theoretical view, or the developmental family life cycle theoretical view. Refer to Chapter 3 for a detailed discussion of working with families from different theoretical perspectives.

Data collection, which is part of assessment, involves both subjective and objective family data that are obtained through direct observation, examination, or in consultation with other health care providers (HCPs). The specific assessment strategies nurses use depend on the reason they are working with the family. In all cases, family assessment begins from the first moment that the family is referred to the nurse. Following are some circumstances in which a family is referred to a nurse:

1. A family is referred by the hospital to a home health agency for wound care on the feet of a client with diabetes.
2. A family calls the Visiting Nurse Association to request assistance in providing care to a family member with increasing dementia.
3. A school nurse is asked to conduct a family assessment by the school psychologist who is investigating potential child neglect issues.
4. A physician requests a family assessment with a child who has nonorganic failure to thrive.

MAKING APPOINTMENTS

As soon as the family is identified, nurses begin to collect data about the family story. Sources of data that can be collected before contacting a family for a home or clinic appointment are listed in Box 4-1. Specifically, the nurse needs to know the following information:

- The reason for the referral or requested visit
- The family knowledge of the visit or referral

BOX 4-1

Sources of Pre-encounter Family Data

- Referral source: includes data that indicated a problem for this family, as well as demographic information
- Family: includes family members' views of the problem, surprise that the referral was made, reluctance to set up the meeting, avoidance in setting up the appointment
- Previous records: in the health care systems or that are sent by having the client sign a release for information form, such as process logs, charts, phone logs, or school records

- Specific medical information about the family member with the health problem
- Strategies that have been used previously
- Insurance sources for the family
- Family problems identified by other health providers
- The need for an interpreter

Before contacting the family to arrange for the initial appointment, the nurse decides whether the most appropriate place to conduct the appointment is in the family's home or the clinic/office. The type of agency where the nurse works may dictate this decision. For instance, home health agencies provide nursing in the home, or mental health agencies require family meetings to occur in the neighborhood clinic office. Advantages and disadvantages of a home setting and a clinic setting are listed in Table 4-1.

Contacting the family for the appointment provides valuable information about the family. It is imperative that the nurse be confident and organized when making the initial contact. Information that is important for the nurse to note is whether the family acts surprised that the referral was made, shows reluctance in setting up a meeting, or expresses openness about working together. The family also gathers important information about the nurse during the initial interaction. For example, family members will notice whether the nurse takes time to talk with them, uses a lot of words they did not understand, or appears organized and open to working with the family. Box 4-2 outlines steps to follow when making an appointment with a family.

USING INTERPRETERS WITH FAMILIES

It is critical for the nurse to determine whether an interpreter is needed during the family meeting, because the number of families who do not speak English is increasing. For 46 million Americans, English is not the primary language spoken in the home, and 21 million of these people speak English poorly or not at all (Khwaja et al., 2006). Language barriers have been found to complicate many aspects of patient care, including comprehension, adherence to plans of care, adverse health outcomes, compromised quality of care, avoidable expenses, dissatisfied families, and increased potential for medical mistakes (Flores, Abreu, Schwartz, & Hill, 2000; Schenker, Wang, Selig, Ng, & Fernandez, 2007). Thus, it is essential that nurses who are not bilingual use interpreters when working with non–English-speaking families.

The types of interpreters that nurses solicit to help work with families have the potential to influence the quality of the information exchanged and the family's ability to follow the suggested plan of

TABLE 4-1	
Advantages and Disadvantages of Home Visits Versus Clinic Visits	
HOME VISIT	**CLINIC VISIT**
Advantages	
- Opportunity to see the everyday family environment.	- Conducting the family appointment in the office or clinic allows for easier access to consultants.
- Observe typical family interactions because the family members are likely to feel more relaxed in their physical space.	- The family situation may be so strained that a more formal, less personal setting will facilitate discussions of emotionally charged issues.
- More family members may be able to attend the meeting.	
- Emphasizes that the problem is the responsibility of the whole family and not one family member.	
Disadvantages	
- Home may be the only sanctuary or safe place for the family or its members to be away from the scrutiny of others.	- May reinforce a possible culture gap between the family and the nurse.
- The nurse must be highly skilled in communication, specifically setting limits and guiding the interaction, or the visit may have a more social tone and not be efficient or productive.	

BOX 4-2

Setting up Family Appointments

- Introduce yourself.
- State the purpose of the requested meeting, including who referred the family to the agency.
- Do not apologize for the meeting.
- Be factual about the need for the meeting but do not provide details.
- Offer several possible times for the meeting, including late afternoon or evening.
- Let the family select the most convenient time that allows the majority of family members to attend.
- Offer services of an interpreter, if required.
- Confirm date, time, place, and directions.

action. One of the most common type of interpreters used are bilingual family members or friends, called *ad hoc family interpreters*. The problems of using family members as interpreters are that they have been found to buffer information, alter the meaning of the content, or make the decision for the person for whom they are interpreting (Ledger, 2002). The ad hoc family member interpreter has been found to lack important language skills, especially when it comes to medical interpretation (Khwaja et al., 2006; Ledger, 2002). If the ad hoc family member interpreter is a child, the information that is being discussed may be frightening or the topic may be too personal and sensitive (Ledger, 2002). Using ad hoc family interpreters also raises confidentially issues (Smettem, 1999). Therefore, it is not recommended that nurses use a family member for interpretation, especially if another choice is available.

If a qualified medical interpreter cannot come to the meeting in the family home, the nurse should plan to bring a speakerphone that can be plugged into the phone outlet in the home so that the professional interpreter can be involved in the conversation with the family. One of the problems with using an interpreter on the phone is that interpreters do not have the advantage of seeing the family members in person and cannot observe nonverbal communication (Bethell, Simpson, & Read, 2006; Herndon & Joyce, 2004). Also, the nurse should be aware that using a telephone interpreter introduces another outside person into the family setting, which

may be perceived as impersonal by the family (Bethell, Simpson, & Read, 2006).

FAMILY MEETING

During the initial interaction with families, it is critical for nurses to introduce themselves to the family, meet all the family members present, learn about the family members not present, clearly state the purpose for working with the family, outline what will happen during this session, and indicate the length of time the meeting will last. By introducing themselves, nurses set the tone for a therapeutic nurse-family client relationship, and send the message that all family members are important and affected by the health event(s) (Wright & Leahey, 2009). The nurse needs to develop a systematic plan for the first and all reoccurring family meetings.

Nurses who use a therapeutic approach to family meetings have found that their focus on family-centered care increased, and that their communication skills with families became more fluid with experience (Martinez, D'Artois, & Rennick, 2007). When nurses use therapeutic communication skills with families, the families report feeling a stronger rapport with the nurse, an increased frequency of communication between families and the nurse occurs, and families perceive these nurses to be more competent (Martinez, D'Artois, & Rennick, 2007).

Conducting family interviews not only requires skilled communication strategies but also requires knowledge of family assessment and intervention models. Nurses use a variety of data collection and assessment instruments to help gather information in a systematic and efficient manner. Therefore, it is important that the instruments be carefully selected so they are family friendly and render information pertinent to the purpose of working with the family.

SELECTING FAMILY ASSESSMENT INSTRUMENTS

Because there are approximately 1,000 family-focused instruments that have been developed and used in assessing family-related variables (Touliatos, Perlmutter, & Straus, 2001), the selection of the appropriate instrument can be complex. Sometimes, a simple questionnaire or instrument can be completed in just a few minutes. One such example is the *Patient/Parent Information and Involvement Assessment Tool (PINT),* which is an instrument that Sobo (2004) designed to assess the family's perspective on shared decision making. Other times, more comprehensive family assessment instruments are necessary, such as the Family Systems Stressor-Strength Inventory (FS³I) (Berkey-Mischke & Hanson, 1991; Hanson, 2001; Kaakinen & Hanson, 2005). The FS³I is an instrument designed by nurses to provide quantitative and qualitative data pertinent to family stressors, family strengths, and intervention strategies (see Appendix A). To select the most appropriate short assessment instrument, be sure the instrument has the following characteristics:

- Written in uncomplicated language at a fifth-grade level
- Only 10 to 15 minutes in length
- Relatively easy to score
- Offers valid data on which to base decisions
- Sensitive to sex, race, social class, and ethnic background

No matter which assessment/measurement instrument is used, families should always be informed of how the information gathered through the instruments will be used by the HCPs.

Two family data-gathering instruments that must always be used in working with families are the family genogram and the family ecomap. Both are short, easy instruments and processes that supply essential family data and engage the family in therapeutic conversation.

FAMILY GENOGRAM AND FAMILY ECOMAP

Genograms and ecomaps actively engage families in their own care and provide care providers with visual diagrams of the current family story and situation (Neufeld, Harrison, Hughes, & Stewart, 2007). The information gathered from both the genogram and ecomap help guide the family plan of action and the selection of intervention strategies (Ray & Street, 2005). One of the major benefits of working with families with these two instruments is that they can feel and visualize the amount of energy they are expending to manage the situation, which in itself is therapeutic for the family (Holtslander, 2005; Rempel, Neufeld, & Kushner, 2007).

FAMILY GENOGRAM

The *family genogram* is a format for drawing a family tree that records information about family members and their relationships over at least three generations (McGoldrick, Schellenberger, & Petry, 2008). This diagram offers a rich source of information for planning intervention strategies because it displays the family visually and graphically in a way that provides a quick overview of family complexities. Family genograms help both nurses and families to see and think systematically about families and the impact of the health event on family structure, function, and processes.

The three-generational family genogram had its origin in Family Systems Theory (Bowen, 1985; Bowen & Kerr, 1988). According to family systems, people are organized into family systems by generation, age, sex, or other similar features. How a person fits into his or her family structure influences his or her functioning, relational patterns, and what type of family he or she will carry forward into the next generation. Bowen incorporates Toman's (1976) ideas about the importance of sex and birth order in shaping sibling relationships and characteristics. Furthermore, families repeat themselves over generations in a phenomenon called the *transmission of family patterns* (Bowen, 1985). What happens in one generation repeats itself in the next generation; thus, many of the same strengths and problems get played out from generation to generation. These include both psychosocial and physical and mental health issues.

Nurses establish therapeutic relationships with families through the process of asking questions while collecting family data. Families become more engaged in their current situation during this interaction and as their family story unfolds. Both the nurse and the family can see the "big picture" historically on the vertical axis of the genogram and horizontally across the family (McGoldrick et al., 2008). The process can help families see connectedness, and help identify potential and missing support people.

The diagramming of family genograms must adhere to specific rules and symbols to assure all parties involved have the same understanding and interpretations. It is important not to confuse family genograms with a family genetic pedigree. A family pedigree is specific to genetic assessments (see Chapter 8), whereas a genogram has broader uses for family HCPs. Olsen, Dudley-Brown, and McMullen (2004) have suggested, however, that given the advancement of genomics in driving health care, nursing should consider blending pedigrees with genograms and ecomaps as a way to offer a more comprehensive holistic nursing care perspective.

Figure 4-3 provides a basic genogram from which a nurse can start diagramming family members over the first, second, and third generations (McGoldrick, Gerson, & Schellenberger, 1999). Figure 4-4 depicts the genogram symbols used to describe basic family membership and structure, family interaction patterns, and other family information of particular importance, such as health status, substance abuse, obesity, smoking, and mental health comorbidities (McGoldrick et al., 2008). The health history of all family members (e.g., morbidity, mortality, and onset of illness) is important information for family nurses and can be the focus of analysis of the family genogram. An example of a family genogram developed from one interview is contained in the Bono family case study in Figure 4-7.

The structure of the interview for gathering the genogram information is based on the reasons why the nurse is working with the family. A suggested format for conducting a concise, focused family genogram interview is outlined in Box 4-3. Most families are cooperative and interested in completing their genogram, which becomes a part of their ongoing health care record. The genogram does not have to be completed at one sitting. As the same or a different nurse continues to work with a family,

---

BOX 4-3
Family Genogram Interview Data Collection

1. Identify who is in the immediate family.
2. Identify the person who has the health problem.
3. Identify all the people who live with the immediate family.
4. Determine how all the people are related.
5. Gather the following information on each family member.
   - Age
   - Sex
   - Correct spelling of name
   - Health problems
   - Occupation
   - Dates of relationships: marriage, separation, divorce, living together, living together/committed
   - Dates and age of death
6. Seek the same information for the family members on the same generational level and for those in the preceding generational level.
7. Add any additional information relative to the situation, such as geographic location and interaction patterns.

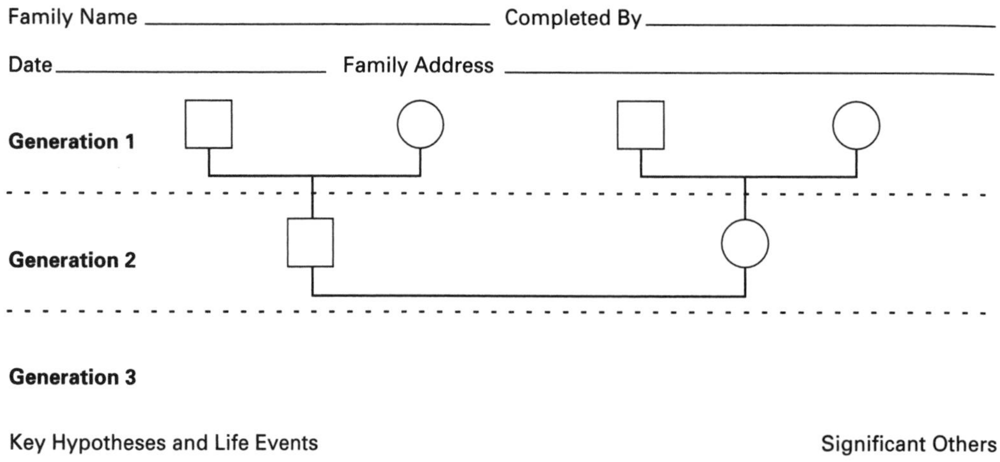

Family Name _____ Completed By _____

Date _____ Family Address _____

Generation 1

Generation 2

Generation 3

Key Hypotheses and Life Events   Significant Others

FIGURE 4-3 Basic genogram format.

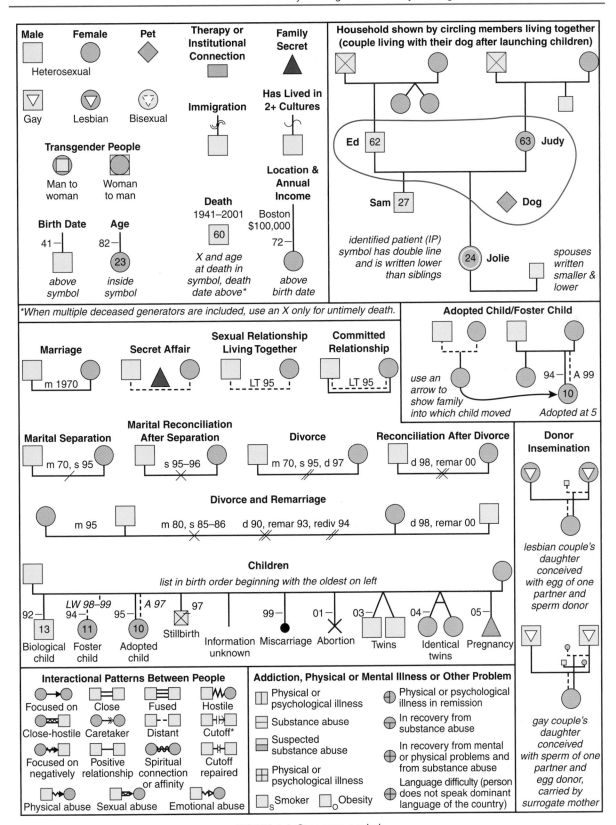

FIGURE 4-4 Genogram symbols.

data can be added to the genogram over time in a continuing process. Families should be given a copy of their own genogram.

FAMILY ECOMAP

A *family ecomap* provides information about systems outside of the immediate nuclear family that are sources of social support or that are stressors to the family (Olsen et al., 2004). The ecomap is a visual representation of the family unit in relation to the larger community in which it is embedded (Kaakinen & Hanson, 2005). It is a visual representation of the relationship between an individual family and the world around it (McGoldrick et al., 2008). The ecomap is thus an overview of the family in its current situation, picturing the important connections among the nuclear family, the extended family, and the community around it.

The blank ecomap form consists of a large circle with smaller circles around it (Fig. 4-5). A simplified version of the family is placed in the center of the larger circle to complete the ecomap. This circle marks the boundary between the family and its extended external environment. The smaller outer circles represent significant people, agencies, or institutions with whom the family interacts. Lines are drawn between the circles and the family members to depict the nature and quality of the relationships, and to show what kinds of energy and resources are moving in and out of the immediate family. Straight lines show strong or close relationships; the more pronounced the line or greater the number of lines, the stronger the relationship is. Straight lines with slashes denote stressful relationships, and broken lines show tenuous or distant relationships. Arrows reveal the direction of the flow of energy and resources between individuals, and between the family and the environment. See the Bono family case study later in this chapter for an example of a completed ecomap (see Fig. 4-8).

The ecomap organizes factual information to provide a more integrated perception of the family situation in relationship to their larger context. Ecomaps not only portray the present situation but also can be used to set goals, for example, to

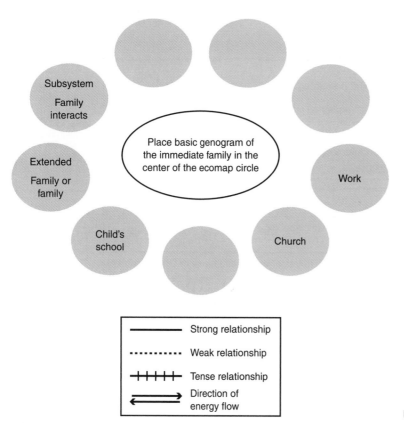

FIGURE 4-5 Blank ecomap.

increase connections and exchanges with individuals and agencies in the community.

The value of using a genogram and ecomap in family nursing practice is expansive. When nurses and families establish an underlying foundation of mutual respect, nurses can ask the family more intimate questions, and thus be more actively involved in their health care management process (Rempel et al., 2007). Through these processes of data collection, patterns of health problems may surface that could benefit from more family education. By creating a visual picture of the system in which the family exists, families are more able to envision alternative solutions and possible social support networks (Ray & Street, 2005; Yanicki, 2005). In addition, the process of this data collection itself helps to expose a clearer picture of the supportive or unsupportive family relationships that are going on in a family system (Neufeld et al., 2007). This information will enhance understanding of the family's social network with their caregivers (Ray & Street, 2005).

FAMILY HEALTH LITERACY

Health literacy is the ability to use health information to make informed decisions through the comprehension of reading material, documents, and numbers. Functional health literacy incorporates all of these elements, but it also implies that the client (family) has the ability to act on health care decisions. Concepts of health literacy include the comprehension of medical words, the ability to follow medical instructions, and the understanding of the consequences when instructions are not followed (Speros, 2005).

Through interactions with the family and when completing the genogram and ecomap, nurses have the opportunity to determine whether there is an issue of health literacy for any member of the family. Health literacy is an important measure for HCPs because lower health literacy is strongly associated with poor health outcomes (DeWalt, Berkman, Sheridan, Lohr, & Pignone, 2004; Sentell & Halpin, 2006; Speros, 2005). Health literacy plays a primary role in people's ability to gain knowledge, make decisions, and take actions that result in positive health outcomes (DeWalt, Boone, & Pignone, 2007; Speros, 2005), especially when managing a chronic illness (Gazmararian, Williams, Peel, & Baker, 2003). Assessment is particularly important when low literacy or low language proficiency exist, because

such individuals are more likely to attempt to hide their inability to read or understand because of shame or embarrassment (Bass, 2005; Dreger & Tremback, 2002).

When nurses design written material for the family, the following common elements make the plan easier to understand from a health literacy perspective (Bass, 2005; Peters, Dieckmann, Dixon, Hibbard, & Mertz, 2007):

- All written information should be in at least 14-point font using high-contrast Arial or sans serif print with plenty of blank space on glossy paper.
- Uppercase and lowercase letters should be used.
- Information is most easily seen when using black ink on white paper. Use short sentences with bullets or lists no longer than seven items (Peters et al., 2007).

Written information presented at the third-grade reading level will reach the largest audience, but it may be necessary to write at the fifth-grade level to retain the meaning of the content (Mayer & Rushton, 2002; Peters et al., 2007). Using multiple forms of communication in working with the family will help families retain the information (Bass, 2005; Dreger & Tremback, 2002). Retention of information and medical teaching were found to be advantageous when visual materials were used in combination with visual instructions (Houts et al., 1998).

Nurses need to tailor their work with families to the level of involvement expressed by the families and their health literacy needs. Building on family strengths together, nurses and families are in the best position to determine the priority family needs, develop realistic outcomes, and design a plan of action that has a high probability of being implemented by the family.

Nurses need to approach assessment of the family health literacy with sensitivity and understanding. It is a crucial element to take into consideration during the analysis of the family story and in the development of the family action plan.

Analysis of the Family Story

One of the challenges of data collection is organizing the individual pieces of information so that the "big picture" or whole family story can be understood. To understand the family picture, the nurse must consolidate the data that were collected into meaningful patterns or categories so that the relationships between and among the patterns of how the family is managing the situation can be visualized. Diagramming the family and the relationships between the data groups assists in the identification of the most pressing issues or problems for the family. If the family and nurse focus on solving these major family problems, the outcome will have a ripple effect by positively influencing the other areas of family functioning.

The Family Reasoning Web (Fig. 4-6) is an organizational tool to help cluster individual pieces of data into meaningful family categories. The components of the Family Reasoning Web have been pulled from various theoretical concepts, such as Family Structure and Function Theory, Family Developmental Theory, Family Stress Theory, and family health promotion models. This systematic approach to collecting and analyzing information helps structure the information collection process to ensure inclusion of important pieces of information. The categories of the Family Reasoning Web are:

1. Family routines of daily living (i.e., sleeping, meals, child care, exercise)
2. Family communication
3. Family supports and resources
4. Family roles
5. Family beliefs
6. Family developmental stage
7. Family health knowledge
8. Family environment
9. Family stress management
10. Family culture
11. Family spirituality

Once the data have been placed into the categories of the Family Reasoning Web template, the nurse assigns a family nursing diagnosis to each category. "A nursing diagnosis is defined as a clinical judgment about individuals, families, or community responses to actual or potential health problems/life processes. Nursing diagnoses link information to care planning. Nursing diagnoses provide the basis for selecting nursing interventions to help achieve outcomes for which nurses are accountable" (Doegnes, Moorhouse, & Murr, 2008, p. 10).

The North American Nurses Diagnosis Association (NANDA; 2007) is the most global nursing classification system. NANDA nursing diagnoses that are specific to families are listed in Box 4-4. If the pattern of family data in the specific category in

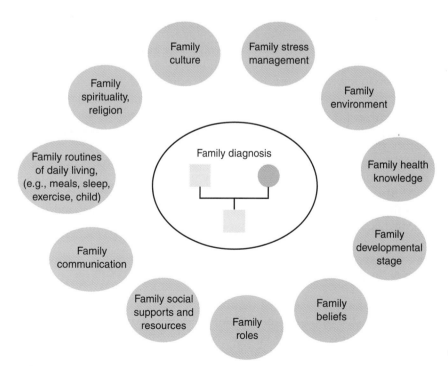

FIGURE 4-6 Family Reasoning Web template.

BOX 4-4

NANDA Nursing Diagnoses Relevant to Family Nursing

- Risk for impaired parent/infant/child attachment
- Caregiver role strain
- Risk for caregiver role strain
- Parental role conflict
- Compromised family coping
- Disabled family coping
- Readiness for enhanced family coping
- Dysfunctional family processes: alcoholism
- Readiness for enhanced family processes
- Interrupted family processes
- Readiness for enhanced parenting
- Impaired parenting
- Risk for impaired parenting
- Relocation stress syndrome
- Ineffective role performance
- Ineffective family therapeutic regimen management

Source: Doegnes, M. E., Moorchouse, M. F., & Murr, A. C. (2008). *Nursing diagnosis manual: Planning, individualizing, and documenting client care* (2nd ed.). Philadelphia: F.A. Davis.

TABLE 4-2

Selected Family-Centered Diagnoses From *Diagnostic and Statistical Manual of Mental Disorders, Fourth Edition, Text Revision*

V61.9	Relational problem related to a mental disorder or general medical condition
V61.20	Parent-child relational problem
V61.10	Partner relational problem
V61.8	Sibling relational problem
V71.02	Child or adolescent antisocial behavior
V62.82	Bereavement
V62.3	Academic problem
V62.4	Acculturation problem
V62.89	Phase-of-life problem

Source: American Psychiatric Association. (2000). *Diagnostic and statistical manual of mental disorders (DSM-IV-TR)* (4th ed.). Washington, DC: Author.

the family reasoning web does not match a NANDA nursing diagnoses, nurses are encouraged to create a family nursing diagnosis that captures the family problem. Nursing diagnoses manuals are extremely important resources for nurses because family nursing diagnoses are readily linked with both the Nursing Intervention Classification (NIC) (McCloskey & Bulechek, 2004) and Nursing Outcomes Classification (NOC) (Moorhead, Johnson, & Maas, 2004) data sets. These resources provide many new ideas for family interventions and suggest focused family outcomes that can be explored with families.

Other diagnostic classification systems that can be used to identify problems include the Omaha System-Community Health Classification System (Martin, 2004), the *Diagnostic and Statistical Manual of Mental Disorders, Fourth Edition* (DSM-IV-TR; American Psychiatric Association, 2000), and the *International Classification of Diseases: Clinical Modifications, Ninth Edition* (ICD-9-CM; American Medical Association, 2007). See Tables 4-2 and 4-3, respectively, for examples of selected family diagnoses from the DSM and ICD-9-CM sources.

After the categories have been assigned a nursing diagnosis, the nurse and family work together to determine the relationships between the categories. Arrows are drawn between the family categories showing the direction of influence if the data in one category influence the data in another category. The important family problems or issues surface by systematically working through all of the relationships because they are the ones that have the most arrows indicating the strongest

TABLE 4-3

Selected Family-Centered Diagnoses From ICD-9-CM

313.3	Relationship problems
313.8	Emotional disturbances of childhood or adolescence
V61.0	Family disruption
V25.09	Family planning advice
V61.9	Family problem
94.41	Group therapy
94.42	Family therapy

Source: American Medical Association. (2007). *International classification of diseases: Clinical modifications (IDC-9-CM)* (10th ed.). Dover, DE: Author.

relationships to all other areas of family functioning. After the primary family problems have been identified and verified with the family, the next step is to work with the family to design a family plan of care.

Designing a Family Plan of Care

The family plan of care is designed by the nurse and the family to focus on the concerns that were identified in the family reasoning web as the most pressing or causing the family the most stress. One of the most crucial aspects of family nursing is encouraging and seeking family involvement in planning care and in the decision-making processes. Universal needs of families include consistency, clarity, comprehensive information, and involvement in shared decision making with HCPs (Claassen, 2000; Salmond, 2008; Schattner, Bronstein, & Jellin, 2006; Whitmer, Hughes, Hurst, & Young, 2005). Nurses, consciously and unconsciously, affect the family stress level by controlling how much (and how fast) they involve the family in the care of their family members (Corlett & Twycross, 2006). Nurses control how much information they share with families, how much they involve the family in the daily routine, visiting hours, and even discussions with/among family members. Families have expressed fears of alienating the HCPs (Taylor, 2006), thus compromising their loved ones' care. All of this may interfere with nurses being able to be effective family advocates (Leske, 2002).

HCPs underestimate the extent that families want to be involved in the care of loved ones (Bruera, Sweeny, Calder, Palmer, & Benisch-Tolly, 2001; Pierce & Hicks, 2001). Although most families prefer a shared decision-making approach (de Haes, 2006; Schattner, Bronstein, & Jellin, 2006; Whitmer et al., 2005), families vary relative to the amount of information they want and their role in the decision-making process (Sobo, 2004). The amount of information families seek or need varies over the course of the health event, varies with the stage of the illness, and varies with the likelihood of a cure (Butow, Maclean, Dunn, Tattersall, & Boyer, 1997).

Sobo (2004) developed the *PINT*, which is a self-administered survey instrument that can be kept in the medical record to facilitate and target information for communication between the health care team and the family. In the challenge to collaborate in the care and meet the needs of individuals and family members, nurses may ask the following two sample questions from the *PINT* tool (Sobo, p. 258):

1. When possible, what level of information would you prefer to receive?
   - The simplest information possible
   - More than the simplest, but want to keep it on everyday terms
   - In-depth information that you can help me understand
   - As much in-depth and detailed information as can be provided
2. When possible, what decision-making role do you want to assume?
   - Leave all decisions to the health care team
   - Have the care team make the decisions about care with serious consideration of our views
   - Share in the making of the decisions with the health care team
   - Make all the decisions about care with serious consideration of the health care team advice
   - Make all decisions about care

Supporting the hypothesis that not all families and family members want full involvement in making health care decisions, Makoul and Clayman (2006) have outlined the following nine options for shared decision making (p. 307):

- Doctor alone
- Doctor led and patient acknowledgment sought or offered
- Doctor led and patient agreement sought or offered
- Doctor led and patient views/option sought or offered
- Shared equally
- Patient led and doctor views/opinions sought or offered
- Patient led and doctor agreement sought or offered
- Patient led and doctor acknowledgment sought or offered
- Patient alone

One of the problems with the implementation of shared decision making is that every HCP has a different definition and understanding of the components of this concept (Makoul & Clayman, 2006). Shared decision making is not just informing the family of the decisions and keeping the lines of communication open, nor is it the HCPs determining what decisions the family can make. Shared decision making requires that HCPs tailor their communication, accommodate their talk to the level of the family, and present information in a way that allows the family to make informed choices. Shared decision making includes the following steps as outlined by Makoul and Clayman (pp. 305–306):

- The family and HCP must define and agree on the health problem that is confronting the family member.
- The HCP presents and discusses options of care in a way that invites family questions.
- The family and HCP discuss pros and cons of options, including cost benefits, convenience, and financial costs.
- The family and HCP discuss values and preferences including ideas, concerns, and outcome expectations.
- The family and HCP discuss ability and confidence to follow through with steps or regimen for each option.
- Both the HCP and family should check and clarify for understanding the discussion and information shared.
- Both the HCP and family should reach a decision or defer decisions until an agreed-on, specified time.
- The HCP should follow up to track the outcome of the decision.

The more specific the family plan of care and the interventions, the more positive are the outcomes. The role of the nurse is to offer guidance to the family, provide information, and assist in the planning process. Working with families from an outcome perspective helps to clarify what information and resources are needed to address the family need. The following four points will help the family break the plan of care into action steps:

1. We need the following type of help.
2. We need the following information.
3. We need the following supplies.
4. We need to involve or tell the following people about our family action plan.

The plan should outline specifically who needs to do what by when. The last step of any family action plan needs to include evaluation.

Family Intervention

Nurses help families in the following ways: (1) providing direct care, (2) removing barriers to needed services, and (3) improving the capacity of the family to act on its own behalf and assume responsibility. One of the important aspects of working with the family is the nurse-family relationship, which is an intervention in and of itself (Friedman, Bowden, & Jones, 2003).

The nurse is responsible for helping the family implement the plan of care. The nurse can assume the role of teacher, role model, coach, counselor, advocate, coordinator, consultant, and evaluator in helping the family to implement the plan of the care they were intimately involved in creating. The types of interventions are limitless because they are designed with the family to meet their needs in the context of their family story.

Family Evaluation

In making clinical judgments, nurses engage in critical thinking to determine whether and to what extent they have met an outcome. Working with the family, decisions are made about whether to proceed as originally planned, to modify the family action plan, or to revisit the family story in total. As indicated previously, the Family Nursing Process is not linear. In practice, a constant flow occurs between the components of the Family Nursing Process model.

If not meeting expected outcomes, nurses should consider whether family apathy and indecision are the barriers. Family apathy may occur because of value differences between the nurse and the family. The family may be overcome with a sense of hopelessness, may view the problems or bureaucracy as too overwhelming, or may have a fear of failure. Nurses also should consider whether they themselves imposed barriers. A more detailed list of possible barriers to family outcomes can be found in Box 4-5.

Aside from evaluating outcomes, another important part of the family evaluation is the decision when to end the relationship with the family. Sometimes care with a family ends suddenly. In this case, it is important for nurses to determine the forces that

BOX 4-5
Barriers to Family Outcomes

- Family apathy
- Family indecision about the outcome or actions
- Nurse-imposed ideas
- Negative labeling
- Overlooking family strengths
- Neglecting cultural or gender implications
- Family perception of hopelessness
- Fear of failure
- Limited access to resources and support
- Limited finances
- Fear and distrust of health care system

brought about the closure. The family may be prematurely seeking to end the relationship, which may require a renegotiating process. The insurance or agency requirements may place a financial constraint on the amount of time nurses can work with a family. Other times, the family-nurse relationship comes to an end more naturally, as when the nurse and family together determine that the family has achieved the intended outcomes. Whatever the reason for the

end of the nurse-family relationship, it is crucial that closure be achieved between the parties.

Building closure into the family action plan will benefit the family by providing for a smooth transition process. Strategies often used in this transition include decreasing contact with the nurse, extending invitations to the family for follow-up, and making referrals when appropriate. If possible, this process should include a summary evaluation meeting where the nurse and family put formal closure to their relationship. Following up with a therapeutic letter can encourage families to continue positive adaptation. The therapeutic letter should include recognition of the family achievement, a summary of the actions, commendations to each family member, and an insightful question for the family to think about in the future that may provide the family a future direction (Wright, Watson, & Bell, 1996). An example of a therapeutic family letter is found in Box 4-6.

NURSE REFLECTION

The final step in the Family Nursing Process is for nurses to engage in critical, creative, and concurrent reflection about the family and their work with the

BOX 4-6
Example of Therapeutic Family Letter

Dear W, H, and T,

First I want to thank all of you for allowing me the opportunity to get acquainted with your family. I appreciated your openness and willingness to talk with me.

During our time together, we discussed several issues that were important to your family. One of these issues was the ongoing possibility of H losing his job because of the seasonal nature of his work. We explored the effects of potential job loss on a personal and family level.

H, you expressed some concern about your ability to provide adequately for your family. You indicated a personal constraining belief that a lack of steady employment meant that you were letting your family down and not providing for them. We discussed the idea that a paying job is only one part of the entire family support system that you provide. We explored some examples of noneconomic means of support, such as specific tasks related to farm chores, household

management, and child care. If your job situation changes again, I hope you will find some of these suggestions helpful.

W, I was so impressed with your ability to juggle your caregiving job with home, farm, kids, and spouse. I can't think of many women who could handle all of that with such strength and grace. With all that you do, it's not surprising that there isn't much time left over for your own personal endeavors. We discussed your constraining belief that you had to be responsible for everything. You envisioned the possibility of letting go of certain tasks and suggesting ways to share other tasks more equitably among family members. If you and your family choose to implement some tasks-sharing ideas, I sincerely hope this will work for all of you.

T, you have mapped out a path to higher education and a future career. You have every reason to expect success. We briefly touched upon what "success" might mean for you and whether success depends

---

BOX 4-6

Example of Therapeutic Family Letter—cont'd

on the university attended. I hope you will consider my thoughts in this regard. Whatever the outcome, you have the love and support of your parents.

Finally, I would like to commend all of you for your deep devotion to each other and for putting family first. You value family time, and you strive to communicate in a way that sustains your close relationship with each other.

I would like to invite W and H to consider a suggestion regarding making time for just the two of you. "Couple time" is easy to overlook when you are focused on creating a loving, stable home for E

and helping to launch T into higher education. Please remember that you two are the solid foundation of your family; the stronger your relationship is, the stronger your whole family can be.

As a result of our time spent together, I came away with the feeling that your family is exceptionally strong, deeply committed to one another, and fully capable of adapting to any of life's challenges. Thank you again for your time.

Best wishes to you and your family,
Suzanne Ahn, R.N., UP_FNP Student

---

family. This step has three distinct parts. One part is for the nurse to reflect on the success of the family outcome. Reflection entails thinking about your thought process relative to this family client. Nurses can link ideas and consequences together in logical sequences using an "if ... then ..." mental exercise. A comparative analysis approach of the family problem can be used to analyze the strengths and weaknesses of competing alternatives. The nurse may decide to reframe the family problem or priority need by attributing a different meaning to the content or context of the family situation based on testing, judgment, or changes in the context or content of the family story (Pesut & Herman, 1999).

The second purpose of reflection is for nurses to build on their expertise by reflecting on client stories and their practice with each family. In essence, nurses create a library of family stories so that each time they come upon a similar family story, they can pull ideas from previous experiences. This aspect of reflection assists nurses with pattern recognition.

The third purpose of reflection is to engage in self-reflection and self-evaluation. By using this critical thinking strategy, nurses learn from mistakes and cement patterns of actions that assist them to advance in their nursing practice from novice to expert family nurse.

Now that we have gone through the nursing process, it is time to apply it to a family.

Family Case Study

In preparation for her appointment with the Bono family, in the mother-baby clinic, Vicki reviews the chart notes written by the nurse midwife about the family and the delivery of Hannah. Vicki sees that the Bono family is coming in for a one week well-baby checkup of newborn infant Hannah and a follow-up with Libby, the mother, after her cesarean section (C-section) delivery 7 days ago. The note from the receptionist indicates that Libby expressed some concerns with her effectiveness in breast-feeding Hannah. The appointment book notes that the whole Bono family is coming for this visit. Vicki notes that the Bonos are a nuclear family that consists of a married

couple with two biological children. Figure 4-7 shows the Bono family genogram.

Knowing that this is a nuclear family coming in for a well-baby checkup, Vicki decides to use a Developmental Family Life Cycle theoretical approach to this family with a new member. (See Chapter 3 for details about this theoretical model.) Based on this approach, Vicki has many questions in her mind as she prepares for her appointment with the Bono family. The questions Vicki has about each family member and the whole family are presented in bulleted lists after a brief description of each family member.

Libby Bono is a 35-year-old mother recovering from a cesarean section delivery 7 days ago. She does not have any existing health problems. Libby's roles in the family

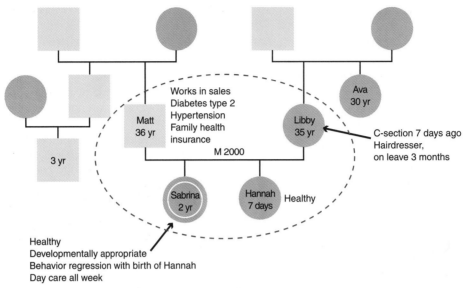

FIGURE 4-7 Bono family genogram.

are primary child-rearer, events planner, disciplinarian, and health expert. Libby is a hairdresser and is independently contracted with a hair salon. She has planned to take off 3 months for maternity leave.

◆ How might Libby's recovery from the cesarean section be affecting her roles in the family, especially with an active 2-year-old and a newborn?

◆ What are Libby's thoughts or plans for returning to work after her maternity leave?

◆ How is Libby is adjusting to her expanded mother role? Assess Libby for postpartum depression.

Matt Bono, 36 years old, works for Frito Lay Company in sales and distribution. His primary roles in the family are decision maker, maintenance person, pioneer, and information provider. He reports feeling little attachment to his occupation and welcomes this new birth as a change in routine and an opportunity to leave his place of employment. His current medical problems include type 2 diabetes and mild hypertension; both are well managed and controlled by oral diabetic and antihypertensive medications. Currently, he is following the Weight Watchers diet to reduce his weight and to control the symptomatology experienced from his health conditions.

◆ How is Matt adjusting to the expanded role of father of two daughters?

◆ What are Matt's plans for employment, specifically about financial support for the family if he leaves

his job? How would this affect health insurance for the family?

Sabrina Bono is a healthy 2-year-old girl who is developmentally appropriate. Psychologically, Sabrina is in the autonomy versus shame-and-doubt developmental stage. Her parents report that she often attempts to try new things on her own, and they frequently praise her efforts to promote independence. She is not yet interested in potty training. Her immunizations are current. She normally goes to a day care center that is close to her mother's work.

◆ How is Sabrina adjusting to the new baby?

◆ Is Sabrina showing any regression in her skills and abilities?

◆ Are each of the parents finding time to spend with Sabrina alone?

◆ How are the parents talking with Sabrina about her role as big sister?

Hannah Bono, 7 days old, was delivered after 42 weeks' gestation and was proved to be adequate for gestational age (AGA; 10th–90th percentile), 53.75 cm and 3,966 g, with APGAR (American Pediatric Gross Assessment Record) scores of 8 at 1 minute and 9 at 5 minutes.

◆ Is Hannah developing on target for her age and gestational age at birth?

◆ How often is Hannah eating, and is she gaining weight?

◆ How is Hannah nursing?

The Bono family is a nuclear family with the addition of second child.

- ✦ What are the major concerns for the family at this time?
- ✦ Who in the family is having the most difficult adjustment to the changes brought about by the addition of a new family member?
- ✦ How is the family adjusting to these changes?
- ✦ Who or what are the support systems for this new family?

FAMILY STORY

During the appointment, Vicki confirms that family life for the Bono family has changed. Hannah was found to be healthy and developmentally appropriate. Libby is healing well from the C-section, but reported occasional discomfort when she "overdoes it." Libby's concerns about breast-feeding were easily relieved as Vicki validated her breast-feeding technique. An assessment for postpartum depression revealed that Libby is not demonstrating any signs of depression at this time. Throughout the examination of Hannah, the parents demonstrated overwhelming signs of bonding, such as talking with the infant, and bragging about her beauty and temperament. During the appointment, Vicki noted that Sabrina was throwing toys and attempting to crawl onto her mother's lap while Libby was nursing Hannah. Sabrina would say "baby back" when she was upset. When Matt attempted to coddle or praise the baby, Sabrina became extremely angry with her father. They were not ignoring Sabrina but were not focused on her during the appointment. The parents' nonverbal actions showed frustration with Sabrina's behaviors. When asked, they reported that Sabrina has been very temperamental and inconsolable at day care. They reported that she had begun to show progress with toilet training before Hannah's birth but had now lost all interest.

ANALYSIS OF BONO FAMILY STORY

To help everyone see the larger family picture, Vicki uses the Family Reasoning Web (see Fig. 4-6). Based on the responses from using the web, the following family information was uncovered for analysis:

- ✦ Family routines of daily living: Matt and Libby are both tired from Hannah's every 3-hour breast-feeding schedule. They share some of the responsibility for comforting Hannah and seeing to her needs. Meals have been challenging as Matt has had to assume this responsibility because Libby has not recovered from her C-section. At this time,

they have do not have extended family support. Sabrina is still going to day care but is evidencing difficulty there.

- ✦ Family communication: Communication has been identified as a strength of the couple. They have a shared decision-making style. They appear nurturing with their children. Sabrina is emotionally up and down. She is clingy with her dad and ignores her mother except when she is breast-feeding Hannah. Sabrina was throwing toys when upset or frustrated. She periodically pointed to Hannah and said, "Take back."
- ✦ Family supports and resources: This family is fully covered under Matt's health insurance through his work. They have some family they can call on to help them. Ava, Libby's sister, volunteered to come for a visit and stay for 2 weeks. Matt's brother, his wife, and their 3-year-old child live in the same city. They have informally talked about sharing some child care. Both parents need to work to sustain their family lifestyle. Libby does not have benefits in her contracted hairdresser job. When she is off work, she does not make money. She does not have paid maternity leave. The couple planned for Libby to take 3 months off from work. The needs that were identified are for some immediate family support with everyday living and some financial concern at the end of the 3 months.
- ✦ Family roles: All of the family members are experiencing role ambiguity with their new roles. Matt and Libby are now parents of two daughters. Sabrina is a big sister, and Hannah is the new infant. Matt expressed some role overload with assuming many of the typical daily household chores of meals, laundry, food shopping, and primary care provider for Sabrina.
- ✦ Family beliefs: They strongly state that "family comes first." This was a planned pregnancy. They see themselves as loving parents. They express some confusion about disciplining Sabrina given her recent behaviors.
- ✦ Family developmental stage: This is a nuclear family in the family with toddler stage. They also have a new infant; therefore, they are in two developmental stages at the same time.
- ✦ Family health knowledge: The family expressed that they needed more help in knowing how to help Sabrina. They do not know how to work with Sabrina to help her adjust to being a big sister. They are confused with Sabrina's changes in

behavior of aggression, behavior swings, clinging, and pointing at the baby and saying "take back." They feel that she has lost some of her skills. Health literacy does not appear to be an issue.

✦ Family environment: At this time, they have enough room in their home for a family of four. They live in a safe neighborhood, but they state they do not know their neighbors well.

✦ Family stress management: They express feeling stressed about Sabrina's behaviors. They are both tired. Sabrina is stressed as evidenced by her behaviors and changes in behavior. They are dealing with the current situation on their own but are open to asking for help from family for the immediate assistance with daily living routines. They are open to learning more about how to help Sabrina.

✦ Family culture: They are white with Italian Catholic background. They are working lower-middle-class socioeconomic status.

✦ Family spiritually: They were both raised Catholic but are not practicing in their religion. They do not belong to a church. They describe themselves as spiritual.

The parents identified that both of them and Sabrina are having difficulty adjusting to the expansion of their family and the shift in their family roles. They state that they are most concerned with Sabrina's adjustment to the new baby. They state that they just do not know the best way to help her. They shared that they thought that since this was the "second time around" they believed they could be even better parents. They have been frustrated thinking about how to cope with what to do with two young children. The nursing diagnosis Readiness for Enhanced Parenting is related to the new role of parents of two children and is evidenced by parents' subjective statements about parenting, Sabrina's reactions to the new baby, and parents asking for information and help on sibling rivalry.

BONO FAMILY ACTION PLAN

Together, the nurse along with Matt and Libby review the family genogram (see Fig. 4-7), which helps the couple visualize their family. The parents decide that Ava is the best person to come to help at this time. They say they will talk later with Matt's brother

and family about sharing some child care. They complete a family ecomap (Fig. 4-8) to help assess what is creating stress and what could help alleviate family stress.

Vicki provides Matt and Libby with several educational packets about toddlers and new infants. She directs them to several online Web sites after she confirms that they have computer skills. They discuss ideas about how both parents can make personal time to spend with each daughter. They brainstorm ways to help Sabrina interact with Hannah but to keep Hannah safe from aggressive toddler behavior to a new sibling. They plan to talk with the day care providers so they can be effective with their help for Sabrina. They will call Ava as soon as they get home to plan for her visit. Vicki makes a follow-up appointment with the Bono family for their next well-baby visit and to see how they are progressing with both children.

EVALUATION

Vicki plans a follow-up phone call to check in with Libby and Matt. At the next visit, Vicki will revisit the family action plan with Libby and Matt to see whether their priority family concerns remain the same, or have decreased/increased or disappeared. Vicki plans to observe Sabrina's behaviors to see how she is coping and whether she is adapting in more positive ways. She will talk with the parents to assess their anxiety level. She will observe the parents and their interactions with both children.

NURSE REFLECTION

Vicki reflects about her work with the Bono family. She determines that her therapeutic communication skills were excellent. She showed empathy and validated the family's concern for the added stresses that a newborn child creates for a family. The 7-day old well-baby visit in the clinic setting presented an ideal time to observe and address parenting techniques and ease parental concerns. Learning how to shift focus from the more medical concern of the well-baby to family dynamics was the most challenging aspect, yet also the most rewarding. The interventions were appropriate and truly empowered their overall ability to cope and function as a family.

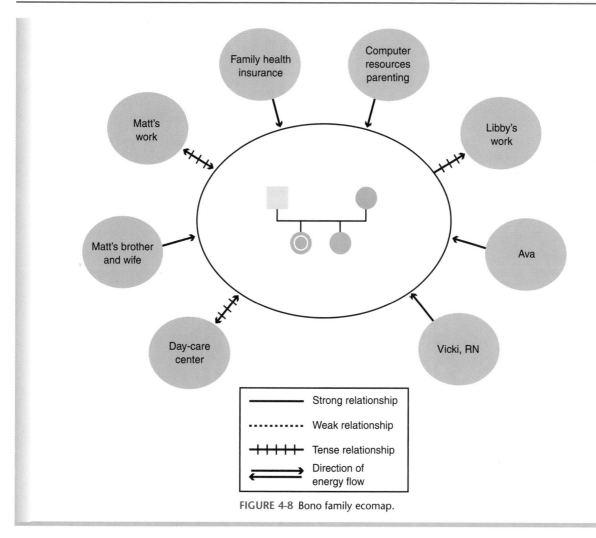

FIGURE 4-8 Bono family ecomap.

FAMILY NURSING ASSESSMENT MODELS

Nurses use a variety of ways to practice family nursing in addition to the family nursing process model presented earlier in this chapter. The following three family assessment models have been developed by family nurses. The Family Assessment and Intervention Model and the FS³I were developed by Berkey-Mischke and Hanson (1991). Friedman developed the Friedman Family Assessment Model (Friedman et al., 2003). The Calgary Family Assessment Model (CFAM) and Calgary Family Intervention Model (CFIM) were developed by Wright and Leahey (2009). These three approaches vary in purpose, unit of analysis, and

level of data collected. Table 4-4 has a detailed comparison of the essential components of these three family assessment models.

Family Assessment and Intervention Model

The *Family Assessment and Intervention Model,* originally developed by Berkey-Mischke and Hanson (1991), is presented in detail in Chapter 3. The model will be briefly reviewed here in the context of this chapter. The Family Assessment Intervention Model is based on Neuman's health care systems model (Kaakinen & Hanson, 2005).

According to the *Family Assessment and Intervention Model,* families are subject to tensions when

TABLE 4-4

Comparison of Family Assessment Models Developed by Family Nurses

Name of model	Family Assessment and Intervention Model and the Family System Stressor-Strength Inventory (FS³I)	Friedman Family Assessment Model	Calgary Family Assessment and Intervention Model
Citation	Berkey-Mischke & Hanson (1991) Hanson (2001)	Friedman, Bowden, & Jones (2003)	Wright & Leahey (2009)
Purpose	Concrete, focused measurement instrument that helps families identify current family stressors and builds intervention based on family strengths	Concrete, global family assessment interview guide that looks primarily at families in the larger community in which they are embedded	Conceptual model and multidimensional approach to families that looks at the fit among family functioning, affective, and behavioral aspects
Theoretical underpinnings	Systems: Family systems Neuman systems Model: Stress-coping theory	Developmental Structural-functional Family stress-coping Environmental	Systems: Cybernetics Communication Change Theory
Level of data collected	Quantitative: Ordinal and interval Qualitative: Nominal	Qualitative: Nominal	Qualitative: Nominal
Settings in which primarily used	Inpatient Outpatient Community	Outpatient Community	Outpatient Community
Unit of analysis	Family as context Family as client Family as system Family as component of society	Family as client Family as component of society	Family as system
Strength	Short Easy to administer Yields data to compare one family member with another family member Assess and measure focused presenting problem	Comprehensive list of areas to assess family	Conceptually sound
Weakness	Narrow variable	Large quantities of data that may not relate to the problem No quantitative data	Not concrete enough to be useful as a guideline unless you study this model and approach in detail

stressed. The family's reaction depends on how deeply the stressor penetrates the family unit and how capable the family is of adapting to maintain its stability. The lines of resistance protect the family's basic structure, which includes the family's functions and energy resources. The family core contains the patterns of family interactions and strengths. The basic family structure must be protected at all costs or the family ceases to exist. Reconstitution or adaptation is the work the family undertakes to preserve or restore family stability. This model addresses three areas: (1) health promotion, wellness activities, problem identification, and family factors at lines of defense and resistance; (2) family reaction and instability at lines of defense and resistance; and (3) restoration of family stability and family functioning at levels of prevention and intervention.

The FS³I is the assessment and intervention tool that accompanies the Family Assessment and Intervention Model. The FS³I is divided into three sections: (1) family systems stressors—general; (2) family stressors—specific; and (3) family system strengths. An updated copy of the instrument, with instructions for administration and a scoring guide, can be found in Appendix A.

Family stability is assessed by gathering information on family stressors and strengths (Curran, 1983, 1985). The nurse and family work together to assess the family's general, overall stressors, followed by an assessment of specific family problems. Family strengths are identified to give an indication of the potential and actual problem-solving abilities of the family system. The nurse and family work together to design a plan of care using the Family Nursing Process.

A strength of the FS³I approach is that both quantitative and qualitative data are used to determine the level of prevention and intervention needed. The family is actively involved in the discussions and decisions. Moreover, this assessment and intervention approach focuses on family stressors and strengths, and provides a theoretical structure for family nursing.

Friedman Family Assessment Model

The *Friedman Family Assessment Model* (Friedman et al., 2003) is based on the structural-functional framework and developmental and systems theory. This assessment model takes a macroscopic approach to family assessment by viewing families as subsystems of the wider society, which includes institutions devoted to religion, education, and health. Family is considered an open social system and focuses on the family's structure, functions (activities and purposes), and relationships with other social systems. The Friedman model is commonly used when the family-in-community is the setting for care (e.g., in community and public health nursing). This approach enables family nurses to assess the family system as a whole, as a subunit of the society, and as an interactional system. The general assumptions of this model are delineated in Box 4-7 (Friedman et al., 2003, p. 100).

Structure refers to how a family is organized and how the parts relate to each other and to the whole. The four basic structural dimensions are role systems, value systems, communication networks, and power structure. These dimensions are interrelated and interactive, and they may differ in single-parent and two-parent families. For example, a single mother may be the head of the family, but she may not necessarily take on the authoritarian role that a traditional man might in a two-parent family. In turn, the value systems, communication networks, and power structures may be quite different in the single-parent and two-parent families as a result of these structural differences.

Function refers to how families go about meeting the needs of individuals and meeting the purposes of the broader society. In other words, family functions are what a family does. The functions of the family historically are discussed in Chapter 1, but

---

BOX 4-7

Underlying Assumptions of Friedman's Family Assessment Model

- A family is a social system with functional requirements.
- A family is a small group possessing certain generic features common to all small groups.
- The family as a social system accomplishes functions that serve the individual and society.
- Individuals act in accordance with a set of internalized norms and values that are learned primarily through socialization.

Source: Friedman, M. M., Bowden, V. R., & Jones, E. G. (2003). *Family nursing: Research, theory & practice* (5th ed.). Upper Saddle River, NJ: Prentice Hall/Pearson Education.

the following specific family functions are considered in this approach:

■ Pass on culture, religion, ethnicity.
■ Socialize young people for the next generation (e.g., to be good citizens, to be able to cope in society through education).
■ Exist for sexual satisfaction and reproduction.
■ Provide economic security.
■ Serve as a protective mechanism for family members against outside forces.
■ Provide closer human contact and relations.

The Friedman Family Assessment Model form consists of six broad categories of interview questions: (1) identification data, (2) developmental stage and history of the family, (3) environmental data, (4) family structure (i.e., role structure, family values, communication patterns, power structure), (5) family functions (i.e., affective functions, socialization functions, health care functions), and (6) family stress and coping. Each category has several subcategories and can be found in the most recent book by Friedman, Bowden, and Jones (2003).

Friedman's assessment was developed to provide guidelines for family nurses who are interviewing a family. The guidelines categorize family information according to structure and function. Friedman's Family Assessment Form exists in both a long form and a short form. The long form is quite extensive (13 pages), and it may not be possible to collect all of the data in one visit. Moreover, all the categories of information listed in the guidelines may not be pertinent for every family. Like other approaches, this model has its strengths and weaknesses. One problem with this approach is that it can generate large quantities of data with no clear direction as to how to use all of the information in diagnosis, planning, and intervention. The strength of this approach is that it addresses a comprehensive list of areas to assess the family, and that a short assessment form has been developed to highlight critical areas of family functioning. The short form, which is included in Appendix B, outlines the types of questions the nurse can ask.

Calgary Family Assessment Model

The CFAM by Wright and Leahey (2009) blends nursing and family therapy concepts that are grounded in systems theory, cybernetics, communication theory,

change theory, and a biology of recognition. The following concepts from general systems theory and family systems theory make up the theoretical framework for this model (Wright & Leahey, 2009, pp. 21–44):

■ A family system is part of a larger suprasystem and is also composed of many subsystems.
■ The family as a whole is greater than the sum of its parts.
■ A change in one family member affects all family members.
■ The family is able to create a balance between change and stability.
■ Family members' behaviors are best understood from a perspective of circular rather than linear causality.

Cybernetics is the science of communication and control theory; therefore, it differs from systems theory. Systems theory helps change the focus of one's conceptual lens from parts to wholes. By contrast, cybernetics changes the focus from substance to form. Wright and Leahey (2009) pull two useful concepts from cybernetics theory:

■ Families possess self-regulating ability.
■ Feedback processes can simultaneously occur at several system levels with families.

Communication theory in this model is based on the work of Watzlawick and colleagues (1967, 1974). Communication represents the way that individuals interact with one another. Concepts derived from communication theory used in the CFAM are as follows (Wright & Leahey, 2009):

■ All nonverbal communication is meaningful.
■ All communication has two major channels for transmission: digital (verbal) and analogical (nonverbal).
■ A dyadic relationship has varying degrees of symmetry and complementarity.
■ All communication has two levels: content and relationship.

Helping families to change is at the very core of family nursing interventions. Families need a balance between change and stability. Change is required to make things better, and stability is required to maintain some semblance of order. A number of concepts from change theory are important to this family nursing approach (Wright & Leahey, 2009):

- Change is dependent on the perception of the problem.
- Change is determined by structure.
- Change is dependent on context.
- Change is dependent on co-evolving goals for treatment.
- Understanding alone does not lead to change.
- Change does not necessarily occur equally in all family members.
- Facilitating change is the nurse's responsibility.
- Change occurs by means of a "fit" or meshing between the therapeutic offerings (interventions of the nurse) and the biopsychosocial-spiritual structures of family members.
- Change can be the result of a myriad of causes.

Figure 4-9 shows the branching diagram of the CFAM (Wright & Leahey, 2009, p. 48). The assessment questions that accompany the model are organized into three major categories: (1) structural, (2) developmental, and (3) functional. Nurses examine a family's structural components to answer these questions: Who is in the family? What is the connection between family members? What is the family's context? Structure includes family composition, sex, sexual orientation, rank order, subsystems, and the boundaries of the family system. Aside from interview and observation, strategies recommended to assess structure include the genogram and the ecomap.

The second major assessment category in the Calgary approach is family development, which includes assessment of family stages, tasks, and attachments. For example, nurses may ask, "Where is the family in the family life cycle?" Understanding the stage of the family enables nurses to assess and intervene in a more purposeful, specific, and meaningful

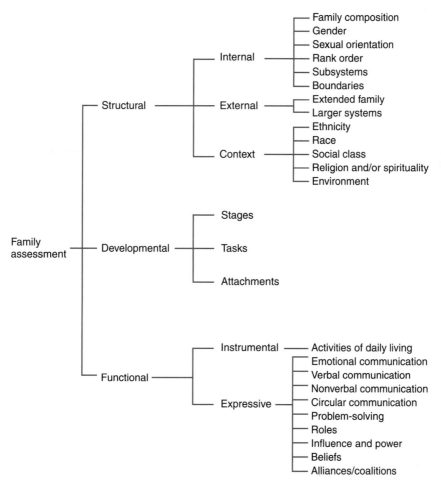

FIGURE 4-9 Calgary assessment model diagram.

way. There are no actual instruments for assessing development, but nurses can use developmental tasks as guidelines.

The third area for assessment in the CFAM is family functioning. Family functioning reflects how individuals actually behave in relation to one another or the "here-and-now aspect of a family's life" (Wright & Leahey, 2009, p. 116). Aspects of family functioning include activities of daily life, such as eating, sleeping, meal preparation, and health care, as well as emotional communication, verbal and nonverbal communication, circular communication, problem solving, roles, influence and power, beliefs, and alliances and coalitions. Wright and Leahey indicate that nurses may assess in all three areas (i.e., structural, developmental, functional) for a macroview of the family, or they can use any part of the approach for a microassessment.

Wright and Leahey (2009) developed a companion model to the CFAM, the CFIM. This intervention model provides concrete strategies by which nurses can promote, improve, and sustain effective family functioning in the cognitive, affective, and behavioral domains. More detail about this assessment model and intervention is available in Wright and Leahey's book, *Nurses and Families: A Guide to Family Assessment and Intervention* (2009).

The strength of the Calgary Assessment and Intervention Model is that it is a conceptually sound model that incorporates multiple theoretical aspects into working with families. The strength of this approach is also its weakness that unless you are intimately knowledgeable of the model and the interventions, it is difficult to implement in the acute care settings.

These three family assessment approaches and instruments offer options to the family nurse.

SUMMARY

This chapter presents the Family Nursing Process model. It describes assessment strategies, including how to select assessment instruments, determine the need for interpreters, assess for family health literacy, and diagram family genograms and ecomaps. This chapter explains intervention strategies to assist nurses and families in shared decision making. A case study is used to demonstrate the Family Nursing Process.

Family nurses must work in partnership with families as they build from a strengths model and not a deficit model. Using the Family Nursing Process approach outlined in this chapter, nurses and families together identify the priority family needs. The Family Reasoning Web is a systematic method used to ensure that families are viewed in a holistic manner, which also helps to keep the interventions oriented to a family strengths orientation. Family interventions need to be tailored to each individual family, with consideration of the family's structure, function, and processes. By subscribing and selecting a theory-based approach to assessment, and formulating mutually derived intervention strategies, families are more likely to be committed and follow through with family plans and interventions. Family nurses serve as the catalyst for the process of assessment, intervention, and evaluation of the Family Nursing Process.

REFERENCES

American Medical Association. (2007). *International classification of diseases: Clinical modifications (ICD-9-CM)* (10th ed.). Dover, DE: Author.

American Psychiatric Association. (2000). *Diagnostic and statistical manual of mental disorders (DSM-IV-TR)* (4th ed. text revision). Washington, DC: Author.

Bass, L. (2005). Health literacy: Implications for teaching the adult patient. *Journal of Infusion Nursing, 28*(1), 15–22.

Berkey-Mischke, K. M., & Hanson, S. M. H. (1991). *Pocket guide to family assessment and intervention.* St. Louis: Mosby Year Book.

Bethell, C., Simpson, L., & Read, D. (2006). Quality and safety of hospital care for children from Spanish-speaking families with limited English proficiency. *Journal for Healthcare Quality, 28*(3), W3.

Bowen, M. (1985). *Family therapy in clinical practice.* Norvale, NJ: Jason Aronson.

Bowen, M., & Kerr, M. (1988). *Family evaluation: An approach based on Bowen's Theory.* New York: W.W. Norton.

Bruera, E., Sweeney, C., Calder, C., Palmer, L., & Benisch-Tolley, S. (2001). Patient preferences versus physician perceptions of treatment decisions in cancer care. *Journal of Clinical Oncology, 19*(11), 2883–2885.

Butow, P. N., Maclean, M., Dunn, S. M., Tattersall, M., & Boyer, M. J. (1997). The dynamics of change: Cancer patients' preferences of information, involvement and support. *Annals of Oncology, 8*(9), 857–863.

Claassen, M. (2000). A handful of questions: Supporting parental decision-making. *Clinical Nurse Specialist, 14*(4), 189–195.

Corlett, K., & Twycross, A. (2006). Negotiation of parental roles within family-centered care: A review of the research. *Journal of Clinical Nursing, 15*(10), 1308–1316.

Curran, D. (1983). *Traits and the healthy family.* Minneapolis, MN: Winston Press.

Curran, D. (1985). *Stress and the healthy family*. Minneapolis, MN: Winston Press.

de Haes, H. (2006). Dilemmas in patient centeredness and shared decision making: A case for vulnerability. *Patient Education and Counseling, 62*(3), 291–298.

DeWalt, D. A., Berkman, N. C., Sheridan, N., Lohr L. L., & Pignone, P. (2004). Literacy and health outcomes. *Journal of General Internal Medicine, 19*(2), 1228–1239.

DeWalt, D. A., Boone, R. S., & Pignone, M. P. (2007). Literacy and its relationship with self-efficacy, trust and participation in medical decision making. *American Journal of Health Behavior, 31*(suppl 3), S27–S35.

Doegnes, M. E., Moorhouse, M. F., & Murr, A. C. (2008). *Nursing diagnosis manual: Planning, individualizing, and documenting client care* (2nd ed.). Philadelphia: F.A. Davis.

Dreger, V., & Tremback, T. (2002). Optimize patient health by treating literacy and language barriers. *Association of Operating Room Nurses Journal, 75*(2), 280–293.

Flores, G., Abreu, M., Schwartz, I., & Hill, M. (2000). The importance of language and culture in pediatric care: Case studies from the Latino community. *The Journal of Pediatrics, 137*(6), 842–848.

Friedman, M. M., Bowden, V. R., & Jones, E. G. (2003). *Family nursing: Research, theory & practice* (5th ed.). Upper Saddle River, NJ: Prentice Hall/Pearson Education.

Gazmararian, J. A., Williams, M. V., Peel, J., & Baker, D. W. (2003). Health literacy and knowledge of chronic disease. *Patient Education and Counseling, 52*(3), 267–275.

Hanson, S. M. H. (2001). Family nursing assessment and intervention. In *Family health care nursing: Theory, practice & research* (2nd ed., pp. 170–195). Philadelphia: F.A. Davis.

Herndon, E., & Joyce, L. (2004). *Getting the most from language interpreters*. American Academy of Family Physicians. Retrieved April 29, 2009, from http://www.aafp.org/fpm/20040600/37gett.html

Holtslander, L. (2005). Clinical application of the 15-minute family interview: Addressing the needs of postpartum families. *Journal of Family Nursing, 11*(1), 217–228.

Houts, P. S., Bachrach, R., Witmer, J. T., Tringali, C. A., Bucher, J. A., & Localio, R. A. (1998). Using pictographs to enhance recall in spoken medical instructions II. *Patient Education and Counseling, 35*(2), 83–88.

Kaakinen, J. R., & Hanson, S. M. H. (2005). Family nursing assessment and intervention. In S. M. H. Hanson, V. Gedaly-Duff, & J. R. Kaakinen (Eds.), *Family health care nursing: Theory, practice & research* (3rd ed., pp. 215–242). Philadelphia: F.A. Davis.

Khwaja, N., Sharma, S., Wong, J., Murray, D., Ghosh, J., Murphy, M. O., Halka, A. T., & Walker, M. G. (2006). Interpreter services in an inner city teaching hospital: A 6-year experience. *Annals of the Royal College of Surgeons of England, 88*(7), 659–662.

Ledger, S. D. (2002). Reflections on communicating with non-English-speaking patients. *British Journal of Nursing, 11*(11), 773–780.

Leske, J. S. (2002). Interventions to decrease family anxiety. *Critical Care Nurse, 22*(6), 61–65.

Makoul, G., & Clayman, M. L. (2006). An integrative model of shared decision making in medical encounters. *Patient Education and Counseling, 60*(3), 301–312.

Martin, K. S. (2004). *The Omaha System: A key to practice, documentation and information management* (2nd ed.). St. Louis, MO: Elsevier Health Sciences.

Martinez, A., D'Artois, D., & Rennick, J. E. (2007). Does the 15 minute (or less) family interview influence family nursing practice? *Journal of Family Nursing, 13*(2), 157–178.

Mayer, B. B., & Rushton, N. (2002). Writing easy-to-read teaching aids. *Nursing, 32*(3), 48–49.

McCloskey, J. C., & Bulechek, G. M. (Eds.). (2004). *Nursing interventions classification (NIC)* (4th ed.). St. Louis, MO: Mosby.

McGoldrick, M., Gerson, R., & Shellenberger, S. (1999). *Genograms in family assessment* (2nd ed.). New York: W.W. Norton.

McGoldrick, M., Shellenberger, S., & Petry, S. S. (2008). *Genograms: Assessment and intervention* (3rd ed.). New York: W.W. Norton.

Moorhead, S., Johnson, M., & Maas, M. (Eds.). (2004). *Nursing outcomes classification* (3rd ed.). St. Louis, MO: Mosby.

Neufeld, A., Harrison, M. J., Hughes, K., & Stewart, M. (2007). Nonsupportive interaction in the experience of women family caregivers. *Health and Social Care in the Community, 15*(1), 530–541.

North American Nursing Diagnosis Association. (2007). *Nursing diagnosis: Definitions and classifications, 2007-2008*. Philadelphia: Nursecom, Incorporated.

Olsen, S., Dudley-Brown, S., & McMullen, P. (2004). Case for blending pedigrees, genograms and ecomaps: Nursing's contribution to the big picture. *Nursing and Health Sciences, 6*(4), 295–308.

Pesut, D. J., & Herman, J. (1999). *Clinical reasoning: The art and science of critical and creative thinking*. Boston: Delmar.

Peters, E., Dieckmann, N., Dixon, A., Hibbard, J., & Mertz, C. K. (2007). Less is more in presenting quality information to consumers. *Medical Care Research and Review, 64*(2), 169–190.

Pierce, P. E., & Hicks, J. D. (2001). Patient decision making behavior. *Nursing Research, 50*(5), 267–274.

Ray, R. A., & Street, A. F. (2005). Ecomapping: An innovative research tool for nurses. *Journal of Advanced Nursing, 50*(5), 545–552.

Rempel, G. R., Neufeld, A., & Kushner, K. E. (2007). Interactive use of genograms and ecomaps in family caregiving research. *Journal of Family Nursing, 13*(4), 403–419.

Salmond, S, (2008). Who is Family? Family and decision making. In S. B. Lewenson & M. Truglio-Londrigan (Eds.), *Decision-making in nursing: Thoughtful approaches for practice* (pp. 89–104). Sudbury, MA: Jones and Bartlett.

Schattner, A., Bronstein, A., & Jellin, N. (2006). Information and shared decision-making are top patients' priorities. *BMC Health Services Research, 6*, 21.

Schenker, Y., Wang, F., Selig, S. J., Ng, R., & Fernandez, A. (2007). The impact of language barriers on documentation of informed consent at a hospital with on-site interpreter services. *Journal of General Internal Medicine, 22*(2), 294–299.

Sentell, T. L., & Halpin, H. A. (2006). Importance of adult literacy in understanding health disparities. *Journal of General Internal Medicine, 21*(8), 862–866.

Smettem, S. (1999). Welcome/Assalaam-u-alaikaam: Improving communications with ethnic minority families. *Paediatric Nursing, 11*(2), 33–35.

Sobo, E. J. (2004). Pediatric nurses may misjudge parent communication preferences. *Journal of Nursing Care Quality, 19*(3), 253–262.

Speros, C. (2005). Health literacy: Concept analysis. *Journal of Advanced Nursing, 50*(6), 633–640.

Taylor, B. (2006). Giving children and parents a voice: The parents' perspective. *Paediatric Nursing, 18*(9), 20–23.

Toman, W. (1976). *Family constellation: Its effect on personality and social behavior* (3rd ed.). New York: Springer.

Touliatos, J., Perlmutter, B., & Straus, M. (2001). *Handbook of family measurement techniques.* Newbury Park, CA: Sage.

Watzlawick, P., Weakland, J. H., & Fisch, R. (1967). *Pragmatics of human communication.* New York: W.W. Norton.

Watzlawick, P., Weakland, J. H., & Fisch, R. (1974). *Change: Principles of problem formulation and problem resolution.* New York: W.W. Norton.

Whitmer, M., Hughes, B., Hurst, S. M., & Young, T. B. (2005). Innovative solutions: Family conference progress note. *Dimensions of Critical Care Nursing, 24*(2), 83–88.

Wright, L. M., & Leahey, M. (2009). *Nurses and families: A guide to family assessment and intervention* (5th ed.). Philadelphia: F.A. Davis.

Wright, L. M., Watson, W., & Bell, J. (1996). *Beliefs: The heart of healing in families and illness.* New York: Basic Books.

Yanicki, S. (2005). Social support and family assets: The perceptions of low-income lone-mother families about support from home visitation. *Canadian Journal of Public Health, 96*(1), 46–49.

CHAPTER 5

Family Social Policy and Health Disparities

Lorraine B. Sanders, DNSc, CNM, FNP-BC, PMHNP, RN

Kristine M. Gebbie, DrPH, RN, FAAN

CRITICAL CONCEPTS

✦ Health disparities arise from complex, deep-rooted social issues, and are directly related to the social and political structure of a society. Many factors determine health status, including educational level, socioeconomic status, and physical surroundings. It is critical for nurses to recognize the link between the determinants of health and health disparities.

✦ The social and political structure of a society influences how health care is delivered and restricted from those in need. Access to quality, affordable health care should be considered a basic human right from a societal perspective and should be designed to minimize disparities.

✦ The policy decisions made by a society or government about families and how they are legally defined, what constitutes a legal relationship, and how the provision of care is delivered have a profound effect on families and their health. Defining families from a legal perspective may contribute to health disparities by restricting access to social and health care services.

✦ In the past, the profession of nursing had a well-defined role in advocating for vulnerable populations. Recently, nurses have not been as involved as they need to be in the development of health policy from either professional organization or individual perspectives.

✦ Nursing professionals can benefit from theoretical and practical education about social policy issues that are broad, complex, and can have resounding effects on the health of a family.

✦ Family nursing practice should be developed to improve the health of all families regardless of definition. Ethical issues arise if we restrict care to families by how they are defined legally.

This chapter exposes the nurse to social issues that affect the health of families. Threaded throughout the chapter is the role of the nurse providing care within the framework of family nursing. At the completion of this chapter, the nurse will have developed a broad understanding of what social policy is, and how it can contribute to the development and maintenance of health disparities. Armed with this knowledge, nurses can assist families to adopt health promotion and disease prevention strategies. When that is not an option and disease or illnesses exist, the nurse will be prepared to assist the family in accessing affordable options to quality care.

The end result of this chapter is not, however, to provide a cookbook or fixed guideline approach to working within a social policy framework to address health disparities for families. Instead, nurses are encouraged to explore issues and alternatives, and to challenge their own biases in understanding disparities. When that is accomplished, nurses will be prepared to apply innovative care to families in the practice setting.

KEY COMPONENTS

It is important first to understand some of the key components of social policy leading to health disparities. We begin with a description of social policy, health determinants, health disparities, definitions of family, and an account of the nurse's role with regard to social policy and health disparities.

Social Policy

An exploration of social policy and its impact on families logically begins with a discussion of what constitutes policy and its process. Policy is defined as a course of action adopted and pursued by government. Social policies are those policies that include social concepts such as health, education, housing, and employment. Some examples of past social policies adopted in the United States that have had resounding effects on the health of families are State Child Health Insurance Program (SCHIP), Medicare Part D, and the Welfare to Work program. These programs, enacted during the 2000s in response to government policy changes, were initiated to address health disparities, improve access to healthcare whereas managing costs, and reduce taxpayer burden, respectively. Social policies are often adopted with the intent to improve access to healthcare while managing costs and reducing taxpayer burden. Unfortunately, such policies do not always reach their goals.

Determinants of Health

The determinants of health are defined as factors that determine the health of individuals, families, and communities (World Health Organization [WHO], 2008). Determinants include a person's characteristics (genetic, sex, race/ethnicity), behaviors (nutrition, smoking, substance use, coping skills), and the physical, social, and economic environment (physical activity, housing, education, access to health care). These factors have a strong, indelible influence on the health of a family and, if unchanged, will continue to contribute to health disparities within family systems. The Social Determinants of Health Model that Dahlgren and Whitehead (1991; Institute of Medicine [IOM], 2002, p. 404) suggested can be used to conceptualize an approach to planning care using a foundation of family nursing theory. This model is depicted in Figure 5-1. The model can assist the nurse in understanding how physical, social, environmental, and psychological components influence and affect the state of health of a family. Historically, nurses have worked closely with vulnerable populations and developed unique solutions to challenging health care problems. Many of these interventions were based in the community setting and focused on the family, not just the individual. As nursing care moved into the hospital setting, much of that changed. Assessing the influence of the determinants of health and evaluating their effects on the overall health of the individual and family lost importance as care became focused on medical diagnosis.

Health Disparities

Health disparities are defined as "population-specific differences in the presence of disease, health outcomes, or access to care" (Health Resources Service Administration, 2001). Health and health status are

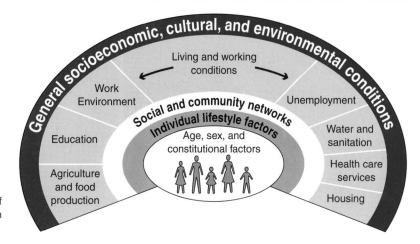

FIGURE 5-1 Social Determinants of Health Model suggested by Dahlgren and Whitehead (1991).

complex concepts, and no universal agreement has been reached on the definition of health. The World Health Organization defines health as a "state of complete physical, mental, and social well-being and not merely the absence of disease or infirmity" (World Health Organization, 2008). This basic definition has not been changed since it was published in 1948.

No single adopted definition of health utilized in the United States can be found despite a thorough search of U.S. government Web sites. Currently, no system exists in the United States to provide universally available health care services to citizens and residents. And although frequently debated, no plan has been implemented yet. At least one proposal for financing universal health care has been presented to, and denied by, Congress every year since 1912 (Chung & Pardeck, 1997).

Lack of a universally available health care system may be a contributing factor to the development and maintenance of health disparities. Lack of access to health care providers can cause a delay in appropriate health screenings. Counseling for health promotion and disease prevention is largely unavailable to the uninsured. Often, illnesses progress to advanced stages before a person accesses health care. This delay of entry into the system is costly on both a financial and a personal level.

Many complex factors contribute to health disparities. Health disparities are such an overwhelming problem in the United States that Congress charged the IOM to investigate and develop a report on the subject. The result describes in detail long-standing and deep-rooted inequalities in health

care directly related to race and ethnicity (IOM, 2003). The data are alarming. For instance, African Americans and Hispanic Americans are two to three times more likely to experience development of diabetes than white Americans (IOM, 2002). Children who live in urban areas are more likely to have asthma than children living in less population dense areas. Health disparities are linked to limited access to health care, exposure to environmental toxins, personal behaviors including substance abuse, inadequate nutrition, lack of physical exercise, and lack of treatment for mental illnesses.

The U.S. Public Health Service has set a target goal to eliminate health disparities among the poor, minority groups, and women; the U.S. Department of Health and Human Services (DHHS) Bureau of Primary Health Care has developed the Health Disparities Collaborative as a mechanism to change the delivery of care to populations at risk (Gillis, 2004, p. 250). The Care Model (Fig. 5-2), initially developed by the Robert Wood Johnson Foundation as a model to deliver quality care to those with chronic illness, has been adapted to assist health care teams change health care delivery systems with a goal of eliminating health disparities.

Components of the Care Model include the health care organization, community resources and policies, decision support, delivery system support, clinical information systems, and self-management support. The Care Model has the potential to frame the work necessary to address this complex problem because it includes the need to form community partnerships to support self-management. Acknowledgment of the importance of family and community

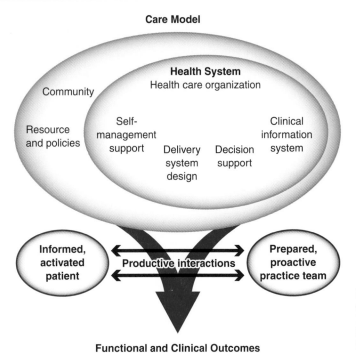

Care Model

Health System
Health care organization

Community

Resource
and policies

Self-
management
support

Delivery
system
design

Decision
support

Clinical
information
system

Informed,
activated
patient

Productive interactions

Prepared,
proactive
practice team

Functional and Clinical Outcomes

FIGURE 5-2 The Care Model. (From Texas Association of Community Health Centers. (2008). *The care model.* Retrieved April 29, 2009, from http://www.tachc.org/HDC/Overview/Care Model.asp, by permission.)

are essential in successful program implementation. Nurses play a crucial role in the implementation of all programs aimed at eliminating health disparities. The effect of social policy and its relationship to health disparities are discussed in depth later in this chapter.

HEALTH LITERACY

Health literacy was included for the first time in the *Healthy People 2010* objectives (National Network of Libraries of Medicine, n.d.). Health literacy is defined in *Healthy People 2010* as "[t]he degree to which individuals have the capacity to obtain, process, and understand basic health information and services needed to make appropriate health decisions" (National Network of Libraries of Medicine, n.d.). Although a relationship between health disparities and health literacy has been established, it is complex. The IOM found that approximately 90 million persons living in the United States, half of the adult population, have difficulty understanding health information (IOM, 2004). Because individuals with low health literacy do not understand health information, it affects their health outcomes such as fewer health

screenings, increased use of urgent or emergency care, errors in medication dosing and scheduling, alternatives in treatment regimens, and the inability to access accurate health-related information. Nurses should consider the health literacy of the patients and families that they serve. Nurses share a particular responsibility as we serve as the educators and advocates for many of the families to whom we provide care. However, the legal definition of family and who the family identifies as family are often different.

Legal Definition of Family

In the United States, the definition of "family" is legally defined by state and local laws and ordinances. The most common element of these definitions is "two or more individuals related by blood, marriage, or adoption." Alternately and more reflective of people's experiences, the definition of family could be: "two or more individuals who depend on one another for emotional, physical, and economical support. The members of the family are self-defined" (Hanson, 2001, p. 6). This definition is contextually quite different from the legal point of view.

TRADITIONAL FAMILIES

In the past, the traditional family, or nuclear family, was defined as persons who were related biologically: the man-woman-biological children image of family. Extended family is another traditional term; it includes the nuclear family and additional family members related either biologically or through marriage. For example, maternal and paternal grandparents would be considered part of the extended family. Laws, regulations, and social expectations may bind us to relatives legally defined as family even when no emotional tie exists. Conversely, relationships may be legally severed although emotional bonds are strong. Grandparents may have no legal relationship to grandchildren after a divorce and may not have access to grandchildren when custodial issues arise.

NONTRADITIONAL FAMILIES

In contrast with the traditional family, nontraditional families include stepfamilies, blended families, chosen families, and foster families. Stepfamilies are defined as two adult individuals who marry and one or both of these adults have children from previous relationships who together form a family unit. The members with a nonbiological link are referred to as step family members. The term *blended family* is used by some to describe families that are not traditional, and may include step relatives, biological relatives, extended family members, and others who are not related by blood or legal means. Many divorced individuals with children remarry, forming step and blended families. By definition, a stepparent or sibling is one who becomes related through marriage but has no relation through genetic or "blood" ties. Legally, few stepparents have a legal right to decision making about and guardianship over a stepchild unless provided by a court of law.

Same-sex partnerships or gay/lesbian couples form families. These families continue to struggle with being legally recognized in the majority of the United States, though they are recognized in Canada and by some U.S. states and state courts. The term *chosen family* is often used as a nontraditional definition of family. A chosen family consists of friends (and possibly relatives) who provide support in a way that the biological family did not. Members of chosen families often cohabitate and celebrate traditional holidays together. In the end,

no right or wrong description of family and no universal shared experience of family exist.

Policy Implications of Family Definitions

The definition of family, rarely challenged until recent times in the United States, has major policy implications. Results from the National Survey of Family Growth are used to "plan health services and health education programs" (U.S. Department of Health and Human Services, 2008a). The family or certain members of a family, within a legal perspective, can be given access to or denied health insurance, housing, and access to social and health programs. The Administration for Children and Families, overseen by the DHHS, "is responsible for federal programs that promote the economic and social well-being of families, children, individuals, and communities in the U.S." (U.S. DHHS, 2009). The 2005 to 2007 budget allotted for these programs, which include Temporary Assistance to Needy Families (TANF), The Healthy Marriage Initiative, and Head Start, was reportedly $46 million annually (U.S. DHHS, 2009). But because of the nature of how families are legally defined, many individuals who consider themselves part of a family unit would be ineligible for some of these programs.

In fact, the limited legal definition of family can have devastating results. In Black Jack City, Missouri, a family composed of two parents and three children was denied an occupancy permit simply because the parents were not legally married and the male parent was not the biological father of the oldest child residing in the household (Coleman, 2006). This legal battle evolved in an attempt to control access to subsidized housing. The city has a financial gain by refusing to provide housing. The family, by not being recognized in legal terms as a family, may lose access to housing.

DEFINITIONS OF FAMILY FROM A POLICY PERSPECTIVE

In 2003, the state of Massachusetts declared the ban on same-sex marriage unconstitutional. This action ignited a debate on how marriage and family are legally defined. One of the many purposes of entering into the legally binding arrangement of marriage is to be recognized as a family and to derive the benefits that married status entails. Government officials, both elected and appointed, quickly joined the debate, both pro and con, about a subject that many would consider personal. The government has long had a role in defining the legality of marriage and what constitutes a family. A policy definition of family will have resounding and long-lasting effects on the health of a family. Many prerequisites determine the ability to enter into a marriage. The persons involved must be of a certain age, must not be first-degree relatives, must be mutually consenting to the arrangement, and in most states and cities, may not be the same sex. From a social perspective, the government may take the position that legal definitions must exist simply to maintain a civil society. Nevertheless, legally naming what a family **is,** also without specifically stating it, defines what a family **is not.**

Legal definitions are grounded in history and the community need for stability, particularly economic and political stability. A genetic or biologic reason for certain definitions or restrictions, however, may or may not exist. Situations that on the surface may appear "illegal" or extremely unusual may, in fact, be extremely functional and positive for those involved. It is critical that nurses who encounter what appears to be an unusual situation be alert to the possibility that judgments based on automatically presumed "normality" can be unhealthy and limiting for the family seeking care and for the nurse.

The Nurse's Role in Facilitating Family Health from a Social Policy Perspective

The nurse in practice today may have little exposure to the world of policy and the legislative process. Nursing leaders have pressed for greater involvement, but nurses in general have difficulty making the link between their clinical practice and social policy. Nurses often do not possess the knowledge and skills to interact with policy makers, an activity that can be learned. Primomo (2007) studied the influence of an educational intervention on political awareness in a group of graduate nursing students and found that perceived competence among the students increased after intervention. The relationship between nursing and political awareness on the undergraduate level is more troubling. Although few studies exist

to describe this complex topic, undergraduate students report no knowledge of how to engage in a dialogue with legislators or how the role of the nurse relates to such activity (Turnock, 2004). Hewison (2007) acknowledges the lack of policy involvement among nurses and concludes that this may be related to the complexity of the policy process. Hewison (2007) recommends an organized method for policy analysis to be used by nurse managers. The method involves a process in which a summary of the policy is developed including its origin and status, its history and link to other policy initiatives, and finally, its themes and elements of nursing practice affected. Once the analysis is concluded, the nurse can take a position on whether this policy will meet the needs of the constituency. Nurses with strong policy analysis skills are critical to improving health for all citizens and to closing the health disparities gap.

The profession of nursing historically has been involved in social issues and has worked tirelessly to advocate and provide a voice to many vulnerable populations. The Henry Street Settlement (HSS) in New York City is an example of this. Lillian Wald, a nurse, founded the HSS in the late 19th century. The mission of the HSS was to provide "health teaching and hygiene to immigrant women" (Henry Street Settlement, 2004). The HSS continues to function as a community center today. Mary Breckinridge established the Frontier Nursing Service (FNS) in Hyden, Kentucky. The FNS introduced community-based midwifery care to the women of Appalachia, a vulnerable population with distinct health care needs; it continues today as a midwifery and family nurse practitioner program. On a professional level, many nursing organizations advocate for vulnerable populations and attempt to solve health disparity issues. Milstead (1999, p. 6), author of one of the seminal works linking the worlds of nursing and policy, *Health Policy & Politics: A Nurse's Guide,* briefly details the history of the American Nurses Association as it moved its national offices in 1992 to Washington, DC, to increase visibility of the profession of nursing among legislators.

Most nurses in the United States function primarily in the acute care setting. This practice breeds a limited perspective on the challenges to individuals, families, and communities, and an associated limitation in advocacy. This limited involvement stands despite such encouragement as the American Nurses Association *Nursing's Social*

Policy Statement (2003), which includes an overview of the nurse's role in social factors within the health care system and society. The means necessary to act on this direction are usually derived from education, both theoretical and practical. Houck and Bongiorno (2006) assert that nurses' roles include taking their influence beyond the bedside and into the health care system.

Professional nurses who have an interest in learning more about their role in the policy arena can find resources through professional associations or can enroll in a policy course. One example is the Washington Health Policy Institute conducted by George Mason University in Arlington, Virginia. Nurses and other health care professionals spend one week learning about health and social policy, and how to advocate for at-risk populations and influence policy makers.

SOCIAL ISSUES AND POLICIES THAT AFFECT FAMILIES

Multiple social issues and policies affect the health of families. In this section, the influence of policy on education, socioeconomic status, and health are explored.

Education

Every child in the United States has a right to an education, up through the completion of high school. This social policy is one of the few guarantees given to residents of the United States. The majority of American children attend a school that is in the same community in which they reside with their family. When a school is community based, it can also serve as a community center providing after school programs for working parents and evening educational programs to community members. Schools can support and improve the lives of children and their families by serving community needs. The school system also serves as a social gatekeeper and may be held accountable for enforcing many public health laws and regulations, such as the requirement for vaccination before children enter the system. Education has moved beyond the 3 R's (reading, writing, and arithmetic), though conflict exists about exactly what else should be a part of the school experience.

The role of the social worker in schools is now established as an integral provider of services for children and families. Psychological testing and services, speech and language, occupational and physical therapy are a right for all children assessed as having "special needs." Additional responsibilities of schools have often been contested from both sides. Dependent on the surrounding community, schools are often called to either limit certain information, such as sexuality, or are challenged to add prayer and alternate theories of evolution to the curriculum. School nurses provide many health-related services including education and counseling to school-aged children; however, they may be constricted by policy in what information they can provide. The school nurse should use evidence of positive impact on children to support programs while avoiding suppression of information because of personal beliefs. The diversity of communities makes it impossible for school districts to satisfy all parents, and a small but growing number of families are deciding to educate their children at home where closer control of content is possible.

School districts may be as small as a single grade school or as large as the million-pupil New York City system; the historic expectation is that a locally elected or appointed school board will determine the way in which the community's children will be educated. Federal funds, often for special education or programs for impoverished students, account for only about 7% of school expenditures (Ramirez, 2002). The reporting about schools without texts, without modern science laboratories or computers, and cutting back on "frills" such as music, art, and gym has stimulated an active search for ways to make equitable funding available, with the expectation that standards can be established and will be met. The shift to national standards, tied to access to funds, is a move away from the long-standing local nature of education in the United States. Given the high positive correlation between health status and level of education, education should be an area of concern to every nurse.

The No Child Left Behind (NCLB) law was enacted in 2001 and was proposed by President George W. Bush. The law is a reauthorization of the Elementary and Secondary Education Act originally made into law in 1965. This educational plan has four "pillars": accountability, flexibility, proven methods, and parental ability to transfer their children out of low-performing schools after 2 years. On paper, the NCLB does not appear to hinder the educational process, but there are many concerns about this law. The title of the law is intentionally inclusive and brings to mind equity in education, but when put into practice, equity was elusive among disabled students and students from ethnic and racial minorities (Thompson & Barnes, 2007, p. 12). The process of grading schools and requiring continuous improvement in test scores as a condition of economic support may prove impossible to manage. Some schools starting with high scores may not be able to make substantial increases, and other schools starting with very low scores may make meaningful improvement without meeting the stated standards.

NURSING ROLE IN SCHOOLS

The National Association of School Nurses (NASN) holds the position that each school nurse plays an active role in assisting children to optimal health, wellness, and development as a foundation to achieve educational success (NASN, 2003). This organization supports the need for a nurse in every school and acknowledges the role of the nurse that extends to family nursing, often the only health care resource in a community. As a resource, the school nurse should function as a case manager with knowledge of available insurance programs, health care providers, and community-based health-related services.

Traditionally, the school nurse has been responsible for managing emergency situations, providing mandatory screenings and immunization surveillance, dispensing prescribed medications, and serving as a resource for health-related information (American Academy of Pediatrics [AAP], 2001). The role of the school nurse, as part of a comprehensive school-based health care team, has expanded into many communities as a source of health care for the uninsured. Many large cities employ registered nurses and advanced practice nurses who provide primary care services in school-based clinics, not only because children lack a source of care but because school-based care is accessible and comfortable for young people.

The variability in the presence or expectations of school nurses is a source of concern. In some districts (and by law in some states), every school has full-time nurses with both knowledge and time to work with children and parents to support or improve physical or mental health. According to the NASN, schools that provide "adequate nursing coverage" have lower dropout rates, higher test scores, and fewer absences, which translates into better outcomes for children and families. The U.S. government recommends 1 nurse for every 750 students as outlined in the *Healthy People 2010* objectives, with adjustment depending on community and student needs (U.S. DHHS, 2000).

The AAP (2001) describes the role of the school nurse as one who provides care to children including acute, chronic, episodic, and emergency. The nurse is also responsible for the provision of health education and health counseling, and serves as the advocate for all students, including those with disabilities. The school nurse should work in collaboration with community-based doctors, organizations, and insurers to assure that each child has access to health care (AAP, 2001). This recommendation is an exceptional expectation especially when many schools function without a full-time nurse. Far too many schools have no nurse, only a part-time nurse, or a nurse whose only role is to assure that children with special health care needs receive their medications, catheter care, or other prescribed services. A nurse in any setting working with a family that includes school-aged children should become familiar with the available school health and school nursing resources.

Socioeconomic Status

Socioeconomic status is determined by income, education level, occupation, and social status. In the United States today, concern exists over a widening income gap. A study conducted at the University of California, Berkeley estimates that the top 300,000 Americans earned the same amount of income as the whole bottom 150 million Americans (Piketty & Saez, 2004). Although the median income grew by $360 for a total of $48,201 in 2006, the poverty level increased to 12.3% (Bernstein, Gould, & Mishel, 2007). Today, more than 4.9 million Americans, including 1.2 million children, live in poverty in the United States. African American families and those with female heads of households disproportionately account for those living at or below the poverty level. African Americans earn 61% ($31,969) of what non-Hispanic white individuals earn ($52,423) Women continue to earn approximately 77% of what men earn overall (DeNavas-Walt, Proctor, & Smith, 2007).

Availability of employment-based health coverage has declined from 64.2% in 2000 to 59.7% in 2006 (Bernstein, Gould, & Mishel, 2007). This decline has left many workers and their dependents without health coverage. Meanwhile, the public debate on an appropriate level of support for families who lack basic housing, food, health services, or social stability continues.

TANF has replaced welfare as a social and financial support program (U.S. DHHS, 2008c). It begun in 1996 during the Clinton administration and is managed by individual states with federal funding. A 5-year lifetime limit exists on assistance. Recipients must work in exchange for assistance, and school attendance is not counted as work. The goals of the program include reducing and eliminating dependency, promoting work, and promoting two-parent families. Requiring work in exchange for assistance is a reasonable goal, but penalizing those who could benefit from attending school only maintains a cycle of poverty.

Poverty, in itself, is a limiting and frightening experience for families. In 1969, 24.2 million Americans lived in poverty; in 1997, the number was 35.6 million, with children overrepresented in that number, and by the beginning of the 21st century, 1 in every 5 children fit this definition (National Center for Children in Poverty, 2008). Many families who live below the poverty level have difficulty acquiring adequate long-term housing. Homeless families often arrive at their situation as a direct result of public policy decisions rather than personal choices. Homeless children are three times more likely to have been born to a single mother than their nonhomeless counterparts (National Center on Family Homelessness, 2008). Education is the ultimate predictor of eventual stability and success, yet education is not (or cannot be) emphasized within homeless communities. In the end, homeless children are more likely to have developmental delays, learning disabilities, and to repeat a grade in school (National Center on Family Homelessness, 2008).

Health and Illness Care

Assuring access to health and illness care services is one way to improve the health of individuals and families. Children should receive necessary immunizations and should be evaluated on a regular basis for normal growth and development. Likewise, it is important that adults be adequately immunized and screened for hypertension, diabetes, and cancer at appropriate ages and intervals. Although much emphasis has been on the roles parents have in assuring that their children receive needed services, many adults also have responsibilities for the health care of aging parents. The absence of a comprehensive commitment to access or assurance of universal health insurance coverage for all makes achieving the desired level of interaction with health professionals extremely difficult. Adults with both children and aging parents dependent for support struggle with access to health care and management of illnesses care, experience a particularly difficult burden in today's world.

Health Insurance Programs

MEDICARE/MEDICAID/STATE CHILD HEALTH INSURANCE PROGRAM

The Center for Medicare and Medicaid Services is a governmental agency with responsibility for Medicare, Medicaid, SCHIP, Health Insurance Portability and Accountability Act (HIPAA), and Clinical Laboratories Improvement Amendment. Medicare is a health insurance program for people older than 65 years, certain disabled individuals younger than 65 years, and those with end-stage renal disease. Medicare covers approximately 40 million persons on an annual basis (U.S. DHHS, 2006a). Medicaid is a federal–state partnership health insurance program for eligible low-income groups and is managed by individual states. SCHIP was enacted in 1997 for a 10-year period to address the lack of health insurance coverage of children who did not qualify for Medicaid. This embattled program has been successful and has provided health insurance to more than 6 million children (U.S. DHHS, 2008d). Currently, it is estimated that 9 million children remain without health insurance in the United States (Kaiser Family Foundation, 2007). The SCHIP program is currently at risk for losing required funding because of disagreements on eligibility requirements.

Prenatal Care Assistance Program (PCAP) targets pregnant women who meet certain income requirements and are eligible for part of the Medicaid system. The PCAP program includes prenatal care, delivery services, postpartum care up to 2 months after the birth of the baby, referral to the Women, Infants, and Children Program (WIC), and infant care for 1 year.

It may appear, after reading about the available government health insurance programs, as though all vulnerable populations have access to health insurance, but that is far from the truth. On an annual basis, it is estimated that more than 45 million residents of the United States have no health insurance (U.S. DHHS, 2005). Those who are younger than 34 years (63%) are more likely to be uninsured. Women and children are disproportionately affected because they are more likely to be living below the poverty level. By not having a payment system, many people delay seeking health care services, which increases the likelihood that illness or need for services will be at a crisis level when they enter the system. When this delay occurs, costs for health care increase.

Because the majority of government health care programs are managed and delivered by individual states with only partial support by the federal program, the burden to state budgets is enormous. Some unique programs have been implemented to address this financial inequity. The state of Massachusetts now mandates that residents have some form of health insurance, similar to the common requirement that anyone with a car have collision insurance. Residents who do not have coverage are at risk for fines and tax penalties. A Massachusetts state-subsidized plan, Commonwealth Care, was established to offer affordable health care to residents, but the potential still exists of posing an additional burden on the poor, especially if they are fined for not enrolling.

Infant Mortality Rates

Infant mortality is defined as the number of deaths of infants 1 year or younger per 1,000 live births. Infant mortality is a leading indicator of the health of a nation. In 2007, the overall infant mortality rate in the United States was 6.37 per 1,000 births (Central Intelligence Agency, 2008). Surprising to many, this U.S. statistic is much worse than other nations such as Sweden at 2.76 per 1,000 and the Czech Republic at 3.86 per 1,000 births. Cuba has better outcomes, with an infant mortality rate of 6.04 per 1,000, than in the United States (Central Intelligence Agency, 2008).

A great disparity exists in infant mortality rates in the United States. The rate is 2.5 times greater for African American infants than it is for white infants (Nurse Family-Partnership [NFP], 2008). The reasons for the greater infant mortality rate are complex, but preventive care may be one of the answers. In the United States, the leading cause of infant mortality is preterm birth and low birth weight. Programs such as the NFP, which encourages early enrollment into prenatal care, home visits by registered nurses over a 2.5-year period, and establishing social support have been successful in improving the health of mothers and children (NFP, 2008).

Obesity

The increasing rates of obesity and diabetes present significant health issues for families. Although the definitions for healthy weight have varied significantly through the last century, the current standard is the body mass index (BMI), or the ratio of weight to height. Overweight people have a BMI of 25 to 29.9; those with a BMI of 30 or greater are obese (U.S. DHHS, 2009). The rate of obesity is startling: 34% of adults older than 20 are considered obese. More than 13.9% of children aged 2 to 5 are overweight. Contributing factors include genetic predisposition, increased portion size, reduced amounts of exercise, reduced school funding for physical activity, and increased television and computer use (U.S. DHHS, 2009). Health consequences include increased risk for heart disease, diabetes, stroke, gallstones, sleep apnea, and some cancers (U.S. DHHS, 2009). Medical expenditures are estimated to be as high as $78.5 billion annually (U.S. DHHS, 2009). Recommendations for the treatment of overweight and obesity include physical exercise and following dietary guidelines for healthy eating.

Family resources and family eating habits have a marked influence on both childhood and adult obesity. Although dietary and exercise recommendations are part of the solution to the obesity epidemic, nurses must consider other contributing factors, including lack of access to healthy foods, unsafe neighborhoods that make physical exercise a challenge, and cultural beliefs and attitudes about weight and health. Fully engaging a family in planning for changes may be a challenge requiring more complex, tailored solutions.

Asthma

According to the American Lung Association (2008), approximately 34.1 million Americans report a diagnosis of asthma, and the incidence of asthma is increasing. Direct health costs for treating asthma are estimated to be $10 billion annually. Asthma is the leading chronic illness among children and is the third leading cause of hospitalization for children younger than 15 (American Lung Association, 2008).

Major asthma attack triggers include second-hand tobacco smoke, as well as first-hand dust, pollution, cockroaches, pets, and mold. Less common triggers include exercise, extremes of weather, food, and hyperventilation (National Center for Environmental Health, 2003). The objective of policy makers now is to create "asthma-friendly communities" by having better access to and quality of treatment for all populations but especially those in poorer communities, increased awareness of asthma and its risks for all, and environmentally safe schools and homes (Lara et al., 2002). New York City began an Asthma Initiative in 1999 that includes an Asthma Institute with a comprehensive program called *Managing Asthma in Schools and Daycare,* Community Integrated Pest Management program, and the Asthma Care Coordinator program that provides follow-up care and support to children hospitalized for asthma. The Asthma Institute provides free education to health care providers, community educators, and homeless shelter workers on asthma signs and symptoms, asthma self-management, and other clinical topics related to asthma. This initiative has helped reduce hospitalizations for asthma by 9% in 2005 (New York City Department of Health and Mental Hygiene, 2008).

HIV/AIDS

HIV was first identified in the United States in the early 1980s (U.S. DHHS, 2008b). Initially, it affected men having sex with men, and women and children were not believed to be at risk for becoming infected. This understanding soon changed, and now approximately 1 million Americans are infected with HIV, and about 25% are unaware of their serostatus (U.S. DHHS, 2008b). Approximately 40,000 newly reported infections of HIV are reported in the United States every year, of which women account for 26%. HIV/AIDS is a disparity illness and is the leading cause of death of African American women aged 25 to 34 (U.S. DHHS, 2008b). The rate of AIDS diagnosis for African American women is 23 times the rate for white women. Unfortunately, HIV/AIDS is a disease of young women of childbearing age, which can greatly affect the decision to become a mother. The use of antiretroviral medications (ARVs) during pregnancy, together with operative delivery, has helped to reduce mother-to-child transmission to approximately 2% in the United States (U.S. DHHS, 2008b).

With the introduction of ARVs in the 1990s, HIV has been treated as a chronic illness, and more and more people are living longer with the infection. In 2007, the HIV vaccine trials were suspended because the vaccine was thought to be ineffective in immunizing participants. Therefore, an increased need for nurses exists to offer prevention education and promote testing for all men and women. The CDC currently recommends routine screening and testing for all adults, adolescents, and pregnant women (U.S. DHHS, 2006b). It is believed that when a person infected with HIV is aware of his or her serostatus, he or she can live a healthy and long life by adopting healthy behaviors and the use of ARVs. Knowing HIV status also helps to reduce transmission by practicing safe sex. Prevention education, screening, and counseling are the priorities for the family nurse.

Aging

The U.S. population is aging. According to the "State of Aging and Health in America 2004," by 2030, more than 70 million people in the United States will be 65 years or older (U.S. DHHS, 2004). This demographic shift will have a pronounced affect on the resources of the government and on individual families. On average, Americans 75 and older have three chronic health conditions and use five prescription medications (U.S. DHHS, 2004). This burden of illness challenges health care resources in planning for the cost of providing care, educating and recruiting a health care workforce to specialize in elder care, and the strain on communities and individual families.

Many chronic and debilitating illnesses in the elderly are preventable. Early adoption of a healthy lifestyle decreases the prevalence of illnesses such as diabetes, cardiovascular disease, and pulmonary disease.

ELDER CARE

The Administration on Aging (U.S. DHHS, 2004) predicts that, by 2020, 19.2% of the 15.2 million persons older than 65 living alone will need help with daily living. The provision of care to the elderly is growing both as a family responsibility and as a profession. More women are caregivers than men. Policies such as the Family and Medical Leave Act are written as gender neutral, but women experience a general expectation that they will be the caregivers regardless of the burden that places on them. Lay caregivers are unpaid, which benefits social programs, especially Medicare and Medicaid. Women who provide lay home health care experience much greater levels of stress than their other family members, as well as more alienation from those outside of the home (Armstrong, 1996).

Women's Reproductive Issues

In 2006, the state of South Dakota banned access to abortion services. This ban was seen as a direct challenge to federal precedent set in *Roe v. Wade*. In South Dakota, it is now a felony for a health care provider to perform an abortion unless there is proof that the mother's life is at risk. At the time of the ban, only one provider of abortion services, Planned Parenthood, operated in the state. The clinic was reliant on physicians who would fly in from other states because no local physician was willing to provide abortions to women. As a result of this law, women do not have access to abortions unless they have the resources to leave the state for care.

On a similar note, some pharmacists across the country have refused to fill prescriptions for contraceptives or emergency contraception, stating that doing so is in direct conflict with their moral and personal beliefs (Stein, 2005). Women, who are often unaware of these reproductive health issues until they are directly affected, are outraged when pharmacists' beliefs override their right to services. Women have a legal right to access to prescription medications. The question is, who decides? According to the Guttmacher Institute (2005), 47 states have a policy that allows health care providers, including nurses and pharmacists, to refuse to participate in the delivery of reproductive health services.

NURSING ROLE IN RELATION TO HEALTH AND ILLNESS CARE

The implications of social policy as a context for nursing care of families are almost limitless. Social policies affect the daily lives of families, contribute to how families are defined, and shape or limit the health and illness services available. Social policies are a contributing factor to the development and maintenance of health disparities. Many social policies may facilitate family strength and effective child rearing. When nurses fail to act on the negative consequences of policies, however, an enormous impact on health results. Professional nurses must develop and use knowledge and information to influence policies that favor families.

The use of family theory to provide a conceptual model for care can help nurses embrace patients' definitions of their family and reject assumptions about family resources available to assist in care. Assumptions that are not based in patient data truncate communication and lead to care that is perceived as unaccommodating. Learning to use open-ended questions that do not assume marital status, gender of partner, relationships with children, and sources of financial support will yield a much more complete assessment. Planning for return to the community should begin with an open exploration of potential support or resources, without assuming that any are automatically available. Opportunities for learning experiences in settings that have established services for vulnerable populations provide the nursing student with clinical situations in which to practice the skills suggested earlier. Homeless shelters, services for gay and lesbian adolescents, shelters for victims of intimate partner abuse, outreach centers for sex workers, street syringe and needle exchange programs all reach a disproportionate share of individuals whose family experiences are not the idealized norm.

Best practices in nursing care with families encountering the negative impact of social policies are yet to be fully explored and described. Nursing research has already developed useful tools and frameworks for providing nursing care across cultural barriers and under difficult circumstances. The recent development of community-based participatory research models (U.S. DHHS, 2001) provides a methodology for studies that is more respectful of the potential different views of family in a community. This approach requires the nurse researcher to establish a relationship with the community in which the study is to occur before the statement of the research question, to share all stages in research with the community, and to work collaboratively toward community improvement based on the results of the study. Adopting this level of respect for potential reshaping of nursing studies of "family" opens the possibility of nursing stepping to the forefront in understanding and changing health care for all kinds of families.

The inclusion of health policy in nursing education has the potential to increase the sensitivity of nurses to social and health policy issues. Nurses understand that it is not sufficient to care in isolation from the forces that increase risk for disease or limit access to medical services. History, economics, and political science inform nurses' understanding of policy and should be introduced in such a way that nurses, at all levels, are better able to understand current affairs, join nursing and other advocacy organizations, and participate in local, state, or national political processes. Nurses are often familiar with the failures of policy, but they need to go a step further by advocating for equity, social justice, and families.

Family Case Study

The following case study of the Powell family is used to demonstrate disparities and the effect of social policies on the family. The Powell family is a nuclear family that is struggling with the after-effects of a hurricane. The Powell family genogram is depicted in Figure 5-3, and the stresses the family currently is experiencing are shown in the family ecomap (Figure 5-4).

FAMILY MEMBERS
+ Tyrone: 38 years old; father, police officer, full-time employed, borderline hypertension
+ Patrice: 35 years old; mother, retail sales manager, recent onset of obesity
+ Keisha: 14 years old; daughter, eighth grader, student-athlete, history of asthma
+ Malik: 12 years old; son, sixth grader, student-athlete, history of asthma

SETTING: Home and community setting

NURSING GOAL: Develop a plan of care using family theory to assist the family in developing health promotion activities, that is, activities to prevent illness and to access services to support life in a postdisaster environment.

POWELL FAMILY STORY
The Powell family is native to New Orleans with strong ties to the area. Tyrone Powell joined the police force after completing an associate's degree in criminal justice at a local community college. He met his wife, Patrice Hughes Powell, in high school, and they married after Patrice graduated. Both Patrice and Tyrone were employed full time and, after 3 years of marriage, had their first child, Keisha. Patrice continued to work full time to help save for the purchase of a home for their growing family. Two years later, Patrice gave birth to a son, Malik. Both children were healthy newborns and thrived. Patrice's mother, Corinne, often helped out caring for her grandchildren while Patrice and Tyrone worked. When Malik was 3, the Powell family purchased its first home in the St. Bernard's parish of New Orleans, close to other family members. Life was uneventful, and the children continued to grow, both entering school as expected and performing well. Both Keisha and Malik were diagnosed with asthma in early childhood. Patrice and Tyrone learned about the disease and incorporated many changes to reduce exposure of asthma triggers to their children. The disease was well managed in both children, who relied on the use of inhalers to treat symptoms and regular visits to the primary care practitioners the family used.

In the late summer of 2005, the inhabitants of the Gulf Coast area of the United States were encouraged to evacuate because a hurricane expected to make landfall in New Orleans. Tyrone, as a New Orleans police officer, was expected to report for duty to assist with disaster-related operations. Patrice, the children, and their extended family made the decision to stay in the area but agreed to relocate to the Superdome (a large en-

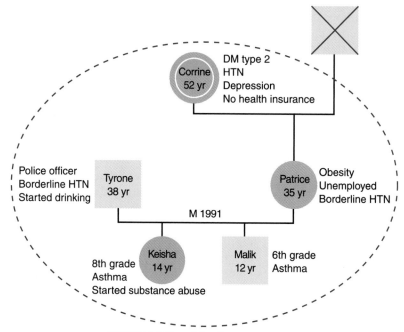

FIGURE 5-3 Powell family genogram.

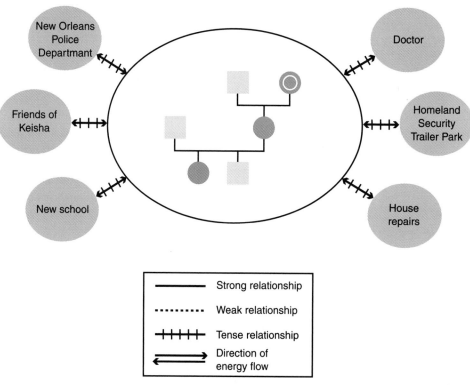

FIGURE 5-4 Powell family ecomap.

closed sports area) for the duration of the storm. They reasoned that they could stay together and return to their homes in the immediate aftermath. Patrice also did not want to leave Tyrone and evacuate farther inland. Unfortunately, the Powell's home was destroyed in the aftermath of Hurricane Katrina as the levee system failed and St. Bernard's parish was flooded.

The family was now homeless. No one in the extended family had housing that was considered livable. Patrice and her children had no choice but to move temporarily to Houston, Texas, where many hurricane survivors were being relocated. Unfortunately, Corinne, Patrice's mother, was not able to secure housing in Houston and was being advised to relocate away from her family in Baton Rouge, the state's capital. Tyrone, as a police officer, was expected to stay in the area to assist with recovery.

After many months of separation, the family was permitted to return to New Orleans and reunite. Expectations were high, and the family knew much work had to be done to restore their home. They were able to secure a trailer from Homeland Security, and Corinne would move in with the family temporarily. On arrival, the family was shocked to see their home and neighborhood. Nothing looked familiar. The odor of mold and rot was pervasive. It was no better in the trailer, which was cramped, leaving little space for living and privacy. The trailer also had a strong odor of chemicals that was not relieved by opening the windows.

FAMILY MEMBERS

Tyrone continues to be employed full time. He works many hours of overtime and has developed anxiety in relation to his experience in the immediate aftermath of the disaster. He feels the response to the disaster was not adequate but does not want to verbalize his feelings because it is not how police officers are expected to function. He also feels that he should be grateful for continued employment, health insurance, and for having a reunited family living together, as housing in a trailer is difficult to secure. His blood pressure is elevated, and he has started taking medication to control it. He finds that he is very short tempered and irritable around his family and coworkers. Before the disaster, when faced with a problem, Tyrone often channeled his energy in a positive way, often working out at the gym. Now he often isolates himself and drinks alcohol to "dull his feelings."

Patrice is now unemployed. Her place of business was destroyed and there are no plans to rebuild. She spends much of her time trying to restore her home, but resources are few and she often feels sick after spending even a short time in the house. She has gained weight and states, "I eat to relieve my stress." It is also difficult to prepare healthy meals in the trailer, because there is little space to store food for her family. Her BMI is now 30, and she is borderline hypertensive. Her fasting blood sugar is also elevated, and her primary care provider has advised her to lose weight to control her symptoms. She is also sad about her life and finds it difficult to find the motivation to work.

Keisha, at 14 years old, never expected her life to be like this. She has no privacy, sharing a trailer with her family and grandmother. She often finds it difficult to breath, and her symptoms of asthma have become more difficult to treat. She feels worse when she is in the trailer. She is often out in the neighborhood with other adolescents, and has started to experiment with drugs and alcohol. She is angry about the response to the disaster and cannot understand why it is taking so long to get back to "normal."

Malik is also suffering from symptoms of asthma. The symptoms are so severe that he has difficulty participating in sports. He also has an increase of symptoms when in the trailer. He is anxious about being separated from his family, and struggles to focus and concentrate on his schoolwork.

Corinne, at 52, has experienced development of type 2 diabetes, hypertension, and depression. She has no health insurance and does not yet qualify for Social Security insurance. The health clinic where she previously received care was destroyed in the hurricane, and her health records were lost. There is no plan to reopen the clinic. Patrice and Tyrone have assumed esponsibility for her bills, but this is a burden to the family. They are seeking some relief but have not received any information at this point. Patrice often accompanies her mother on her many visits to health care providers. No central location for treatment exists, and it often appears that each provider is unaware of her other diagnosis. The fragmentation of care is a stress to both Corinne and Patrice.

The Powell family faces many issues that are related to both health and social policies. These problems are both a direct and indirect result of a natural disaster. Although the Powells had some risks for health disparities, these had not surfaced until Hurricane Katrina devastated the Gulf Coast.

SUMMARY

The impact of health disparities affects every individual and all families on both a national and a global level. Health disparities are complex issues that threaten to overwhelm many of the families nurses care for. Many families have difficulty accessing quality, cost-effective health care in a timely manner. Nurses have an important role in developing effective solutions that derive from planning care using family nursing theory. Nursing must care beyond the personal delivery of care and act as the advocate for vulnerable families. Family nursing theory provides nurses a framework to conduct assessments and plan care by maximizing the rules and policies of the health care and legislative systems to favor families and improve health outcomes.

The development of social policies is dependent on the accurate interpretation of the needs of society. Nurses must understand the effect that existing social systems and public policies have on families. Many of the families with whom nurses work are not in a position to advocate for necessary changes. *Nurses can give voice to the concerns of the under-represented* and assist in devising creative alternatives to social policies that limit access to quality care.

Finally, nurses contribute to the development of new knowledge. The call to incorporate evidence-based practice must include family nursing interventions. Much research is needed about families and how to help them achieve higher levels of health within complex social systems. Studies of the effects of social policy on families must draw on a range of disciplines and theories, and should involve an interdisciplinary approach.

REFERENCES

American Academy of Pediatrics. (2001). *The role of the school nurse in providing school health services.* Retrieved March 2, 2008, from http://www.nasn.org/Portals/0/statements/aapstatement.pdf

American Lung Association. (2008). *What is asthma?* Retrieved March 10, 2008, from http://www.lungusa.org/site/apps/s/content.asp?c=dvLUK9O0E&b=4061173&ct=5314727

American Nurses Association. (2003). *Nursing's social policy statement* (2nd ed.). Washington, DC: American Nurses Association.

Armstrong, P. (1996). Resurrecting the family: Interring the state. *Journal of Comparative Family Studies, 27*(2), 221–248.

Bernstein, J., Gould, E., & Mishel, L. (2007). *Poverty, income and health insurance trends 2006.* Retrieved February 21, 2008, from http://www.epi.org/content.cfm/webfeatures_econindicators_income20070828

Central Intelligence Agency. (2008). *The world factbook.* Retrieved March 13, 2008, from https://www.cia.gov/library/publications/the-world-factbook/rankorder/2091rank.html

Chung, W. S., & Pardeck, J. T. (1997). Explorations in a proposed national policy for children and families. *Adolescence 32*(126), 426–436.

Coleman, T. (2006). *Eye on unmarried America. Column one.* Retrieved February 28, 2008, from http://www.unmarriedamerica.org/column-one/2-27-06-definition-of-family.htm

Dahlgren, G., & Whitehead, M. (1991). *Policies and strategies to promote social equity in health*, Institute of Futures Studies, Stockholm.

DeNavas-Walt, C., Proctor, B., & Smith, J. (2007). *U.S. Census Bureau: Income, poverty, and health insurance coverage 2006.* Retrieved March 3, 2008, from http://www.census.gov/prod/2007pubs/p60-233.pdf

Gillis, L. (2004). The Health Disparities Collaborative. In J. O' Connell (Ed.), The healthcare of homeless persons; A manual of communicable diseases & common problems in shelters & on the streets. Boston, MA: Guthrie Nixon Smith Printers.

Guttmacher Institute. (2005). Striking a balance between a provider's right to refuse and a patient's right to receive care. Retrieved March 13, 2008, from http://www.guttmacher.org/media/presskits/2005/08/04/index.html

Hanson, S. (2001). *Family health care nursing: Theory, practice, and research* (2nd ed.). Philadelphia: F.A. Davis.

Health Resources and Services Administration. (2001). *Eliminating Health Disparities in the United States.* Retrieved April 29, 2009, from http://archive.hrsa.gov/newsroom/NewsBriefs/2001/eliminatingdisparities.htm

Henry Street Settlement. (2004). *About our founder, Lillian Wald.* Retrieved March 10, 2008, from http://www.henrystreet.org/site/PageServer?pagename=abt_lwald

Hewison, A. (2007). Policy analysis: A framework for nurse managers. *Journal of Nursing Management, 15*(7), 693–699.

Houck, N., & Bongiorno, A. (2006). Innovations in the public policy education of nursing students. *Journal of the New York State Nurses Association, 37*(2), 4–8.

Institute of Medicine. (2002). *The future of the public's health in the 21st century.* Washington, DC: The National Academies Press.

Institute of Medicine. (2003). *Unequal treatment: Confronting racial and ethnic disparities in health care.* Washington, DC: The National Academies Press.

Institute of Medicine. (2004). *Health literacy: A prescription to end confusion.* Washington, DC: The National Academies Press.

Kaiser Family Foundation. (2007). *Medicaid and the uninsured.* Retrieved February 12, 2008, from http://www.kff.org/uninsured/upload/7698.pdf

Lara, M., Nicholas, W., Morton, S., Vaiana, M. E., Genovese, B., & Racelefsky, G. (2002). *Improving childhood asthma outcomes in the United States: A blueprint for policy action.* Washington, DC: RAND.

Milstead, J. (1999). *Health policy & politics: A nurse's guide.* Gaithersburg, MD: Aspen.

National Association of School Nurses. (2003). *Access to a school nurse.* Retrieved February 29, 2008, from http://www.nasn.org/Portals/0/statements/resolutionaccess.pdf

National Center for Children in Poverty. (2008). *Child poverty.* Retrieved March 3, 2008, from http://www.nccp.org/topics/childpoverty.html

National Center for Environmental Health. (2003). *Basic facts about asthma.* Atlanta, GA: Air Pollution and Respiratory Health Branch, Centers for Disease Control and Prevention.

National Center on Family Homelessness. (2008). *America's homeless children.* Retrieved March 3, 2008, from http://www.familyhomelessness.org/pdf/fact_children.pdf

National Network of Libraries of Medicine. (n.d.). *Health literacy.* Retrieved May 9, 2008, from http://nnlm.gov/outreach/consumer/hlthlit.html

New York City Department of Health and Mental Hygiene. (2008). *Asthma initiative.* Retrieved March 3, 2008, from Nhttp://www.nyc.gov/html/doh/html/asthma/asthma.shtml

Piketty, T., & Saez, E. (2004). *Income inequality in the United States, 1913–2002.* Retrieved February 7, 2008, from http://elsa.berkeley.edu/~saez/piketty-saezOUP04US.pdf

Primomo, J. (2007). Changes in political astuteness after a health systems and policy course. *Nurse Educator 32*(6), 260–264.

Ramirez, A. (2002). The shifting sands if school finance. *Educational Leadership 60*(4), 54–58.

Stein, R. (2005). Pharmacists' rights at front of new debate. *Washington Post.* Retrieved March 12, 2008, from http://www.washingtonpost.com/wp-dyn/articles/A5490-2005Mar27.html

Texas Association of Community Health Centers. (2008). *The care model.* Retrieved April 29, 2009, from http://www.tachc.org/HDC/Overview/CareModel.asp

Thompson, T. G., & Barnes, R. E. (2007). *Beyond no child left behind.* The Aspen Institute. Retrieved February 14, 2007, from http://www.aspeninstitute.org/site/c.huLWJeMRKpH/b.938015/

Turnock, B. (2004). *Public health: What it is and how it works* (3rd ed.). Subury, MA: Jones & Bartlett.

U.S. Department of Health and Human Services. (2000). *Healthy people 2010: Understanding and improving health objectives for improving health* (2nd ed., 2 vol). Washington, DC: U.S. Government Printing Office.

U.S. Department of Health and Human Services. (2001). *Comunity-Based Participatory Research: Conference Summary.* Agency for Healthcare Research and Quantity. Retrieved October 9, 2009, from http://www.ahrq.gov

U.S. Department of Health and Human Services. (2004). *State of aging and health in America 2004.* Centers for Disease Control and Prevention. Retrieved March 15, 2008, from http://www.cdc.gov/aging/pdf/State_of_Aging_and_Health_in_America_2004.pdf

U.S. Department of Health and Human Services. (2005). *Overview of the uninsured in the United States.* Retrieved March 1, 2008, from http://aspe.hhs.gov/health/reports/05/ uninsured-cps/ib.pdf

U.S. Department of Health and Human Services. (2006a). *Medicare enrollment—All beneficiaries: As of 2006.* Centers for Medicare and Medicaid Services. Retrieved October 9, 2009, from http://www.cms.hhs.gov/MedicareEnRpts/Downloads/06All.pdf

U.S. Department of Health and Human Services. (2006b). *Revised recommendations for HIV testing of adults, adolescents, and pregnant women in health care settings.* Centers for Disease Control and Prevention. Retrieved March 15, 2008, from http://www.cdc.gov/mmwr/preview/mmwrhtml/rr5514a1.htm

U.S. Department of Health and Human Services. (2008a). *National survey of family growth.* Centers for Disease Control and Prevention. Retrieved February 28, 2008, from http://www.cdc.gov/nchs/nsfg.htm

U.S. Department of Health and Human Services. (2008b). *History of HIV in the U.S.* Centers for Disease Control and Prevention. Retrieved March 15, 2008, from http://www.cdc.gov/hiv/topics/basic/index.htm#history

U.S. Department of Health and Human Services. (2008c). *Welcome to the Office of Family Assistance.* Administration for Children & Families: Office of Family Assistance. Retrieved March 3, 2008, from http://www.acf.hhs.gov/programs/ofa/

U.S. Department of Health and Human Services. (2008d). *National SCHIP Policy Overview.* Centers for Medicare & Medicaid Services. Retrieved March 4, 2008, from http://www.cms.hhs.gov/NationalSCHIPPolicy/downloads/SCHIPEverEnrolledYearGraph.pdf

U.S. Department of Health and Human Services. (2009). *About ACF.* Administration for Children & Families. Retrieved on October 9, 2009, from http://www.act.hhs.gov

World Health Organization. (2008). *The determinants of health.* Retrieved January 8, 2008, from http://www.who.int/hia/evidence/doh/en/index.html

CONTACTS

- *Centers for Medicare and Medicaid Services:* http://www.cms.hhs.gov/
- *Children's Defense Fund:* http://www.childrensdefense.org/site/PageServer?pagename=homepage
- *George Mason University Washington Health Policy Institute:* http://www.gmu.edu/departments/chpre/policyinstitute/home_whpi.html
- *Guttmacher Institute:* http://www.guttmacher.org
- *Henry Street Settlement:* 265 Henry Street, New York, NY 10002. http://www.henrystreet.org/site/PageServer?pagename=cnt_home
- *Kaiser Family Foundation:* http://www.kff.org/
- *Nurse Family Partnership:* http://www.nursefamilypartnership.org/index.cfm?fuseaction=home
- *Office of Minority Health and Health Disparities:* http:// www.cdc.gov/omhd/About/about.htm

Families Across the Health Continuum

CHAPTER 6

Culturally Sensitive Nursing Care of Families

Deborah Padgett Coehlo, PhD, RN, PNP

Margaret M. Manoogian, PhD

CRITICAL CONCEPTS

- ✦ Cultural diversity includes not only differences in race and ethnicity, but also differences in socioeconomic status, family structure, abilities, sex, age, and hierarchy from the normative culture.

- ✦ Culture begins with shared values, beliefs, knowledge, and practices within families, and extends to larger groups within a community to progressively larger groups that influence individuals and families from a societal level.

- ✦ Cultural diversity includes understanding the different beliefs about the causes (i.e., biological vs. psychological or spiritual causes) and treatment of disease (i.e., westernized vs. alternative treatments) within a cultural group.

- ✦ Family nursing includes cultural competency that embraces cultural awareness, sensitivity, and critical thinking when caring for a family different from the nurse's personal or professional culture, or both.

- ✦ Health disparities are evident for most minority groups within United States, including lack of a medical home, longer waits for care, more emergency department visits, decreased health care coverage through insurance, and a greater incidence of many chronic illnesses.

- ✦ Two theories and one perspective that assist in providing culturally competent family nursing care include the Bowman's Family System Theory, Duvall's Family Development Theory, and the life course perspective.

- ✦ Nursing care of families includes being familiar with generalizations (common beliefs of any one culture), whereas avoiding stereotyping families (believing all families automatically share all cultural beliefs, values, knowledge, and practices of a cultural group).

- ✦ Nursing care includes hearing the voices of family members and accommodating differences, with the ultimate goal of having a culture of caring.

(continued)

The terms *culture* and *diversity* typically are linked to describe the phenomenon of caring for patients with different beliefs, values, backgrounds, traditions, behavior, or practices. For nurses, learning more about culturally diverse families has grown from the awareness of the mounting gap in culture between patients and professionals, and the real and potential harm that can result when professionals lack cultural competence when caring for diverse families. The definition of cultural diversity, by itself, has expanded beyond race and ethnic differences to include differences from the *majority culture* in the areas of race, ethnicity, socioeconomic status, abilities, age, developmental stage, education, language, religion, sexual orientation, gender, and family structure. This expanded view has brought to light the importance of professionals learning how to care effectively for individuals, families, and communities who are outside the definition of "normative." In the United States, the long-held belief is that the normative family includes two heterosexual, white, middle-aged, middle-class parents with two biological children, with the primary breadwinner being the husband. This normative view has been studied and challenged, and has directed the growing emergence of studies on diverse populations.

Culture, by itself, refers to the shared values, worldview, language, jargon, and norms held by a group of people. Culture contains the environmental, social, and economic influences that form the nurse's *and* the client's beliefs and values, sense of identity and self-worth, and expectations of behavior and family roles (Cortis, 2003; Leeder, 2003). Understanding culture is an important part of understanding family roles, responses, adaptation, and organization (Mercer, 1989). Therefore, cultural competency is a requirement for safe and effective family nursing care (de Villiers & Tjale, 2000).

The smallest unit of culture is the family, as the members within the family form specific values and beliefs, establish traditions, and agree on familial practices, such as health care. This unit of culture is then expanded to include the surrounding community and identified groups chosen by the family to expand their identity, such as religious and ethnic groups and/or groups with similar family structures (i.e., single parents). The largest cultural group is represented by the human species, recognizing that some characteristics extend beyond smaller cultural groups leading to similarities among humans across continents. For example, women across time and across cultures rock their newborn infants at the same cadence of 80 beats per minute (Blum, 2002). Figure 6-1 illustrates the connection from family cultures to broader cultures.

The expanded view of cultural diversity beyond race and ethnicity has prompted studies that demonstrate a stark and growing health disparity between culturally diverse populations and the majority European-white populations in westernized countries. For example, the National Health Care Disparities Report (2007) indicates that Hispanic/Latino populations had fewer identified primary health care providers or medical homes, more average wait time for health care, and decreased appointment times when compared with similar white populations. Because of this growing health disparity with diverse populations, professional nursing organizations have emphasized the need for enhanced education and competency with cultural diversity. Care of individuals from diverse backgrounds is improved with awareness, training, and critical thinking skills. Yet, care of individuals without considering family as

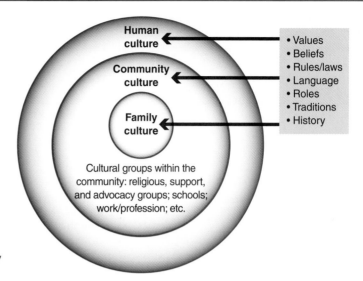

FIGURE 6-1 Connection between family and larger culture.

the context for cultural learning both for the client and the nurse can decrease the effectiveness of health care (Kozulin, Gindis, Ageyev, & Miller, 2005). This chapter explores nursing care of diverse families using the Family System's Theory, Family Developmental Theory, and life course perspective as guiding frameworks.

REVIEW OF LITERATURE

Much has been written, mandated, and taught in recent years on cultural diversity. The growing numbers of diverse populations in the United States have challenged all stages of health care, from acute hospital care to community care for chronic illnesses. Using the expanded view beyond race and ethnicity, we conclude that growing diverse populations include:

- Families with English as a second language, or emerging English speakers
- Families living in poverty
- Families without a stable or affordable home, or both
- Aging populations
- Adolescent populations
- Families coping with a family member with a physical or chronic mental illness, or both

- Families with nontraditional structures, including single-headed households, grandparents raising grandchildren, same-sex parents, or blended families
- Groups oppressed by race, ethnicity, religion, sexual orientation, ability, geographic location, sex, or any combination thereof

This expanded view has heightened our awareness of how differences from the identified norm in any culture can have a measurable impact on the incidence of health conditions and outcomes, and on the quality of health care provided to individuals and families from diverse backgrounds. Table 6-1 provides a list of the expanded view of diverse populations with incident rates now studied to guide competent, culturally diverse nursing care. As explained in the table, diverse families continue to face health care disparities in the incidence of illness, delay in health care, and shortened life expectancy for adults and children. Notable is the growing incidence of psychological distress and mental illness in diverse family members, at a time when mental health services are harder to find. This is true for same-sex couples, grandchildren raised by grandparents, and children and adults with disabilities (National Health Care Disparities Report, 2007). This trend underlines why the expanded view of diversity is needed to encourage health care equality across all groups.

TABLE 6-1

Expanded List and Incidence of Culturally Diverse Populations with Identified Health Disparities

CATEGORY OF CULTURAL DIVERSITY	INCIDENCE IN THE UNITED STATES	HEALTH DISPARITIES (NATIONAL HEALTH CARE DISPARITIES REPORT, 2007)
Families living in poverty	12.3% of the population; 36.5 million people (U.S. Census Bureau, 2006)	Poor individuals received poorer care than high-income individuals in more than 85% of items measured,* including communication problems, increased wait for care, and lack of dental care.
Families considered homeless	3.5 million people, with 1.5 being children younger than 18 years (National Coalition for the Homeless, 2007)	Mortality rates for the homeless are 3 to 5 times greater than those with stable housing, with heart disease being the leading cause of death for young and old adults (McCary & O'Connell, 2005).
Aging families, or those with the head of household older than 65 years	35.5 million adults older than 65 years (Centers for Disease Control and Prevention, 2007)	Diversity in the older population is growing, with an estimate of whites decreasing from 83% of the population of older adults in 2003 to 72% in 2030, with an increase of the Hispanic population from 6% in 2003 to 18% in 2030 (Centers for Disease Control and Prevention, 2007). Diverse populations of older adults, particularly Hispanic populations, have greater numbers of and poorer outcomes from chronic illness than white populations, especially in rural, poor areas of the United States (Centers for Disease Control and Prevention, 2007).
Families with same-sex parents	Approximately 1–3% of families have same-sex parents, with 22% of lesbian families having children younger than 18 years and 6% of gay families having children younger than 18 years (Ambert, 2005)	Gay, lesbian, and bisexual individuals have higher levels of psychological and physical chronic conditions reported than heterosexual individuals. The psychological conditions are related to depression and anxiety, and physical conditions related to HIV infection in men (Cochran & Mays, 2007).
Families with changing roles: Parents Grandparents	4 million children are currently living with their grandparents (RAND Corporation, 2000)	A study of 99,890 children showed that those children living with grandparents had poorer physical and mental health than those living in other family structures (Bramlett & Blumberg, 2007).
Families faced with behavioral/emotional problems in one or more members	It is estimated that one in five children and adolescents have a mental health disorder that requires medical treatment (National Mental Health Information Center, 2003). In the United States, 19.1 million individuals are currently using illicit medications. Native Americans and families living in poverty have the greatest rates of substance abuse (National Health Care Disparities Report, 2007).	African American, Hispanic, Native American/Alaskan Native, poor, uneducated, and rural families received less mental health services than white families (National Health Care Disparities Report, 2007).

TABLE 6-1

Expanded List and Incidence of Culturally Diverse Populations with Identified Health Disparities—cont'd

CATEGORY OF CULTURAL DIVERSITY	INCIDENCE IN THE UNITED STATES	HEALTH DISPARITIES (NATIONAL HEALTH CARE DISPARITIES REPORT, 2007)
Families with one or more members with a chronic illness	5.6 million individuals younger than 65 years had one or more disabling conditions in 2006; 14 million individuals older than 65 had limitations in one or more activities of daily living and/or instrumental activities of daily living (National Health Care Disparities Report, 2007). The most commonly reported chronic health conditions reported in children were asthma, allergies, learning disabilities, and attention-deficit disorder from 2003–2006 (National Health Care Disparities Report, 2007).	Parents of children with special needs consistently report that their children receive less complete health care services than those without a disability (National Health Care Disparities Report, 2007).
Families in oppressed groups: Non-Christian		Although the group of non-Christians is growing in America, there are no studies yet indicating how this shift affects health care. Non-Christians include those that follow a non-Christian religion and those stating they do not or no longer follow a Christian religion of their parents.
Native American		Native American individuals received poorer care than whites in more than 40% of items measured, including less prenatal care and high level of communication difficulties between professional and patient.
Hispanic and Latino		Hispanic individuals received poorer care than whites in more than 50% of items measured, including AIDS diagnoses, communication problems between professional and patient, and increased wait time for care.
African American		African Americans received poorer care than whites in more than 40% of items measured, including AIDS diagnoses, children being hospitalized for asthma, and families being left unseen in emergency departments.

*"Poor" is defined as having family income less than 100% of the Federal poverty level, and "high income" is defined as having family income 400% or more of the Federal poverty level. The complete table for federal poverty guidelines (2008) can be found at http://aspe.hhs.gov/poverty/08Poverty.shtml.

Historical Perspective

The understanding of cultural diversity began as a broad appreciation of the meaning of culture. Culture was initially defined as the beliefs, values, knowledge, and behaviors of an identified group. Many limited this definition to distinct ethnic groups, such as Mexican Americans, or races, such as African Americans. This limited view ignores the commonality of several groups who share language, customs, traditions, heritage, history, and relationships. Today, the definition of culture is largely unchanged, but the application of this definition is expanded to include a variety of groups who share beliefs, values, knowledge, and behaviors. Established in the past as the dominant cultural model of family life, the view of the normative culture, that of white, heterosexual, middle-class adults raising biological children, with the husband being the primary breadwinner, is now considered just one of many diverse family structures across society.

Take, for example, the culture of nurses. Nurses use linguistically shared jargon and abbreviations rarely used by other groups. Nurses co-create a culture together when they share stories among each other that others outside the culture of nurses would not understand or even want to hear. Nurses share the history of nursing and the heritage of famous nurses making a difference in our world (e.g., Florence Nightingale). Nurses share common knowledge about health, standardized by the National Board of Nurses. Nurses share customs and traditions, such as morning report, Nurses' Day, and pinning ceremonies. Nurses often share health beliefs centered on prevention, compassion, and holistic care. Are any of these shared beliefs, values, knowledge, and behaviors wrong because they are different than other cultural groups? Should nurses give up their language, beliefs, knowledge, or behaviors because they do not match larger groups' customs or the normative culture? Instead, nurses offer a breadth of knowledge and added compassion to health care of individuals and families that augments the care provided by other professionals. Nurses' diversity is what makes the profession unique and valuable rather than replaceable.

Nursing Perspective on Cultural Diversity

Two important concepts to consider with any current discussion on cultural diversity are the distinctions between cultural *awareness* and cultural *sensitivity*. Cultural *awareness* begins with a self-exploration of personal cultural beliefs, values, knowledge, and behaviors, whereas cultural *sensitivity* is the awareness of others and an understanding that others may view health beliefs, values, knowledge, and behaviors differently. Sensitivity strives to capture the importance of differences between the nurse's culture and client's culture (Sawyer et al., 1995). It requires compassion for clients, and adaptation and accommodation to

their beliefs and behaviors whenever possible. Determining what is possible for adaptation and accommodation requires knowledge about different cultures and an understanding as to what is the same or similar to the nurse's culture, followed by informed critical thinking to enhance the ways the two cultures may work together. Cultural sensitivity starts with an open dialogue between clients and nurses (Martin & Henry, 1989). Understanding the nature of both cultural awareness and cultural sensitivity is a start, but merely understanding these terms is insufficient to change nursing care to competent nursing care. Leininger (1996), in developing the Cultural Care Theory, further enhances understanding of the different terms and concepts related to cultural diversity. Leininger conceptualizes the concepts of culture, care, diversity, and cultural and social structural dimensions in this theory. Leininger was one of the first nursing theorists to develop a theory based on culture and care emphasizing the interaction among cultural dimensions, including religion or spirituality, economics, kinship, education, technology, and family values and beliefs taught within and external to the culture across generations. Table 6-2 includes the definitions of these concepts that Leininger proposes.

TABLE 6-2
Leininger's Cultural Care Theory Definitions
Culture: the lifeways of a particular group with its values, beliefs, norms, patterns, and practices that are learned, shared, and transmitted intergenerationally
Care: the abstract and manifest phenomena and expressions related to assisting, supporting, enabling, and facilitating ways to help others with evident or anticipated needs to improve health, a human condition, or a lifeway
Diversity: refers to cultural variability or differences in care meanings, patterns, values, symbols, and lifeways among and between cultures
Cultural and Social Structure Dimensions: refers to the dynamic, holistic, and interrelated patterns or features of culture (or subculture), related to religion (spirituality), kinship (social), political (and legal), economic, education, technology, cultural values, language, and ethnohistorical factors of different cultures

Source: From Leininger, M. (1996). Cultural care theory, research, and practice. *Nursing Science Quarterly, 9*(2), 71–78, by permission.

Cultural competency was expanded by including an understanding of values, beliefs, knowledge, and behavior in the context of age, developmental stage, geographic location, socioeconomic status, environment, and experiences (Yearwood, 2006). Cultural competency was identified as an aspiration for many health care providers. Campina-Bacote (2007) has suggested a dynamic model for becoming culturally competent, entitled the Process of Cultural Competence in the Delivery of Healthcare Services. This model includes five constructs for health care providers toward becoming culturally competent, emphasizing that this is a changing, ongoing process rather than an end point. The five constructs include:

- **Awareness:** the process of examining personal beliefs, biases, and knowledge about identified diverse individuals, groups, and communities
- **Knowledge:** the knowledge about different cultures' worldview and the field of biocultural ecology
- **Skill:** the ability to conduct a cultural assessment in a sensitive manner
- **Encounters:** the exposure to diverse cultures, with meaningful, in-depth interactions
- **Desire:** the motivation to understand, know, and work with diverse individuals and groups, and to decrease cultural conflicts

This view has led us to a deeper understanding of competent assessment and care of diverse clients. A growing body of literature, however, emphasizes that stereotyping groups may be misleading, and potentially harmful, if individual differences are not carefully considered. It is equally important to gain knowledge about cultural groups, and ask why any family within the context of a larger culture has individual differences. For example, a second-generation Latino man may share values and beliefs about how illness emerges as a result of psychological trauma but may reject his parents' ideas on how to treat the illness because of his geographic residence, access to education, and developmental stage that influences his understanding differently than his parents (Willies-Jacobo, 2007).

Many health care agencies mandate cultural competency training. This mandate grew out of an increased awareness of the gap between health professionals' cultures, including nurses' and clients' cultures (Yearwood, 2006). This view is illustrated by comments typically found in nursing textbooks,

such as "We are convinced that nurses will be able to provide culturally competent and contextually meaningful care for clients from a wide variety of cultural backgrounds" (Andrews & Boyle, 2003). Simply learning about different cultures is not enough! Nurses today are encouraged instead to consider how to use their cultural knowledge and critical thinking skills in everyday practice, research, education, and scholarly writing (Yearwood, 2006). The ultimate goal is to transcend individual cultures into one culture of caring. Rosen (2007) summarizes this goal in stating, "A fundamental belief and practice around creating a culture of caring also dissolves some of the differences we might otherwise focus on" (p. 9). The National Standards for Culturally and Linguistically Appropriate Services in Health Care (2001), listed in Table 6-3, were developed to assist health care agencies and professionals to provide more culturally and linguistically appropriate services.

Common Cultural Differences

DEFINITION OF HEALTH. The definition of health has expanded over the last several decades to be more than the absence of disease. Rather, health is now the state of well-being considering physical, mental, emotional, and spiritual aspects (World Health Organization, 2003). Health is also no longer limited to the health of any one individual. Rather, the health of the individual is intertwined with the health of the family, the community, and the larger culture and environment in which the individual lives. Health defined by one cultural group may be different than that for another cultural group. For example, a child with a seizure disorder may be described as healthy and protected by higher powers in the H'mong culture, whereas the same child may be described as ill and disabled in a Western culture (Fadiman, 1997).

DEFINITION OF ILLNESS AND DISEASE. The client's sociocultural explanation of illness or disease addresses the off balance or disequilibrium between the body, the environment, and the believed influences of God or a god, spirits, ancestors, sorcery, environment, stress, and/or vectors (i.e., bacteria, cancerous cells, viruses) as causes of the presenting symptoms or situation (de Villiers & Tjale, 2000). This definition conflicts with a strict

TABLE 6-3

National Standards for Culturally and Linguistically Appropriate Services in Health Care (CLAS)

Standard 1
Health care organizations should ensure that patients/consumers receive from all staff members effective, understandable, and respectful care that is provided in a manner compatible with their cultural health beliefs and practices and preferred language.

Standard 2
Health care organizations should implement strategies to recruit, retain, and promote at all levels of the organization a diverse staff and leadership that are representative of the demographic characteristics of the service area.

Standard 3
Health care organizations should ensure that staff at all levels and across all disciplines receive ongoing education and training in culturally and linguistically appropriate service delivery.

Standard 4
Health care organizations must offer and provide language assistance services, including bilingual staff and interpreter services, at no cost to each patient/consumer with limited English proficiency at all points of contact, in a timely manner during all hours of operation.

Standard 5
Health care organizations must provide to patients/consumers in their preferred language both verbal offers and written notices informing them of their right to receive language assistance services.

Standard 6
Health care organizations must assure the competence of language assistance provided to limited English-proficient patients/consumers by interpreters and bilingual staff. Family and friends should not be used to provide interpretation services (except on request by the patient/consumer).

Standard 7
Health care organizations must make available easily understood patient-related materials and post signage in the languages of the commonly encountered groups and/or groups represented in the service area.

Standard 8
Health care organizations should develop, implement, and promote a written strategic plan that outlines clear goals, policies, operational plans, and management accountability/oversight mechanisms to provide culturally and linguistically appropriate services.

Standard 9
Health care organizations should conduct initial and ongoing organizational self-assessments of CLAS-related activities and are encouraged to integrate cultural and linguistic competence-related measures into their internal audits, performance improvement programs, patient satisfaction assessments, and outcomes-based evaluations.

Standard 10
Health care organizations should ensure that data on the individual patient's/consumer's race, ethnicity, and spoken and written language are collected in health records, integrated into the organization's management information systems, and periodically updated.

Standard 11
Health care organizations should maintain a current demographic, cultural, and epidemiologic profile of the community, as well as a needs assessment to accurately plan for and implement services that respond to the cultural and linguistic characteristics of the service area.

Standard 12
Health care organizations should develop participatory, collaborative partnerships with communities, and utilize a variety of formal and informal mechanisms to facilitate community and patient/consumer involvement in designing and implementing CLAS-related activities.

TABLE 6-3
National Standards for Culturally and Linguistically Appropriate Services in Health Care (CLAS)

Standard 13
Health care organizations should ensure that conflict and grievance resolution processes are culturally and linguistically sensitive and capable of identifying, preventing, and resolving cross-cultural conflicts or complaints by patients/consumers.

Standard 14
Health care organizations are encouraged to regularly make available to the public information about their progress and successful innovations in implementing the CLAS standards and to provide public notice in their communities about the availability of this information.

Source: National Standards for Culturally and Linguistically Appropriate Services in Health Care (2001). *Executive Summary.* Washington, D.C.: U.S. Department of Health and Human Services Office of Minority Health. Retrieved September 16, 2009, from www.omhrc.gov/Assets/pdf/checked/executive.pdf.

biomedical perspective. Some cultures emphasize the biomedical cause and cure, whereas other cultures emphasize illness caused by other sources including spiritual, environmental, relational, and historical factors.

HEALTH PRACTICES. Cultures that emphasize the biomedical causes of disease and illness, and minimize other causes tend to turn to Westernized medical models for care and cure of their illnesses. In contrast, cultures that emphasize other than biomedical causes of disease tend to turn to such things as alternative healers (Latin cuanderismo, herbalists, lay midwives), witch doctors (ancient tribal sorcerers who for centuries have used poisons and body parts to bring about healing or punishment by death), ancestor worship (endeavoring to honor and satisfy the spirits of those who have died through sacrifices of food, animals, and children), prayer (prayer to one god during individual prayer or prayer circles within many major religious groups), or the worship of multiple gods deemed to oversee health, marriage selection, fertility, and harvest yield.

In addition to alternative healers and spiritual approaches to health practices, many cultures combine herbal or pharmaceutical practices with other alternative health practices, such as acupuncture, biofeedback, physical exercise, nutritional changes, and meditation.

Theoretical Framework

Working with families from diverse cultures can be complex because of the dynamic nature of any one individual, family, and community, as well as the broader cultural beliefs, values, and knowledge. Two theories enhance our understanding of nursing care with diverse families: Family Systems Theory (Bowen, 2004) and the Family Development Theory (Duvall, 1967; Bengtson & Allen, 1993). Many authors have viewed family care from a systems approach that recognizes that the beliefs, actions, and experiences of one family member affects all family members, and that each family functions based on internal and external systems. Chapter 3 reviews the key concepts within family system theories. Bowen's Family Systems Theory has been used by family professionals and builds on family system theories by presenting eight primary concepts to facilitate understanding of family functioning across time and across cultures:

- **Triangulation:** Tension is relieved through triangulation of sharing tension among three rather than two people. Triangulation strengthens the system but often leaves two people stronger and one person, the outsider, weaker. The family feels stronger with three members, but tensions increase as energy flows from dyad to dyad, often leaving a third member feeling like an outsider. An example is when a child is born: mothers and infants often form strong dyads, resulting in some fathers feeling like outsiders.
- **Differentiation:** This is the ability to differentiate individual thoughts and feelings from group thoughts and feelings. A loner is differentiated too much, whereas a follower is not differentiated enough. Differentiation from the larger culture is more likely with physical separation, length of time within a cultural group, and membership in other cultural groups.

- **Nuclear family emotional system:** This refers to the tendency to take on the emotions of other family members. For example, if a young mother is anxious about parenting, the infant will feel anxious as well. In families from diverse cultures, fear of the larger culture experienced by parents may be communicated and felt by the children, leading to similar emotional responses among all family members.
- **Family projection:** This is the process of a family member projecting emotions and opinions onto another family member. For example, if a parent is fearful of members outside the family's culture and communicates that fear verbally to his or her child, then he or she will project those feelings onto a child, and model and teach the child to be fearful of members outside his or her cultural group.
- **Multigenerational transmission:** This is the process of transmitting thoughts, feelings, values, beliefs, and behaviors across generations. For example, health and illness routines are passed down from parents to children across several generations within a cultural group.
- **Emotional cutoff:** This is the process of cutting off family members because of unresolved conflict. This occurs often as individuals leave or change long-held cultural practices.
- **Sibling position:** This refers to characteristics that are commonly seen as dependent on sibling position of parents and children. This can vary across cultural groups depending on the value placed on sibling order. For example, several cultural groups honor the oldest male member. Other groups expect the youngest female member to remain single to care for aging parents.
- **Societal emotional process:** This is the transmission of societal emotions to individual families. For example, if a society feels fearful or threatened, then individual families often feel fearful or threatened.

Each of these concepts is influenced by how a family adapts to internal and external tensions, as well as the strength of their connections to family members, and the external culture and society within their network. As such, each family may differ depending on their family of origin, which may include the surrounding culture, family structure, family tensions, sibling order of the parents and children and the meaning of that hierarchy within the broader culture, unresolved conflicts and emotional reactions to those conflicts, and the function of the broader society and culture.

Family Case Study Family Systems Theory

Shani was a 26-year-old Native American born on an Indian Reservation. She was one of seven children, and the oldest girl in her family. When Shani was 7 years old, she went to live with her maternal grandparents because of her parents' divorce and chronic alcoholism. Two younger brothers continued to live with her mother, and the remaining four children were dispersed among paternal relatives. Shani never saw her father or four of her siblings again. Her grandparents raised her off the reservation in what she described as a "middle-class home." She attended and received her diploma from a public school when she was 18 years old. Meanwhile, her two brothers living with her mother continued to live in extreme poverty. They both started using drugs and alcohol during middle school, and failed to complete high school. Because she felt uncomfortable about the privileges she received in comparison with her two brothers, Shani felt it was her responsibility to return to the Reservation to help her mother and brothers. She obtained a job as a preschool teacher, which included simple housing for herself and her family members. Her brothers continued to struggle with drug addiction, which also included troubles with the local authorities regarding illegal activities. Her mother continued to drink and could not work because of chronic diabetes and obesity. Shani tried to build new relationships and start a family of her own but had several failed relationships because of her brothers' and mother's behaviors, and their growing dependency on her. At age 26, Shani began experiencing "anxiety attacks." Several times per month, she would feel heart palpitations that would last from several minutes to several hours. Because she could not figure out a way to help her family and take care of herself, Shani began to show signs of depression and started thinking about suicide. Worried about her health, Shani's grandparents encouraged her to leave the Reservation and return to her previous stable life. Shani responded to their concern by stating that she was unable to face the guilt of leaving her family one more time. Shani also was influenced by the stories she heard from her family and the conditions she encountered on the Reservation. Her mother and brothers shared stories about the oppression they experienced within the white culture and the distrust they developed as a consequence of their experiences. As a young girl, Shani's mother had been sent to boarding school where she was restricted from speaking her language or engaging in tribal rituals and practices. Her mother relayed a story to Shani about an incident at the boarding school where a teacher held her mother's hands on a frozen flag pole for not stating the Pledge of Allegiance correctly. Shani's brothers also described incidents of not being able to find employment, being attacked by groups of young men from other cultures, being harassed by white police, and being denied services outside the Reservation. Her mother cried with frustration at not being allowed into treatment programs for her alcoholism. Shani started to fear white people and became more anxious about leaving the Reservation.

Using Bowmen's Family Systems Theory, develop nursing care for this family:

+ *Triangulation.* Shani's family began to triangulate during the parents' divorce, with a divide between the parents and their respective relatives. The children were divided into three groups, including the mother, the father's relatives, and the maternal grandparents. Although this move separated the children, the family was stronger through triangulation than it was together. The culture allowed the family to remain with family relatives rather than strangers but did not allow regular contact between all family members.

+ *Differentiation.* Shani initially became differentiated from thinking like her parents or the larger culture. When she returned to the Reservation and lived with her mother and brothers, however, she found it hard to differentiate her thoughts from the group thoughts. Even when she talked to her grandparents, she could not differentiate what thoughts and opinions were hers versus what were her grandparents' thoughts. Her anxiety increased as she tried to differentiate individual thought from group thought.

+ *Nuclear family emotional system.* Primary family emotions included helplessness, hopelessness, and anger toward treatment from the larger society. Shani did not share this emotion until she returned to live with her mother and brothers. She

then found herself feeling emotions similar to her mother and brothers.

+ *Family projection.* Shani's mother projected her feelings onto Shani and her brothers. Her mother's helpless, hopeless, and angry feelings led her to alcohol as a primary coping mechanism. She shared these feelings with her children. Her sons followed a similar path. Because Shani observed other coping strategies while living with her grandparents, she did not want to use drugs and alcohol as coping mechanisms but felt uncomfortable and guilty about the differences she observed between herself and her family members.

+ *Multigenerational transmission.* Experiences of physical and mental abuse often occur across several generations. Inadequate housing, poverty, substance abuse, unemployment, and lack of educational opportunities have been typical features of Reservation life across our nation. Tribal groups have lost homes, languages, cultural traditions, and lives. In many current cases, cultural helplessness, hopelessness, and anger remain today because of multigenerational transmissions and the continued oppression of tribal members. Health disparity, as one example of oppression, continues with many Native Indians struggling with greater rates of several chronic illnesses and shorter life expectancies. Shani absorbed the emotional feelings of her family across previous generations. She could repress these feelings when living away from the Reservation but could not ignore these feelings when surrounded by the evidence of abuse and the continued oppression of her family members.

+ *Emotional cutoff.* Shani eventually severed the relationship with her grandparents. She decided to decrease her internal tension because of confusion about how she could best support her family members, take care of herself, and manage her internal guilt. Her father and other siblings were emotionally unavailable to Shani, her mother, and her brothers.

+ *Sibling position.* Because Shani was raised as an only child in her grandparents' home, she developed characteristics of a leader or overly responsible person. Her brothers and mother were younger siblings, and developed characteristics of dependency. When she joined her mother and brothers, Shani assumed responsibility for their needs.

◆ *Societal emotional process.* The overall emotion of the surrounding society of the Reservation where Shani lived reflected oppression and impoverishment. This made it more difficult for Shani to see and develop healthy and positive coping strategies for herself and her family members.

Nursing Care Using the Family Systems Model

Nursing care for Shani and her family would begin with a thorough family assessment, focusing on:

1. *Family structure.* Structures includes a family genogram (Fig. 6-2), ecomap (Fig. 6-3), and clear description of cultural values influencing this family's ecologic systems (individuals, family as a whole, and the surrounding community). The ecomap would illustrate support and resources utilized by this family and the perception of the quality of that support.

2. *Family development.* This includes the developmental stages of Shani and her family members, the family as a whole, and attachments within this family. For example, it would be important to explore Shani's perception of attachment to her grandparents, her mother, and her father.

3. *Family function.* Function includes current and past roles and responsibilities of family members, outside influences on those roles and responsibilities, and family communication, including problem solving, support, and passing on of family culture and traditions.

The family assessment would provide information that would assist the nurse in making clinical judgments that would guide interventions. The nurse would aid this family in outlining their strengths and challenges, including strength in loyalty to their culture and to their family, willingness to share multigenerational stories to clarify beliefs and values, and desire to form stronger and

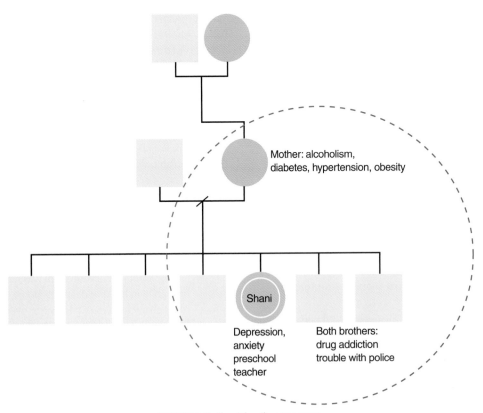

Mother: alcoholism, diabetes, hypertension, obesity

Shani

Depression, anxiety preschool teacher

Both brothers: drug addiction trouble with police

FIGURE 6-2 Shani family genogram.

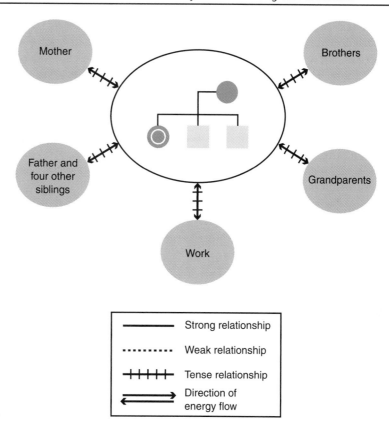

FIGURE 6-3 Shani family ecomap.

healthier relationships. Challenges include mental health disorders within and surrounding the family, including depression, anxiety, and multigenerational trauma, leading to disruptions in family development, limited coping strategies, and limited support from the community.

Based on this clinical judgment, nursing interventions would center on the family's strengths whereas addressing challenges (for further reading on strength-based transcultural nursing care, refer to Lind & Smith, 2008):

1. *Mental health:* Recommendations would include referral for mental health services for Shani and her immediate family members. Shani would benefit from one-on-one counseling from a professional with expertise in tribal care to address Shani's internal conflict and multigenerational sense of oppression. An appropriate counselor also could assist Shani in building healthy relationships with her mother and brothers, including healthy boundaries, to allow energy for her own growth and development, and movement toward healthy adult relationships. Shani's

mother and brothers also would benefit from advocacy provided by the nurse to assist them in obtaining addiction treatment.

2. *Coping strategies:* The nurse would outline priority goals for this family, and help them identify coping strategies and resources that could assist them in reaching these goals. For example, if addiction treatment was identified as a priority, then the nurse would help each family member develop a plan to obtain treatment and obtain support to succeed in that treatment. Likewise, if the family stated that they wanted to regain healthy tribal relationships, the nurse could help the family identify strategies to reach this goal, such as participation in healthy community activities that did not include drug use. The nurse also would refer this family to other community support resources, such as financial assistance, educational services, and health services.

3. *Family communication:* It is important to address family communication patterns that may hinder the healthy development of individual family members and the family as a whole.

Having each family member recognize and verbalize the needs of other family members would help break the cycle of overdependency on Shani. Discussing Shani's conflict between her relationship and experiences with her grandparents versus her mother and brothers would help the family see their role in helping Shani to develop relationships across family boundaries. Referral to a counselor who could help Shani strengthen her own identity would improve family communication patterns.

The evaluation of this family would be based on identified challenges and the expected outcomes following the interventions outlined. Expected outcomes would include improved and clarified boundaries between all family members, stronger and clearer relationships within and outside the family structure, successful use of outside support and resources, and evidence of sobriety of all family members. Identified mental health disorders would be treated and stabilized by appropriate health care professionals. Expected timelines for each of these outcomes would be outlined with the family and guide timelines for follow-up services.

A family such as Shani's may be encountered in a variety of health care settings, ranging from mental health outpatient clinics to inpatient acute or chronic care. Shani may encounter nursing care related to her increasing symptoms of anxiety, her family's struggles with addiction, or an acute illness in a clinic or emergency department. Shani may be seeking family care, or this concept may be new to her, resulting in initial resistance and mistrust. The nurse has the challenge of identifying timing for a family assessment, appropriateness of the depth of interventions based on the health care setting and the expertise of the nurse, and building a trusting relationship to allow strength-based interventions. This case study illustrates the importance of looking beyond the individual, because without an understanding of family within the context of culture, the care for Shani would be incomplete and ineffective (Yurkovich & Lattergrass, 2008).

Family Developmental Theory

The Family Developmental Theory was developed in the 1950s and 1960s in response to the growing awareness of changes occurring in families regarding member roles and functions across time. Evelyn Duvall (1967) shifted the work of the 1950s from describing family roles over time to describing family stages, emphasizing the developmental tasks of individual family members and the family group as a whole. Because this theoretical model was developed more than 40 years ago, it has received some criticism because of its lack of inclusiveness of diverse family structures. This theory, however, is useful when implementing care for families as family member roles, developmental stages, and tasks change over time. Despite today's increasing diversity of family experiences and structures, it is still critical to address family adaptation to changes and attention to the developmental needs of family members within a larger cultural context. The eight family stages outlined in Duvall's Family Development Theory include:

- Stage 1: Married couples. The primary tasks for married couples are to leave the home of origin and establish a new home by developing positive relationships with a spouse and a peer network, as well as sharing mutually satisfying goals. The place within the broader family network or kinship is begun.
- Stage 2: Childbearing families. The primary tasks are adjusting to new parental roles, maintaining the marital couple, and encouraging the development of the infant.
  • Age of oldest child is newborn to 30 months.
- Stage 3: Families with preschool children. The primary tasks are continuing to define family member roles and encouraging the development of the child(ren).
  • Age of oldest child is 2.5 to 6 years.
- Stage 4: Families with schoolchildren. The primary tasks are to move beyond the family culture and into the larger culture, including schools, to enhance child development and learning.
  • Age of oldest child is 6 to 13 years.
- Stage 5: Families with teenagers. The primary tasks are to establish trust and guidance of an adolescent whereas allowing increasing responsibility and freedom. The parents, at the same time, begin to explore interests outside of parenting and reconnect to a strong couple dyad.
  • Age of oldest child is 13 to 20 years.
- Stage 6: Families as launching centers. The primary tasks are to launch young adults into the

broader culture whereas maintaining a stable and predictable homefront.

- First child being gone to last child leaving home is covered.

■ Stage 7: Middle-aged parents. The primary tasks are to strengthen the marital relationship and build extended kinship relationships across the younger and older generations.

- "Empty nest" to retirement is covered.

■ Stage 8: Aging family members. The primary tasks are to maintain close kinship ties whereas coping with repeated losses, including health, home, and death of loved ones.

- This stage refers to retirement to death of both spouses.

To adapt this theory to families within diverse structures (i.e., single-headed households, same-sex parents, or blended families) or to diverse cultural practices (i.e., cultural groups where adult children co-reside in multigenerational residences), you must consider developmental tasks and coping strategies that assure healthy development of all family members and the family as a whole. For example, for families experiencing divorce, the task of strengthening the marital couple shifts to strengthening the mutually agreed-on goals for parenting. For blended families, a new task emerges that includes establishing realistic expectations for attachment and family roles, and addressing individual differences from merging family cultures. This approach is often blended with the life course perspective to view families across time, considering their culture, developmental stages, life events, and changes in family structure from a historical viewpoint.

Family Case Study

FAMILY DEVELOPMENT THEORY

Jethra and Benyamin have been married 35 years and have successfully raised two daughters, 29 and 26 years old. Although their marriage has been difficult for several years because of ongoing conflict between Jethra and Benyamin, they have both committed to staying together "for the sake of their children and for a stable financial base." Jethra has worked 35 years part-time as a pharmacist, and Benyamin has worked 35 years as a computer specialist for a large company. This family's culture is Orthodox Jewish, including strict adherence to kosher foods, Jewish traditions and culture, and Jewish values and beliefs. This family is considered upper middle class, and they have a large support group of other Jewish families within a large urban community. Several changes occurred to this family over the span of 2 years:

- ✦ Benyamin lost his job, including his health insurance.
- ✦ Benyamin was in a bike accident resulting in a head injury, resulting in his inability to return to the workforce, and more than $100,000 in medical bills.
- ✦ This couples' oldest daughter, Rivka, gave birth to her first child 2 years ago. This child was recently diagnosed with autism and is just now beginning early intervention services. At this point, this child does not speak and has serious temper tantrums that last more than an hour two to three times per day. Rivka is in denial and is furious at her mother for thinking her child has autism, despite the diagnosis being given to this family after a full interdisciplinary evaluation at a university-affiliated child development center.
- ✦ This couple's youngest child, Yitra, is planning her wedding, which will occur in 9 months. She would like a wedding like her older sister's wedding, which cost the family more than $20,000. Jethra and Benyamin cannot afford this type of wedding at this point.
- ✦ Jethra had planned to retire within 2 years but now has to increase her hours at work to full-time to obtain health benefits and cannot retire for at least 5 years.
- ✦ Jethra discovered Benyamin has been having an affair with another woman. She is now considering divorce, which is unacceptable within her cultural and support group.

It is useful to use the Family Developmental Theory as part of the assessment of this family. Considering the developmental stage Jethra and Benyamin are facing, including families as launching centers, with the primary tasks including launching young adults into the broader culture whereas maintaining a stable and predictable homefront, and middle-aged parents, with the primary tasks being strengthening the marital relationship and building extended kinship relationships across the younger and older generations, it is clear successful navigation through these stages is being threatened by life events. Rivka's tasks for childbearing families is to adjust to her new parenting roles, maintaining her roles within a marital couple, and encouraging the development of her young child. These tasks are being threatened by the diagnosis of autism and the related strain on the parents because of delayed speech development, and frequent and intense temper tantrums. The journey through these family developmental stages are further complicated by membership within a cultural group that has strong religious values including adherence to religious practices, sexual and procreation rules, differences in male and female roles within the family and the culture, and dietary rules, including consumption of only kosher foods, and the strict adherence to dietary restrictions including the absence of pork and shellfish from the diet. Within the Orthodox Jewish communities throughout the United States, there are diverse practices, especially regarding interaction with the secular communities, and roles and practices of women. (For further reading about the Orthodox Jewish religion and culture, refer to *Orthodox Jews in America* [Gurock, 2009].) Nursing care for this family includes the assessment of cultural beliefs and practices, and how their beliefs and practices influence their decisions about family health across different family stages. For example, some Orthodox Jews believe that God punishes those who do not follow God's word; therefore, any negative life event is viewed as a punishment. Others do not believe this and, in contrast, believe God will guide humans through hard circumstances. Understanding how religious beliefs influence meaning to the event of the diagnosis of autism can assist the nurse in determining support needed and probable health care reactions. Nurses are in the position to assess beliefs of the individual *and* within the family and broader culture. Determining whether the family's beliefs fit with their surrounding community and source of support can also help determine the level of support versus separation this family is facing. The family culture fits into the assessment of developmental tasks, because certain religious groups have strong feelings about the timing and adherence to family developmental stages. Many families face the challenge of dissolving an unhappy marriage to maintain health whereas being rejected by the support group and traditions the family has been surrounded by for generations. Likewise, obtaining certain treatments for a disability, such as autism, may or may not fit with religious teachings and traditions. It may be easier to deny problems and maintain support, rather than challenge long-held traditions.

Family developmental theory can be helpful in guiding the nurse through the assessment of a family. Family

culture can be assessed for each family developmental stage. This theory, taken across time, can add even more insight into how families adapt to changes in their family culture given the diagnosis of a chronic condition. This assessment can lead to more effective and culturally sensitive interventions, rather than applying generalized interventions that are likely to be rejected by the family.

Life Course Perspective

The life course perspective (Bengtson & Allen, 1993; Elder, 1974, 1994) focuses on the family as the unit of analysis and, when applied, encourages a family-focused approach to working with clients in health care. Multidisciplinary in nature, the life course perspective falls under the theoretical umbrella of individual life span, family development, and life course theories (see White & Klein, 2008). This perspective highlights individual development and normative expectations that occur across the life span, and calls attention to the linked lives of family members who interact within shifting social and cultural contexts (Bengtson & Allen, 1993). For instance, an understanding of clients' health expectations and behaviors must acknowledge the multiple influences of individual developmental change, family interactions and transitions over time, and the broader sociohistorical context. This perspective promotes a deeper understanding of individual and family diversity by highlighting how social norms, social class, and social meanings shape lives over time and across generations. As an example, the experience of becoming a parent, a common transition for most women and men, may be distinctly different across families as reflected by such contextual factors as cultural traditions, gender role expectations, and economic resources.

Key concepts in the life course perspective include:

- Families consist of individual members who forge connections, share stories, and create meanings. With time, these family ties may shift and change as sociohistorical changes occur. For instance, an older widow may become dependent on adult children when chronic illness compromises her abilities to perform typical daily activities and formal care providers are unavailable to her.

- Individual family members, their relationships with others inside and outside of the family, their family structure, and the set of expectations or norms about family life change with time. Time is multifaceted and includes: (1) ontogenetic time—the life course and development of an individual family member; (2) generational time—the transitions, stages, and events that families move through over time; and (3) historical time—events that occur within a broad social context that influence individual and family lives.

- How family members experience life course transitions, events, and relationships shapes their development and related outcomes over time.

- Family members are influenced by their location within the broader social structure. Perceptions of health care may be shaped by whether a family has economic resources or has established cultural practices of healing.

- As family members encounter particular life course events, they give them specific cultural meanings. Social norms shape behaviors and expectations about the timing of life events such as obtaining an education, becoming a parent, or retiring from paid work. These expectations may vary across race, ethnicity, sex, religion, sexual orientation, and class continuums.

- How family members act and respond to temporal contexts reflects both change and continuity over time. Particular health routines learned in earlier generations may remain central in families, whereas other health routines may alter because of developing medical technology and knowledge.

- Family members create their life courses, as they respond actively to both the opportunities and obstacles they encounter. Their expression of agency implies that they have choices and diversity in the life paths they forge. As family members age, social context shifts, and demographic changes increase the diversity of experiences and outcomes for development. Simply, heterogeneity, or differences in changes based on different experiences across time, is associated with aging.

Family Case Study

LIFE COURSE PERSPECTIVE

Joe, a 59-year-old retired veteran, lives with his wife, Linda, in rural West Virginia. Diagnosed with type 2 diabetes 4 years earlier, Joe has difficulties managing his illness and also takes medication for both high cholesterol and blood pressure. Typical of the Appalachian region, Joe and Linda own a small hillside home, located miles from their neighbors. They grow much of their own food, participate in local Grange activities, and have family members who live in the vicinity. Joe is close to one adult daughter, and reports that the other is "too busy with her own life." He is estranged from his five siblings with the exception of one older sister. He and his older sister were both raised by two aunts when his parents were unable to manage their large family economically. Joe has a strong interest in "putting away" food for the winter months. He often has large groups over for a meal or helps cook at large community events and his wife's family reunions.

Joe confesses that he has troubles managing his daily routines that would help him better manage his diabetes. Enjoying his large garden, Joe spends hours outside. He typically forgoes both breakfast and lunch, eating a large dinner once he comes inside, with continued snacking into the evening. He checks his blood sugar "maybe once a week," and has lost interest in testing and recording his results "because the doctor don't really look at it." Joe also expresses frustration at his diagnosis interfering with his retirement plans. Smoking, a habit he started while in the military, is an activity he shares with his wife. Joe knows that he needs to manage his weight, control portion sizes, and stay vigilant regarding his diabetes management. Joe admits that he is concerned about future complications because of his disease, but he states, "I don't dwell on it. I am hoping like everyone else that it don't get no worse. The only thing you can do whatever comes along is take it and go on."

By using a life course perspective, nursing care for Joe can help him manage his disease better. Without a clear understanding of Joe's family experiences over time, a nurse may miss the opportunity to help Joe establish realistic and healthier diabetes management activities on a daily basis. In addition, because most of Joe's health routines occur at home outside the purview of the medical community, a nurse will need to probe deeper in understanding the unique and diverse practices of Joe and other patients similar to him who are challenged with this serious, chronic disease.

The life course perspective suggests that Joe's health and his attempts at diabetes management need to be addressed within the context of his family relationships. Using the concepts highlighted earlier, nurses expand their abilities to understand illnesses within families, provide support that addresses health behaviors and expectations that extend across a life course, and initiate interventions for care that have potential for not only the patient, Joe, but his entire family network.

◆ Joe and his family members, particularly his wife, Linda, have established health routines and daily practices that inevitably influence Joe's ability to manage his disease. Together, they hold an understanding of type 2 diabetes that is deeply influenced by the experiences of older family members. A nurse may find, with attention to the generational experiences of Joe and Linda's families of origin, that both Joe and Linda have family members who have diabetes. Joe's mother died of complications after losing her sight and her leg, and his sister struggles with her sight as well. Linda's sister shares information with Joe about strategies for managing his weight and exercise programs from her own experiences. Because both Joe and Linda grew up in families with limited economic resources, as is true for many Appalachian families, they were less able to access health care services and relied on home remedies. Joe's and Linda's perceptions about diabetes are shaped by the extreme and painful experiences of older family members at a time when little was known about the serious complications of diabetes in this community.

◆ Because Joe and Linda are both retired from paid work, their fixed incomes provide little security. They are concerned about the cost of their medications and worry about their future health needs. Combined with a lifetime of limited economic resources, the life course perspective would suggest that their current expectations and experiences of health were shaped by earlier experiences. Joe is less likely to see a physician, works hard to produce food, and has multiple storage strategies to maintain food security over the winter months. As a retired veteran, Joe has access to medical care but must drive 2 hours to receive it. The financial constraints, combined with his reticence and lack of practice in accessing preventative medical care support, leave Joe and Linda vulnerable to future health issues and provide a backdrop in which a nurse may work with this family.

◆ Appalachian families often rely on informal support resources to help in times of need. Joe and Linda have family in the area, but Joe's family relationships with his siblings and one of his adult daughters are strained. Understanding the cultural context of families in the region would suggest that strong family ties exist. It would be critical to evaluate Joe's social support resources to determine whether his family experience fits within typical cultural patterns and behaviors.

◆ Joe and Linda both lived through periods of war, where Joe served active duty in Vietnam. His military and generational experiences suggest that he is conservative with his resources, may be less likely to express pain and other health concerns, and may feel frustrated with medical practitioners who approach him in a manner that appears disrespectful of his age, culture, and sex. At the same time that he is aging and experiencing other health concerns, he has less economic security but more time to devote to his health care needs.

◆ Linda, the only other family member in the household, plays a critical role in providing support to Joe. Understanding their relationship, the gender roles and expectations they have established across their married years, and the ways that family labor are performed has ramifications for Joe's care. Appalachian families tend to hold traditional family values with distinct roles for women and men in families. Understanding these roles, such as Linda's responsibility for cooking the household meals, suggests that she needs to be part of diabetes education and health care appointments with Joe.

◆ Joe expressed frustration that his retirement years will be influenced by his illness. Expectations of a healthy retirement and his current reality leave him angry and shape his attitude about managing his disease. It would be critical to understand how Joe's life course transition into retirement is shaping his daily experiences and family relationships.

◆ Joe takes great pride in helping out at Grange events and family reunions. He is viewed as a community chef at these activities in a cultural context that traditionally involves food. The regional cuisine challenges healthy eating, and

Joe may need help to evaluate his current food practices. He readily admits that he grew up in a time where "cleaning my plate every meal was important. You didn't know when the next one would come!" Understanding these long-standing patterns across Joe's life course will aid the nurse in developing effective strategies with Joe.

✦ A nurse may work with Joe and his family in understanding how the health routines he learned as a child and currently practices may be thwarting his diabetes management activities. He and Linda also will need help in examining how family stories and generational memories about health issues may be less applicable to today's health care realities.

✦ Joe expresses concern and fear as he responds to both the opportunities and challenges presented to him once he was diagnosed with diabetes. A nurse may help Joe and Linda understand their choices and reinforce their abilities to build their family life course, with diabetes management strategies across time integrated within that plan.

✦ Joe and Linda's experiences are unique to their family situations. The Appalachian cultural context that shapes their family experiences may suggest avenues for creating health care protocols for Joe and Linda, as well as other families in the region. For instance, the emphasis on family ties, the isolation from others because of geographic terrain, and the traditional family values held by many may suggest specific health strategies that could involve menu adaptations; programs through churches, schools, and small community centers; and exercise options that focus on small community centers.

NURSING CARE HONORING CULTURAL DIVERSITY

Acknowledging the client's voice is the first step in providing culturally diverse competent care. This process can be enhanced by obtaining cultural knowledge before the encounter. Sought from reliable sources, cultural knowledge provides the nurse with valuable generalizations about the broader culture experienced by the family (Cortis, 2003). An important distinction is to clarify the difference between *generalizations* and *stereotyping*.

Generalizations are a beginning point of reference (e.g., "Women from Japan tend to be quiet and stoic. I wonder if this woman from Japan is not complaining of pain because of this cultural tradition rather than a true lack of pain."). Stereotyping yields judgment and finality (e.g., "This woman is from Japan, so she must be quiet and stoic and not telling me the truth about her pain. How can she hope to get care for her pain with this behavior?"), and the nurse becomes vulnerable to misinterpretation and failure. Nurses are especially at risk for stereotyping families if they practice with the false assumptions and expectations that all families from a given culture have identical expectations and behaviors. (For an overview of cultural generalizations, refer to D'Avanzo & Geissler, 2003). Kleinman (1980) has developed eight simple yet insightful questions to help clarify generalizations and give personal meaning to the illness or condition (Table 6-4). In an effort to learn the family's perception, Campbell, McDaniel, and Cole-Kelly (2003) have added the following family-focused questions:

▪ Has anyone else in your family had this problem?

▪ What do your family members believe caused the problem or could treat the problem?

▪ Who in your family is most concerned about the problem?

▪ How can your family be helpful to you in dealing with this problem?

TABLE 6-4

Cultural Assessment: Eight Questions to Ask Yourself and Then Your Client

Questions to Include in a Cultural Assessment

1. What do you think caused your illness?
2. Why do you think your illness started when it did?
3. What do you think your illness does to you?
4. How severe is your illness?
5. What are the chief problems your illness has caused you?
6. What do you fear most about your illness?
7. What kind of treatment do you think you should receive?
8. How do you hope to benefit from treatment?

Source: From Kleinman, A. (1980). *Patients and healers in the context of culture.* Berkley, CA: University of California Press, by permission.

Prior cultural knowledge encourages nurses to rephrase questions into the present context. One example is the care of a pregnant woman. Pregnancy is not an illness, yet learning how a woman and her family feel about the pregnancy, labor, birth, and early parenting is central to the quality cultural nursing care of this client.

Diagnosis and Clinical Judgment

It is critical that nursing diagnoses and clinical judgments are adjusted to match the cultural values and beliefs of clients as guided by cultural practices. For example, each culture has distinct responses to particular illnesses, and applies meaning based on cultural and spiritual beliefs. Asking a family to articulate its understanding of a particular diagnosis and what it means is important, because the response to this question can help guide effective interventions.

Interventions

Interventions for culturally diverse families are based on an assessment of critical differences and similarities between the nurse and the family. The interventions also are based on critically evaluating what is beneficial to the family versus what is harmful. Literature on nursing interventions with culturally diverse families provides mixed opinions as to the approach when cultural practices are deemed potentially or already harmful to one or more family members by the nurse. For example, if a mother from Southeast Asia brings her infant in with a fever and a bilateral ear infection, and has been using coining, the process of rubbing coins on the skin to treat illness (Yonemitsu & Cleveland, 1992), rather than having the child evaluated for an infection and treated with antibiotics, cultural conflict may emerge for the nurse and the family. Past use of North American Nursing Diagnosis Association's nursing diagnosis guidelines would suggest this family fell into the category of "knowledge deficit." Current recommendations include recognizing reciprocal knowledge deficits between the nurse and the family, and working with the family to accommodate both cultural beliefs. As a result, many families are willing to incorporate Western medicine practices, given sufficient information about the rationale, adverse effects, and expected outcomes within the context of their cultural practices. This is a workable solution in most cases, and becomes a problem only when cultural practices have negative outcomes, such as mixing prescription medications with herbal remedies, or causing physical or psychological harm (e.g., female genital mutilation or son preference) (Office of the High Commissioner on Human Rights, 1979).

Evaluations

The evaluation of nursing care for diverse families is dependent on the culturally competent assessment, diagnosis, and plan of care that includes the families' history, developmental changes, and cultural beliefs and values. If culturally competent care is initiated throughout the nursing process, the evaluation will show evidence of improved well-being based on the combined definition from the nurse and the family.

International Nursing

Cultural encounters can be interesting and challenging but are enhanced when the nurse crosses borders to live and work within a new cultural environment. In these situations, nurses are isolated from their personal cultural norms, values, practices, and resources. For instance, practicing within a new cultural context may create differing expectations for 8-hour shift practices and hold challenges for all activities of daily living. In the new international setting, the nurse must relearn, if not come to reunderstand and revalue, new units of intervention that define identity, health care promotion, disease prevention, and healing. A new process of prioritizing family needs, resources, and actions is required (Long, 2000). Regarding international nursing, Long (2000) describes three units of intervention as relationship to self, relationship to others, and relationship to the environment. Relationship to self includes hygiene and personal caregiving, risk behaviors, identity, worth, and efficacy. Relationship to others is the interaction within the family and community. Interactions include relating to the larger population, community agencies, and groups outside the health care arena. Relationship to the environment addresses the patterns of exposure to the land, economic structures, and employment, and all cultural practices, values, and beliefs.

Anthropologists Spradley and Phillips (1972) used the Cultural Readjustment Rating Questionnaire to rate the adaptation of Peace Corps and international students in their stress-related adjustment to a new international environment. The readjustment questionnaire items listed in Table 6-5 demonstrate various conditions and situations the international nurse of today may face. According to the authors, "Cultural practices of every sort are reported to induce stress: toilet training, puberty rites, residential change, polygamous households, belief in malevolent gods, competition, and discontinuities between childhood socialization and adult roles" (Spradley & Phillips, 1972, p. 518). Two unexpected findings emerged from this classic study. First, neither previous intercultural experience nor a similar cultural background to the new culture influenced the appraisal and adaptation process needed within the new environment. Second, knowing the language alone did not prove significant in cultural adaptation. It remains necessary to understand the cultural definitions of the words and the issues (Spradley & Phillips, 1972).

Case Study

INTERNATIONAL NURSING

Three young American nurses met in a small African nation ready for volunteer service within a mission hospital. The hospital bedded 250 patients and had a medical staff of only 5 physicians. The nationals spoke both their tribal language and British English, and the nursing roles and titles were defined by the British system. As the nurses had received their baccalaureates in nursing and were educated in the American Western health care system, it required an immediate practice and autonomy paradigm shift to practice independently in this new country. These nurses faced challenges of catching newborns without midwifery skills, suturing without experience, diagnosing and treating tropical ailments without related education and training, and striving to understand the role of the witch doctor within the hospital system. The change crisis was

---

TABLE 6-5

Cultural Readjustment Items

1. The type of food eaten	18. How free and independent women seem to be
2. The type of clothes worn	19. Sleeping practices such as amount of time, time of day, and sleeping arrangement
3. How punctual people are	
4. Ideas about what offends people	20. General standard of living
5. The language spoken	21. Ideas about friendship, that is, the way people act and feel toward friends
6. How ambitious people are	
7. Personal cleanliness of most people	22. The number of people of your religious faith
8. The general pace of life	23. How formal and informal people are
9. The amount of privacy I would have	24. You own opportunities for social contacts
10. My own financial state	25. The degree to which your good intentions are misunderstood by others
11. Type of recreation and leisure-time activities	
12. How parents treat their children	26. The number of people who live in the community
13. The sense of closeness and obligation felt among family members	27. Ideas about what is funny
	28. Ideas about what is sad
14. The amount of body contact such as touching and standing close	29. How much friendliness and hospitality people express
15. The subjects that should not be discussed in normal conversation	30. The amount of reserve people show in their relationships to others
	31. Eating practices such as amount of food, type of eating, and ways of eating
16. The number of people of your own race	
17. The degree of friendliness and intimacy between unmarried women and men	32. Type of transportation used
	33. The way people take care of material possessions

Source: From Spradley, J., & Phillips, M. (1972). Culture and stress: A quantitative analysis. *American Anthropologist, 74*(3), 518–529, by permission.

enhanced by being assigned to supervisory positions, within an unknown health care system.

Two of the nurses adapted well through active interaction with the nationals and missionary workers. Daily discussions allowed for expression of likes, dislikes, questions, and emotions. These nurses completed their overseas commitment and continued to have other international service experiences. The third nurse struggled with her placement. The cultural crisis and progressive culture shock precipitated an early return home, and she required counseling to aid her recovery. She continued to practice nursing but only within the borders of the United States.

The risk for cultural maladaptation and culture shock is a real possibility for international health care workers. Unresolved culture shock may result not only in ineffective and nonproductive nursing care of new patients and their families, but also compromised health for the nurse including depression, psychosis, withdrawal, abnormal and disruptive behaviors, menstrual irregularities, eating disorders, insomnia, stress-induced cardiac and hormonal crisis, and suicide. Whether the international nurse is leaving Western civilization to serve in another country or the reverse, mechanisms for support during cultural adaptation are essential for the health and well-being of the nurse, and in turn, the patient and family.

Throughout the literature and international service preparation materials, the stages of culture shock typically are outlined for any nurse traveling to and arriving in a new country. Initial shock and adjustment are common. Fellow travelers, with their sights and smells, as well as local customs, language, perceived safety, and weather changes, may cause the nurse to question the decision of international service. When a nurse has prior knowledge of the culture, has made detailed and firm arrangements, and has a welcoming committee present, early adjustment often proceeds without significant physical and emotional distress (Jones, 2001). The World Health Organization (2003) provides guidelines and suggestions for international travel preparation and process (refer to *International Travel and Health* [World Health Organization, 2003] for these guidelines and suggestions).

After recuperation from the physical symptoms (jet lag) associated with crossing multiple time zones within a short period (World Health Organization, 2003), the first days and weeks in a new host country often are described as the "honeymoon" phase. This is a common euphoria experienced by the temporary traveler to a region. This phase is followed by a more realistic view of the culture as the traveler encounters more in-depth experiences.

When the new culture does not conform to the expectations of the nurse, conflict often emerges (Spradley & Phillips, 1972). It is common for progressive negative attitudes and emotions toward the people and the culture to formulate. The very people who could serve to help the nurse adjust become threatening: "The first step in critical contextualization is to study the culture phenomenologically. If, at this point, the [nurse] shows any criticism of the customary beliefs and practices, the people will not talk about them for fear of being condemned" (Hiebert, 1994, p. 174).

The risk for a cycle of anger, hostility, and mutual isolation can occur for some nurses unless active and dynamic intervention is found. Ideally, the nurse will serve internationally with a home support system with which the nurse remains bonded, and to whom the nurse can discuss the areas of conflict. This alone is inadequate, however. Those at home have no insight into what the nurse is experiencing. Therefore, it also is recommended that the nurse immediately seek host nationals or others from the home nation living in the host county. Establishing friendships and mentorship relationships to instruct, guide, and assist in the transition helps prevent culture shock in the nurse and validates the importance of the new culture and people.

This pattern of cultural shock can and does occur with nurses who come to live and work in the United States. A study of Korean nurses revealed that feelings of depression, isolation, and physical impairments were more common than among American nurses. The Korean nurses expressed feelings of exhaustion from trying to learn the new culture while completing expected duties as a nurse. The cultural shock is greatest among nurses learning English after arriving to the United States, and those with little support from other nurses in the workplace or host family arrangement.

SUMMARY

Cultural diversity is a welcome yet challenging aspect of nursing care of families. Knowledge of diversity, while avoiding stereotyping, can enrich the nurse's experience while working with families different from the nurse's experiences and beliefs, knowledge, practices, and behaviors. Understanding and using cultural diversity competency concepts can lead to a deeper understanding of how family members maintain well-being in the midst of health, illness, and disability. True cultural sensitivity is an art and a science that goes a long way in helping families from diverse backgrounds. The theories outlined here provide a framework that can help nurses provide quality family nursing care that avoids stereotyping, but rather addresses family and community cultural differences in a manner that promotes health.

REFERENCES

Agency for Healthcare Research and Quality (2007). *National Health Care Disparities Report: 2007.* Retrieved March 15, 2008, from http://www.ahrq.gov/qual/qrdr07.htm

Ambert, A. M. (2005). *Changing families: Relationships in context.* Toronto, Ontario Canada: Pearson.

Andrews, M., & Boyle, J. (2003). *Transcultural concepts in nursing care* (4th ed.). Philadelphia: Lippincott.

Bengtson, V. L., & Allen, K. R. (1993). The life course perspective applied to families over time. In P. G. Boss, W. J. Doherty, R. LaRossa, W. R. Schumm, & S. K. Steinmetz (Eds.), *Sourcebook of family theories and methods* (pp. 469–498). New York: Plenum.

Blum, D. (2002). *Love at Goon Park.* Cambridge: Perseus.

Bowen, M. (2004). Bowen Theory from the Bowen Center for the Study of Families at Georgetown University retrieved on March 1, 2008, at http://www.thebowencenter.org/pages/conceptds.html

Bramlett, M. & Blumberg, S. (2007). Family structure and children's physical and mental health. *Health Affairs, 26*(2), 549–558.

Campbell, T., McDaniel, S., & Cole-Kelly, K. (2003). Family issues in health care. In R. Taylor (Ed.), *Family medicine principles and practice* (6th ed., pp. 24–32). New York: Springer.

Campinha-Bacote, J. (2007). *The process of cultural competence in the delivery of healthcare services: The journey continues* (5th ed.). Cincinnati, OH: Transcultural C.A.R.E Associates.

Centers for Disease Control and Prevention. (2007). *The state of aging and health in America: 2007.* Whitehouse Station, NJ: Merck Company Foundation.

Cochran, S. D., & Mays, V. M. (2007). Physical health complaints among lesbians, gay men, and bisexual and homosexually experienced heterosexual individuals: Results from the California Quality of Life Survey. *American Journal of Public Health, 97*(11), 2048–2055.

Cortis, J. (2003). Culture, values and racism: Application to nursing. *International Nursing Review, 50*(1), 55–64.

D'Avanzo, C., & Geissler, E. (2003). *Pocket guide to cultural health assessment* (3rd ed.). St. Louis: Mosby.

de Villiers, L., & Tjale, A. (2000, November). Rendering culturally congruent and safe care in culturally diverse settings. *Africa Journal of Nursing and Midwifery,* 21–24.

Duvall, E. M. (1967). *Family Development.* Philadelphia: Lippincott.

Elder, G. H., Jr. (1974). *Children of the Great Depression: Social change in life experience.* Chicago: University of Chicago Press.

Elder, G. H., Jr. (1994). Time, human agency, and social change: Perspectives on the life course. *Social Psychology Quarterly, 57,* 4–15.

Fadiman, A. (1997). *The spirit catches you and you fall down.* New York: Farrar, Straus, and Giroux.

Gurock, J. S. (2009). *Orthodox Jews in America.* Bloomington: Indiana University Press.

Hiebert, P. (1994). *Anthropological reflections on missiological issues.* Grand Rapids, MI: Baker Books.

Jones, N. (2001). *The rough guide to travel health.* London: Penguin Group.

Kleinman, A. (1980). *Patients and healers in the context of culture.* Berkley: University of California Press.

Kozulin, A., Gindis, B., Ageyev, V. S., & Miller, S. M. (2005). *Vygotsky's educational theory in cultural context (Learning in doing: Social, cognitive and computational perspectives).* Cambridge: Cambridge University Press.

Leeder, E. (2003). *The Family in Global Perspective: A Gendered Journey.* Thousand Oaks, CA: Sage.

Leininger, M. (1996). Cultural care theory, research, and practice. *Nursing Science Quarterly, 9*(2), 71–78.

Lind, C., & Smith, D. (2008). Analyzing the state of community health nursing: Advancing from deficit to strengths-based practice using appreciate inquiry. *Advances in Nursing Science, 31*(1), 28–41.

Long, W. (2000). *Health, healing, and God's kingdom.* Harrisonburg, VA: R.R. Donnelly and Co.

Martin, M., & Henry, M. (1989). Cultural relativity and poverty. *Public Health Nursing 6*(1), 28–33.

McCary, J. M., & O'Connell, J. J. (2005). Health, housing, and the heart cardiovascular disparities in homeless people. *Circulation, 111,* 2555–2556.

Mercer, R. (1989). Theoretical perspectives on the family. In C. Gillis (Ed.), *Toward a science of family nursing.* Menlo Park, CA: Addison-Wesley.

National Coalition for the Homeless. (2007). *How many people experience homelessness.* Retrieved March 15, 2008, from http://www.nationalhomeless.org

National Standards for Culturally and Linguistically Appropriate Services in Health Care. (2001). *Executive Summary.* Washington, D.C.: U.S. Department of Health and Human Services Office of Minority Health. Retrieved September 16, 2009, from www.omhrc.gov/Assets/pdf/checked/executive.pdf.

Office of the High Commissioner on Human Rights. (1979). *Fact sheet no. 23, harmful traditional practices affecting the health of women and children.* Retrieved March 15, 2008, from http://www.unhchr.ch/html/menu6/2/fs23.htm#i

RAND Corporation. (2000). *Grandparents caring for grandchildren: What do we know?* Retrieved March 28, 2008, from http://rand.org/pubs/research_briefs/RB5030/index1.html

Rosen, E. (2007). *The culture of collaboration.* San Franciso: Red Ape.

Sawyer, L., Regeu, H., Proctor, S., Nelson, M., Messias, D., Barnes, D., & Meleis, A. (1995). Matching versus cultural competence in research: Methodological considerations. *Research in Nursing and Health, 18,* 557–567.

Spradley, J., & Phillips, M. (1972). Culture and stress: A quantitative analysis. *American Anthropologist, 74*(3), 518–529.

U.S. Census Bureau. (2006). *Income, poverty, and health insurance coverage in the United States: 2006.* U.S. Department of

Commerce Economics and Statistics Administration. Washington D.C.: Author.

White, J. M., & Klein, D. M. (2008). *Family theories*, (3rd ed.). Los Angles: Sage.

Willies-Jacobo, J. (2007). Susto: Acknowledging patients' beliefs about illness. *Virtual Mentor, 9*(8), 532–536.

World Health Organization. (2003). *International travel and health*. Geneva: Author.

Yearwood, E. L. (2006). The problem with diversity. *Journal of Child and Adolescent Psychiatric Nursing 19*(3), 161–162.

Yonemitsu, D. M., & Cleveland, J. O. (1992). *Culturally competent service delivery: A training manual for bilingual/ bicultural case managers*. Culturally and Linguistically Appropriate Services, Childhood Research Institute. Retrieved March 12, 2008, from http://clas.uiuc.edu/ fulltext/ cl00147/cl00147.html

Yurkovich, E. E., & Lattergrass, I. (2008). Defining health and unhappiness: Perceptions held by Native American Indians with persistent mental illness health. *Mental Health, Religion & Culture, 11*(5), 437–459.

CHAPTER 7

Canadian Context of Family Nursing

Colleen Varcoe, PhD, RN

Gweneth Hartrick Doane, PhD, RN

CRITICAL CONCEPTS

✦ Families, health, and family nursing are shaped by the historical, geographic, economic, political, and social diversity of Canada. By understanding this diversity, when providing care, nurses are prepared to take into account the contextual nature of families' health and illness experiences, and how their lives are shaped by their circumstances. This helps with conveying understanding and providing more appropriate care.

✦ "Context" is not something outside or separate from people; rather, contextual elements (e.g., socioeconomic circumstances, family and cultural histories) are quite literally embodied in people and within their actions and responses to particular situations.

✦ Similar to other Western developed countries, Canada has an overall level of prosperity accompanied by a significant and growing gap between rich and poor, and has a biomedical- and corporate-oriented health care system. These influences shape Canadians' health, their experiences of family, and their experiences of health care and nursing care. By understanding how these economic and political influences shape family experiences, nurses respond more effectively toward the promotion of health.

✦ Dominant expectations and discourses about families in Canada are also similar to other Western countries. These expectations and discourses shape Canadians' health, their experiences of family, and their experiences of health care and nursing care. By examining how families and nurses themselves draw on these expectations and discourses, nurses can improve their responsiveness to families.

✦ Multiculturalism is part of Canada's national identity and is enshrined in Canadian state policy. Multiculturalism is understood in Canada to promote equality and tolerance for diversity, especially as it relates to linguistic, ethnic, and religious diversity. Tensions exist between this

(continued)

CRITICAL CONCEPTS   (continued)

understanding and the lived experiences of families, however, particularly those who are racialized, those who do not have French or English as their first language, and those from nondominant religions. *Racialization* refers to the social process by which people are labelled according to particular physical characteristics or arbitrary ethnic or racial categories, and then dealt with in accordance with beliefs related to those labels (Agnew, 1998). Nurses who understand these tensions and how they shape families and experiences are better prepared to provide responsive nursing care.

✦ As a colonial country, Canada has an evolving history of oppressive and genocidal practices against Canada's indigenous people, and an evolving history of varied immigration practices. Understanding how migration and colonization affects both indigenous and newcomer families, and the health and lives of people within those families is fundamental to providing effective family nursing care.

✦ Competent, safe, and ethical family nursing involves taking the context of families' lives into account. In addition, nurses need to consider the ways in which their own contexts shape their understandings and responses to particular families and situations. Together, these actions enable nurses to tailor their understanding and care to the specific circumstances of families' lives and mitigate the possibility of making erroneous assumptions about the families they serve. Without this careful consideration of context and its impact on families' health and illness experiences, nurses typically draw uncritically on stereotypes in ways that limit possibilities for families they serve. By inquiring into the context of families' and nurses' own lives, nurses are able to provide responsive, ethical, and appropriate care.

*U*nderstanding the context of families, health, and family nursing in Canada provides a key resource and strategy for responsive health promoting family nursing practice. Having an appreciation for the range of diverse experiences and how the dynamics of geography, history, politics, and economics shape those experiences allows nurses to provide more effective care to particular families, better understand the stresses and challenges families face, and better support families to draw on their own capacities. Developing such an appreciation requires that nurses consider how the varied circumstances of their own lives shape their understanding. The purpose of this chapter is to consider the significance of context and the importance of attending to context in family nursing practice. Specifically, we highlight the interface of sociopolitical, historical, geographic, and economic elements in shaping the health and illness experiences of families in Canada. This chapter begins by discussing why consideration of context is important to nursing. We then discuss some of the key characteristics of Canadian society,

and how those characteristics shape health, families, health care, and family nursing. Finally, we propose ways that nurses might practice more responsively and effectively based on this understanding.

CONTEXTUAL FOUNDATIONS FOR THE NURSING OF FAMILIES

"Context" is often conceptualized as a sort of container of people—something that surrounds people but is somewhat distinct and separate from people themselves. This encourages us to think of contexts as something outside of people's health and illness experiences—as something they might leave, something over which they have control, or both. This chapter encourages you to think of context as something that is integral to the lives of people, as something that shapes not only people's external circumstances and opportunities but their physiology at the cellular level. For example, if a person is born into a middle-class, English-speaking, Euro-Canadian family, the very way that person speaks—accent, intonation, vocabulary—is shaped by that context. The way that person's body grows is influenced by the nutritional value of the food and quality of water available, the level of stress in the family, the quality of housing the family has, the opportunities for rest and physical activity, and so on. Similarly, the person's sense of self and expectations for her life are shaped by the circumstances into which the person is born. The individual's success in education will depend not only on what educational opportunities are available, but on how the person comes to that education—for example, how well fed or hungry, well rested or tired, confident and content he or she is—and the economic resources available that shape which school the person attends. Thus, a person's multiple contexts cannot be "left" or understood as being outside or separate from one's self or necessarily under one's control. Rather, although circumstances change, people embody their circumstances, and although people have some influence over their circumstances, such influence generally is more limited than we would like to imagine. Moreover, the contextual elements and the experiences those elements give rise to live on in people. That is, past contexts go forward with people, shaping how they experience present and future contexts.

Throughout your nursing career, you will be providing care in specific contexts, and families will live in their own diverse contexts. Consciously considering the interface of these differing contexts and how they are shaping families' health and illness experiences is vital to providing responsive, health-promoting care. Also foundational to this process is the necessity to inquire into the contexts shaping your own life and practice. This enables you to choose more intentionally how to draw on those influences to enhance your responsiveness to families.

DIVERSE CANADIAN CONTEXTS

As noted at the beginning of this chapter, Canada is diverse in multiple ways. This section considers five key areas of diversity that are significant to families and family nursing, including geographic, economic, ethnocultural, linguistic, and religious diversity. These contextual elements overlap and intersect, shaping health, experiences of family, and experiences of health care and nursing.

Geographic Diversity

Canada's varied geography, encompassing differing terrains and climates, and ranging from dense urban settings to sparsely populated remote rural areas, shapes Canadian life. Across the prairies, the various coastal regions, the remote areas of the north, and the different mountain ranges are varied resources and climatic conditions that shape the lives of Canadians in differing ways. The population of Canada is concentrated primarily in urban centers in the south. In 2006, Statistics Canada reported that just less than 20% of Canadians (about 6 million people) were living in rural areas (areas located outside urban centers with a population of at least 10,000) (Statistics Canada, 2006a). A continuing trend exists toward urbanization as more people move from less to more urban settings (Statistics Canada, 2002). In 2006, more than 25 million Canadians (80%) lived in urban areas, a reversal from more than a century ago (Human Resources and Social Development Canada, 2006). The three largest urban areas in Canada—Toronto, Vancouver, and Montreal—made up just more than one-third (34.4%) of Canada's entire population. Geographic differences influence other aspects of life. For example, incomes in rural settings are lower than in urban settings (Singh, 2004), and health indicators are generally poorer in rural settings. In 2001, a lower proportion of Canadians living in small towns, rural regions, and northern regions rated their health as "excellent" compared with the national average and had a greater prevalence of being overweight and smoking (Mitura & Bollman, 2003). People living in northern regions had greater unmet health care needs compared with the national average, whereas people in major urban regions had lower unmet health care needs. Life expectancy is lower and mortality rates are greater, particularly from diabetes, injuries, suicide, and respiratory disease, in rural settings compared with urban settings (Canadian Population Health Initiative, 2006). Geographic diversity shapes health through multiple pathways, including different access to food, housing, and other health resources; the kinds of employment available; environmental conditions and hazards; and social patterns.

Economic Diversity

Although Canada is a wealthy, developed nation, a large and steadily widening income gap exists between rich and poor (Statistics Canada, 2006d), with many Canadians living in poverty. Statistics Canada estimated that in 2006 3.4 million Canadians (10.5%) lived in low-income families (Statistics Canada, 2008). About 760,000 children younger than 18 years (11.3%) lived in low-income families. About 307,000, or 40%, of these children lived in a lone-parent family headed by a woman. Canadian families with low incomes needed, on average, $7,000 Canadian to climb above the low-income cutoff.

Despite the economic prosperity in Canada in recent years, the benefits of that prosperity are disproportionately distributed, and the inequities between those who are wealthy and those who are poor, and between those who are healthy and those who are not continue to grow (Coburn, 2006). For example, a study analyzing the Canadian Community Health Survey found that, compared with white people, although people who were identified as visible minorities were more likely to have achieved secondary or postsecondary education, they were also more likely to earn less than $30,000 Canadian per year (Quan et al., 2006). A study of Aboriginal[1] people in urban settings found that approximately 30% of Aboriginal households are headed by a lone parent compared with 13.4% for non-Aboriginal households in the same communities (Canada Mortgage and Housing Corporation, 2006). More than 50% of urban Aboriginal children in the Prairie and Territories Regions live in single-parent households versus 17% to 19% for non-Aboriginal children.

Income is a key determinant of health, affecting multiple dimensions of well-being. People who are racialized, are new immigrants, live in rural settings, and have disabilities are more likely to be poor, and are thus more affected by the health consequences of poverty.

The term *Aboriginal* refers to First Nations, Métis, and Inuit peoples (Royal Commission on Aboriginal Peoples, 1996, p. xii), reflecting "organic political and cultural entities that stem historically from the original peoples of North America, rather than collections of individuals united by so-called 'racial' characteristics" (p. xii).

Ethnocultural Diversity

Canada is one of the most ethnically diverse countries in the world, and the ethnic diversity of the Canadian population is increasing (Statistics Canada, 2003a). In 2001, 1.3 million people reported Aboriginal ancestry, comprising 4.4% of the total Canadian population. Of the non-Aboriginal population aged 15 years and older, nearly half (46%), or about 10.3 million people, reported only British or French ethnic or cultural origins, or reported as "Canadian" only. After this group, the next largest proportion of Canada's population was composed of the descendants of other Europeans. People of non-European descent accounted for 13% of the population aged 15 years and older, or 2.9 million people. This group includes people with origins in places such as Asia, Africa, Central and South America, the Caribbean, Australia, and Oceania. The most frequent origins were Chinese and East Indian.

Approximately 250,000 people immigrate to Canada annually. Of the more than 13.4 million immigrants who came to Canada during the 20th century, the largest number arrived during the 1990s. The 2001 census shows that 18.4% of the population was born outside Canada, the highest proportion since the 1930s. The origins of immigrants to Canada have changed in recent decades, with increasing numbers coming from non-European countries.

Although Canada has an official state policy that advocates equality and promotes tolerance through multiculturalism, many argue that the rhetoric of multiculturalism masks inequities and discrimination based on ethnicity and racism (Abu-Laban & Gabriel, 2002; Ng, 1995). Although Canadians often pride themselves on valuing diversity, and "multiculturalism" is official Canadian policy, in 2003, the Ethnicity Diversity Survey (Statistics Canada, 2003a) found that 2.2 million people, or 10%, reported that they felt uncomfortable or out of place sometimes, most of the time, or all of the time because of their ethnocultural characteristics. Those people who were identified as "visible minorities" were most likely to feel out of place. Henry, Tator, and Mattis (2006) argue that, in Canada, liberal democratic racism is widely practiced, wherein Canadian policies and rhetoric simultaneously promote equity and justice while tolerating widespread discrimination.

Racism has significant health effects (Cain & Kington, 2003; Nazroo, 2003). Discrimination based on race has been linked with health outcomes such as hypertension and other chronic diseases (Krieger, Chen, Coull, & Selby, 2005; Krieger & Sidney, 1996; Young et al., 1999), mental health problems such as depression and suicide (Borrell, Kiefe, Williams, Diez-Roux, & Gordon-Larsen, 2006), and low birth weight (Krieger, 2000; Mustillo et al., 2004; Rich-Edwards et al., 2001).

The changing immigration patterns and increasing ethnic diversity coupled with discriminatory policies and attitudes have an influence on families' experiences and health. Migration processes are stressful, and this stress is intensified when combined with language barriers and downward economic mobility (Beiser, Hou, Hyman, & Tousignant, 2002). The health of people after migration is complex, however, being shaped by their experiences and the sociocultural environment in which they live (Beiser, 2005).

Linguistic Diversity

Consistent with Canada's history as a colonial nation and a destination for immigrants from around the globe, the country is linguistically diverse. Of the more than 50 Aboriginal languages spoken before contact with Europeans, many are still spoken, but as of 1996, only three—Cree, Inuktitut, and Ojibway—had large enough populations to be considered truly secure from the threat of extinction (Statistics Canada, 1998). Most Canadians speak one or both of the official languages French and English, but in 2001, about 1 of every 6 people reported having a mother tongue other than English or French, an increase of 12.5% from 1996 (Statistics Canada, 2001). The 2001 census shows that 61% of immigrants who came to Canada in the 1990s used a "nonofficial" language as their primary home language. Between 1996 and 2001, language groups from Asia and the Middle East increased in number, and Chinese is now the third largest language group after English and French.

Language affects health in many ways. First, language is connected to identity. Language loss is, therefore, related to loss of cultural identity, something that is experienced in an ongoing manner by Aboriginal peoples and by immigrants to Canada whose first language is neither French nor English. Second, language barriers have a profound effect on access to social and health resources, including employment. Finally, language barriers can prevent the provision of ethical and adequate health care.

Some people who speak the dominant languages of Canada presume that everyone should learn French or English, without considering the resources it requires to do so and the barriers (such as poverty, transportation, discrimination) to doing so. Very limited supports are available for language acquisition, and in the case of immigrant families, the priority for language classes is often the person who is most likely to be able to obtain employment.

Religious Diversity

Canada is also a country of considerable religious diversity. Although Canada is predominantly Roman Catholic and Protestant, with 7 of every 10 Canadians identifying themselves as either Roman Catholic or Protestant (Statistics Canada, 2003b), this pattern is changing. Over the past few decades, fewer people are identifying as Protestant and more are identifying with religions such as Islam, Hinduism, Sikhism, and Buddhism. Most of this shift is the result of the changing sources of immigrants. In addition, major Protestant denominations dominant in the country, such as Anglican and United Church, have declined in numbers since the 1930s, in part because their members are aging and fewer young people are identifying with these denominations. Despite this changing profile, Christianity continues to dominate many Canadian public institutions, including health care.

Religious affiliation affects health in multiple ways, including fostering social inclusion and community support, and depending on the religion, serving as a basis for discrimination. Despite Canada's professed tolerance for diversity, acts of anti-Semitism and discrimination against other non-Christian religious groups are not uncommon. In particular, since 2001, discrimination against Muslims and those presumed to be Muslim have escalated (Helly, 2003; Mojab & El-Kassem, 2008).

HOW FAMILY IS UNDERSTOOD IN CANADA

Given this incredible geographic, economic, ethnocultural, and religious diversity, what constitutes "family" in Canada, and how family is lived and experienced varies greatly. Despite this diversity, however, particular ideas and taken-for-granted assumptions about family continue to dominate. These ideas shape our expectations about families (e.g., that families are "normally" nuclear and comprise a mother, father, and two kids), shape policies (e.g., that people receiving social assistance should turn to extended family and "exhaust" family resources before accepting social assistance), and also shape health care providers' expectations and practices (e.g., that families should provide care to elderly family members). Exploring and critically scrutinizing these dominant ideas in light of the diverse contextual elements that shape any particular family assists nurses to understand better both their own and families' expectations, the differences between those expectations, and the tensions that might arise between different stakeholders.

Three key elements to understanding families in Canada are especially useful for nurses to examine. First, similar to other industrialized western countries, families are generally assumed to be "nuclear," that is, to consist of two generations, including parents (generally assumed to be heterosexual) and children. Second, and again similar to other industrialized countries, women are generally expected to do the majority of parenting and caregiving, and certain views of motherhood and women are upheld as ideals. Third, family is generally held to be a safe and nurturing experience. Although these ideas dominate, considerable variations in people's experiences exist, and many people's experiences are in tension with these ideas.

Heterosexual Nuclear Family as the Norm

The idea that the heterosexual nuclear family is the norm is belied by statistics; for example, in 2006, 16.5% of families with children in Canada's metropolitan areas and 13.3% of families in rural areas and small towns were lone-parent families (Statistics Canada, 2006b). Statistics Canada notes that throughout the 20th century and into the 21st century, the proportion of large households has decreased with each successive census, and there has been a steadily increasing trend toward smaller households. The 2006 census found that there were more than three times as many one-person households as households with five or more persons.

Of the 12,437,500 private households, 26.8% were one-person households, whereas 8.7% were households of five or more persons. Furthermore, in 2001, Statistics Canada counted same-sex couples for the first time and identified a total of 34,200 same-sex common-law couples, representing 0.5% of all couples. Some of these couples have children living with them. About 15% of the 15,200 female same-sex couples were living with children, compared with only 3% of male same-sex couples. The 2006 census enumerated 45,300 same-sex couples. Of these, about 7,500, or 16.5%, were married couples, although same-sex marriage only became legal in Canada in 2005.

Although some people misconstrue living in households with larger numbers of people as a "cultural" preference, doing so primarily reflects economic considerations. For example, the Longitudinal Survey of Immigrants to Canada (LSIC) (Statistics Canada, 2005) notes that, although the 2001 census reported that the average size of a Canadian household was 2.6 persons, the average household size for LSIC immigrants was 3.4 persons, ranging from 3.1 for skilled worker immigrants to 4.0 persons for refugees. Most LSIC immigrants reported living in two- (21%), three- (24%) or four-person (22%) households, and were more likely to report living in a household of six or more people (12%) as compared with the Canadian average (3%). Aboriginal households were somewhat more crowded than the general population, with an average of 2.9 occupants and 2.6 bedrooms, compared with 2.5 and 2.8, respectively, for non-Aboriginal households.

Rather than simply assuming a "norm," or assuming that "nontraditional" families are a reflection of culture, it is important for nurses to understand the economic and social influences that shape housing for families. For example, the number of lone mothers heading families is, in part, a reflection of the prevalence of violence against women and the social expectation for women to "leave" abusive partners.

Ideals of Motherhood and Women

In Canada, dominant ideas about mothering and women shape families' experiences, their health, and health care provider expectations. Despite the diversity of family structures and roles, the "gold standard" continues to be mothering within a two-parent family with primary attention to the children (Ford-Gilboe, 2000), the ideal of exclusive mothering. Family caregiving for dependent elders or those who are ill or have disabilities continues to be a social expectation, especially in the wake of changes to the health care and social services systems that include deinstitutionalization of care. These expectations are at odds with other social forces, however. Women, including mothers, increasingly are expected to work outside the home (Statistics Canada, 2000a). As of 1999, 61% of women with children younger than 3 years were employed, a figure that doubled over the preceding two decades. Social policy, such as "work fare" social assistance policies, increasingly forces women with dependent children into waged labor, even when the work available is not adequate to cover the costs of safe child care. At the same time, policies such as cuts to minimum wage levels have deepened women's poverty even as they attempt to participate in the waged labor force (Morrow, Hankivsky, & Varcoe, 2004; Ricciutelli, Larkin, & O'Neill, 1998).

As described earlier, women are increasingly lone parents, often living below the poverty line and often on social assistance (Statistics Canada, 2000b, 2006e). But influences such as changing expectations of men as fathers mean that fathers are somewhat more actively engaged in child care and somewhat more likely to be the head of lone-parent families than in previous decades. Of the 15.2% single-parent households, 12.7% of single-parent families were headed by women, compared with 3.2% headed by men (Statistics Canada, 2006a). At least partly because of gender economics, many children are not being raised by their mothers. For example, the 2001 Canadian Census reported that 56,790 grandchildren younger than 18 years were living with their grandparents without parents in the home, with implications for the health of older men and women. Based on federal and provincial and territorial reports from 2000, Farris-Manning and Zandstra (2004) estimate that approximately 76,000 children in Canada were under the protection of Child and Family Services across the country. These trends, juxtaposed against ideals of good mothering and fathering, have produced new discourses, such as those regarding the "working mother," the "welfare mom," and the "deadbeat dad," that convey negative judgments.

When families are judged against the ideal of "exclusive" mothering, or against the ideals of family caregiving, they are often found wanting. That is, when women do not devote themselves to mothering exclusively or take up caregiving for a parent, spouse, or other dependent person and forego labor force participation, they are often judged as inadequate. Paradoxically, exclusive mothering implies economic dependence. Still, the economic and social conditions do not exist for most women to care for children and other dependents without also participating in waged work. In Canada, the "typical" mother is working outside the home and is often the lone head of a household and may also be living under or near the poverty line.

Family as Safe and Nurturing

In Canada, as in many Western countries, family is portrayed generally as positive, supportive, and safe. Yet, Canada is similar to other Western countries in the levels of violence perpetrated within families and levels of substance use. According to the most conservative estimates, 7% of female individuals and 6% of male individuals in current or previous spousal relationships reported having experienced some form of spousal violence during the previous 5 years (Statistics Canada, 2006c). Violence against women tends to be much more severe. Between 1995 and 2004, male individuals perpetrated 86% of one-time incidents, 94% of repeat (two to four) incidents, and 97% of chronic incidents (Statistics Canada, 2006c). In that same time frame, the rate of spousal homicide against female individuals was three to five times greater than the rate of male spousal homicide. Clark and Du Mont (2003) reexamined prevalence studies in Canada, suggesting that as many as 23% of women experience intimate partner violence each year. Lifetime rates of physical assault by an intimate partner have been estimated at 25% to 30% in Canada and the United States (Johnson & Sacco, 1995; Jones et al., 1999). Physical assault is often accompanied by sexual violence or emotional abuse, and many women experience intimate partner violence in more than one relationship over their lifetime (Johnson, 1996).

Estimates of child abuse rely primarily on *reported* cases and are thus underestimates. Based on data from child welfare authorities, the Canadian Incidence Study (CIS) of Reported Child Abuse and

Neglect estimated a rate of 21.52 investigations of child maltreatment per 1,000 children (Public Health Agency of Canada, 2001). Importantly, the greatest proportion of reported and substantiated child abuse cases involved neglect, which often overlaps with the social conditions created by poverty. Socioeconomic status has been shown consistently to be related to parenting effectiveness (Wekerle, Wall, Leung, & Trocmé, 2007). Despite the prevalence of neglect, less attention is paid to neglect in research, policy, and practice than to severe physical abuse and child sexual abuse, possibly in part because those forms of abuse are more sensational (McLean, 2001). Child welfare authorities tend to focus on risk assessment and urgent intervention for severe cases of child physical abuse, rather than on the more frequent situations of neglect. Trocmé, MacMillan, Fallon, and De Marco (2003) argue that because the CIS found severe physical harm (severe enough to warrant medical attention) in about 4% of substantiated cases, assessment and investigation priorities need to be revised and include consideration of long-term needs for housing, income, child care, and so on. Health care providers should focus on helping families access longer-term and broader social support.

Although it is difficult to estimate the extent of elder abuse in Canada, it is purported to be a significant problem. Almost 2% of older Canadians indicated that they had experienced more than one type of abuse (Canadian Centre for Justice Statistics, 2002). Elder abuse and neglect encompasses intimate partner violence that continues into older adulthood, and forms of abuse and neglect that arise as persons become more vulnerable with age. As with any form of intimate partner violence, in older adults it is gendered—that is, older women are at greater risk than men. Statistics Canada (1999) reported that, in the 1999 General Social Survey on Victimization, approximately 7% of the sample of more than 4,000 adults older than 65 years reported that they had experienced some form of emotional or financial abuse by an adult child, spouse, or caregiver in the 5 years before the survey, with most abuse committed by spouses. Emotional abuse was more frequently reported (7%) than financial abuse (1%). The two most common forms of emotional abuse reported were being put down or called names, or having contact with family and friends limited. Only a small proportion of older adults (1%) reported experiencing physical or sexual abuse.

Substance abuse is another factor that may make the experience of family less than safe and nurturing. Most problematic use in Canada involves alcohol. The Canadian Addiction survey found that, although most Canadians drink in moderation, 6.2% of past-year drinkers engaged in heavy drinking (five drinks or more in a single sitting for male individuals and four or more drinks for female individuals) at least once a week and 25.5% at least once a month (Collin, 2006). Using the Alcohol Use Disorder Identification Test, which identifies hazardous patterns of alcohol use and indications of alcohol dependency, Collin identified 17% of current drinkers as high-risk drinkers. Although most heavy and hazardous drinkers were male individuals younger than 25, this pattern suggests that harmful alcohol use is fairly common. According to the 2002 Canadian Community Health Survey, 2.6% of Canadians aged 15 and older (3.8% male and 1.3% female) reported symptoms consistent with alcohol dependence at some time during the 12 months before the survey. Rehm et al. (2006) estimate that 9% of disease and disability in Canada is caused by alcohol use. A range of problems are associated with problematic alcohol use, including violence and neglect.

Given the statistics on violence and substance abuse, although many families are safe and nurturing, this cannot be assumed. Indeed, in light of the levels of violence against women, children, and older persons, and the levels of substance use, nurses can anticipate that many of the families they meet are experiencing some form of violence or problematic substance use. In Canada, it is mandatory to report child abuse, but no reporting requirements exist for other forms of abuse, including elder abuse. In Canada, it is not recommended to screen for child abuse. Because of the high rate of false-positive results in screening tests for child maltreatment and the potential for incorrectly labeling people as child abusers, the possible harms associated with screening outweigh the benefits (MacMillan, 2000). Similarly, insufficient evidence of benefit has been reported to warrant screening for other forms of violence (Chalk & King, 1998; Coker, 2006; Ramsey, Richardson, Carter, Davidson, & Feder, 2002). Nevertheless, nurses need to be aware that family is not always a safe and nurturing experience for people, and to be responsive to indications of harm.

CANADIAN HEALTH CARE CONTEXT

The funding and structure of the Canadian health care system influences families, health, and family nursing. Although Canada has "universal" health care, and all Canadian citizens have access to what are termed *medically necessary* services, considerable inequities are present in access to health care, and these inequities are deepening as the health care system is increasingly privatized. Currently, the health care system in Canada is approximately 70% publically funded and 30% privately funded. This means that many important elements of health care are paid for by individuals or by private insurance. Therefore, in most provinces, medications outside of hospital, many types of treatments such as physiotherapy, and services such as home care are paid for privately in whole or in part.

Thus, despite commitment to universal access to health care, access to health care in Canada is inequitable along many dimensions (Adelson, 2005; Asada & Kephart, 2007; Ouellette-Kuntz et al., 2005; Shah, Gunraj, & Hux, 2003; Sin, Svenson, Cowie, & Man, 2003; Wilson & Rosenberg, 2002). Families living in rural settings have access to fewer services (Buske, 2000) and must pay for their own transportation, accommodation, and loss of income to access services. Families without private insurance and those with lower incomes face more financial hardship associated with illness. Because some groups of people are more likely to have lower incomes, such as those who are elderly, those with disabilities, and women, families from such groups are more likely to face greater barriers.

Although the Canadian health care system has been dominated by hospital care, over the past several decades fiscal concerns have stimulated shifts to decrease hospital care and increase the care provided at home. From mental illness, to surgery, to maternity care, to elder care, to end-of-life care, the trend has been to deinstitutionalize care, shorten length of stay, and shift to care "in the community." Such care mostly means care by family members, primarily women (Gregor, 1997; Stobert & Cranswick, 2004), which affects families, their health, and family nursing (Williams, Forbes, Mitchell, & Corbett, 2003). All of this serves to shape families' experiences of health and affect the health care they receive.

FAMILY NURSING PRACTICE: ATTENDING TO CONTEXT

To this point, this chapter has outlined the context of family nursing in Canada. As the discussion earlier has highlighted, families in Canada live diverse lives that are shaped by the interface of geography, economics, culture, language, and religion. Similarly, their lives and their health and illness experiences are shaped by differing understandings and forms of "family." Yet the health care system, including policies and norms that dominate health care practices, has been built on limited understandings of family, understandings that reflect Eurocentric, post–World War II notions of the nuclear two-parent, heterosexual family. *It is the discrepancies between the realities of families' lives and the normative expectations and understandings of family that often dominate health care settings and practices that make attending to context not only important but ethically essential.*

Overall, attending to context requires taking a stance of inquiry as a family nurse. It involves listening carefully to families, inquiring into their health/illness situations, and paying attention to, observing, and critically considering the way in which contextual elements are shaping their experiences and how those contextual elements might be addressed to promote health. An essential aspect of this inquiry process is reflexive consideration of your own contextual location, including the values, norms, and assumptions of family, health, and nursing that you act both from and within.

The following story illustrates the significance of context to families' health experiences and how attending to context enhances family nursing practice. As you read Sharon's story, look for the contextual elements that seem to be shaping the experiences of the two families she meets. Pay attention to how the elements we discussed in the earlier part of the chapter (e.g., geography, economics, culture, language, religion, understandings of family, health care policies, and normative practices) are shaping the experience and responses of the different family members and of Sharon as a nurse. Also pay attention to how Sharon is or is not attending to those elements as she engages with the families. Ask yourself how your own context is similar or different from Sharon's, and from the two families in the story. Furthermore, reflect on how those similarities and differences might affect how you would respond as a nurse.

Sharon's Story

After several years of experience on a pediatric medical unit, Sharon has begun to work in a pediatric diabetic teaching clinic. She just completed her 1-week orientation, and this morning is about to do an "intake" on two families new to the clinic. It is clinic policy to have a half-hour appointment for "intake" and 15 minutes for subsequent appointments. Families usually attend the clinic for about three or four sessions, biweekly, depending on their needs. The referral information Sharon has on the two families is as follows:

Family 1: Justin Henderson, 11 years old, is from Stony Life Reservation. Justin has been newly diagnosed with diabetes. He began an insulin regimen on Tuesday (3 days ago) that was ordered by the general practitioner in a walk-in clinic close to where he lives; Justin was referred to the clinic for diabetic teaching and counseling. This is his first visit to the clinic.

Family 2: Greg Stanek, 12 years old, is from Belcarra. Greg has been newly diagnosed with diabetes. His insulin regimen was started yesterday by the family's general practitioner, who referred Greg to the clinic for diabetic teaching and counseling. This is his first visit.

Justin's appointment was scheduled for 9:00, but he does not arrive on time. At 9:15, Sharon decides to see her other new client, Greg Stanek, first because he and his father arrived early. Greg seems small for his age; he is thin and looks quite pale. He is very quiet and barely looks at Sharon. Greg's father speaks with heavily accented English that Sharon recognizes as Czechoslovakian, in part because she associates Belcarra with the large community of people who emigrated from Czechoslovakia. Sharon does a brief physical assessment, noting that Greg is 4' 8", but weighs only 41 kg (about 90 pounds). Sharon attempts to take the family history as outlined on her intake form, but Greg's father wants to deal with the fact that he cannot bring his son to clinic. Greg's father tells Sharon that he was just laid off from his job as a carpet layer and is required by unemployment insurance policies to be searching for work. Mr. Stanek says bitterly that

when he came to Canada he had been promised he could find work in his field as a mining engineer. Greg lives with his mother, who works in a local meat processing plant, and she cannot take time off to bring Greg to the clinic without risking the loss of her job. Sharon reinforces with the father how important it is for Greg to learn about his diabetes and how to manage it, and how important supportive family is. Mr. Stanek increasingly becomes annoyed and insists that they cannot come to clinic again. As Greg's father becomes more frustrated, Sharon finds it more difficult to understand what he is saying because of his heavy accent and rapid talking. Sharon tries to engage Greg by asking him how he is feeling and how it is going at school, but Greg answers Sharon's questions by shrugging his shoulders and saying "OK." Greg's father attempts to return the conversation back to his own concerns. Eventually, Sharon says that she will "see what she can do." The half-hour clinic visit ends with little of the intake form completed, all parties feeling frustrated, and no follow-up appointment scheduled. As Sharon walks out of the room, the clinic receptionist lets her know Justin and a woman who turns out to be his grandmother have been waiting to see her for their appointment.

Sharon reviews what she knows about Justin from reading his intake information. She remembers that the Stony Life Reservation is located several hours from the hospital in which her clinic is located, and that Jackson is a small town near the reservation. Sharon wonders how Justin and his grandmother got to the clinic today. As she walks in the room, Sharon apologizes for keeping them waiting and asks if they drove to the appointment. Justin's grandmother says one of her brothers drove them because the appointment was too early to be able to come by bus. She also shares that she had to borrow money to pay her brother gas money. Sharon does a brief physical assessment on Justin. Justin, like Greg, barely looks at Sharon, even when she is addressing him specifically. Justin appears somewhat overweight, as does his grandmother, and on assessment Sharon notes that he is 4' 5" and weighs 55 kg (121 pounds). With Justin and his grandmother, who introduces herself as Rose Tarlier, the intake assessment goes more smoothly for Sharon. Mrs. Tarlier tells her that she has had custody of Justin and his two younger sisters since he was 4 years old and the sisters were infants. She shares with Sharon that Justin's mother, her daughter, has had problems with alcohol for many years, is now living in Montreal, and has not seen her children for several years. Mrs. Tarlier makes it a point to tell Sharon that she herself has been "clean and sober" for more than 20 years. Having heard about recent residential school settlements, Sharon asks if Mrs. Tarlier had experience with residential school. Mrs. Tarlier says yes but does not seem to want to say more. As Sharon continues with the intake assessment, she finds out that Justin's grandmother gives Justin his insulin and helps him check his blood sugar. Sharon listens as the grandmother describes what she has been doing, and Sharon provides positive feedback and encouragement. Although Sharon tries to bring Justin into the conversation, he does not look at her and does not answer her questions. Sharon reviews what subsequent appointments will cover, and thinking about the distance and gas money, inquires if it would be better to have one longer appointment next week rather than the usual two short ones a week apart. She schedules the next appointment at the conclusion of the office visit.

Taking a Stance of Inquiry

Attending to context begins by taking a stance of inquiry to understand what is meaningful and significant to a particular family, and inquire into their current experience and the contextual intricacies shaping the family's life. In taking this stance with the two families in the earlier story, what becomes immediately apparent is the way that contextual forces have contributed to and are shaping each of the family's situations. For example, although Justin's family may want to live in their Aboriginal community (for cultural and social reasons), they may have little choice but to live on the Reservation for economic reasons. Justin's grandmother may well be one of many Aboriginal women living on low income or in poverty. At the time of the 2001 census, based on before-tax incomes, more than 36% of Aboriginal women, compared with 17% of non-Aboriginal women, were living in poverty (Townson, 2005). High rates of poverty among Aboriginal people have overwhelming effects on health, with the life expectancy of Aboriginal people being 7 years less than that of the overall Canadian population. Also, as Townson notes, there are almost twice as many infant deaths among Aboriginal peoples, a greater rate than the poorest neighborhoods in

Canada. Campaign 2000 notes in the Report Card on Child Poverty that Statistics Canada data show that 40% of off-reserve Aboriginal children live in poverty (2006).

The fact that Justin lives on the Reservation may be significant given his diabetes. The matrix of policies related to Aboriginal people in Canada has insured that many Reservation communities have been denied access to traditional foods (fish, game, naturally growing plants) and have substandard housing, poor water supplies, and insufficient income opportunities for their members. Justin's grandmother's attendance at residential school, both his mother's and grandmother's experiences with alcohol, and the current situation with Justin's grandmother being his primary caregiver present a clear example of the impact colonization of Aboriginal people has on family well-being. Historical colonizing policies and practices in Canada included the creation of the Indian Act; removal of entire communities onto reserves, often with insufficient resources to sustain the community, government appropriation of Aboriginal lands, forced removal of children into residential schools, outlawing of cultural and spiritual practices; and widespread discriminatory attitudes toward Aboriginal peoples. The effects of colonization continue to exert their influence on peoples' health, social, and economic status today (Adelson, 2005; Bourassa, McKay-McNabb, & Hampton, 2004), and colonizing practices continue as Aboriginal people are racialized by wider society and governed by race-based policies, including those related to land ownership, banking, and health care.

Although it is important to emphasize that these are general statistics, and Justin and his grandmother's situation may not reflect any or all of these contextual challenges, this historical and current contextual backdrop shapes their situation and their responses to health care providers, including their willingness and desire to attend clinic. Moreover, the complexities and challenges they face accessing the clinic (e.g., appointment times that are out of sync with bus schedules, having younger children to care for, the cost of travel) may make coming to clinic seem less than positive in terms of the effect on Justin's and the families' overall health.

Similarly, Greg's family experience has been shaped by multiple factors. Both parents are facing significant job insecurity. The family has experienced immigration laws and policies that limit employment opportunities and contribute to the "downward mobility" experienced by many well-educated immigrants. Beiser, Hou, Hyman, and Tousignant (2002) have found that foreign-born children were more than twice as likely to live in poverty. Using Statistics Canada 2001 census data, the 2006 Canadian Report Card on Child Poverty (Campaign 2000, 2006) reports that 49% of children in recent immigrant families and 34% of children in racialized families are poor. The Report Card notes that these rates are caused by an overrepresentation of racialized groups in low-paying jobs, market failure to recognize international work experience and credentials, and racial discrimination in employment.

Canada is a country of considerable ethnic diversity, but despite national commitment to tolerance and multiculturalism, racialized groups experience considerable discrimination both in policies and institutions, and in the attitudes expressed toward them at an interpersonal level. Was this playing out during the clinic visit? Although nurses cannot assume what families' experiences will have been, taking a stance of inquiry and attending to context enables nurses to be aware of the likelihood of discriminatory experiences and of the potential health effects.

Listening and Paying Attention to Experience and Context

Attending to context involves listening carefully to families, and to what is meaningful and significant within the current context of their lives. For Justin and his grandmother who live in a rural setting and for Greg's family in which both parents need to work, it becomes apparent that geography, economics, and health are intricately intertwined. For example, although for Sharon what is most significant is getting Greg's family to attend clinic so Greg's diabetes can be monitored and addressed, for Greg's father, finding employment is of greatest concern. Moreover, the experience of being told that he would be able to work in his profession and then finding that this was not the case may well be influencing his response and willingness to engage with yet another authority and institution that does not seem to be recognizing the importance of his employment or interested in what is most pressing for him. Although Sharon cannot address the employment concern directly within her current role (i.e., she cannot help find him a job), it is obvious

that those concerns will ultimately affect Greg's experience and management of diabetes. Thus, listening to and recognizing the interrelationship of those concerns regarding how the family will be able and willing to care for Greg and his diabetes is crucial. For example, in listening and paying attention to experiences and context, what stands out is the way in which the well-intended clinic may actually be heightening health challenges for families by not taking these contextual elements into consideration. Even the way in which the clinic appointments have been structured as short, frequent sessions affects both families' ability to attend clinic and ignores the socioenvironmental elements that profoundly affect families' health on a day-to-day basis. Attending to context would involve acknowledging the distress Greg's father is experiencing about his employment and inviting him to talk about what it has been like for different family members as they have sought employment and attempted to build a life with limited resources, support, or both. As part of this process, it would be important to communicate respect and genuine interest and concern, asking what from their perspective might be helpful, that is, how the clinic could assist them in caring for Greg's diabetes in light of the many other challenges they are currently experiencing as a family. Although on the surface focusing on the father's concerns might not seem to be the top nursing priority, doing so might have reduced frustration for both Sharon and Greg's father, made better use of the time, and possibly allowed both of them to turn attention more effectively to Greg.

Listening and paying attention to experience and context with Justin's family brings attention to the geographic distance between the family's home and the clinic, and raises questions about other possibilities for supporting the family in diabetes care. For example, knowing the economic statistics for Aboriginal women, one wonders about the impact the cost of travel to the clinic might have on the family. If they are on a limited income, frequent travel may be impossible and may take money from other essential needs. If this were the case, Sharon might look into resources at the local level such as a community health representative or local community health nurse who might be able to provide the face-to-face care to the family while liaising with the clinic so that the family does not need to travel such a great distance so frequently.

Overall, attending to context sets one up to be curious, interested, and to inquire rather than assume a knowing stance to and make judgments and assumptions based on surface characteristics and behaviors. For example, both Greg and Justin were quiet and did not make eye contact or respond much to Sharon. Rather than making assumptions about the children based on her own location and context, Sharon might intentionally reflect on the contexts the children come from and have been living over the past while. In so doing, their responses might be viewed through a range of possibilities including everything from wondering about the physiologic effect of diabetes, to the immediate effect of the diagnosis of diabetes, to the experience of coming to the clinic for the first time, to the multiple contextual experiences and challenges they and their families have been living. Attending to context can cue us to stay open to questions, whereas gently and thoughtfully reaching out to connect with people and families as they are in the moment. Rather than focusing on behavior or lack of response as a problem or frustration, any response is viewed contextually—people and families are not measured against any norms, but rather the goal is to understand their reaction contextually to respond in a meaningful and relevant manner.

Attending to context also moves us beyond the immediate situation of particular patients to question how the larger policies and structures governing our practice and agency are affecting families. That is, the contextual particularities of these families reveal the limitations of the policies and structures of the clinic more generally. It becomes apparent that the clinic policies and structures might need to be changed to be more responsive to families. For example, offering home visits, evening appointments, or both for families who have both parents working and are unable to make daytime appointments might enhance the clinic's responsiveness. Similarly, seeing the family in context draws attention to the importance of working with the contexts within which the families live. This could include everything from intentionally establishing relationships with government departments and community agencies that are part of the family's context and that might liaise with the clinic in providing services and resources, to lobbying for increased access and resources for particular groups or particular services and supplies.

Reflexivity

Reflexivity, meaning intentional and critical reflection on one's own understanding and actions in context, is central to using contextual knowledge. Reflexivity draws attention to a nurse's own contextual background, including taken-for-granted assumptions, stereotypes, and knowledge one draws on when engaging with families. Examining how one's context and social location shapes and structures one's nursing is a first step to attending to families' contexts. For example, if Sharon had grown up in a rural setting or in poverty, it would be important for her to consider reflexively how those experiences influence her when working with families who share that context and social location. Her background might lead her to see herself as successful despite those constraints, and to overlook how the challenges she faced and privileges she enjoyed might differ from the experiences of the families with whom she is working. Or, if she had grown up in a middle-class urban setting, she may find that she is somewhat oblivious to or does not think to consider the challenges that poverty and geography raise in accessing health care. Similarly, as a nurse working within the diversity of the Canadian milieu, it would be important for Sharon to consider how her own family history might be shaping her attitudes toward immigrants, people whose first language is not English, racialized groups, Aboriginal people, and other groups. Perhaps she herself is an immigrant, perhaps she is a member of a racialized group, or perhaps she is a member of dominant groups—English speaking, Euro-Canadian, middle class. It would be important to ask herself how her religious affiliations (or lack thereof) shape the extent to which she thinks religion is relevant to health and to her nursing practice.

Although each aspect of Sharon's social location may shape her thinking, as Applebaum (2001) notes, one's social location "does not imply that we are inevitably locked within a particular perspective. White feminists can be anti-racist, men can be feminists, and heterosexuals can be 'straight but not narrow.'" (p. 416). That is, by reflexively scrutinizing our own social locations, we can examine our understandings and make explicit decisions about how to draw on (or not) various views and assumptions.

Interestingly, examining our own contexts and social locations to see how we are limiting our views of families can be challenging. Often, we tend to see more easily our own disadvantages than our privileges. For example, Sharon might have to work harder to see how her privilege as a securely employed, fluent English-speaking health care provider gives her an advantage that Greg's father does not have. If she has experienced employment disadvantages based on her sex, she might see him as a privileged man and have difficulty recognizing the challenges he faces.

Overall, reflexivity in family nursing involves developing a critical awareness of our own context and social location, scrutinizing how that context/location is shaping our view of a particular family, and intentionally looking *beyond* that location to consider the family within their own context. In the earlier situation, this would involve Sharon examining the ways in which the rural context, economics, language, ethnicity, and religion, and her understandings of these shape how she is engaging with the families. She might ask herself how her own experiences of family are shaping her ability to see and accept the differing forms of family—for example, a separated family, such as Greg's, and a grandmother-led family such as Justin's. How does her own location enable or limit her ability to understand how difficult it might be for Greg's father and mother to get him to the clinic appointments given their current family situation?

Engaging in such reflexive examination also enables consideration of the wider sociopolitical elements that are shaping a family's experiences—for example, contextual factors that may have contributed to Greg's parents separating, how the stress of immigration might have contributed to the family's experiences, among other elements. At the same time approaching her work in this reflexive manner highlights areas of knowledge that she may need to learn more about. For example, how well does Sharon understand the history of the Aboriginal people with whom she will be working? How well does she understand the relationship between historical trauma and diabetes?

SUMMARY

One of a few predictable characteristics of Canadian families is diversity. By understanding this diversity when providing care, nurses are prepared to take into account the contextual nature of families'

health and illness experiences, and how their lives are shaped by their circumstances. Contexts are literally embodied in people; both nurses and families live their contexts and circumstances. To work responsively with a range of different families requires understanding the particular families, and this requires taking a stance of inquiry, listening and paying attention to the particular experiences of particular families, reflexively attending to one's own understandings, and continuously developing new knowledge and cultural awareness.

REFERENCES

Abu-Laban, Y., & Gabriel, C. (2002). *Selling diversity: Immigration, multiculturalism, employment equity and globalization.* Toronto: Broadview.

Adelson, N. (2005). The embodiment of inequity: Health disparities in aboriginal Canada. *Canadian Journal of Public Health. Revue Canadienne De Santé Publique, 96*(suppl 2), S45–S61.

Agnew, V. (1998). *In search of a safe place: Abused women and culturally sensitive services.* Toronto: University of Toronto Press.

Applebaum, B. (2001). Locating one's self, I-dentification and the trouble with moral agency. *Philosophy of Education Year Book,* 412–422.

Asada, Y., & Kephart, G. (2007). Equity in health services use and intensity of use in Canada. *BMC Health Services Research, 7,* 41.

Beiser, M. (2005). The health of immigrants and refugees in Canada. *Canadian Journal of Public Health, 96*(Mar/Apr), S30–S44.

Beiser, M., Hou, F., Hyman, I., & Tousignant, M. (2002). Poverty, family process, and the mental health of immigrant children in Canada. *American Journal of Public Health, 92*(2), 220–228.

Borrell, L. N., Kiefe, C. I., Williams, D. R., Diez-Roux, A. V., & Gordon-Larsen, P. (2006). Self-reported health, perceived racial discrimination, and skin color in African Americans in the CARDIA study. *Social Science & Medicine, 63*(6), 1415–1427.

Bourassa, C., McKay-McNabb, K., & Hampton, M. R. (2004). Racism, sexism, and colonialism: The impact on the health of Aboriginal women in Canada. *Canadian Woman Studies, 24*(1), 23–29.

Buske, L. (2000). Availability of services in rural areas. *CMAJ: Canadian Medical Association Journal, 162*(8), 1193.

Cain, V. S., & Kington, R. S. (2003). Investigating the role of racial/ethnic bias in health outcomes. *American Journal of Public Health,* 191–192. Retrieved April 29, 2009, from http://search.ebscohost.com/login.aspx?direct=true&db=aph&AN=9036654&site=ehost-live

Campaign 2000. (2006). *Oh Canada! Too many children in poverty for too long: 2006 report card on child and family poverty in Canada.* Retrieved April 29, 2009, from http://www.campaign2000.ca/rc/rc06/06_C2000NationalReportCard.pdf

Canada Mortgage and Housing Corporation. (2006). *Urban Aboriginal households: A profile of demographic, housing and* economic conditions in Canada's prairie and territories region. Retrieved September 18, 2008, from http://dsp-psd.pwgsc.gc.ca/Collection/NH18-23-106-024E.pdf

Canadian Centre for Justice Statistics. (2002). *Family violence in Canada: A statistical profile*. Ottawa, Ontario, Canada: Statistics Canada.

Canadian Population Health Initiative. (2006). *How healthy are rural Canadians? An assessment of their health status and health determinants—A component of the initiative Canada's rural communities: Understanding rural health and its determinants*. Ottawa, Ontario, Canada: Canadian Institute for Health Information.

Chalk, R., & King, P. A. (1998). *Violence in families: Assessing prevention and treatment programs*. Washington, DC: National Academy Press.

Clark, J., & Du Mont, J. (2003). Intimate partner violence and health: A critique of Canadian prevalence studies. *Canadian Journal of Public Health, 94*(1), 52–58.

Coburn, D. (2006). Health and health care: A political economy perspective. In D. Raphael, T. Bryant, & M. Rioux (Eds.), *Staying alive: Critical perspectives on health, illness and health care* (pp. 59–85). Toronto: Canadian Scholar's Press.

Coker, A. L. (2006). Preventing intimate partner violence: How we will rise to this challenge. *American Journal of Preventive Medicine*, 528–529.

Collin, C. (2006). *Substance abuse and public policy in Canada: Alcohol and related harms*. Ottawa, Ontario, Canada: Political and Social Affairs Division, Library of Parliament, Canada.

Farris-Manning, C., & Zandstra, M. (2004). *Children in care in Canada: A summary of current issues and trends with recommendations for future research*. Ottawa, Ontario, Canada: Child Welfare League of Canada, Foster LIFE Inc.

Ford-Gilboe, M. (2000). Dispelling myths and creating opportunity: A comparison of the strengths of single-parent and two-parent families. *Advances in Nursing Science, 23*(1), 41–58.

Gregor, F. (1997). From women to women: Nurses, informal caregivers and the gender dimension of health care reform in Canada. *Health and Social Care in the Community, 5*(1), 30–36.

Helly, D. (2003). *Canadian multiculturalism: Lessons for the management of cultural diversity?* Paper presented at the Canadian and French perspectives on diversity, Gatineau, Quebec, Canada.

Henry, F., Tator, C., & Mattis. (2006). Racism and human-service delivery. *The colour of democracy: Racism in Canadian society*. Toronto: Harcourt Brace.

Human Resources and Social Development Canada. (2006). *Indicators of well being in Canada: Canadians in context—geographic distribution*. Retrieved September 18, 2008, from http://www4.hrsdc.gc.ca

Johnson, H. (1996). *Dangerous domains: Violence against women in Canada*. Scarborough, Ontario, Canada: International Thomson Publishing.

Johnson, H., & Sacco, V. (1995, July). Researching violence against women: Statistics Canada's national survey. *Canadian Journal of Criminology*, 281–304.

Jones, A. S., Gielen, A. C., Campbell, J. C., Schollenberger, J., Dienemann, J. A., Kub, J., et al. (1999). Annual and lifetime prevalence of partner abuse in a sample of female HMO enrollees. *Women's Health Issues, 9*(6), 295–305.

Krieger, N. (2000). Epidemiology, racism, and health: The case of low birth weight. *Epidemiology, 11*(3), 237–239.

Krieger, N., Chen, J. T., Coull, B. A., & Selby, J. V. (2005). Lifetime socioeconomic position and twins' health: An analysis of 308 pairs of United States women twins. *PLoS Medicine, 2*(7), 0645–0653.

Krieger, N., & Sidney, S. (1996). Racial discrimination and blood pressure: The CARDIA study of young Black and White adults. *American Journal of Public Health, 86*(10), 1370–1378.

MacMillan, H. L. (2000). Preventive health care, 2000 update: Prevention of child maltreatment. *Canadian Medical Association Journal/Journal De L'association Medicale Canadienne, 163*(11), 1451–1458.

McLean, C. (2001). Less sensational but more dangerous. *Report/Newsmagazine (National Edition), 28*(22), 44.

Mitura, V., & Bollman, R. D. (2003). The health of rural Canadians: A rural-urban comparison of health indicators. *Rural and Small Town Canada Analysis Bulletin, 4*(6), 1–23.

Mojab, S., & El-Kassem, N. (2008). Cultural relativism: Theoretical, political and ideological debates. *Canadian Muslim women at the crossroads: From integration to segregation?* Gananoque, Ontario, Canada: Canadian Council of Muslim Women.

Morrow, M., Hankivsky, O., & Varcoe, C. (2004). Women and violence: The effects of dismantling the welfare state. *Critical Social Policy, 24*(2), 358–384.

Mustillo, S., Krieger, N., Gunderson, E. P., Sidney, S., McCreath, H., & Kiefe, C. I. (2004). Self-reported experiences of racial discrimination and Black-White differences in preterm and low-birthweight deliveries: The CARDIA Study. *American Journal of Public Health, 94*(12), 2125–2131.

Nazroo, J. Y. (2003). The structuring of ethnic inequalities in health: Economic position, racial discrimination, and racism. *American Journal of Public Health, 93*(2), 277–284.

Ng, R. (1995). Multiculturalism as ideology: A textual analysis. In M. Campbell, & A. Manicom (Eds.), *Knowledge, experience, and ruling relations: Studies in the social organization of knowledge*. Toronto: University of Toronto Press.

Ouellette-Kuntz, H., Minnes, P., Garcin, N., Martin, C., Lewis, M. E. S., & Holden, J. J. A. (2005, March/April). Addressing health disparities through promoting equity for individuals with intellectual disability. *Canadian Journal of Public Health, 96*, S8–S22.

Public Health Agency of Canada. (2001). *The Canadian Incidence Study of reported child abuse and neglect: Highlights*. Retrieved April 15, 2008, from http://www.phac-aspc.gc.ca/cm-vee/cishl01/

Quan, H., Fong, A., De Coster, C., Wang, J., Musto, R., Noseworthy, T. W., et al. (2006). Variation in health services utilization among ethnic populations. *CMAJ: Canadian Medical Association Journal, 174*(6), 787–791.

Ramsey, J., Richardson, J., Carter, Y. H., Davidson, L. L., & Feder, G. (2002). Should health professionals screen women for domestic violence? Systematic review. *British Medical Journal, 325*(7359), 314–318.

Rehm, J., Baliunas, D., Brochu, S., Fischer, B., Gnam, W., Patra, J., et al. (2006). *The Costs of Substance Abuse in Canada 2002*. Ottawa: Canadian Centre on Substance Abuse.

Ricciutelli, L., Larkin, J., & O'Neill, E. (1998). *Confronting the cuts: A sourcebook for women in Ontario*. Toronto: Inanna.

Rich-Edwards, J., Krieger, N., Majzoub, J., Zierler, S., Lieberman, E., & Gillman, M. (2001). Maternal experiences of racism and violence as predictors of preterm birth: Rationale and study design. *Paediatric and Perinatal Epidemiology, 15*(suppl 2), 124–135.

Royal Commission on Aboriginal Peoples. (1996). *Report of the Royal Commission on Aboriginal Peoples.* Ottawa, Ontario: Canada Communications Group-Publishing.

Shah, B. R., Gunraj, N., & Hux, J. E. (2003). Markers of access to and quality of primary care for Aboriginal people in Ontario, Canada. *American Journal of Public Health, 93*(5), 798–802.

Sin, D. D., Svenson, L. W., Cowie, R. L., & Man, S. F. (2003). Can universal access to health care eliminate health inequities between children of poor and nonpoor families? A case study of childhood asthma in Alberta. *Chest, 124*(1), 51–56.

Singh, V. (2004). The rural-urban income gap within provinces: An update to 2000. *Rural and Small Town Canada Analysis Bulletin, 5*(7).

Statistics Canada. (1998, December 14). *Statistics Canada—The daily: Canada's Aboriginal languages, 1996.* Ottawa, Ontario, Canada: Statistics Canada.

Statistics Canada. (1999). *Family violence in Canada: A statistical profile 1999.* Ottawa, Ontario, Canada: Canadian Centre for Justice Statistics.

Statistics Canada. (2000a). *Statistics Canada—The daily: Women in Canada.* Ottawa, Ontario, Canada: Statistics Canada.

Statistics Canada. (2000b). *Women in Canada: A gender-based statistical report.* Ottawa, Ontario, Canada: Statistics Canada.

Statistics Canada. (2001). *Profile of languages in Canada.* Retrieved April 12, 2007, from http://www12.statcan.ca/english/census01/Products/Analytic/companion/lang/canada.cfm

Statistics Canada. (2002). *Canadian population by mobility status: Canada, a nation on the move.* Retrieved September 15, 2008, from http://www12.statcan.ca/english/census01/Products/Analytic/companion/mob/provs.cfm#3

Statistics Canada. (2003a). *Ethnic diversity survey: Portrait of a multicultural society.* Ottawa, Ontario, Canada: Statistics Canada.

Statistics Canada. (2003b). *Religions in Canada.* Ottawa, Ontario, Canada: Statistics Canada.

Statistics Canada. (2005). *Longitudinal Survey of Immigrants to Canada (LSIC): A portrait of early settlement experiences.* Retrieved September 15, 2008, from http://www.statcan.ca/bsolc/english/bsolc?catno=89-614-X

Statistics Canada. (2006a). *Family portrait: Continuity and change in Canadian families and households in 2006: Families and households, 2006 Census.* Retrieved August 31, 2007, from http://www12.statcan.ca/english/census06/analysis/popdwell/Subprov7.cfm

Statistics Canada. (2006b). *Family portrait: Continuity and change in Canadian families and households in 2006: Subprovincial changes.* Retrieved August 31, 2007, from http://www12.statcan.ca/english/census06/analysis/popdwell/Subprov7.cfm

Statistics Canada. (2006c). *Family violence in Canada: A statistical profile 2006.* Ottawa, Ontario, Canada: Canadian Centre for Justice Statistics.

Statistics Canada. (2006d, March 30). *Statistics Canada—The daily. Income of Canadians.* Retrieved July 14, 2007, from http://www.statcan.ca/Daily/English/030623/d030623c.htm

Statistics Canada. (2006e, March 7). *Statistics Canada—The daily. Women in Canada.* Retrieved November 23, 2006, from http://www.statcan.ca/Daily/English/030623/d030623c.htm

Statistics Canada. (2008). *Income of Canadians—The Daily.* Retrieved May 3, 2009, from http://www.statcan.gc.ca/daily-quotidien/080505/dq080505a-eng.htm

Stobert, S., & Cranswick, K. (2004). Looking after seniors: Who does what for whom? *Canadian Social Trends* (74), 2–6.

Townson, M. (2005). *Poverty issues for Canadian Women.* Ottawa, Ontario, Canada: Status of Women Canada.

Trocmé, N., MacMillan, H., Fallon, B., & De Marco, R. (2003). Nature and severity of physical harm caused by child abuse and neglect: Results from the Canadian Incidence Study. *Canadian Medical Association Journal/Journal De L'association Medicale Canadienne, 169*(9), 911–915.

Wekerle, C., Wall, A.-M., Leung, E., & Trocmé, N. (2007). Cumulative stress and substantiated maltreatment: The importance of caregiver vulnerability and adult partner violence. *Child Abuse & Neglect, 31*(4), 427–443.

Williams, A., Forbes, D., Mitchell, J., & Corbett, B. (2003). The influence of income on the experience of informal caregiving: Policy implications. *Health Care for Women International, 24*(4), 280–292.

Wilson, K., & Rosenberg, M. W. (2002). The geographies of crisis: Exploring accessibility to health care in Canada. *Canadian Geographer, 46*(3), 223–234.

Young, T. K., O'Neil, J. D., Elias, B., Leader, A., Reading, J., & McDonald, G. (1999). Chronic diseases. In First Nations and Inuit Regional Health Survey National Steering Committee (Ed.), *First Nations and Inuit Regional Health Survey: National report 1999.* Ottawa, Ontario, Canada: Assembly of First Nations.

CHAPTER 8

Genomics and Family Nursing Across the Life Span

Janet K. Williams, PhD, RN, CGC, PNP, FAAN

Heather Skirton, PhD, MSc, RGN, Registered Genetic Counsellor

CRITICAL CONCEPTS

- Biological members of a family may share the risk for disease because of genetic factors.
- Genomics refers to the study of all genes in the human genome and their interactions with each other, the environment, and other factors.
- Genetic refers to the study of individual genes and their effect on clinical disorders.
- Results of genetic tests are private and cannot be disclosed to other family members without the person's consent.
- Families are unique and respond to genetic discoveries differently based on personal coping styles, family values, beliefs, and patterns of communication. Even within the same family, members react differently.
- The two major nursing responsibilities when a genetic risk is identified are to help families understand that the risk is present and to help the families make decisions about management and surveillance.
- Nurses apply genetic and genomic knowledge in obtaining a minimum of a three-generation pedigree in the family history as a component of a nursing assessment.
- In every case, it is the nurse's role to support families to make decisions that are most appropriate for their particular circumstances, cultures, and beliefs.
- Nurses identify accurate information and access to resources for families with concerns regarding genetic and genomic health risks.
- Nurses evaluate the effect of interventions on family health outcomes.

Some illnesses "run in families" and people commonly wonder if they, or their children, will develop a disease that is present in their parents or grandparents. The ability to apply understanding of genetics in the care of families is a priority for nurses and for all health care providers. As a result of genomic research and the resultant rapidly changing body of knowledge regarding genetic influences on health and illness, more emphasis has been placed on involving all health care providers in this field. This integration of genetic knowledge, attitudes, and skills is especially important for nurses, and is reflected in the Essential Nursing Competencies and Curriculum Guidelines for Genetics and Genomics (Consensus Panel, 2006), hereafter referred to in this chapter as "Essential Nursing Competencies." It is important for family nurses to be aware of the effect of genetics on families because biological family members share genetic risk factors. In addition, families function as systems with shared health risks that affect the whole family, and family processes mediate the coping and adaptation of both individual family members and the family unit as a whole (Walsh, 2003).

Family members inevitably have an effect on each other's lives, and in many cases, they support each other in seeking and maintaining healthy growth and development, regardless of their biologic kinship. Much of what is known about health care needs of persons with genetic conditions has focused on the individual, with less attention directed toward the persons' biological and socially defined family. This chapter describes nursing responsibilities for families of persons who have, or are at risk for having, genetic conditions. These responsibilities are described for families before conception, with neonates, teens in families, and families with members in the middle to elder years. All nurses, regardless of their areas of practice, apply an understanding of the effects of genetic risk factors when conducting assessments, planning, and evaluating nursing interventions. The purpose of this chapter is to describe the relevance of genetic information within families when there is a question about genetic aspects of health or disease for members of the family. Family nursing knowledge is incomplete without attention to the effects of genetic factors on health and functioning of individuals, as well as family units.

GENETICS AND GENOMICS

The human genome consists of approximately 3 billion nucleotides of DNA sequence, some of which is unique to each person (Christensen & Murray, 2007). Individuals inherit genetic material from their parents and pass it on to their children. Some conditions result from a change or mutation in a DNA sequence known as a gene. For example, Huntington disease (HD) results from a specific change within the DNA sequence in a particular gene. This is an example of a condition traditionally referred to as a "Mendelian" or "single-gene disorder" and is one that follows an identified pattern of traditional inheritance, in this case, an autosomal dominant inheritance pattern. Persons who are biologically related may have inherited many of the same DNA sequences in addition to having shared common environments with other family members; this combination ultimately increases risks for specific illnesses.

Researchers also identify common genetic variations known as single nucleotide polymorphisms. These may not cause an actual disruption in the DNA coding but can often be used as tools that help scientists and clinicians recognize DNA variations that may be associated with disease. These conditions include common disorders such as diabetes that are observed to occur more frequently in families but do not follow a traditional pattern of inheritance. The term *genomics* is commonly used to reflect the study of all genes in the human genome, as well as interactions among genes and with environmental and other psychosocial or cultural factors (Feetham & Thomson, 2006).

A core competency for nurses is to maintain knowledge of the relationships of genetic and genomic factors to the health of individuals and their families. Cancer provides an example of the relationships between genes, environment, and health. The development of a malignant tumor is the result of a complex series of changes at the cellular level. A number of genes protect against cancer by regulating cell division (during mitosis), and mutations in those genes can occur over the course of a person's lifetime, affecting his or her predisposition to cancer. A person may be at increased risk of developing cancer if he or she inherited a mutation in one of those genes or if exposed to environmental factors that influence genetic mutations. For example, tumor suppressor genes help protect against the development of breast cancer. If a woman inherits a mutation in a tumor suppressor gene (such as the *BRCA1* gene), she has lost some of her protection against breast cancer from birth, but she will not necessarily develop cancer unless other cellular changes (some of which are influenced by factors such as her reproductive history) occur during her lifetime (Gulati & Domchek, 2008). Others in her family may also have inherited the same mutation and are similarly at risk. If she subsequently becomes a smoker, she has an additional increased risk for lung cancer because of the environmental influence of smoking on cell division in the lungs. In families where smoking is the norm, there may be a perceived "familial" condition because of the shared environmental influences on a number of members of the family. Essential nursing competencies include both the ability to apply genetic and genomic knowledge in conducting a nursing assessment and the ability to assess responses to genetic and genomic information (Consensus Panel, 2006). These competencies are also identified in documents for general practitioners in the UK (National Genetics Education and Development Centre, 2008).

FAMILY DISCLOSURE OF GENETIC INFORMATION

Access to genetic information raises a host of questions regarding confidentiality, who to tell and what and when to tell them, and maintaining secrets within families.

Confidentiality

The nurse must maintain the confidentiality of each family member's decision regarding privacy relative to genetic risks, testing, disease, or management. Results of genetic tests are private, and in the United States, they cannot be disclosed to other family members without the person's consent (United States Department of Health and Human Services, 1996). Confidentiality rights do differ in other countries. For example, in the United Kingdom, it might be permissible in rare cases to disclose test results if the health of other family members would be seriously

jeopardized by secrecy (Royal College of Physicians, Royal College of Pathologists and British Society for Human Genetics, 2005). In most cases, the choice of disclosure of genetic information is an individual decision that is made in the context of the family.

Discovery of health problems in more than one family member should be accompanied by a discussion with family members regarding their understanding of risks for potentially inherited disorders. Disclosure can be a challenging task, as the person with the genetic mutation must decide who to inform, what to say, and when to talk about this finding (Gaff et al., 2007).

Family members may prefer to maintain privacy regarding their decision about predictive testing, even within the family. This decision may reflect an attempt to avoid disagreements within the family, or an attempt to protect others in the family from sadness or worry. People who have predictive HD testing may be reluctant to share this information with their primary care provider. This reluctance may be because they fear that any notation in their medical record may be accessed by an employer or insurance provider, which may lead to loss of employment or insurance. Although laws have been passed that prohibit insurance or employment discrimination based on a person's genotype, some individuals may be concerned that revealing their genotype may place them at risk for discrimination (Penziner et al., 2008).

When one person in a family has a condition that is caused by an alteration in a single gene, such as a gene associated with hereditary breast or ovarian cancer, the person with the mutation is asked to notify others in the family that they too may have this same DNA mutation. In general, the family passes on this information, but occasionally, with the consent of all concerned, direct conversations can occur between the nurse and other family members. Because families vary in their adaptability regarding health challenges (McDaniel, Rolland, Feetham, & Miller, 2006), families vary in how they decide to share information.

The family communication style will affect disclosure and sharing of genetic information. For example, a family with a disengaged communication pattern may share affection for each other but speak relatively infrequently (McDaniel et al., 2006). For these families with this style of communication and lack of closeness, sharing information about one's personal medical history may be especially difficult (Stoffel et al., 2008). In contrast, families with an enmeshed style of family communication frequently talk with others in the family about personal health matters (McDaniel et al., 2006).

In some families, it has been found that it is more difficult for women to communicate genetic information to older parents, brothers, or fathers (Patenaude et al., 2006). Men have been noted to have difficulty disclosing genetic information to all family members (Gaff, Collins, Symes, & Halliday, 2005). Box 8-1 depicts an example of family communication of genetic information.

BOX 8-1
Family Communication of Genetic Information

Brian, a 46-year-old man, is the oldest of three siblings. He is married but has no biological children. Brian was aware that his mother died of bowel cancer at the age of 38 years, and although this worried him, he hid his anxiety from both friends and relatives. He never discussed his mother's death with his wife or siblings. Brian had been experiencing abdominal pain for some months when he collapsed at work one day and was taken to his local hospital emergency department. He was found to be anemic and suffering a bowel obstruction. A tumor located near the hepatic flexure of the large colon was removed successfully. Brian was informed that his family and medical history indicated that it was likely he inherited a mutation in an oncogene that predisposed him to bowel cancer. He was advised to share this finding with his siblings, and recommend they seek advice and screening for themselves. Brian was reluctant to discuss the issue with his siblings but did tell his wife what the doctor had told him. Brian did not disclose this information to his siblings. Several months later, at the encouragement of his wife, they met with the cancer nurse to discuss the situation. The cancer nurse helped Brian decide what information to share with his siblings, and they created a plan for how and when to share the information. Subsequently, both Brian's sister and brother had genetic testing. Brian's sister was found to carry the mutation. She was screened, and she worked with the nurse to devise a plan to tell her children about their possible risk when they reached 18 years of age.

Parents: To Tell or Not to Tell

When communication is between parents and their minor age children with genetic disorders, the parents take into consideration what to tell their child about the condition based on their developmental level and their extent of interest in knowing about their genetic condition. Parents whose children had a single gene disorder described sharing genetic information with their children as an unfolding process that was not a one-time occurrence but continued throughout childhood (Gallo, Angst, Knafl, Hadley, & Smith, 2005).

Parents usually believe that they are the most appropriate people to inform their offspring of genetic risks, but when no current effective treatment or cure exists, they may wonder whether "the right" of the individual to know about their potential genetic risks overrules their natural instinct as parents to spare their children from undue anxiety (Tercyak et al., 2007). In some cases, individuals delay telling other adults in the family because they are worried that they will accidently say something to the child or that may be overheard by the child (Speice, McDaniel, Rowley, & Loader, 2002).

Parents of children with genetic conditions may not share information because they have concerns about school issues, obtaining health care for their children, and insurability or employability of their children. School concerns can include worry that their child could feel different from other children because of food or activity restrictions, or visible signs of their child's condition (Gallo, Hadley, Angst, Knafl, & Smith, 2008).

Concealing Information: Family Secrets

Some families are quite open, whereas others choose to keep the genetic information a secret, even from other family members, possibly to avoid stigmatization (Peters et al., 2005). Families choose to keep genetic formation secret for a variety of reasons. Sometimes information is kept a secret out of a desire to protect other family members. Some keep a secret because they feel shame. For example, there have been times when HD was misdiagnosed as alcoholism and dementia (Williams & Sobel, 2006). Families may choose to keep information secret because the exploration of inheritance may reveal other information that is personal. For example, consider a family with four sisters who want health advice because their father has a form of familial colon cancer. In the course of obtaining the family history, the mother confides to the nurse that her husband is not the biologic parent of their oldest daughter, and that others in the family do not know this history. In this situation, the nurse recognizes that the oldest daughter does not share the same risk for this disease as her sisters. But the nurse would not be permitted to reveal that information to any family member without the mother's permission. This family secret can create conflict for the nurse, because the lack of disclosure might mean the eldest daughter is exposed to unnecessary procedures, such as a colonoscopy (which carries a risk for morbidity) that is advised for those who are at risk. The nurse should discuss the issue of risks for procedures with the mother so that the she can consider telling her daughter the family secret to avoid unnecessary anxiety and the risks of the procedures. Of course, the benefits of disclosure may be outweighed by the distress caused to the daughter by having information about her parentage. In the United States, the Health Insurance Portability and Accountability Act (HIPAA) allows for permitted disclosures of health information if there is an immediate and serious threat to the person and if the disclosure could reasonably lessen or prevent the threat (United States Department of Health and Human Services, 1996). However, in other countries, the requirement to do no harm could outweigh the mother's right to confidentiality.

FAMILY REACTIONS TO DISCLOSURE OF GENETIC INFORMATION

Families are unique and respond to genetic discoveries differently. Even within the same family, the family members will respond differently. Some members will seek predictive testing to determine whether they have inherited the genetic condition. Some members will react with grief, loss, and denial. Others will choose not to seek testing. The nurse's role is to support all family members in their choices.

Minor age children in a family may wonder if they will have the condition present in a parent. For example, this may be the case for teens who have a parent or grandparent with HD, an autosomal dominant condition. Although guidelines do not recommend predictive testing until a teen is old enough to provide informed consent, teens with parents who have HD may wonder about their own futures, and when given the opportunity may express their questions and concerns (Sparbel et al., 2008). Teens may wish to protect their parents from the knowledge that they are thinking about the condition or preserve their own confidentiality and seek discussion and support with a knowledgeable health care provider. Nurses can provide opportunities for teens and parents to talk about the teens' questions.

Elders in the family may have questions regarding genetics, as well as serve as a source of family history information. Research has shown that elders are aware of advances in genetics and are keen to contribute to genetic studies to help their offspring (Skirton, Frazier, Calvin, & Cohen, 2006). Advances in genomics will make susceptibility testing for common diseases of middle and old age (such as coronary artery disease or cancer) more commonly used.

Pre-selection Beliefs

Family members have ideas and beliefs about who in the family will develop a genetic condition, these beliefs are termed *pre-selection* (Kessler, 1988). Pre-selection beliefs are often based on the family's previous experience. For example, if only male relatives have been affected by an autosomal dominant condition that could affect either sex, female members in the family may believe they are not at risk. Sometimes pre-selection is based on the fact that the person thought to have inherited the condition physically resembles the affected parent or shares a physical characteristic (such as hair color) with other affected relatives. A pre-selection belief may influence the person's self-image and overall functioning. Those who believe they will develop the condition may, for example, make different career choices, avoid long-term relationships, or decide not to have children.

Predictive or Presymptomatic Testing

When family members want to know the likelihood that they will develop the condition in the future, they can request genetic testing for the same mutation as that identified in the affected family member. This action may be referred to as either *predictive* or *presymptomatic testing,* and is offered through geneticists or specialists in the diagnosis and management of that disease.

Family members seek further testing for a variety of reasons. Some will elect to know so they can make life choices, such as having their own children, choice of a career, or to reduce their fear of the unknown.

These issues are illustrated using an example of three siblings whose father has HD. The genetic mutation for HD has been identified, and adults who have a parent or grandparent with HD may have predictive testing. HD is an inherited, progressive, neurodegenerative disorder characterized by involuntary motor movements, dementia, mood disturbances, and affective disorders. Although the age of onset can occur in childhood through old age, the average age at diagnosis is middle thirties. This condition is inherited in an autosomal dominant manner (Fig. 8-1), which means that each offspring of a person with HD has a 50% or one in two chance of inheriting the gene that has the mutation associated with HD.

Given these statistics, one sibling elected not to undergo predictive testing, but to avoid passing on the gene to future generations, decided not to have children. One sibling who elected to have the predictive testing found that she did not inherit the disease but decided to keep the results private in order not to put pressure on the other siblings. A third sibling chose not to have the predictive testing but

wanted information about purchasing a long-term care insurance policy as a way to not burden the family in the future.

Genetic testing can be performed for several purposes, including prenatal diagnosis, detection of carrier status, predictive testing for familial disorders, and presymptomatic testing (Burke, 2002). For example, family members may seek testing if they are at greater risk for familial colon cancer (Madlensky, Esplen, Gallinger, McLauglin, & Goel, 2003). In some cases, clinical practice guideline criteria recommend that genetic testing be done to determine whether a person is at risk. For example, the National Comprehensive Cancer Network (2008) continually updates guidelines that specify what kind of screening is indicated for a person who has a gene mutation that increases her chances of cancer developing. In the pediatric health care arena, failure in achieving developmental milestones is one common reason for genetic referrals.

Several types of genetic tests exist; these are listed in Box 8-2. The specific potential benefits, risks, and limitations are unique to each test. Nurses should understand the differences in the types of genetic tests that families may consider (see Box 8-2) and the potential advantages or disadvantages of predictive genetic tests (Box 8-3). Nurses who participate in discussions about genetic testing must maintain current knowledge about these tests, as well as new technology for testing and interpretations of results.

Genetic tests have limitations that vary according to the specific test. For some tests, not all persons

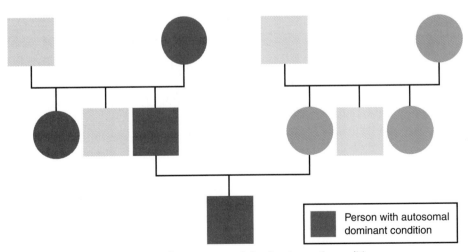

Person with autosomal dominant condition

FIGURE 8-1 Pedigree autosomal dominant genetic condition.

BOX 8-2
Types of Genetic Tests

Diagnostic	Performed when signs, symptoms, or both of a genetic condition are present. Confirms that the person has the suspected condition.
Carrier	Detects whether a person is a carrier of either an autosomal recessive or an X-linked disorder.
	A carrier of an autosomal recessive condition usually has no signs of the condition and will be at risk for having an affected child if the other parent is also a carrier. He or she has one normal copy of the gene in question and one mutated copy.
	A female carrier of an X-linked condition has one normal copy of the gene on the X chromosome and one mutated copy of the gene on the other X chromosome, and generally has no signs or very mild signs of the condition. Her sons have a 50% chance of having the condition, and her daughters have a 50% chance of being carriers.
Predictive or presymptomatic	Performed on healthy individuals; detects whether they inherited a mutation in a gene and, therefore, whether they will or may develop the condition in the future.
Prenatal diagnosis	Genetic test performed on the fetus. Indicates whether the fetus has inherited the gene mutation that causes a specific condition and, therefore, whether they will develop that condition.

---

who want the test may qualify, which occurs when their family history does not suggest that the disease has a major genetic component, or where the genetic mutation that causes the disease has not been identified. For some tests, it is possible that a result may be difficult to interpret. These are complex issues, and nurses who participate in genetic testing should become thoroughly prepared to provide education and assess understanding of the potential benefits, risks, and limitations of genetic testing. For some conditions, genetic mutations have been discovered that are associated with the

---

BOX 8-3
Potential Advantages and Disadvantages of Predictive Genetic Tests

Potential advantages of testing are:
- Opportunity to learn whether one has an increased likelihood of developng an inherited disease; in those who prefer certainty, this can help resolve feelings of discomfort, even if the result shows the person has inherited the condition
- Relief from worry about future health risks for a specific disease if the test is negative
- Information that can be used for making reproductive decisions
- Information to inform lifestyle choices (e.g., food choices, smoking, alcohol use, contraceptive choice)
- Information to guide clinical surveillance or management of the condition
- Information for other family members about their own status
- Confirmation of a diagnosis that has been suspected (i.e., that early or nonspecific signs and symptoms are due to a specific condition)

Potential disadvantages are that the test results may provide:
- A source of increased anxiety about the future
- Guilt at having survived when others in the family are affected, if the result is negative ("survivor's guilt")
- Concern about potential discrimination based on genetic test results
- Regret about past life decisions (such as not having children)
- Changes in family attitudes toward the person who has been tested (such as less reliance on them for support)

disease in that family. Because many genes may be associated with one condition, or a number of different mutations may be possible in a gene, it is often necessary to test an affected family member first to try to identify which gene is involved and which type of mutation is causing the disease in that family. A sample is taken from the affected person to determine whether a genetic mutation can be identified that is associated with that disease.

When a genetic condition, such as cystic fibrosis, is identified through newborn screening, parents receive a large amount of information in a relatively short period, and much of this information is overwhelming and complex. For example, a test result may be in the positive range for a screening test, but screening tests must be differentiated from diagnostic tests, and a positive screening test simply means a diagnostic test is required to determine whether the infant has the condition. It is important for parents to understand that, in some infants, a diagnostic test result can indicate that the infant has a genetic condition and will need further evaluation and treatment, and in other cases, subsequent tests will be normal. When an infant has further evaluation, and is found not to have the condition, the first test result is sometimes referred to as a false positive, or an out-of-range result that requires further testing. Parents who understand the reason for the repeated testing tend to experience less stress than those who do not. When a family has received an abnormal newborn screening test result, it is important for the nurse to determine the family's understanding that abnormal results from a screening test do not necessarily mean that the child is ill, but that all infants with an abnormal test result need further evaluation (Hewlett & Waisbren, 2006). The waiting period between the newborn screening result and the diagnostic testing can be especially difficult for parents (Tluczek, Koscik, Farrell, & Rock, 2005). Some parents may not be aware of what conditions are included in the newborn screening programs and likely have no knowledge or experience with the particular conditions that are included in screening programs.

Reactions to Predictive Testing Outcomes

The majority of conditions are inherited in an autosomal recessive pattern, and it is a common experience that no one else in the family will inherit the condition. Still, adjustment to a negative (i.e., no mutation) result can be difficult. For example, people at risk for HD who learn that they will not have the condition in the future sometimes find it difficult to "give up" the expectation that they would become ill, because that is what they and their family had believed (Williams, Schutte, Evers, & Holkup, 2000). In addition, those family members who have not inherited the condition may experience "survivor guilt." Therefore, those who have a good result may require significant psychological support after testing.

Although a test result provides certainty of one kind, the onset of symptoms is uncertain, and hypervigilance in searching for symptoms may follow a positive test result (Soltysiak, Gardiner, & Skirton, 2008). Not everyone who has testing will completely understand the chances that they will have the genetic condition. In the example of cancer, some people do not understand what they can do to decrease the chances of developing cancer or know how to identify cancer early (Beery & Williams, 2007).

Evidence exists that when individuals have a genetic test that indicates they will develop the condition, others in the family may rely on them less than previously, in an emotional sense. They may feel they have lost their place in the family well before they develop symptoms (Williams & Sobel, 2006). Some experience a deep sense of grief and loss of a potential future. For example, when families have not worked through the stages of grief associated with HD, other coping mechanisms, such as denial, may be important (Skirton, 1998).

ROLES OF THE NURSE

When a genetic risk is identified, nurses, together with others on the health care team, have two major responsibilities: (1) to help families understand that the risk is present, and (2) to help family members make decisions about management or surveillance. In every case, the nurse's role is to support families to make decisions that are most appropriate for their particular circumstances, cultures, and beliefs (International Society of Nurses in Genetics Position Statement; International Society of Nurses in Genetics, 2003). Seeking testing for determining one's potential to have a genetic condition evokes many strong emotions. Nurses are important sources of information and encouragement for those who may need to undergo more frequent screening. In any situation, giving what can be regarded as bad news is difficult, and nurses have a role in offering families support during this period and providing accurate written information that can be provided to relatives.

Personal Values: A Potential Conflict

Nurses must become aware of cultural values that differ from their own family cultural values, and how their personal values might influence the decisions families make about genetic health topics. Attitudes that reflect Western values, such as assuming that individuals (rather than family or community leaders) make health care decisions, require continued awareness by all health care providers. Cultural awareness allows nurses to tailor their practices to meet the needs of the family. Box 8-4 demonstrates how a nurse who does not understand a family's cultural value could have caused a poor outcome.

It is a difficult emotional situation when nurses' personal values conflict with those of families. One example of this type of conflict occurs when the nurse personally does not agree with the family decisions relative to the potential risks of having a child that is genetically predisposed to having a terminal disease. It is unethical for nurses to try to influence the decisions of the family or family members because of their personal views.

Another type of conflict occurs when opinions within the family vary. In this type of situation, the role of the nurse is to facilitate the family members in expressing their views. Genetic testing is discussed with an individual or with the person's family if the testing can offer useful information to the person. In clinical genetics, more than one family member may be involved in decision making, and nurses should respect each person's autonomy.

Although it is not possible for health professionals to have current knowledge about every condition, nurses exhibit competence in this area by having an awareness of their limitations, being open to discussion, finding appropriate resources, and referring to specialists when required. It is essential that nurses working in all types of settings be prepared with an adequate knowledge base to explain the basis and implications of the tests, and to ensure that patients understand the issues before consenting.

Conducting a Genetic Family History

All nurses should be able to conduct a risk assessment that includes obtaining a genetic family history (Consensus Panel, 2006). In Chapter 4, a genogram is used to collect useful information about family structure and relationships. For the purposes of making an accurate genetic risk assessment, a three-generation family pedigree is the instrument nurses use to provide information about a potential inheritance pattern and recurrence risks. The genetic risk assessment enables health professionals to identify those family members that may be at risk for disorders with a genetic component so that they can be provided appropriate lifestyle advice, screening recommendations, and possibly reproductive options. Information on standardized pedigree symbols and the construction of a genetic family pedigree is available to the public through the U.S. Surgeon General's Family History Initiative (http://www.hhs.gov/familyhistory; U.S. DHHS, 2005), and resources are available through the National Genetics Education and Development Centre (2008, http://www.geneticseducation.nhs.uk/).

BOX 8-4
Cultural Awareness

Kate is a genetic nurse working in a pediatric clinic for children with inherited metabolic conditions. She was scheduled to see a family whose son had a rare inherited metabolic disorder to discuss future reproductive options including prenatal diagnosis. When the family entered the room, she noted with surprise that the parents and the child were accompanied by both sets of grandparents. She quickly arranged for more chairs to be brought into the room. Kate was quite disconcerted to find that the paternal grandfather repeatedly answered questions that were directed to the parents, and she continued to address the parents. Eventually, the child's father explained that, according to his culture, the oldest male relative on the father's side was responsible for making the decision that would affect the family; therefore, it was critical that the grandfather be fully involved in all discussions. While reflecting with her mentor, Kate realized that, in the future, she would ask the family at the beginning of the family conference to share any specific cultural needs she should know about, to help meet their family needs.

The purpose of drawing the family tree using a genetic family pedigree is to enable medical information to be presented in context of the family structure. Obtaining a genetic family history in this systematic manner helps assure that no critical information is missed in the analysis (Skirton, Patch, & Williams, 2005). The process of obtaining a detailed health history and causes of family deaths is as follows:

- Start with the client
- Client's immediate family members
- Client's mother's side of the family
- Client's father's side of the family
- Relatives who have died, including their cause of death

Relatives who are not biologically related, such as those joining the family through adoption or marriage, should also be noted with the appropriate pedigree symbol. Obtaining a family genetic history is a nursing skill that requires technical expertise and knowledge of what needs to be asked, as well as sensitivity to potentially personal or distressing topics, and an awareness of the ethical issues involved. Box 8-5 outlines the components of a genetic nursing assessment. Information given by the patient is considered part of their personal health record, and should be treated as personal and private information (U.S. Department of Health an-Human Services, 1996).

BOX 8-5
Genetic/Genomic Nursing Assessment

A genetic nursing assessment includes the following information:
- Three-generation pedigree using standardized symbols
- Health history of each family member
- Reproductive history
- Ethnic background of family members (as described by the family)
- Documentation of variations in growth and development of family members
- Individual member and family understanding of causes of health problems that occur in more than one family member
- Identification of questions family members have about potential genetic risk factors in the family
- Identification of communication of genetic health information within the family

---

Drawing the genetic family pedigree or family tree for at least three generations often provides important data about the potential inheritance pattern. When a condition affects both male and female members, and is present in more than one generation, a dominant condition is suspected (see Fig. 8-1). Conditions that affect mainly male relatives, with no evidence of male-to-male transmission, increase suspicion of an **X-linked recessive** condition (Fig. 8-2). When more than one child is affected of only one set of parents, it may be evidence of an autosomal **recessive** condition (Fig. 8-3).

Nurses should not assume that a condition is genetic merely because more than one family member has it. Family members who are subject to similar environmental influences may have similar conditions without a genetic basis. One such example is a family with a strong history of lung cancer. Bob, a 62-year-old man, was affected by lung cancer. His two brothers and father all died of lung cancer. Bob expressed deep concern about having a genetic predisposition that he could pass on to his grandsons. The family history revealed that Bob's father and every male member of his family worked underground as coal miners from the age of 14 years. In addition, they all smoked at least 40 cigarettes a day from when they were teenaged. None of the women was a smoker, none ever worked in the mines, and none developed lung cancer. In this family, the cancer could likely be attributed to environmental rather than inherited causes.

Preconception Education

It is ideal when a family has the opportunity to discuss difficult genetic decisions before a pregnancy. During a pregnancy, the emotional ties to the existing fetus often make decision making extremely difficult for the parents. Preconception counseling enables the members of the couple to explore their options without time pressures.

Preconception counseling is an intervention that includes providing information and support to individuals before a pregnancy to promote health and reduce risks (Pillitteri, 2007). Part of this intervention is the identification of a health risk profile that includes family history, prescription drug use, ethnic background, occupational and household exposures, diet, specific genetic disorders, and habits such as smoking, alcohol, or street drug

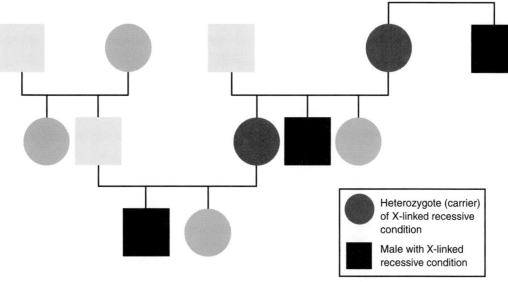

FIGURE 8-2 Pedigree of X-linked recessive condition.

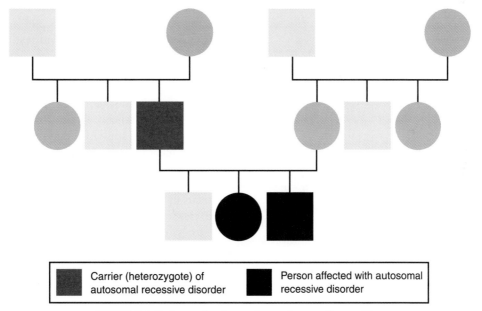

FIGURE 8-3 Pedigree of autosomal recessive genetic condition.

use. When nurses identify information that may present a health risk in future offspring, they should explore whether the woman or family wants a more extensive evaluation from a genetic specialist. Box 8-6 provides an example of preconception education for a couple for whom genetic risk exists for their offspring.

In addition to identifying inherited conditions, preconception counseling includes education regarding other risk factors that could change the outcome of a pregnancy. During preconception counseling, family nurses explain the importance of taking an adequate amount of folic acid, one of the B vitamins, which is known to a decrease the number of babies born with neural tube defects (NTD) (Centers for Disease Control and Prevention, 2006). NTDs are congenital abnormalities that result from the failure of the closure of the neural tube in the fourth week of gestation.

BOX 8-6
Preconception Education

Jay and Sara are college students who are planning to be married. Both are of Ashkenazi Jewish ancestry. Although both have heard about Tay–Sachs disease, and the availability of carrier testing, neither has had the carrier test. When Sara visited the student health office, she talked with the nurse about her fears that she may not be able to have healthy babies. She knew that Tay–Sachs disease, a degenerative neurologic condition, is more common in Ashkenazi Jewish families, and that no treatment will alter the course of the disease. Sara was interested in learning more about what a carrier test is, and the nurse offered to refer Sara to a genetics specialist, who would help the couple explore childbearing options, such as:

- Decide against having children
- Have a pregnancy with no form of genetic testing
- Have preimplantation genetic diagnosis
- Have a pregnancy and have prenatal genetic diagnosis with an option to terminate an affected fetus
- Have a pregnancy using donor gamete from a noncarrier donor
- Adopt a child

BOX 8-7
Folic Acid Recommendations to Prevent Neural Tube Defects

In 1992, the U.S. Public Health Service recommended that all women capable of becoming pregnant take 0.4 mg/400 µg folic acid daily, which is the amount of folic acid in most multivitamins. A daily intake of folic acid does not completely rule out the possibility that an infant will have NTDs. Studies have reported an 11% to 20% reduction in cases of anencephaly and a 21% to 34% reduction in cases of spina bifida after this recommendation was issued (Mosley et al., 2009).

These deficits include anencephaly, spina bifida, and encephalocele. The risk for this condition varies according to ethnic background, with greater rates among British and Irish populations (Jorde, Carey, Bamshad, & White, 2005). A combination of genetic and environmental factors is believed to contribute to the risk for NTDs. Box 8-7 provides more information about NTDs.

Risk Assessment in Adult-Onset Diseases

Genetic history taking is important in the adult population to assess for risk factors that are pertinent to common diseases such as cancer and coronary heart disease. The basic risk assessment is based on the genetic family pedigree, but additional genetic or biochemical testing may be used to clarify the potential risk to each individual. Consent is required from all living relatives to access their medical records and confirm relevant medical history to ensure privacy. Family members who are seeking information are advised of their risks and options for clinical screening and follow-up. One example is the assessment of risk for cancer when there is a strong history of cancer in the family (Gammon, Kohlmann, & Burt, 2007). Individuals who find through counseling and testing that they have an increased risk for cancer may experience psychological difficulties (Kenen, Ardern-Jones, & Eeles, 2006). Nurses must explore feelings of grief and anxiety about the future, as well as beliefs about the inheritance pattern. Providing explanations enables the family to understand the information and helps them learn about possible options to reduce the risk for cancer in their family members.

Increasingly, women with a family history of breast or ovarian cancer, or both, are seeking to reduce their risks for these conditions. This is especially true for women whose own mothers died at a relatively young age from breast or ovarian cancers (van Oostrom et al., 2006). All women have a risk for breast cancer (a lifetime risk of about 1 in 11 in the U.S. population) and may be offered mammography screening according to the standards of care or regional health policy (National Institute for Clinical Excellence, 2006). For women with a genetic family history that is consistent with familial breast and ovarian cancer, earlier and more frequent screening will be discussed by genetic and familial cancer specialists. Because of the density of the breast tissue, however, mammography is not as reliable at detecting tumors in women before menopause. Therefore, other methods of screening, such as magnetic resonance imaging, may be recommended for high-risk premenopausal women.

With appropriate treatment, some health problems with a major genetic component may improve or at least remain stable. But many genetic conditions lead to increasing loss of health and function throughout the person's life span. These genetic conditions require increasingly more complex care from both health care providers and the family. In the chronic phase of a genetic condition, individuals and the family not only come to terms with the permanent changes that come with the onset of illness symptoms (Rolland, 1994), but also must adapt their family routines and roles, and locate needed resources to meet increasingly complex health care needs.

Providing Information and Resources

An essential nursing competence includes the need for nurses to be able to identify resources that are useful, informative, and reliable for patients and families. Knowledge of genetics is rapidly changing, and Web-based resources may provide the most current information. Patients value the recommendations of health professionals on suitable sources of information (Skirton & Barr, 2008). It is the role of the nurse to ensure that recommended Web sites include relevant and evidence-based information. Web sites associated with government-funded bodies (such as National Institutes for Health) are generally reliable, as are those associated with institutions of higher education or national patient or lay support groups. When recommending Web sites hosted by patient support groups, it is important to confirm that the organization has a medical advisor

and the information has been assessed by a knowledgeable person. Patients and families have a need for psychosocial and medical information; therefore, any information that is prepared for distribution should include material on both types of issues (Lewis, Mehta, Kent, Skirton, & Coviello, 2007).

Evaluation of Genetic and Genomic Nursing Interventions

Genetics and genomics are relatively new fields in nursing, but some work has assessed the value of genetic services, including nursing input, for patients and their families. A study to define nursing outcomes relative to genetics was conducted in both the United States and the United Kingdom (Williams et al., 2001). The views of nurses indicated that enhancing patient knowledge of the disease and the genetic risks associated with the disease were important aspects of care. Nurses also believed that offering families psychosocial support was an integral part of their practice. In Skirton's study (2001), patients report that they gained peace of mind from the care they received, and that increasing their knowledge about the condition, being treated as an individual, and having a warm relationship with the health professionals caring for them were important to the overall outcome of the consultation. Nurses should aim not only to be knowledgeable about genomics but also provide individualized care, and address the needs and specific agendas of each family. Box 8-8 provides an example of a nurse's evaluation of interventions with a family whose child has a genetic condition.

BOX 8-8
Evaluation of Nursing Intervention

Fiona is a 5-year-old child who is attending kindergarten. Her teacher is concerned that she does not appear to be progressing as well as expected, and asks the school nurse, Cindy, to check her hearing. Cindy arranges for Fiona's parents to bring her for a hearing test. She asks Fiona's mother about her medical history; the mother says she has always been a well child and has not had any ear infections but has developed some "funny patches" on her skin. They have not caused a problem, but the mother has wondered what they are and if they could turn cancerous. Cindy checks these and notes that they seem to be café-au-lait patches—small, pale brown pigmented areas of the skin. She reassures the parents that the café-au-lait patches are not harmful but could indicate an underlying cause for Fiona's slight learning problems. She draws a genetic family pedigree or family tree (Fig. 8-4) and notes that Fiona's father and his mother (Fiona's paternal grandmother) had unusual skin lumps, but no other medical problems.

Continued

BOX 8-8
Evaluation of Nursing Intervention—cont'd

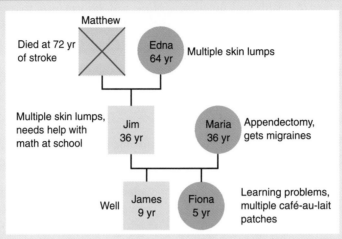

FIGURE 8-4 Genetic pedigree: Fiona's family tree.

When the pediatrician sees the family, she measures Fiona's head circumference and examines her skin. She confirms that the skin marks are café-au-lait patches and Fiona has eight of these. Fiona's head circumference is larger than average, on the 97th percentile for her age. A diagnosis of neurofibromatosis type 1 is made. The pediatrician explains that this is a genetic condition, but that it could have arisen for the first time in Fiona or may have been inherited from one of her parents. Neither parent is aware of the condition in the family. The pediatrician examines both parents and finds that Fiona's father has a large head circumference and has several raised lumps on the skin, called *neurofibromas.* He tells the pediatrician he needed extra help with math at school, but he finished college and works teaching French. He has never been concerned about the lumps because his own mother had dozens of them, and apart from having one removed because her shoe was rubbing against it, they did not cause her a problem.

The pediatrician is aware that children with this condition may have learning problems. She recommends that Fiona be evaluated to identify whether Fiona would benefit from extra help at school. As high blood pressure and malignancies can occur as a result of the condition, she also makes arrangements for Fiona and her father to have an annual checkup. Fiona's brother, James (9 years old), is also examined but has no signs of the condition and does not require any further checkups.

When Cindy is informed of the diagnosis, she helps the family to identify reliable sources of information on the Web and provides Fiona's parents with information about neurofibromatosis organizations.

SUMMARY

Families share both social and biological ties. Identifying biologic risk factors is an essential component of professional nursing practice, and a nursing assessment is incomplete without identifying biological factors that may place individuals or their offspring at risk for genetic conditions. Nurses providing care to families across all health care settings and throughout the life span must maintain current knowledge of genomic aspects of health and risk for illness to assist families to obtain information and further evaluation if needed. Interventions with families include assessment, identification of issues influencing family members' health, facilitating appropriate referrals, and evaluating the effect of these activities on the family's health and well-being. Family values, beliefs, and patterns of communication are integral components of how families will cope with and respond to the opportunity to identify and promote health of family members with medical conditions that have a genetic component.

REFERENCES

Beery, T., & Williams, J. K. (2007). Risk reduction and health promotion behaviors following genetic testing for adult-onset disorders. *Genetic Testing, 11*(920), 111–123.

Burke, W. (2002). Genetic testing. *New England Journal of Medicine 347*(23), 1867–1875.

Centers for Disease Control and Prevention. (2006). *Recommendations to improve preconception health and health care: United States. MMWR Recomm Rep 55*(RR-6), 1–23.

Christensen, K., & Murray, J. C. (2007). What genome-wide association studies can do for medicine. *New England Journal of Medicine, 356*(11), 1094–1097.

Consensus Panel. (2006). *Essential Nursing Competencies and Curricula Guidelines for Genetics and Genomics.* Retrieved May 5, 2008, from http://www.genome.gov/Pages/Careers/HealthProfessionalEducation/geneticscompetency.pdf

Feetham, S. L., & Thomson, E. J. (2006). Keeping the individual and family in focus. In S. M. Miller, S. H. McDaniel, J. S. Rolland, & S. L. Feetham (Eds.), *Individuals, families, and the new era of genetics* (pp. 3–33). New York: W.W. Norton.

Gaff, C. L., Clarke, A. J., Atkinson, P., Sivell, S., Elwyn, G., Iredale, R., et al. (2007). Process and outcome in communication of genetic information within families: A systematic review. *European Journal of Human Genetics, 15,* 999–1011.

Gaff, C. L., Collins, V., Symes, T., & Halliday, J. (2005). Facilitating family communication about predictive genetic testing: Probands' perceptions. *Journal of Genetic Counseling, 14*(2), 133–139.

Gallo, A. M., Angst, D., Knafl, K. A., Hadley, E., & Smith, C. (2005). Parents sharing information with their children about genetic conditions. *Journal of Pediatric Health Care, 19*(5), 267–275.

Gallo, A. M., Hadley, E. K., Angst, D. B., Knafl, K. A., & Smith, C. A. M. (2008). Parents' concerns about issues related to their children's genetic conditions. *Journal of the Society for Pediatric Nursing, 13*(1), 4–14.

Gammon, A., Kohlmann, W., & Burt, R. (2007). Can we identify the high-risk patients to be screened? A genetic approach. *Digestion 76*(1):7–19.

Gulati, A. P., & Domchek, S. M. (2008). The clinical management of BRCA1 and BRCA2 mutation carriers. *Current Oncology Reports, 10*(1):47–53.

Hewlett, J., & Waisbren, S. E. (2006). A review of the psychosocial effects of false-positive results on parents and current communication practices in newborn screening. *Journal of Inherited and Metabolic Diseases, 29,* 677–682.

International Society of Nurses in Genetics. (2003). *Position statement: Access to genomic healthcare: The role of the nurse.* Retrieved April 20, 2008, from http://www.isong.org/about/ps_genomic.cfm

Jorde, L., Carey, J., Bamshad, M., & White, R. (2005). *Medical genetics updated edition for 2006-2007 with student online access.* New York: Elsevier Health Sciences.

Kenen, R., Ardern-Jones, A., Eeles, R. (2006). "Social separation" among women under 40 years of age diagnosed with breast cancer and carrying a BRCA1 or BRCA2 mutation. *Journal of Genetic Counseling, 15*(3), 149–162.

Kessler, S. (1988). Invited essay on the psychological aspects of genetic counseling. V. Preselection: A family coping strategy in Huntington disease. *American Journal of Medical Genetics, 31*(3), 617–621.

Lewis, C., Mehta, P., Kent, A., Skirton, H., & Coviello, D. (2007). An assessment of written patient information relating to genetic testing from across Europe. *European Journal of Human Genetics, 15,* 1012–1022.

Madlensky, L., Esplen, M. J., Gallinger, S., McLauglin, J. R., & Goel, V. (2003). Relatives of colorectal cancer patients: Factors associated with screening behavior. *American Journal of Preventive Medicine, 25*(3), 187–194.

McDaniel, S., Rolland, J., Feetham, S., & Miller, S. (2006). "It runs in the family": Family systems concepts and genetically linked disorders. In S. M. Miller, S. H. McDaniel, J. S. Rolland, & S. L. Feetham (Eds.), *Individuals, families, and the new Era of genetics* (pp. 118–138). New York: W.W. Norton.

Mosley, B. S., Cleves, M. A., Siega-Riz, A. M., Shaw, G. M., Canfield, M. A., Waller, D. K., et al; for the National Birth Defects Prevention Study. (2009). Neural tube defects and maternal folate intake among pregnancies conceived after folic acid fortification in the United States. *American Journal of Epidemiology, 169*(1), 9–17.

National Comprehensive Cancer Network. (2008). *NCCN Clinical Practice Guidelines in Oncology.* Retrieved May 5, 2009, from http://www.nccn.org

National Genetics Education and Development Centre. (2008). *A competence framework for general practitioners with a special interest in genetics.* Retrieved May 26, 2008, from http://www.geneticseducation.nhs.uk

National Institute for Clinical Excellence. (2006). *CG41 familial breast cancer—full guideline (the new recommendations and the evidence they are based on).* Retrieved April 23, 2008, from http://www.nice.org.uk/nicemedia/pdf/CG41fullguidance.pdf

Patenaude, A. F., Dorval, M., DiGianni, L. S., Schineider, K. A., Chiteenden, A., & Garber, J. E. (2006). Sharing BRCA1/2 test results with first-degree relatives: Factors predicting who women tell. *Journal of Clinical Oncology, 24*(4), 700–706.

Penziner, E., Williams, J. K., Erwin, C., Wallis, A., Bombard, Y., Beglinger, L., et al. (2008). Perceptions of genetic discrimination among persons who have undergone predictive testing for Huntington disease. *American Journal of Medical Genetics Part B, 147B,* 320–325.

Peters, K., Apse, K., Blackford, A., McHugh, B., Michalic, D., & Biesecker, B. (2005). Living with Marfan syndrome: Coping with stigma. *Clinical Genetics 68*(1), 6–14.

Pillitteri, A. (2007). Assessing fetal maternal health: Prenatal care. In A. Pillitteri, *Maternal & Child Health Nursing.* Philadelphia, PA: Lippincott, Williams, & Wilkens.

Rolland, J. S. (1994). *Families, illness, and disability: An integrative treatment model.* New York: Basic Books.

Royal College of Physicians, Royal College of Pathologists and British Society for Human Genetics. (2005). *Consent and confidentiality in genetic practice: Guidance on genetic testing and sharing genetic information.* Report of the Joint Committee on Medical Genetics. London: RCP, RCPath, BSHG. Retrieved May 1, 2008, from http://www.bshg.org.uk/documents/official_docs/Consent_and_confid_corrected_21[1].8.06.pdf

Skirton, H. (1998). Telling the children. In A. Clarke (Ed.), *The genetic testing of children* (pp. 103–111). Oxford: Bios Scientific Publishers.

Skirton, H. (2001). The client's perspective of genetic counseling—a grounded theory study. *Journal of Genetic Counseling, 10*(4), 311–329.

Skirton, H., & Barr, O. (2008). Antenatal screening: Informed choice and parental consent. Retrieved May 5, 2009, from http://www.learningdisabilities.org.uk/publications

Skirton, H., Frazier, L. Q., Calvin, A. O., & Cohen, M. Z. (2006). A legacy for the children: Attitudes of older adults in the United Kingdom to genetic testing. *Journal of Clinical Nursing, 15,* 565–573.

Skirton, H., Patch, C., & Williams, J. (2005). *Applied genetics in healthcare: A handbook for specialist practitioners.* New York: Taylor & Francis Group.

Soltysiak, B., Gardiner, P., & Skirton, H. (2008). Exploring supportive care for individuals affected by Huntington disease and their family caregivers in a community setting. *Journal of Clinical Nursing, 17*(7B):226–234.

Sparbel, K. J. H., Driessack, M., Williams, J. K., Schutte, D. L., Tripp-Reimer, T., McGonigal-Kenney, M., et al. (2008). Experiences of teens living in the shadow of Huntington disease. *Journal of Genetic Counseling, 17*(4), 327–335.

Speice, J., McDaniel, S. H., Rowley, P. T., & Loader, S. (2002). Family issues in a psychoeducation group for women with a BRCA mutation. *Clinical Genetics, 62*(2), 121–127.

Stoffel, E. M., Ford, B., Mercado, R. C., Punglia, D., Kohlmann, W., Conrad, P., et al. (2008). Sharing genetic test results in Lynch syndrome: Communication with close and distant relatives. *Clinical Gastroenterology & Hepatology, 6*(3), 333–338.

Tercyak, K. P., Peshkin, B. N., Demarco, T., Patenaude, A. F., Schneider, K. A., Garber, J. E., et al. (2007). Information needs of mothers regarding communicating BRCA1/2 cancer genetic test results to their children. *Genetic Testing, 11*(3), 249–255.

Tluczek, A., Koscik, R. L., Farrell, P. M., & Rock, M. J. (2005). Psychosocial risk associated with newborn screening for cystic fibrosis: Parents' experience while awaiting the sweat-test appointment. *Pediatrics, 115*(6), 1692–1704.

U.S. Department of Health and Human Services. (1996). Office for Civil Rights-HIPAA. *Medical Privacy: National standards to protect the privacy of personal health information.* Retrieved May 5, 2009, from http://www.hhs.gov/ocr/privacy/index.html

U.S. Department of Health and Human Services. (2005). *Surgeon General's family history initiative.* Retrieved May 5, 2009, from http://www.hhs.gov/familyhistory

Van Oostrom, I., Meijers-Heijboer, H., Duivenvooden, H. J., Brocker-Vriends, A. H., van Asperen, C. J., Sijmons, R. H., et al. (2006). Experience of parental cancer in childhood is a risk factor for psychological distress during genetic cancer susceptibility testing. *Annals of Oncology, 17*(7), 1090–1095.

Walsh, F. (2003). *Normal family processes* (3rd ed.). New York: Guilford.

Williams, J. K., Schutte, D. L., Evers, C., & Holkup, P. A. (2000). Redefinition: Coping with normal results from presymptomatic gene testing for neurodegenerative disorders. *Research in Nursing and Health, 23,* 260–269.

Williams, J. K., Skirton, H., Reed, D., Johnson, M., Maas, M., & Daack-Hirsch, S. (2001). Genetic counseling outcomes validation by genetics nurses in the UK and US. *Journal of Nursing Scholarship, 33*(4), 369–374.

Williams, J. K., & Sobel, S. (2006). Neurodegenerative genetic conditions: The example of Huntington disease. In S. M. Miller, S. H. McDaniel, J. S. Rolland, & S. L. Feetham (Eds.), *Individuals, families, and the new era of genetics* (pp. 231–247). New York: W.W. Norton.

CHAPTER 9

Family Health Promotion

Yeoun Soo Kim-Godwin, PhD, MPH, RN

Perri J. Bomar, PhD, RN

CRITICAL CONCEPTS

✦ Family health promotion refers to activities that families engage in to strengthen the family unit and increase family unity and quality of family life.

✦ Health promotion is learned within families, and patterns of health behaviors are formed and passed on to the next generation.

✦ A major task of the family is to teach health maintenance and health promotion.

✦ The role of the family nurse is to help families attain, maintain, and regain the highest level of family health possible.

✦ The national economy directly affects the family's ability to promote health in its family members.

✦ Positive, reinforcing interaction between family members leads to a healthier family lifestyle.

✦ Different cultures define and value health, health promotion, and disease prevention differently. Clients may not understand or respond to the family nurses' suggestions for health promotion because the suggestions conflict with their health beliefs and values.

✦ Family health promotion should become a regular part of taking a family history and a routine aspect of nursing care.

Fostering the health of the family as a unit and encouraging families to value and incorporate health promotion into their lifestyle are essential components of family nursing practice. Family health promotion refers to the activities that families engage in to strengthen the family as a unit. Family health promotion is defined as achieving maximum family well-being throughout the family life course and includes the biological, emotional, physical, and spiritual realms for family members and the family unit (Bomar, 2004a; Loveland-Cherry & Bomar, 2004). Health promotion is learned within families, and patterns of health behaviors are formed and passed on to the next generation. Families are primarily responsible for providing health and illness care, being a role model, teaching self-care and wellness behaviors, providing for care of members across their life course and during varied family transitions, and supporting each other during health-promoting activities and acute and chronic illnesses. A major task of families is to teach health maintenance and health promotion, regardless of age.

The purpose of this chapter is to introduce family health and the family health models, and examine internal and external factors that influence family health promotion. This chapter includes a case study of a family, to apply models for family assessment and interventions. In addition, this chapter discusses the role of nurses, and intervention strategies in maintaining and regaining the highest level of family health. The Research Brief section later in this chapter suggests the strategies that families typically utilize to keep themselves healthy.

WHAT IS FAMILY HEALTH?

Definitions of *family health* have evolved from anthropologic, biopsychosocial, developmental, family science, cultural, and nursing paradigms. The concept of family health is often used interchangeably with the terms *family functioning, healthy families, resilient families,* and *balanced families* (Kaakinen & Birenbaum, 2008; Soubhi, Potvin, & Paradis, 2004; Walsh, 2006). Refer to Chapter 1 for the explanations of family health. Family scientists define healthy families as resilient (Walsh, 2006), and as possessing a balance of cohesion and adaptability that is facilitated by good communication (Olson, 2000). Chapter 1 has a detailed section on family communication and its relation to family health.

In terms of defining family health, family therapy definitions often emphasize optimal family functioning and freedom from psychopathology (Goldenberg & Goldenberg, 2007; McGoldrick, Gerson, & Petry, 2008). Within the developmental framework, healthy families complete developmental tasks at appropriate times (Carter & McGoldrick, 2005; Duval & Miller, 1985).

Other definitions of family health focus on the totality, or *gestalt,* of the family's existence, and include the internal and external environment of the family. A holistic definition of family health encompasses all aspects of family life, including interaction and health care function. A healthy family has a sense of well-being. Family health care function includes family nutrition, recreation, communication, sleep and rest patterns, problem solving, sexuality, use of time and space, coping

with stress, hygiene and safety, spirituality, illness care, health promotion and protection, and emotional health of family members (Bomar, 2004a; Friedman, Bowden, & Jones, 2003). According to Hanson (2005), family heath is "a dynamic changing relative state of well-being which includes the biological, psychological, spiritual, sociological and cultural factors of the family system" (p. 7). In summary, and for purposes of this chapter, *family health* is a holistic, dynamic, and complex state. Family health is more than the absence of disease in an individual family member or the absence of dysfunction in family dynamics. Rather, it is the complex process of negotiating and solving day-to-day family life events and crises, and providing for a quality life for its members (Bomar, 2004a).

Preliminary results of the "Healthy Family Inventory," by the Psychological Studies Institute (2004), found that 83% of a family's health appears attributable to 14 sets of behaviors: problem solving, affirmation, open communication, clear boundaries, family rituals and traditions, trust, healthy sexuality, healthy family of origin relationships, religious/faith core, community connection, time together and shared interests, physical and financial well-being, adaptation to stress and loss, and behavior control (Association of Operating Room Nurses, 2004). Box 9-1 lists the characteristics of healthy families showing how families promote health.

COMMON THEORETICAL PERSPECTIVES

Many models and theories are applicable to family health and family health promotion. This section briefly describes the selected models of family health and family health promotion.

Model of Family Health

Building on Smith's (1983) models of health, Loveland-Cherry and Bomar (2004) suggest that there are four views of family health:

1. *Clinical model.* Examined from this perspective, a family is healthy if its members are free of physical, mental, and social dysfunction.

BOX 9-1
Characteristics of Healthy Family

UNITY

Commitment	Time Together
Has a sense of trust traditions	Shares family rituals and traditions
Teaches respect for others	Enjoys each other's company
Exhibits a sense of shared responsibility	Shares leisure time together
Affirms and supports all of its members	Shares simple and quality time

FLEXIBILITY

Ability to Deal with Stress	Spiritual Well-Being
Displays adaptability	Encourages hope
Sees crises as a challenge and opportunity	Shares faith and religious core
Shows openness to change	Teaches compassion for others
Grows together in crisis	Teaches ethical values
Seeks help with problems	Respects the privacy of one another
Opens its boundaries to admit and seek help	

COMMUNICATION

Positive Communication	Appreciation and Affection
Communicates well and listens to all members	Cares for each other
Fosters family table time and conversation	Exhibits a sense of humor
Shares feelings	Maintains friendship
Displays nonblaming attitudes	Respects individuality
Is able to compromise and disagree	Has a spirit of playfulness/humor
Agrees to disagree	Interacts with each other and a balance in the interactions is noted among the members

Source: Modified from Hanson, S. M. H., Gedaly-Duff, V., & Kaakinen, J. R. (Eds.). (2005). *Family health care nursing: Theory, practice & research* (3rd ed.) Philadelphia: F.A. Davis; Olson, D. H. L., & Defrain, J. (2003). *Marriage and the family: Diversity and strengths* (4th ed.). NewYork: McGraw-Hill; and Psychological Studies Institute. (2004, September 15). New study identifies specific behaviors linked to family health. *Physican Law Weekly.* Retrieved April 16, 2008, from http://www.newsrx.com/newsletters/Physican-Law-Weekly/2004-09-15/091320043331272PLW.html, by permission.

2. *Role-performance model.* This view of family health is based on the idea that family health is the ability of family members to perform their routine roles and achieve developmental tasks.
3. *Adaptive model.* In this model, families are adaptive if they have the ability to change and grow and possess the capacity to rebound quickly after a crisis.
4. *Eudaimonistic model.* Professionals who use this model as their philosophy of practice focus on efforts to maximize the family's well-being and to support the entire family and individual members in reaching their greatest potential.

Table 9-1 defines the four models of family health. According to Loveland-Cherry and Bomar (2004), these family health models are useful in three ways: (1) they provide frameworks for understanding the level of health that families are experiencing; (2) they may be useful in designing interventions to assist families in maintaining or

TABLE 9-1

Four Models of Family Health

MODEL	DEFINITION OF FAMILY HEALTH
Clinical model	Lack of evidence of physical, mental, or social disease or deterioration, or dysfunction of family system
Role-performance model	Ability of the family system to conduct family functions effectively and to achieve family developmental tasks
Adaptive model	Family patterns of interaction with the environment characterized by flexible, effective adaptation or ability to change and grow
Eudaimonistic model	Ongoing provision of resources, guidance, and support for realization of family's maximum well-being and potential throughout the family life span

Source: Modified from Bomar, P. J. (2004a). Introduction to family health nursing and promoting family health. In P. J. Bomar (Ed.), *Promoting health in families: Applying family research and theory to nursing practice* (3rd ed., pp. 3–37). Philadelphia: WB Saunders, by permission.

regaining good health, or in coping with illness; and (3) they may facilitate organization of the family nursing literature and serve as a focus for family research.

FAMILY HEALTH MODEL

Based on family health studies with Appalachian families (Denham 1997, 1999a, 1999b, 1999c), and a broad base of literature and existing research about family health, Denham (2003a) has proposed The Family Health Model. Family health is viewed as a process over time of family members' interactions and health-related behaviors, and strives to enhance the process of becoming. In the Family Health Model, family health includes the systems, interactions, relationships, and processes that have the potential to maximize well-being. The model emphasizes the biophysical, holistic, and environmental factors that influence health.

In her Family Health Model, Denham (2003a, 2003b) suggests that family health routines offer the means of connecting with health promotion for changes. Family routines are behavior patterns related to events, occasions, or situations that are repeated with regularity and consistency. Family routines have been identified as key structural aspects of family health that can be assessed by nurses, provide a focus for family interventions, and have potential for measuring health outcomes (2003a). Routines supply information about behaviors and their predictability, member interactions, family identity, and specific ways families live.

Denham (2003a) makes the following propositions about family health routines (p. 191):

- Families that tend toward moderation in family health routines are healthier than families who are highly ritualized and those who lack rituals.
- Families with clearer ideas about their goals are more likely to accommodate health needs effectively through their family routines than families who are less certain about their goals.
- Families and individuals are more likely to accommodate changes related to health concerns when family routines are supported over time by embedded contextual systems than families who are not supported.
- Family routines that support individual health care needs are more likely to achieve positive care outcomes in the individual with the health concern than families who do not have routines that support the needs of family members with health concerns.
- Children who are taught routines in the home and are supported by the embedded context are more likely to practice health routines in the home than those not supported by the embedded context.

Kushner's (2007) study reports that routines are the means by which family members deal with everyday health needs in the household context, the way that they teach children health behaviors, and the way they support stress management. Kushner's study is presented in more detail in the Research Brief section later in this chapter.

Denham lists the diverse types of routines, including individual routine, family routine, family health routine, family ritual, family tradition, and family celebration (Denham, 2003a). Health routines are described as interactions affected by biophysical, developmental, interactional, psychosocial, spiritual, and contextual realms, with implications for the health and well-being of members and family as a whole. Heath routines include self-care routines, safety and prevention, mental health behaviors, family care, illness care, and member caregiving. Kusher (2007) has found additional routines to monitor or keep track of family health. Table 9-2 presents the types of health routines that Denham (2003a) proposes.

TABLE 9-2

Types of Family Health Routines

FAMILY HEALTH ROUTINE	ASPECTS OF THE ROUTINE	DESCRIPTION OF THE ROUTINES
Self-care routines	Dietary Hygiene Sleep-rest Physical activity and exercise Gender and sexuality	These routines involve patterned behaviors related to usual activities of daily living experienced across the life course.
Safety and prevention	Health protection Disease prevention Smoking Abuse and violence Alcohol and substance abuse	These routines pertain to health protection, disease prevention, avoidance and participation in high-risk behaviors, and effort to prevent unintended injury across the life course.
Mental health behaviors	Self-esteem Personal integrity Work and play Stress levels	These routines have to do with the ways individuals and families attend to self-efficacy, cope with daily stresses, and individuate.
Family care	Family fun (e.g., relaxation, activities, hobbies, vacations) Celebrations, traditions, special events Spiritual and religious practices Pets Sense of humor	These routines include daily activities, traditional behaviors, and special celebrations that give meaning to daily life, and provide shared enjoyment, pleasure, and happiness for multiple members.
Illness care	Decision making related to medical consultation Use of health care services Follow-up with prescribed medical regimens	These routines are the various ways members make decisions related to health-care needs; choose when, where, and how to seek supportive health services; and determine ways to respond to medical directives and health information.
Member caregiving	Health teaching (i.e., health, prevention, illness, disease) Member roles and responsibilities Providing illness care Support of member actions	These routines pertain to the ways family members act as interactive caregivers across the life course as they socialize children and adolescents about a wide variety of health-related ideals, participate in specific health and illness care needs, and support members' individual routine patterns.

Source: From Denham, S. A. (2003a). *Family health: A framework for nursing.* Philadelphia: FA Davis, by permission.

Models for Family Health Promotion

In the past, most of the attention of health professionals focused on individuals, family subsystems (marital and parent-child dyads), and community health problems. A great need exists to encourage health promotion of the whole family unit because health behaviors, values, and patterns are learned within a family context. Family health promotion activities are crucial both during wellness and during illness of a family member. Family health promotion increases family unity and quality of life. According to Pender, Murdaugh, and Parsons (2006), family health promotion involves the family's lifelong efforts to nurture its members, to maintain family cohesion, and to reach the family's greatest potential in all aspects of health.

FAMILY HEALTH PROMOTION MODEL

Most models of health promotion focus on the individual. Adapting Pender's (1996) health promotion model, Loveland-Cherry and Bomar (2004) present a family health promotion model. In this model, the likelihood of a family engaging in health-promoting behaviors is influenced by the following general, health-related, and behavioral specific factors:

1. *General influences*
   - Family systems patterns such as values, communication, interactions, and power
   - Demographic characteristics such as family size, structure, income, and culture
   - Biological characteristics
2. *Health-related influences*
   - Family health socialization patterns
   - Family definition of "health"
   - Perceived family health status
3. *Behavior-specific influences*
   - Perceived barriers to health-promoting behavior
   - Perceived benefits to health-promoting behavior
   - Prior related behavior
   - Family norms regarding health-promoting behavior
   - Intersystem support for behavior
   - Situational influences
   - Internal and environmental family cues

For example, a family who lives in poverty would be less likely to be involved in health promotion. From a survey of a convenience sample of 67 mothers (ages 27–44) with preschool children (3–5 years of age) in Canada, Monteith and Ford-Gilboe (2002) report that family income significantly predicted 11% of the variance in the mother's health-promoting lifestyle practices, but individual factors (i.e., the mother's resilience) also explained 17% of the variance in health-promoting lifestyle practices. In addition, if a family defines "health" as the absence of disease, it is also less likely to engage in a health-promoting lifestyle. All of these variables are interrelated and affect the quality of family health-promoting outcomes. Although similarities exist in families in each of these variables, families also have unique differences that affect health outcomes. For example, family health beliefs, religion, social support, and gender roles affect health promotion. Figure 9-1 depicts the Family Health Promotion Model.

DEVELOPMENTAL MODEL OF HEALTH AND NURSING

The Developmental Model of Health and Nursing (DMHN) constructed by Canadian scholar F. Moyra Allen in the mid-1970s and 1980s (Allen & Warner, 2002) has a goal of increasing the capacity of families and individuals in health promotion in everyday life situations. In this interaction model, the nurse's role changes at each phase of the health promotion process, thereby empowering clients toward improving their health status. Examples of the nursing functions include:

- Focuser, stimulator, and resource producer who involves the client in such tasks as clarifying concerns and goals, and thinking about his or her learning style
- Integrator and awareness raiser who assists clients with analyzing the situation, identifying additional resources, and seeking potential solutions
- Role model, instructor, coach, guide, and encourager as clients make decisions on alternatives and try new behaviors
- Role "reinforcer" and reviewer as clients review and evaluate outcomes (Allen & Warner, 2002, p. 122)

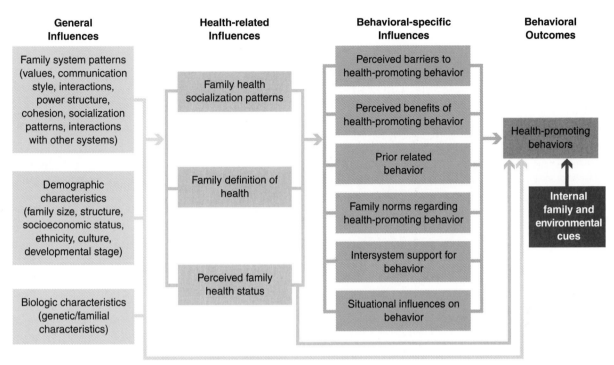

| General Influences | Health-related Influences | Behavioral-specific Influences | Behavioral Outcomes |

FIGURE 9-1 Family Health Promotion Model. (Reproduced from Bomar, P. J. [2004a]. Introduction to family health nursing and promoting family health. In P. J. Bomar [Ed.], *Promoting health in families: Applying family research and theory to nursing practice* [3rd ed., pp. 3–37]. Philadelphia: WB Saunders, by permission.)

Ford-Gilboe (2002) summarizes six studies that tested the propositions of Allen's DMHN. The studies tested four concepts: health potential, health work, competence in health behavior, and health status. Results indicate significant relationships between health potential and health work. The level of family health potential, health work, and health competence all were found to be significant predictors of family functioning. Monteith and Ford-Gilboe (2002) also report that health work predicted 24% of the variance in the mother's health-promoting lifestyle practices.

MODEL OF THE HEALTH-PROMOTING FAMILY

The primary concern of the Model of the Health Promoting Family that Christensen (2004) proposes is the "health practices of the family." The model addresses how families can play a part in promoting both the health of children and their capacities as health-promoting actors, which explains how families, in their everyday life, engage in promoting the health of their members. The model draws on contemporary social science approaches to health, the family, and children, suggesting a new emphasis on the family's ecocultural pathway, family practices, and the child as a health-promoting factor.

As shown in Figure 9-2, this model is analytically divided into two parts to distinguish factors external to the family and factors internal to it. The external factors are further divided into societal and community level factors. The societal factors provide the material base for the family and will, therefore, to a large degree shape the resources available to the family. These include, for example, income and wealth, education and knowledge, family structure and housing, ethnicity, social networks, and time. The community level is the configuration of social spheres that contribute to child health. These include the consumer society, the local community, schools, the health services, the mass media, peer groups, and day care institutions.

The components of the model central to the conception of the family and the processes that may be thought of as going on "inside" it are indicated with a semipermeable boundary—the circle. These are

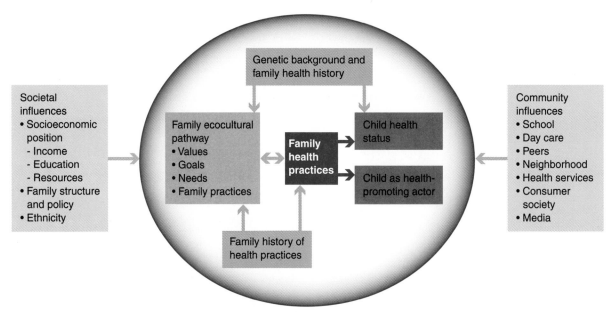

FIGURE 9-2 Model of the Health Promoting Family. (Reproduced from Christensen, P. [2004a]. The health promoting family: A conceptual framework for future research. *Social Science & Medicine, 59,* 377–387, by permission.)

linked to and influenced by the processes and factors "outside" of the family. The internal level has the "family ecocultural pathway" and "family health practices" as the main elements. By interacting with each other, these elements lead to collective patterns of health action, practice, and forms of knowledge. An important feature of the model is that it will allow differences between families to be revealed by identifying the conditions for a family to act in an optimal way for health. It also highlights the obstacles for families in promoting the health and well-being of children, and the barriers to enabling the child's development as a health-promoting actor during his or her growth.

Family health practices fall into the center of the circle (internal factors), and include all those activities of everyday life that shape and influence the health of family members. These consist of the traditional health practices around food and healthy eating, physical activity, alcohol and smoking, and care and connection, as well as other key factors that can be shown to affect young people's health and well-being.

Although family health promotion has received considerable emphasis in nursing in the past decade, reports on the effectiveness of family-focused health promotion continue to be scanty. Therefore, contin-

ued research is required using family health promotion models to evaluate the effectiveness of interventions to promote family health.

ECOSYSTEM INFLUENCES

Family health promotion is a multidimensional construct that is the by-product of family interactions with factors outside the home and internal family processes (Bomar, 2004a). This section shows how the ecosystem influences the quality of family life.

External Influences

External ecosystem influences include such things as the national economy, family and health policy, societal and cultural norms, media, and environmental hazards such as noise, air, soil, crowding, and chemicals.

ECONOMIC RESOURCES

The national economy directly affects the family's ability to promote health. The availability of jobs directly affects the quality of a family's lifestyle. Clear disparities exist between health promotion initiatives geared toward middle-class families and those geared toward low-income families. In economic downturns, health promotion initiatives tend to take a backseat to other more pressing needs. Until the mid-1980s, little attention was given to the health of minorities and people of low income (U.S. Department of Health and Human Services [U.S. DHHS], 1985). The U.S. Office of Minority Health was created in 1985 to address the specific health needs of African Americans, Asians and Pacific Islanders, Hispanics, and Native Americans. With the adoption of *Healthy People 2000* and *Healthy People 2010,* the health promotion and disease prevention focus has moved more toward decreasing health disparities between socioeconomic classes (DHHS, 1990, 2000). What this suggests is that socioeconomic class is related to health promotion.

Likewise, when a family has economic health, it has the resources needed for family health promotion. Adequate family income contributes to emotional well-being and supplies resources for adequate family space, recreation, and leisure. Socioeconomic class is a crucial ingredient in family health promotion. Middle- and upper-class families are more likely than poor families to engage in health-promoting and preventive activities (Bomar, 2004b). The cost of buying recreational and exercise equipment, for example, is often beyond the means of low-income families. The activities of low-income families are often directed toward meeting basic needs—providing for food, shelter, and safety, and curing acute illness—rather than preventing illness or promoting health.

GOVERNMENTAL HEALTH AND FAMILY POLICIES

Health and family policies at all governmental levels also affect the quality of individual and family health. Many of the objectives in *Healthy People 2010* are couched in terms of the individual; many of these objectives, however, can be attained only by providing access to health care (Chowdhury, Balluz, Okoro, & Strine 2006; Stasko & Neale, 2007) and require changing family health lifestyles (Bulwer, 2004). Local communities provide water and monitor its quality, maintain sanitation, develop and maintain parks for recreation, and provide health services to low-income and elderly families. Such local services enhance the health of individuals and enhance family

health. At the state level, services include assistance with medical care through Medicaid, the maintenance of state recreational areas and parks, health promotion and prevention programs, and economic assistance for low-income families and children (Anderson, Ward, & Hatton, 2008).

Additional federal level policies and fiscal support are needed to improve the quality of family health; in particular, there is a need for policy supporting the following programs: (1) primary care for individuals across the life span, (2) child care, (3) economic support for vulnerable families, (4) more national parks and recreation areas, and (5) research on families and family health-promoting lifestyle practices (Bomar, 2004b).

Because of the number of different government agencies involved in health care and family issues, a need exists for collaboration among these policy-making bodies. Box 9-2 summarizes the brief historical perspectives of family health promotion.

ENVIRONMENT

According to Bomar (2004c), awareness of the quality of the family living environment is crucial because the family and its members are exposed to public, occupational, and residential hazards. Environmental health is one of the areas of emphasis of the *Healthy People 2010 Objectives*. Box 9-3 lists the major objectives specific to families. Many environmental hazards are not monitored consistently by families or organizations. Therefore, it is imperative to increase the capacity of families to recognize environmental hazards and to teach strategies to prevent, remove, or cope with environmental hazards such as pollution of air, water, food, and soil from numerous chemicals, occupational hazards, and violence (Bomar, 2004c; Cowan, 2008; Sattler & Lipscomb, 2003). For instance, to prevent exposure to lead and pesticides, families could be taught to wash fruits and vegetables before eating. Workers should be taught to monitor chemicals and infectious materials that might be transmitted to them and their families on work clothing or their skin, or both. In addition, paint in older homes and outside play areas should be inspected for lead contamination. Families with young children and workers who work around metals and chemicals need to be especially cautious of lead poisoning, and should consult Web sites such as the Centers for Disease Control and Prevention for additional information.

BOX 9-2
Historical Perspectives of Family Health Promotion

Although the majority of health care professionals continue to focus their activities on prevention and treatment of illness in individuals and dysfunctional families, key social forces, including the wellness and self-care movement since 1979, continue to stimulate the nursing profession to focus on health promotion for families. The 1980 White House Conference on Families pointed out the need to improve family functioning and encourage healthy family lifestyles. The conference brought to light the importance of disease prevention and health promotion for improving the quality of family life in the United States. Three documents from the DHHS—*Healthy People: The Surgeon General's Report on Health Promotion and Disease Prevention* (1979); *Promoting Health/Preventing Disease: Objectives for the Nation* (1980); and *Healthy People 2000: National Health Promotion and Disease Prevention Objectives* (1990)—provided overall goals for the nation regarding health promotion for individuals and families.

Although there are many improvements in the health status of the nation as a whole, *Healthy People 2010* (U.S. DHHS, 2000) builds on the lessons learned from the three previous initiatives. The goals for 2010 through 2020 are to eliminate health disparities and to increase the quality and years of life. Major objectives for the millennium include promoting healthy behaviors, promoting healthy and safe communities, improving systems for personal and public health, and preventing and reducing diseases and disorders.

Since the first report by the surgeon general in 1979 and the continued national interest in health promotion in the 1990s, health professionals, family scientists, sociologists, psychologists, religious leaders, and social workers have made considerable strides in understanding and intervening to improve the quality of family health. Another example of this continuing national interest in health promotion is the increasing use of parish nurses, who provide health care and health promotion to individuals and families in faith communities (Solari-Twadell, McDermott, & Matheus, 1999).

BOX 9-3
Healthy People 2010 Environmental Objectives Specific to Families

Objective Short Title	
OUTDOOR AIR QUALITY	
8-1	Reduce harmful air pollutants
8-2	Increase alternative modes of transportation
8-3	Increase the use of cleaner alternative fuels
WATER QUALITY	
8-5	Increase access to safe drinking water
8-6	Reduce waterborne disease outbreaks
8-7	Increase water conservation
8-8	Reduce surface water health risks
8-10	Reduce human consumption of contaminated fish
TOXICS AND WASTE	
8-11	Reduce increased blood lead levels in children
8-12	Reduce risks posed by hazardous sites
8-13	Reduce pesticide exposures
8-14	Reduce toxic pollutants in the environment

BOX 9-3
Healthy People 2010 Environmental Objectives Specific to Families—cont'd

Healthy Homes and Healthy Communities

8-16	Reduce indoor allergens
8-17	Improve office building air quality
8-18	Increase homes tested for radon
8-20	Implement school policies to protect against environmental hazards
8-21	Increase disaster preparedness plans and protocols
8-22	Increase lead-based paint testing
8-23	Reduce the number of occupied substandard housing

Others Environmental Objectives Specific to Children

24-2a	Reduce asthma-related hospitalizations of children younger than 5
27-9	Reduce the percentage of children regularly exposed to secondhand smoke

Source: U.S. Department of Health and Human Services. (2000). *Healthy People 2010* (Vol.1). Washington, DC: U.S. Government Printing Office. Retrieved March 26, 2008, from http://www.health.gov/healthypeople/Document/tableofcontents.htm

MEDIA

Another influence on family health is the visual and print media. According to the American Academy of Pediatrics (AAP), "Children are influenced by media—they learn by observing, imitating, and making behaviors their own" (2001, p. 1224). Media influence on children has steadily increased as new and more sophisticated types of media have been developed and made available to the American public. Consistent evidence has been reported that violent imagery in television, film and video, and computer games has substantial short-term effects on arousal, thoughts, and emotions, increasing the likelihood of aggressive or fearful behavior in younger children, especially in boys (Browne & Hamilton-Giachritsis, 2005).

Many advertisements advocate drinking alcohol, using tobacco products, and consuming foods that are high in sugar, salt, and fat. Increasingly, tobacco, alcohol, and illicit drugs have been glamorized in the media. Tobacco manufacturers spend $6 billion per year, and alcohol manufacturers $2 billion per year in advertising that appeals to children ("Influence on Children Media," 2008). Movies and television programs often show the lead character or likeable characters using and enjoying tobacco and alcohol products.

The Office of the Surgeon General (2001) and the AAP (2001) have offered recommendations to address the issue of media influence on children. Included in these recommendations are suggestions for parents, educators, and health care professionals to advocate for a safer media environment for children through media literacy. In addition, they urge media producers to be more responsible in their portrayal of violence. They advocate for more useful and effective media ratings. Specifically, they recommend proactive parental involvement in children's media experiences. By monitoring what children hear and see, discussing issues that emerge, and sharing media time with their children, parents can moderate the negative influences and increase the positive effects of media in the lives of their children (AAP, 2001; Office of the Surgeon General, 2001).

The readily available and rapidly increasing amounts of health information in the media put more emphasis on health (Lee, 2008). Relatively recent tobacco advertising regulations take a small step in the right direction toward promoting healthier families. For example, in the 1990s, laws were passed that prohibit tobacco advertisements near schools, on T-shirts, and in magazines for teens. Many states require that cigarettes not be in the reach of minors in retail stores.

SCIENCE AND TECHNOLOGY

Advances in science and technology have increased the life span of Americans, decreased the length of hospital stays, and contributed to our understanding of how to prevent, reduce, and treat disease. The development of more effective medications and advanced medical equipment technology has greatly increased the feasibility of home health care for chronically ill family members of all ages. Families are often the caregivers for ill members, and they provide the majority of care to older adults. Many valuable sources of information on health promotion for families and individuals are now available. The Internet and the use of the World Wide Web is one forum that has come of age in the areas of family life education and nutrition education (Silk et al., 2008; Välimäki, Nenonen, Koivunen, & Suhonen, 2007).

Other technologic advances are changing how we provide health care. For example, telehealth permits families to transmit heart rates via telemedicine to health care providers and for specialists to consult with family physicians, making it easier for individuals to access health care and for practitioners to provide it. McCarthy and Fox (2006) report that telehealth has the potential to improve health care access, quality, and efficiency; cost savings are shared by the telehealth's patient (through reductions in waiting time, time away from work, and travel time), third-party payers (through reduced reimbursement for travel, and more timely and appropriate treatment that averts costly complications), and providers (through efficiencies in the care process).

Internal Influences

Internal ecosystem influences include family type and developmental stage, family lifestyle patterns, family processes, the personalities of family members, power structure, family role models, coping strategies and processes, resilience, and culture. All of these factors are interrelated. For example, a family's lifestyle cycle stage influences a family's structural pattern (Carter & McGoldrick, 2005), and family structures affect the family interaction process and relationship. Therefore, nurses working with families in the area of health promotion must be sensitive to these various factors to recommend successful family health promotion interventions.

FAMILY TYPE AND DEVELOPMENT

Family structure, whether healthy or dysfunctional, affects the health and well-being of the family. Families who are flexible and able to adjust to change are more likely to be involved in health-promoting activities (Olson, 2000). Soubhi, Potvin, and Paradis (2004) examined the relationships between family environment and parents' leisure-time physical activity, and found that balanced families consistently received the highest scores of physical activity, family rules, and family support compared with traditional, disconnected, and emotionally strained families.

When families experience transitions, changes in their health-promoting lifestyles are often required. Thus, when a family member becomes ill, the health-promoting activities of the caretakers are generally curtailed. In addition, the stage of family development (including childbearing, school-age launching, retirement, and the accomplishment of developmental tasks) also significantly influences a family's ability to be healthy. For example, Carter (2005) has found that divorce rates are very high in families with young children, suggesting that families have difficulty coping with all the transitions required in this family developmental stage.

FAMILY STRUCTURE

Families in this millennium are quite different from the families of the 1970s. Family structures are more diverse; there are more dual-career/dual-earner families, blended families, same-sex couples, and single-parent families (Kaakinen & Birenbaum, 2008). Recently, increasing numbers of grandparents raising grandchildren have been reported (Leder, Grinstead, & Torres, 2007). Families in both the middle and lower class are in such economic strain that they both struggle with health promotion. The number of vulnerable families has also increased, including low-income traditional families, low-income migrant families, homeless families, and low-income older adults. Included in the vulnerable population are low-income, single-parent families and single-parent teen families. Vulnerable families are coping with a pileup of stressors and may be unable to focus on activities to enhance health (Wuest, Ford-Gilboe, Merrit-Gray, & Bernman, 2003).

Health promotion for these different families presents various challenges. For example, a single, working parent may lack parent-child time, experience role stress, and have poor lifestyle patterns and poor life satisfaction (Moriarty & Wagner, 2004; Wuest et al., 2003). As stated earlier, low-income families may focus less on health promotion and more on basic needs of obtaining shelter, adequate food, and health care.

FAMILY PROCESSES

Family processes are continual actions, or a series of changes, that take place in the family experience. Essential processes of a healthy family include functional communication (Crawford & Tarko, 2004) and family interaction (Denham, 2003a). Through both verbal and nonverbal communication, parents teach behavior, share feelings and values, and make decisions about family health practices. It is through communication that families adapt to transitions and develop cohesiveness (Olson & DeFrain, 2003). Positive, reinforcing interaction between family members leads to a healthier family lifestyle. In addition, families must utilize their natural support systems to achieve optimal health promotion (Bullock, 2004; Heitman, 2004).

FAMILY CULTURE

Cultures define and value health, health promotion, and disease prevention differently (Leininger & McFarland, 2006; Meyer, Toborg, Denham, & Mande, 2008). A mounting trend is toward a global society with ever-increasing diversity among the populations; therefore, an expanded worldview is necessary for health care students and providers (Purnell & Paulanka, 2005). Clients may not understand or respond to the family nurse's suggestions for health promotion because the suggestions conflict with their health beliefs and values. Hence, it is crucial to assess and understand the family culture and health beliefs before suggesting changes in health behavior (McGoldrick, Giordano, & Garcia-Preto, 2005; Spector, 2008).

FAMILY LIFESTYLE PATTERNS AND ROLE MODELS

Lifestyle patterns affect family health. In North America, hundreds of thousands of unnecessary deaths occur each year that can be directly attributed to unhealthy lifestyles. These deaths can be traced back to heart disease, hypertension, cancer, cirrhosis of the liver, diabetes, suicide, mental health, and homicide.

When family members engage often in leisure activities, recreation, and exercise, they are able to cope with day-to-day problems better (Fomby, 2004; Soubhi, Potvin, & Paradis, 2004). Time together also often promotes family closeness. Healthy lifestyle practices such as good eating habits (James & Flores, 2004), good sleep patterns (Langford, 2004), proper hygiene, and positive approaches to stress management (Boss, 2003) are passed from one generation to another (McGoldrick, Gerson, & Petry, 2008). In addition, when one family member initiates a health behavior change, other family members often make a change too. For example, when an individual family member changes eating patterns, perhaps by going on a diet, other family members often change their eating patterns.

Family members provide both negative and positive role models (Friedman, Bowden, & Jones, 2003). For example, smoking, use of drugs and alcohol, poor nutrition, and inactivity are often intergenerational patterns (McGoldrick et al., 2008). Stress management, exercise, and communication are learned from parents, siblings, and extended family members such as grandparents (McGoldrick et al., 2008). By health teaching in the community, faith-based centers, homes, and the workplace, nurses promote positive role modeling.

FAMILY NUTRITION

Family nutrition is a crucial aspect of 21st century family health promotion and health protection. A major issue today for American families is tendency toward overweight and lack of exercise among family members of all ages. Major factors that influence nutritional health are societal trends (technology, media, fast food, status), the family system (rituals, mealtime, environment, culture, values, communication, finances, marital status), and individual characteristics (self-concept, age, activity levels) (James & Flores, 2004). According to James and Flores (2004), because of the hurried family lifestyle and frequent unhealthful restaurant meals, "over nutrition" in American families is often the issue rather than malnutrition. A result of societal and family changes is that obesity in children and adolescents is a key 21st-century issue. Effective parenting, health teaching about nutrition, physical activity, and consideration of the family context are reported to be essential to reducing childhood obesity (Kitzmann, 2008). The nurses' role in family nutrition is to assess the quality of nutrition for individuals and the family system, provide anticipatory guidance, teach about nutrition, and support changes in the individual and family nutritional lifestyle (James, 2005; James & Flores, 2004). For example, one of the primary issues for people is large portion size. To promote weight loss and control, the family cook and members could be taught the appropriate portion size according to age and nutritional guidelines. A nurse can become familiar with the most current guidelines for infants, children, adolescents, breast-feeding, women, adults, aging, and vegetarians by the *Dietary Guidelines for Americans* published every 5 years by U.S. Department of Agriculture (2005).

RELIGION AND SPIRITUALITY

Another factor that influences the quality of family life is religion and spirituality (Warner & Bomar, 2004). The positive effect of spirituality is pervasive in health care for the lives of many families; therefore, a need exists to integrate spiritual assessment and interventions in total family care (Tanyi, 2006). Although often used interchangeably, the terms *religion* and *spirituality* are different. Religion tends to relate to the expression of beliefs and includes a relationship with God or some supernatural power (Warner & Bomar, 2004). Spirituality provides transcendence, meaning, and compassion for others. Pivotal life events such as births, marriage, life-threatening illness, tragedy, and death are situations that may spark a family's interest in spirituality (Ingersoll-Dayton, Krause, & Morgan, 2002).

Family spirituality provides the basis for harmony, communication, and wholeness among family members (Warner & Bomar, 2004). Two common nursing diagnoses related to family spiritual health are spiritual well-being and spiritual distress (Carpenito, 2005). Spiritual well-being is transcendence and connection with self, others, nature, life, and the universe. Spiritual distress is a disruption in the harmony of life and pervades the entire person's or family's universe. Religion is a significant factor in family resilience, health, and healing (Walsh, 2006). Religion also shapes family health values, practices, and beliefs, and may be a positive

force in family life because it has the following characteristics:

1. Provides a source of social support and belonging
2. Encourages family togetherness through family activities and recreation
3. Provides a sense of meaning in family life
4. Promotes love, hope, faith, trust, forgiveness, forbearance, goodness, self-control, morality, justice, and peace
5. Encourages a belief in divine assistance during times of family stress and crisis
6. Teaches reverence for family life (Warner & Bomar, 2004)

The social support of religion and the clergy is often particularly helpful during family transitions (Warner & Bomar, 2004). Many faith communities sponsor support groups that are a valuable resource for single parents, stepfamilies, single adults, the bereaved, widows and widowers, the unemployed, and parents of young children. Religion aids in family coping responses (Friedman, Bowden, & Jones, 2003) and is reported to provide support for selected caregivers (Heitman, 2004). To provide holistic care, clinicians should assess a family's spiritual health (Tanyi, 2006) in a nonjudgmental manner by supporting the family's spiritual beliefs, assisting families to meet their spiritual needs, providing spiritual resources for family transitions and lifestyle changes, and assisting families to find meaning in their circumstances (Carson & Koenig, 2002). Lastly, to foster a family's spiritual well-being, the health professional should listen, be encouraging and empathetic, show vulnerability, and demonstrate commitment. Research on the dimensions of religion and spirituality and family health are sparse. Sample topics for research on religion and family life include punitiveness, coping and family stress, religion and family life satisfaction, and marital satisfaction.

NURSING PROCESS FOR FAMILY HEALTH PROMOTION

Family nurses have a crucial role in facilitating health promotion and wellness within the family context across the life span. Enhancing the well-being of the family unit is essential during periods of wellness, as well as during illness, recovery, and stress. A primary goal of nursing care for families is empowering family members to work together to attain and maintain family health; therefore, family promotion should focus on strengths, competencies, and resources (Wright & Leahey, 2009).

When working with families in the realm of health promotion, the nurse makes assumptions about families. Family health promotion needs and interventions, which differ for each family, will be influenced by the nurse's assumptions and actions. According to Bomar (2004b), the following assumptions are a useful guide for family health promotion and nursing practice:

- Families have a right to health information to make informed decisions about behaviors and lifestyle choices.
- Families have the capacity to change in constructive and destructive directions.

- The health-seeking process occurs in the context of interpersonal and social relationships.
- Families will use only health behaviors that they find relevant and compatible with their family lifestyle and structure.
- Families have the potential for improvement in their health, and a nurse who is caring and culturally competent can enhance this.
- Families are ultimately responsible for their own health.

Family nursing that focuses on health promotion should be logical, systematic, and include the client(s). The following case study of the Budd family is used throughout the remainder of the chapter to demonstrate how different theoretical approaches can be used for assessing and intervening in family for health promotion.

Family Case Study

SETTING: Prenatal clinic (regular prenatal checkup)

FAMILY NURSING GOALS: Work with the family to assist them in successful family transition and balance

FAMILY MEMBERS:
- ✦ James: father; 32 years old; full-time but temporarily employed without benefits, expected to be promoted to a permanent position soon with benefits (married Eleanor 3 years ago)
- ✦ Eleanor: mother; 33 years old; full-time employed, a school teacher at an elementary school with benefits, considering being a "stay-at-home" mother after giving birth (six months' pregnant); first marriage, married to James after giving birth to Dustin
- ✦ Hanna: oldest child; 8 years old; daughter (from James's first marriage), third grade, usually a good student
- ✦ Dustin: son; 3.5 years old; all-day preschool (private day care facility), developmentally on target
- ✦ The couple is expecting a baby girl.

FAMILY STORY

James (32 years old) and Eleanor (33 years old) have one daughter, Hanna (8 years old), and one son, Dustin (3.5 years old). James is a full-time worker in a sales business. (See the Budd family genogram in Figure 9-3.)

Currently, he is a full-time employee but under temporary status; he is expected to have a permanent position soon (date is not sure) that provides benefits and covers health insurance. Eleanor has a full-time position as an elementary-school teacher. She wants to be a stay-at-home mother but is afraid of losing health insurance and family income if she quits now, so she wants to wait until James gets a permanent full-time position with benefits.

The couple married 3 years ago; they recently moved from an apartment to a house because the family needs additional space for the new baby. Although the house is spacious, it is old and needs some renovation.

This is the first marriage for Eleanor and second marriage for James (James divorced 5 years ago). Eleanor stated that the family has been successfully going through the remarriage cycle, and Hanna and Eleanor have a pretty good relationship. Hanna is usually withdrawn after visiting her biological mother (summer and winter school vacations, and several holidays—generally five times a year), who is also married and gave Hanna a new stepbrother (age 2) from her current marriage. Hanna is attending an after-school program at the same school where Eleanor works and returns home with Eleanor. On the way home, Eleanor picks up Dustin from the daycare where Dustin attends from 7:30 a.m. to 4:30 p.m. during the weekdays. Hanna attends a piano lesson on Tuesdays and ballet class on Thursday.

Because of the family's busy schedule, they often eat at fast-food restaurants during the evenings (at least

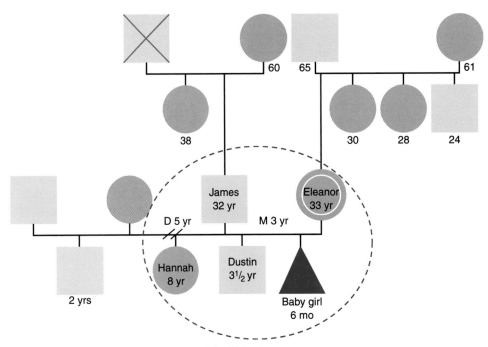

FIGURE 9-3 Budd family genogram.

twice a week), and meals at home are usually rushed and often eaten in front of the television. Although the family tries to eat meals together, they cannot do so because James's job requires frequent traveling, so they often end up eating meals without James. When James is at home, he does outdoor chores, whereas Eleanor usually does indoor chores. The children usually watch television and play video games when the couple is working at home. The couple tries to do family activities on each Sunday, and all family members attend a local Presbyterian church. But James is generally not home one Sunday for each month because of the travel requirements for his job. With the exception of family vacations, holidays, and Sundays, the Budds rarely spend time together enjoying each other's company.

James and Eleanor seldom agree on parenting practices: whereas Eleanor is firm and detailed, James is laid-back. James has some guilty feelings toward Hanna, thus making him very lenient toward her. Hanna usually goes to her dad to escape her regular duties and whenever Eleanor asks Hanna to complete her tasks. James usually accepts Hanna's request because of his guilty feelings, and this makes Eleanor uncomfortable and frustrated.

Eleanor was seen by a nurse in the OB/GYN clinic for her regular prenatal checkups. She is going through a normal pregnancy, but she has been experiencing serious fatigue recently. Her additional concern is that she

has a difficult time putting Dustin to bed each night. Dustin used to go to bed easily when they lived in the apartment, where he shared a room with Hanna. After moving to the new house 3 months ago, where he has his own room, he has not been the same. Eleanor notices that he is more energetic at night and wants to stay with her before going to bed. In addition, Dustin has recently been visiting the parents' bed at night, and staying with them during the night, when he should be sleeping in his own bed. Dustin has recently complained about his tummy being upset, and Eleanor is not sure whether he is sick or is just faking to get attention. Dustin is excited to have a baby sister, but he has also showed some jealousy. For example, Dustin acted like an infant baby when his parents decorated the baby's room and bed with pink colors.

Although James is helping Hanna at night, putting Dustin to bed is Eleanor's job, and she is overwhelmed with her son's behavior. Eleanor says that James is a good husband, but she feels that James considers parenting as a mother's role, which sometimes makes her overwhelmed and angry. Eleanor perceives that all family members are healthy and that they are just a busy family. Her additional concern is the family finances after she quits her job. The nurse sees only Eleanor during this time, and requests that James and the children come for the next visit. (See the Budd family ecomap in Figure 9-4.)

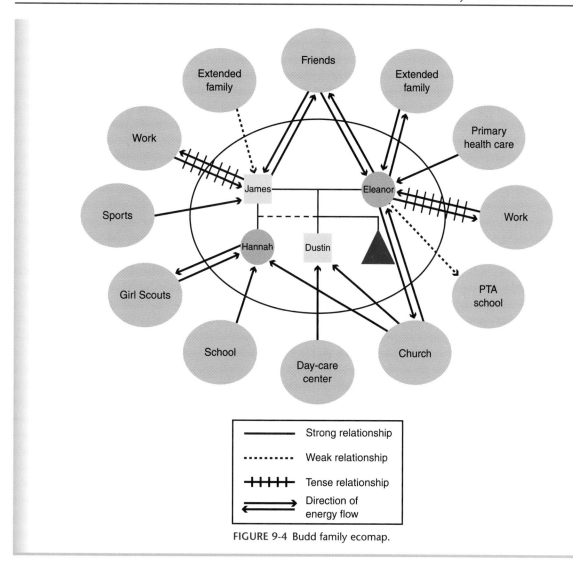

———————	Strong relationship
··············	Weak relationship
+++++	Tense relationship
⇄	Direction of energy flow

FIGURE 9-4 Budd family ecomap.

Assessment

As explained in Chapter 3, models that nurses use to assess family health differ. The following illustrates how different assessments and options for interventions vary based on the theoretical perspectives of the family.

FAMILY SYSTEMS THEORY. The focus of the nurses' practice from this perspective is family as client; therefore, assessments of family members are focused on the family as a whole. In the case study, all members of the Budd family are affected when the mother gives birth. Eleanor currently feels that

her husband considers parenting as a mother's role. If James continues to be passive in his parenting role, it would cause a difficult family transition when the baby is born. In addition, the arrival of the new baby could make going to bed even more difficult for Dustin at night, if not resolved.

DEVELOPMENTAL AND FAMILY LIFE CYCLE THEORY. The family is a blended family and is in the stage of the "families with young children" (infancy to school age) because their oldest daughter, Hanna, is an elementary-school child. The family is experiencing an additional normative developmental stressor of adding a new family member. The tasks required for this family include adjusting to the addition of a new family member, defining and sharing childrearing, financial and household tasks, and realigning relationships with extended family, parents, and grandparents. In addition, although Dustin is developmentally on target, the family is experiencing a challenge to make Dustin go to bed each night, and may face a challenge with potential sibling rivalry.

FAMILY CYCLE OF HEALTH AND ILLNESS. In Danielson, Hamel-Bissell, and Winstead-Fry's (1993) Family Health and Illness Life Cycle Theory, the family is in the first phase of health promotion and risk reduction, which indicates that the family and its members engage in activities to foster family health and attain optimal levels of functioning. The Budd family generally engages in a variety of activities to improve and maintain the health of individual members and promote family functioning. For example, each of the family members sees a doctor annually for regular checkups. Also, Hanna's and Dustin's immunizations are up-to-date. Nevertheless, there is an indication of moving to phase two (family vulnerability and the symptom experience phase). For example, the couple does not have much couple time, and the family is not frequently spending evenings together as a family. In addition, the family does not have regularly scheduled family meetings to problem-solve for family risk reduction. Eleanor's increasing fatigue and feeling of role overload as a mother could also lead to the second phase of vulnerability if James is not actively involved in parenting and older children do not share age-appropriate chores. Moreover, because of their busy schedule, the couple seldom exercises regularly. James has been a smoker since he was 18, and he generally smokes about 10 cigarettes per day. He has tried to quit smoking several times but failed.

BIOECOLOGICAL THEORY. In the bioecological model, nurses need to assess the microsystem (i.e., family composition and home environment), mesosystem (i.e., external environment), exosystem (i.e., job and income), and macrosystem (i.e., community). The Budd family consists of two parents, two children, and a baby on the way. The couple has a white European heritage. The family lives in an old one-story house with four bedrooms in an older suburban section of town. During further interviews, the nurse found that the Budd's house was built before 1950 and is still under renovation.

The extended family (grandparents and siblings of Eleanor's side) live nearby, and Eleanor has a close relationship with them. The extended family gets together for most holidays; James and Hanna seem to have a tenuous relationship with Eleanor's family. After divorcing his ex-wife, James moved to the current town, where he met Eleanor. The town is largely composed of white ethnicity with 30% African American. None of the parents or siblings of James lives nearby. James's dad passed away 10 years ago in a car accident; his mother remarried 7 years ago and lives 500 miles away. The Budds and James's mother usually meet once a year and talk once or twice a month via telephone. James has an older sister who lives out of the country because of her husband's military service.

FAMILY ASSESSMENT AND INTERVENTION MODEL. Using the Family Systems Stressor-Strength Inventory (FS^{3}I) of the Family Assessment and Intervention Model, the major family stressors include: (1) Dustin's bedtime problem, (2) Eleanor's upcoming birth, (3) insufficient couple time and family playtime, (4) insufficient "me time" (specifically Eleanor), (5) inadequate time with the children and watching television too much (children), (6) overscheduled family calendar, and (7) parenting conflict and lack of shared responsibility. Some job stress exists because James is still in a temporary position and his work requires traveling.

Family strengths include: (1) shared religious core, (2) family values and encouragement of individual values, (3) affirmation and support of one another, (4) successful family transition into a new blended family, (5) trust between members, (6) support from extended family (specifically Eleanor), (7) adequate income (current-dual career family), (8) and ability to seek help.

Through assessment, nurses identify family strengths that foster health promotion and stressors that impede on health promotion (Pender, Murdaugh, & Parsons, 2006). Integration of the family perspective into assessment and planning facilitates more effective plans for health promotion (Wright & Leahey, 2009).

Family Nursing Interventions

Family health promotion is a family nursing area in which tremendous opportunities exist for the development and testing of family interventions (Wright & Leahey, 2009). A myriad of strategies and interventions facilitate family health promotion, such as empowerment, promotion of family integrity, maintenance of family process, exercise promotion, environmental management, mutual goal setting, parent education, offering information, drawing forth family support, and anticipatory guidance (Denham, 2003a; Wright & Leahey, 2009).

The family and nurse must collaborate and set mutual goals by establishing a nursing contract. The nursing contract is a working agreement that is continuously renegotiable and may or may not be written depending on the situation (Anderson, Ward, & Hatton, 2008). The premise of contracting is that it is under the family's control. Their ability to make healthy choices is increased, and this process facilitates family empowerment by collaborating with a health professional (Anderson et al., 2008).

Once the nurse and family have identified family strengths and areas for growth and change, the family should prioritize its goals. The commitment of all family members directed toward achieving a goal is crucial to the family's success. Nurses can also assist a family to develop a self-care contract to improve health behaviors, independently or with a nurse. Table 9-3 provides components and sample items of a family self-care contract. The contracts are more effective when the components are negotiated and signed by all family members (Bomar, 2005).

Family nurse scholars (Bomar, 2004b; Denham, 2003a; Hanson, 2005) have identified the following areas in which nurses can provide family support, anticipatory guidance, family education, and family enrichment:

TABLE 9-3

Components of a Family Self-Care Contract

COMPONENT OF THE CONTRACTING PROCESS (MUTUALLY AGREED ON BY FAMILY MEMBERS AND HEALTH PROFESSIONAL OR BY FAMILY ALONE)	EXAMPLE OF ITEM IN A FAMILY CONTRACT
Family assessment of wellness and identification of area for improvement	Our family feels a sense of always being hurried with no time to relax, and we are irritable with each other.
Set the goal, environmental planning, and reinforcement	We want to have more relaxing time together as a family and to enjoy our time together.
Develop a plan	Have a family meeting to evaluate barriers and create a plan. The outcome might be to reduce sports activities for children. Specify a family fun night/afternoon.
Assign responsibilities	Plan an evening game night with no television or phone calls allowed.
	All members agree on the game or recreation activity. No one else but the family should participate. Evaluate the budget for games. The family nurse will assist the family to create the plan. Family members will agree to take part in the family fun time.
Determination of time frame	We plan to do this for 2 months one night a week on Sunday evening from 4:00 p.m. to 7:00 p.m.
Evaluate the outcomes	After each week, we will spend 5 minutes talking about what was good and what could be improved. How are we relating to each other the remainder of the week?
Modify, renegotiate, or terminate	We will evaluate the family fun time after 2 months and mutually agree on changes.

Source: Bomar, P. (2005). Family health promotion. In S. M. H. Hanson, V. Gedaly-Duff, & J. R. Kaakinen (Eds.), *Family health care nursing* (3rd ed.). Philadelphia: F.A. Davis.

- Coping with family transitions (both normative and non-normative, such as births, acute or chronic illnesses, or both, separations, launching children, divorce, death, and retirement)
- Family and individual dietary patterns
- Family and individual recreation and exercise
- Family sexuality
- Family sleep and rest patterns
- Family environmental practices
- Transition from illness to wellness
- Socialization and rearing of children
- Risk reduction and socialization of individual family members in health care practices (prevention and promotion)
- Encouraging a balance between togetherness and individuation
- Providing for family systems and household maintenance
- Encouraging family spirituality

FAMILY EMPOWERMENT. The nurse collaborates with the family and provides information, encouragement, and strategies to help the family make lifestyle changes. This process is termed *empowerment*. Empowerment requires a viewpoint that often conflicts with the views of nurses. The underlying assumption of empowerment is one of a partnership between the professional and the client as opposed to one in which the professional is dominant. Families are assumed to be either competent or capable of becoming competent (Anderson et al., 2008).

The primary emphasis in family empowerment is involvement of the family in goal setting, planning, and acting, not on having the nurse do this for the family. A key role of family nurses in family health promotion is to empower family members to value their "oneness," to appreciate family togetherness (Denham, 2003b), and to plan activities to foster their unity.

One way of empowering a family is the use of commendation because it enables families to view the family problems differently and move toward solutions that are more effective. Wright and Leahey (2009) recommend that nurses routinely commend family and individual strengths, competencies, and resources observed during the family interview. Often, a family has unique strengths that are temporarily overshadowed by the health needs, so these strengths lie outside of the family's awareness (Arnold, 2003). Specifically, reinforcement and

amplification of family strengths in times of crisis can both enhance and maintain behavioral changes needed in recovery (Arnold, 2003). By commending a family's competence and strengths, and offering them a new opinion of themselves, a context for change is created that allows families to discover their own solutions to problems (Wright & Leahey, 2009). In addition, by offering opportunities for family members to express feelings about family experiences, the nurse can enable the family to draw forth its own strengths and resources to support one another (Wright & Leahey, 2009). Drawing forth family support is especially important in primary health care settings (Wright & Leahey, 2009).

ANTICIPATORY GUIDANCE AND OFFERING INFORMATION. During their life course, families inevitably experience crises and either normative or non-normative stress. The family's resilience, unity, and resources influence how they cope with crisis and stress (Boss, 2003). The goal of the family nurse is to facilitate family adaptation by empowering the family to promote resilience, reduce the pileup of stressors, make use of resources, and negotiate necessary changes to enhance the family's ability to rebound from stressful events or crises. The nurse can teach families to anticipate life changes, make the necessary adjustments in family routines, evaluate roles and relationships, and cognitively reframe events. For example, in military families, changes occur in family decision making, roles, responsibilities, communication patterns, and power when a military member is deployed. Anticipatory guidance by health professionals could help military families anticipate economic changes, maintain the household, maintain communication, and parent the children long distance.

Offering information should be based on family abilities and should encourage family members to seek resources independently (Wright & Leahey, 2009). Families usually desire information about developmental issues and health promotion. For example, helping parents to understand and help their children is a common but important intervention for families (Wright & Leahey, 2009).

Nurses working with well families can teach family awareness, encourage family enrichment, and provide information on community agencies and Web sites that are resources for strengthening and enriching families. Although beginning family nurses may not be skilled in all these areas, they can seek out community resources such as Web sites for well families and individual members. The family could be encouraged to agree on a goal to attend or find out more about such a program. In some cases, the nurse may need to review Web sites, call an agency, or visit and observe an agency in action to determine its appropriateness (also see the Chapter Web Sites listed at the end of this chapter). The beginning family nurse is prepared to intervene by teaching about healthy processes (e.g., basic nutrition, exercise routines, hygiene, and preventive health practice). Awareness of family life education, family enrichment, and marriage enrichment are interventions that are more appropriate for advanced practice nurses.

USE OF RITUALS/ROUTINES AND FAMILY TIME.

Fomby (2004) emphasizes the use of family rituals and routines for health promotion: "Family routines are observable and repeated activities by family members that occur with expected regularity, family rituals are actions intentionally performed by multiple family members with great consistency that can be recalled, discussed and taught" (Fomby, 2004, p. 451). Family ritual may be perceived as being a fairly reliable index of family collaboration, accommodation, and synergy (Denham, 2003b). According to Fomby (2004), ritual provides cohesiveness among family members, that is, a sense of family pride, continuity, understanding, closeness, and love. The findings of previous research also indicated that predictable routines and meaningful rituals are related to healthier outcomes (Griswold, 2002), and that establishing routines was vital to managing demands in households with many extended family members (Hall, 2007).

Rituals are best introduced when there is an excessive level of confusion, and they provide clarity in a family system (Imber-Black, 2005; Imber-Black, Roberts, & Whiting, 2003). For example, parents who cannot agree on parenting practices commonly give conflicting messages to their children, which could result in chaos and confusion for the children. The introduction of a ritual can typically assist the family. The parents could experiment with being responsible for the children alternately (Wright & Leahey, 2009).

The most important family ritual is family mealtime (Fomby, 2004). Research on family mealtime reveals that families who take time to eat together are twice as likely to eat five servings of fruits and vegetables, and are less likely to consume excessive amounts of fried food and carbonated beverages (Fomby, 2004). Wiley (2007) identifies the following outcomes from families eating together:

- Teenagers who eat meals with their families frequently are less likely to be depressed or use drugs than those who do not eat with their families as frequently. They are also less likely to be violent, to have sex, and to experience emotional stress. These adolescents who eat meals with their families frequently also are likely to be more highly motivated in school and have better peer relationships.
- Regular shared mealtimes can increase children's sense of belonging and stability, and the entire family's feeling of group connection. Many adolescents in a large national study reported that they want to be with their parents for most evening meals.
- Teenagers who share meals with their families on a regular basis tend to eat healthier foods than those who do not. They consume fewer high-fat, high-sugar prepared and packaged foods, and more fruits and vegetables and other foods high in important nutrients and fiber.

In addition, family mealtimes facilitate improving family communication, fostering family tradition, and teaching life skills to children. Encouraging shared meals when possible is a way to enhance family bonding because this gives families an opportunity to be together and enhance communication.

The family needs to plan "family time," when the sense of belonging and "oneness" or "togetherness" can be experienced. Healthy families have both together family time and provide for individual family member alone time (Olson & DeFrain, 2003). Nurses can encourage families to schedule weekly family time. Each member would make that family time a priority and let no other activity interfere with it. The nurse could help by consulting local newspapers, family magazines, and community agencies for activities that might interest the entire family, and afterward encouraging them to continue these activities themselves. Families may require help in meeting both the needs of the family as a whole and members' individual needs. To find a balance, each family member should have time alone to develop a sense of self and to focus on spiritual growth.

IMPLICATIONS OF HEALTH PROMOTION IN FAMILY NURSING

Family health promotion is an important component of nursing practice, nursing education, family policy, and nursing research.

Nursing Practice

As resources changed in the 1990s and into the new millennium, individuals and families assumed more responsibility for the care and support of their families in the area of health promotion. Major tasks of nursing with families are: (1) to work in partnership with families, (2) to empower and increase the capacity of families to find ways to achieve their lifestyle and health care goals, (3) to illuminate the importance of family health promotion, (4) to serve as a family advocate, and (5) to be an expert in family health promotion matters. The goal is for families to attain, maintain, or regain the highest possible level of family health.

The advanced practice nurse, particularly the family nurse practitioner who practices in a primary care setting, has the opportunity to interact with the family, initiate family health promotion, and assist families to identify risks to their well-being. The continuing shift in health care from the hospital to community settings means that nurses will have more direct interactions with families in ambulatory health care settings and homes. The increase in family empowerment for providing care for ill family members requires in-depth evaluation and creative interventions to focus on family health, family protection, and family health promotion. At all stages of the family health and illness cycle, the goal is to return the family, as a whole, to its highest health potential. To do so, nurses provide programs for promoting family health and reducing risks for dysfunction in a variety of settings. Selected topics include parenting from infancy to old age; role changes during family and individual transitions such as retirement, birth of a new baby, bereavement, and so forth; and coping with individual and family stressors.

Single-parent and blended families often need anticipatory guidance, family enrichment activities, and parenting and stepparenting education. The nurse can encourage all family members to monitor their family for its unity, strengths, and a sense of belonging. In any setting, nurses can advocate for families by writing and voting on family issues, supporting a philosophy of practice that encourages family nursing, volunteering in community activities for families, and supporting family programs. In general, health promotion assessment should become a regular part of taking a family history and a routine aspect of nursing care.

Nursing Education

In addition to traditional content on family theoretical frameworks, illness, stress and coping, and crisis; curricula at the undergraduate and graduate level should include content on family health promotion. Currently, however, few students are prepared in family health promotion. Most curricula continue to focus primarily on acute and chronic physical illness, psychosocial problems, and community nursing; the primary focus is on the individual in the context of the family. Limited attention is paid to groups of families in the community or to maintaining healthy families.

If nurses are to be a part of the efforts to meet the national health goals for the year 2020, undergraduate and graduate curricula in schools of nursing will need to include content on the family as the unit of care, and on family health promotion and disease prevention. Although the individual might be the patient, students should be taught that assessments and interventions should include the family. For example, diabetic teaching should include all family members, particularly the person who prepares meals. Schools of nursing will need to use learning-service community partnership models and create innovative sites for clinical practice where students can provide nursing care to well families (Kataoka-Yahiro, Cohen, Yoder, & Canham, 1998). Such sites might include a nursing clinic in a low-income housing project, a senior center, a family exercise center, a faith community, a work site, a rural health clinic, or a school or nurse-managed primary care clinic.

Family Policy

The document *Healthy People 2010* and the current emphasis on eliminating disparities in health care for all citizens will help shape local, state, and national policies toward improving family health. The goals for *Healthy People 2020* are in development. The passage of the 1993 Family and Medical Leave Act marked a beginning in the effort to implement policies to improve the quality of family health. To reach the goals for the nation, families must be empowered to assume more responsibilities in the realm of health promotion and disease prevention for family members. Family issues most frequently reviewed by policy makers include marriage, divorce, family violence, abortion, child care, child health care, and family health insurance coverage. Continuing 21st-century family health policy issues are family poverty and economic well-being (Bogenschneider, 2002; Hildebrandt, 2002). The family nurse needs to be aware of policies advancing family health throughout the family life course and should support them. Nurses can support family policy legislation by keeping informed about issues, voting, communicating with policy makers about family needs, giving expert testimony, maintaining membership in and supporting professional nursing organizations, and financially supporting the political advocacy activities of health professional organizations (Briar-Lawson, Lawson, Hennon, & Jones, 2001).

Examples of U.S. Congressional legislation reviewed in 2003 include Family and Medical Leave Act enhancement, family life span respite care, tax credits for family caregivers, adult stem cell research, and genome research. Such legislative policies would support families and would improve the quality of family life, but they do not address the epidemic proportions of underinsured or uninsured people in this nation.

Family Nursing Research

Many regional and national nursing research societies and organizations sponsor family research interest groups, but research on family health promotion is still needed. The National Institute of Nursing Research (NINR) agenda for nursing research includes developing and testing community-based programs to promote family health using nursing models and assessing the effectiveness of nursing interventions for families during the chronic illness of a family member. Specific research for family health promotion that needs to be explored includes the following:

- Design of research that strengthens family health promotion, well-being, economic development, and environment
- Creation, testing, and dissemination of intervention and evidence-based, family-focused studies
- Testing and development of family health promotion theories on diverse families and their issues, processes, and challenges
- Design of international research intervention evidence-based, qualitative studies to illuminate and provide solutions to improve the health of families and their members
- Design of intervention research that tests family-centered health promotion strategies to reduce obesity, violence, substance abuse, smoking cessation, and so forth
- Research focused on vulnerable families and individuals
- Design of intervention research to assess issues of health care technology and telehealth with ethnic families (Bomar, 2004b, p. 646)

BOX 9-4
Research Brief

Kushner, K. E. (2007). Meaning and action in employed mother's health work. *Journal of Family Nursing, 13*(1), 33–55.

Family health meanings and family health work among women explain significant proportions of mothers' health promoting lifestyle practices. Previous research lacked attention to the ways in which women, when they are mothers and paid workers, along with their families, manage everyday health choices about family and health work.

PURPOSE OF THE STUDY
The purpose of the study was to examine employed mothers' meanings of family and personal health as they frame the context of daily experience in caring for their families' and their own health.

METHODS
A sample of 22 mothers employed in support staff positions at a large institution in Western Canada participated in repeated interviews over 2 years.

Continued

Women were asked four questions about their health and health actions: What does being healthy mean to you? What do you do to take care of your health? What does having a healthy family mean to you? What do you do to take care of your family's health?

RESULTS

Women's work that promotes family health included keeping track, constructing routines, facing challenges, setting priorities, being there for each other, finding joy and fulfillment, and fostering personal development. The researchers suggest a preliminary typology of four orientations

to family health work: ensuring order, feeling strong, keeping up, and making changes.

IMPLICATIONS

Study findings suggest that nurses should support activities that strengthen family health work. The findings also suggest the importance of family routines as a means of connecting with health promotion strategies for change. Recognized family health routines provide a basis for developing acceptable and workable modifications to individuals and family behaviors that serve to strengthen health-promoting family health routines.

SUMMARY

A synopsis of family health promotion is provided in this chapter. Definitions of family health and family health promotion are discussed. Selected models of family health and family health promotion are introduced. The diverse internal and external factors influencing family health promotion are described. Family assessment and intervention strategies as well as nursing implications for family health promotion are also discussed.

- Fostering the health of the family as a unit and encouraging families to value and incorporate health promotion into their lifestyle are essential components of family nursing practice.
- Health promotion is learned within families, and patterns of health behaviors are formed and passed on to the next generation.
- A major task of the family is to teach health maintenance and health promotion.
- The role of the family nurse is to help families attain, maintain, and regain the highest level of family health possible.
- Family health is a holistic, dynamic, and complex state. It is more than the absence of disease in an individual family member or the absence of dysfunction in family dynamics. Instead, it is the complex process of negotiating day-to-day family life events and crises, and providing for quality of life for its members.

- Family health promotion refers to activities that families engage in to strengthen the family unit, and increase family unity and quality of family life.
- Health and family policies at all governmental levels affect the quality of individual and family health.
- The national economy directly affects the family's ability to promote health in its family members.
- Health promotion advertisements have generally targeted the more health-conscious middle class, rather than the vulnerable and underserved who are often the targets for alcohol and tobacco advertising campaigns.
- Families who are flexible and able to adjust to change are more likely to be involved in health-promoting activities.
- Vulnerable families are coping with a pileup of stressors and may be unable to focus on activities to enhance family health.
- Low-income families may focus less on health promotion and more on basic needs such as obtaining shelter, adequate food, and health care.
- Middle-class families are skimping on health promotion, such as dental care, as they face current economic struggles.
- Positive, reinforcing interaction between family members leads to a healthier family lifestyle.
- Through verbal and nonverbal communication, parents teach behavior, share feelings and

values, and make decisions about family health practices.

- Different cultures define and value health, health promotion, and disease prevention differently. Clients may not understand or respond to the family nurses' suggestions for health promotion because the suggestions conflict with their health beliefs and values.
- A primary goal of nursing care for families is empowering family members to work together to attain and maintain family health by focusing on family strengths, competencies, and resources.
- Health behaviors must be relevant and compatible with the family structure and lifestyle to be effective and useful to the family.
- The goal of the family nurse is to facilitate family adaptation by empowering the family to promote resilience, reduce the pileup of stressors, make use of resources, and negotiate necessary change to enhance the family's ability to rebound from stressful events or crises.
- Family health promotion should become a regular part of taking a family history and a routine aspect of nursing care.

REFERENCES

Allen, F. M., & Warner, M. (2002). A developmental model of health and nursing. *Journal of Family Nursing, 8*(2), 96–135.

American Academy of Pediatrics (AAP). (2001). Media violence. *Pediatrics, 108*, 1222–1226.

Anderson, D. G., Ward, H., & Hatton, D. (2008). Family health risks. In M. Stanhope & J. Lancaster (Eds.), *Public health nursing: Population-centered health care in the community* (7th ed., pp. 578–601). Mosby: St. Louis.

Arnold, E. (2003). Communicating with families. In E. Arnold & K. U. Boggs (Eds.), *Interpersonal relationships* (4th ed., pp. 332–364). St. Louis, MO: Saunders.

Association of Operating Room Nurses (AORN). (2004, November). Specific behaviors may influence family health. *AORN Journal.* Retrieved April 13, 2008, from http://findarticles.com/p/articles/mi_m0FSL/is_/ai_n6365091

Bogenschneider, K. (2002). *Family policy matters: How policy-making affects families.* Mahwah, NJ: Lawrence Erlbaum Associates.

Bomar, P. J. (2004a). Introduction to family health nursing and promoting family health. In P. J. Bomar (Ed.), *Promoting health in families: Applying family research and theory to nursing practice* (3rd ed., pp. 3–37). Philadelphia: WB Saunders.

Bomar, P. J. (Ed.). (2004b). *Promoting health in families: Applying family research and theory to nursing practice* (3rd ed.). Philadelphia: WB Saunders.

Bomar, P. J. (2004c). Family environmental health. In P. J. Bomar (Ed.), *Promoting health in families: Applying family research and theory to nursing practice* (3rd ed., pp. 534–580). Philadelphia: WB Saunders.

Bomar, P. (2005). Family health promotion. In S. M. H. Hanson., V. Gedaly-Duff, & J. R. Kaakinen (Eds.), *Family health care nursing: Theory, practice and research* (3rd ed., pp. 243–264). Philadelphia: F.A. Davis.

Boss, P. (Ed.). (2003). *Family stress: Classic and contemporary readings.* Thousand Oaks, CA: Sage.

Briar-Lawson, K., Lawson, H. A., Hennon, C. B., & Jones, A. R. (2001). *Family-centered policies and practices.* New York: Columbia University Press.

Browne, K., & Hamilton-Giachritsis, C. (2005). The influence of violent media on children and adolescents: A public health approach. *Lancet, 365*, 702–710.

Bullock, K. (2004). Family social support. In P. J. Bomar (Ed.), *Promoting health in families: Application of research and theory to nursing practice* (3rd ed.). Philadelphia: WB Saunders.

Bulwer, B. E. (2004). Sedentary lifestyles, physical activity, and cardiovascular disease: From research to practice. *Critical Pathway Cardiology, 3*(4), 184–193.

Carpenito, L. J. (2005). *Nursing diagnosis: Application to clinical practice source* (11th ed.). Philadelphia: Lippincott Williams & Wilkins.

Carson, V. B., & Koenig, H. G. (2002). *Parish nursing.* Philadelphia: Templeton Foundation Press.

Carter, B. (2005). Becoming parents: The family with young children. In B. Carter & M. McGoldrick (Eds.), *The expanded family life cycle: Individual, family and social perspectives* (3rd ed., pp. 249–273). New York: Allyn & Bacon, Pearson Education.

Carter, B., & McGoldrick, M. (2005). *The expanded family life cycle: Individual, family and social perspectives* (3rd ed.). New York: Allyn & Bacon, Pearson Education.

Chowdhury, P. P., Balluz, L., Okoro, C., & Strine, T. (2006). Leading health indicators: A comparison of Hispanics with non-Hispanic whites and non-Hispanic blacks, United States 2003. *Ethnicity & Disease, 16*(2), 534–541.

Christensen, P. (2004). The health promoting family: A conceptual framework for future research. *Social Science & Medicine, 59*, 377–387.

Cowan, M. K. (2008). Child and adolescent health. In M. Stanhope & J. Lancaster (Eds.), *Public health nursing: Population-centered health care in the community* (7th ed., pp. 602–630). St. Louis, MO: Mosby.

Crawford, J., & Tarko, M. A. (2004). Family communication. In P. J. Bomar (Ed.), *Promoting health in families: Applying family research and theory to nursing practice* (3rd ed.). Philadelphia: WB Saunders.

Danielson, C. B., Hamel-Bissell, B., & Winstead-Fry, P. (1993). *Families in health and illness.* St. Louis, MO: Mosby.

Denham, S. A. (1997). *An ethnographic study of family health in Appalachian microsystems.* Unpublished doctoral dissertation, University of Alabama at Birmingham.

Denham, S. A. (1999a). The definition and practice of family health. *Journal of Family Nursing, 5*(2), 133–159.

Denham, S. A. (1999b). Family health: During and after death of a family member. *Journal of Family Nursing, 5*(2), 160–183.

Denham, S. A. (1999c). Family health in an economically disadvantaged population. *Journal of Family Nursing, 5*(2), 184–213.

Denham, S. A. (2003a). *Family health: A framework for nursing.* Philadelphia: FA Davis.

Denham, S. A. (2003b). Relationships between family rituals, family routines, and health. *Journal of Family Nursing, 9*(3), 305–330.

Duval, E. M., & Miller, B. C. (1985). *Marriage and family development* (6th ed.). New York: Harper & Row.

Fomby, B. W. (2004). Family routines, rituals, recreation, and rules. In P. J. Bomar (Ed.), *Promoting health in families: Application of research and theory to nursing practice* (3rd ed., pp. 450–475). Philadelphia: WB Saunders.

Ford-Gilboe, M. (2002). Developing knowledge about family health promotion by testing the developmental model of health and nursing. *Journal of Family Nursing, 8*(2), 140–156.

Friedman, M. M., Bowden, V. R., & Jones, E. G. (2003). *Family nursing: Research, theory and practice* (5th ed.). Upper Saddle River, NJ: Prentice Hall.

Goldenberg, H., & Goldenberg, I. (2007). *Family therapy: An overview* (7th ed.). Belmont, CA: Wadsworth.

Griswold, A. (2002). *Reduce stress with family routines and rituals.* Parenting again. University of Illinois Extension. Retrieved April 16, 2008, from http://www.urbanext.uiuc.edu/grandparents/0202b.html

Hall, W. (2007). Imposing order: A process to manage day-to-day activities in two-earner families with preschool children. *Journal of Family Nursing, 13*(1), 56–82.

Hanson, S. M. (2005). Family health care nursing: An introduction. In S. M. H. Hanson, V. Gedaly-Duff, & J. R. Kaakinen (Eds.), *Family health care nursing: Theory, practice and research* (3rd ed., pp. 3–37). Philadelphia: F.A. Davis.

Hanson, S. M. H., Gedaly-Duff, V., & Kaakinen, J. R. (Eds.). (2005). *Family health care nursing: Theory, practice and research* (3rd ed.) Philadelphia: F.A. Davis.

Heitman, L. K. (2004). Social support and cardiovascular health promotion in families. *Journal of Cardiovascular Nursing, 19*(1), 86–91.

Hildebrandt, E. (2002). The health effects of work-based welfare. *Journal of Nursing Scholarship, 34*(4), 363–368.

Imber-Black, E. (2005). Creating meaningful rituals for new life cycle transitions. In B. Carter & M. McGoldrick (Eds.), *The expanded family life cycle: Individual, family and social perspectives* (3rd ed., pp. 202–214). New York: Allyn & Bacon, Pearson Education.

Imber-Black, E., Roberts, J., & Whiting, R. A. (2003). *Rituals in families and family therapy* (Revised Ed.). New York: Norton.

Influence on children media: History of media for children, general considerations, studies of media influence, domains of influence, recommendations. (2008). Retrieved March 18, 2008, from http://education.stateuniversity.com/pages/2212/Media-Influence-on-Children.html

Ingersoll-Dayton, B., Krause, N., & Morgan, D. (2002). Religious trajectories and transitions over the life course. *International Journal of Aging and Human Development, 56*(1), 51–70.

James, K. (2005). *Dr. Kathy's Health and Weight Loss Guide.* Bloomington, IN: Author House.

James, K., & Flores, E. A. (2004). Family nutrition. In P. J. Bomar (Ed.), *Promoting health in families: Applying family research in theory to nursing practice* (3rd ed., pp. 339–371). Philadelphia: Saunders.

Kaakinen, J. R., & Birenbaum, K. L. (2008). *Family development and family nursing assessment.* In M. Stanhope & J. Lancaster (Eds.), *Public health nursing: Population-centered health care in the community* (7th ed., pp. 547–577). St. Louis, MO: Mosby.

Kataoka-Yahiro, M., Cohen, J., Yoder, M., & Canham, D. (1998). A learning-service community partnership model. *Nursing and Health Care Perspectives, 19*, 274–277.

Kitzmann, K. I. (2008). Beyond parenting practices: Family context and treatment of pediatric obesity. *Family Relations, 57*, 13–23.

Kushner, K. E. (2007). Meaning and action in employed mother's health work. *Journal of Family Nursing, 13*(1), 33–55.

Langford, D. (2004). Family health protection. In P. J. Bomar (Ed.), *Promoting health in families: Applying family research and theory to nursing practice* (3rd ed.). Philadelphia: WB Saunders.

Leder, S., Grinstead, L., & Torres, E. (2007). Grandparents raising grandchildren. *Journal of Family Nursing, 13*(3), 333–352.

Lee, C. (2008). Does the internet displace health professionals. *Journal of Health Communication, 13*, 450–464.

Leininger, M., & McFarland, M. (2006). *Culture care diversity and universality: A worldwide nursing theory.* New York: Jones & Bartlett.

Loveland-Cherry, C. J., & Bomar, P. J. (2004). Family health promotion and health protection. In P. J. Bomar (Ed.), *Promoting health in families: Applying research and theory to nursing practice* (3rd ed., pp. 61–89). Philadelphia: WB Saunders.

McCarthy, D., & Fox, K. (2006). *Case study: University of Tennessee Health Science Center's telehealth network in improving quality for rural residents through telehealth. Health policy, health reform, and performance improvement.* Retrieved April 21, 2008, from http://www.commonwealthfund.org/publications/publications_show.htm?doc_id=360830

McGoldrick, M., Gerson, R., & Petry, S. (2008). *Genograms: Assessment and interventions* (3rd ed.). New York: W.W. Norton.

McGoldrick, M., Giordano, J., & Garcia-Preto, N. (2005). Overview: Ethnicity and family therapy. In M. McGoldrick, J. Giordano and J. Pearce (Eds.), *Ethnicity and family therapy* (pp. 1–30). New York: Guilford Press.

Meyer, M. G., Toborg, M. A., Denham, S. A., & Mande, M. J. (2008). Cultural perspectives concerning adolescent use of tobacco and alcohol in the Appalachian mountain region. *Journal of Rural Health, 24*(1), 67–74.

Monteith, B., & Ford-Gilboe, M. (2002). The relationships among mother's resilience, family health work, and mother's health promoting lifestyle practices in families with preschool children. *Journal of Family Nursing, 8*(4), 383–407.

Moriarty, P. H., & Wagner, L. D. (2004). Family rituals that provide meaning for single-parent families. *Journal of Family Nursing, 10*(2), 190–210.

Office of the Surgeon General. (2001). *Youth violence: A report of the Surgeon General.* Retrieved March 18, 2008, from www.surgeongeneral.gov/library/youthviolence

Olson, D. H. (2000). Circumplex model of marital and family systems. *Journal of Family Therapy, 22*(2), 144–167.

Olson, D. H. L., & DeFrain, J. (2003). *Marriage and the family: Diversity and strengths* (4th ed.). New York: McGraw-Hill.

Pender, N. J. (1996). *Health promotion in nursing practice* (3rd ed.). Norwalk, CT: Appleton & Lange.

Pender, N. J., Murdaugh, C. L., & Parsons, M. A. (2006). *Health promotion in nursing practice* (5th ed.). Upper Saddle River, NJ: Prentice Hall.

Psychological Studies Institute. (2004, September 15). New study identifies specific behaviors linked to family health. *Physician Law Weekly*. Retrieved April 16, 2008, from http://www.newsrx.com/newsletters/Physician-Law-Weekly/2004-09-15/091320043331272PLW.html

Purnell, L. D., & Paulanka, B. J. (2005). *Transcultural health care: A culturally competent approach* (3rd ed.). Philadelphia: F.A. Davis.

Sattler, B., & Lipscomb, J. (Eds.). (2003). *Environmental health and nursing practice*. New York: Springer.

Silk, K. J., Sherry, J., Winn, B., Keesecker, N., Horodynski, M. A., & Sayir, A. (2008). Increasing nutrition literacy: Testing the effectiveness of print, web site, and game modalities. *Journal of Nutrition Educational Behaviors, 40*(1), 3–10.

Smith, J. (1983). *The idea of health: Implications for the nursing profession*. New York: Teachers College Press.

Solari-Twadell, P. A., McDermott, M., & Matheus, R. (1999). Educational preparation. In P. A. Solari-Twadell & M. McDermott (Eds.), *Parish nursing: Promoting whole person health within faith communities*. Thousand Oaks, CA: Sage.

Soubhi, H., Potvin, L., & Paradis, G. (2004). Family process and parent's leisure time physical activity. *American Journal of Health Behaviors, 28*(3), 218–230.

Spector, R. E. (2008). *Cultural diversity in health and illness* (7th ed.). Upper Saddle River, NJ: Prentice Hall.

Stasko J. C., & Neale, A. V. (2007). Health care risks and access within the community of Michigan over-the-road truckers. *Work, 29*(3), 205–211.

Tanyi, R. A. (2006) Spirituality and family nursing: Spiritual assessment and interventions for families. *Journal of Advanced Nursing, 53*(3), 287–294.

U.S. Department of Agriculture. (2005). *Dietary guidelines for Americans*. Retrieved March 4, 2008, from http://www.cnpp.usda.gov/DietaryGuidelines.htm

U.S. Department of Health and Human Services. (1979). *Healthy people: The Surgeon General's report on health promotion and disease prevention* (U.S. Public Health Service, Publication No. PHS 79–55071). U.S. Department of Health, Education, and Welfare. Washington, DC: U.S. Government Printing Office.

U.S. Department of Health and Human Services. (1980). *Promoting health/preventing disease: Objectives for the nation*. Washington, DC: U.S. Government Printing Office.

U.S. Department of Health and Human Services. (1985). *Black and Minority Health: Report of the Secretary's Task Force*. Washington, DC: U.S. Government Printing Office.

U.S. Department of Health and Human Services. (1990). *Healthy people 2000: National health promotion and disease prevention objectives* (Department of Health and Human Services, Publication No. PHS 91–50213). Washington, DC: U.S. Government Printing Office.

U.S. Department of Health and Human Services. (2000). *Healthy people 2010* (Vol. 1). Washington, DC: U.S. Government Printing Office. Retrieved March 26, 2008, from http://www.health.gov/healthypeople/Document/tableofcontents.htm

Välimäki, M., Nenonen, H., Koivunen, M., & Suhonen, R. (2007). Patients' perceptions of Internet usage and their opportunity to obtain health information. *Med Inform Internet Med, 32*(4), 305–314.

Walsh, F. (2006). *Strengthening family resilience* (2nd ed.). New York: Guilford Press.

Warner, C. G., & Bomar, P. J. (2004). Family spirituality. In P. J. Bomar (Ed.), *Promoting health in families: Applying research and theory to nursing practice* (3rd ed.). Philadelphia: WB Saunders.

Wiley, A. (2007). *Reclaiming the family table*. Retrieved May 23, 2008, from http://parenting247.org/article.cfm?ContentID=597&strategy=2&AgeGroup=4

Wright, L., & Leahey, M. (2009). *Nurses and families: A guide to family assessment and intervention* (5th ed.). Philadelphia: F.A. Davis.

Wuest, J., Ford-Gilboe, M., Merrit-Gray M., & Bernman, H. (2003). Intrusion: The central problem for family health promotion among children and mothers after leaving an abusive partner. *Qualitative Health Research, 13*(5), 597–622.

CHAPTER WEB SITES

Government Web Sites

- Dietary guidelines for Americans—*U.S. Department of Agriculture:* www.cnpp.usda.gov/DietaryGuidelines.htm
- Dietary guidelines for Americans 2005—*Healthy People:* http://www.health.gov/dietaryguidelines/dga2005/document/default.htm
- Low cost insurance for children and teens—*Healthy Families- California:* www.healthyfamilies.ca.gov/
- Services for Families—*Administration for Children and Families:* http://www.acf.dhhs.gov/acf_services.html
- Providing health information to prevent harmful exposures and diseases related to toxic substances—*Agency for Toxic Substance and Disease Registry:* www.atsdr.cdc.gov
- Preventing or controlling those diseases or deaths that result from interactions between people and their environment—*National Center for Environmental Health:* www.cdc.gov/nceh/
- Understanding how the environment influences the development and progression of human disease—*National Institute of Environmental Health:* www.niehs.nih.gov

Institution Web Sites

- *International Institute for Health Promotion:* www.american.edu/academic.depts/cas/health/iihp
- *International Union for Health Promotion and Education:* http://www.iowapublichealth.org/xr/ASPX/RecordId.10305/rx/IphiRecordDetails.htm
- *Institute of Medicine, Board on Health Promotion and Disease Prevention:* www.iom.edu/lOM/lOMHome.nsf/Pages/Health+Promotion+and+Disease+Prevention
- *Research and Training Center on Family Support and Children's Mental Health:* www.rtc.pdx.edu/
- *Berkeley Center for Working Families:* http://wfnetwork.bc.edu/berkeley/outreach.html
- *Family Support America:* www.familysupportamerica.org
- *National Council on Family Relations:* www.ncfr.com
- *National Center for Families:* www.nationalcenter.com/

Other Resources

- Health Promotion in Ontario, across Canada and other parts of the world—*Health Promotion Bookmarks/Hot Links:* www.web.net/~stirling

- Effective family programs for prevention of delinquency—*Strengthening America's Families-Office of Juvenile Justice and Delinquency Prevention:* www.strengtheningfamilies.org
- *National Clearinghouse on Families & Youth-NCFY:* www.ncfy.com
- *Families First: Making Families Last:* www.familiesfirst.org/
- *Managing Your Dual Career Family:* www.dr-jane.com/chapters/Jane133.htm
- *The National Partnership for Women and Families:* www.nationalpartnership.org/

- *Parents without Partners:* www.parentswithoutpartners.org/
- Helping to support and educate stepfamilies—*Stepfamily Network Inc.:* www.stepfamily.net
- *Parenting and Family:* home.about.com/parenting/
- *Campaign for Tobacco-Free Kids:* www.tobaccofreekids.org
- Family mealtime—*West Virginia University Extension Service:* http://www.wvu.edu/~exten/infores/pubs/fypubs/wlg129.pdf

CHAPTER 10

Families with Chronic Illness

Sharon A. Denham, DSN, RN

Wendy Looman, PhD, RN, CPNP

CRITICAL CONCEPTS

✦ Three conceptual frameworks are useful for nurses to consider chronic illness management from family perspectives: the Chronic Care Model, the Family Health Model, and the Family Management Style Framework.

✦ Chronic illness presents family and individual challenges throughout the life span; knowledge about disease self-management and adherence to a therapeutic medical regimen are essential for prevention of additional complications and comorbidities.

✦ Chronic illnesses that occur at birth or early childhood are most likely to be genetic and require special attention during developmental changes and across the life span.

✦ Although family history can cause greater risks for a chronic condition, healthy lifestyle behaviors and early detection or screening may prevent the disease.

✦ Family-focused care is important when chronic illness occurs; this implies careful attention to assessing and planning for family needs when a member has a chronic illness.

✦ Nurses must use evidence-based practice to empower families with the information, skills, and abilities needed for optimal disease management and prevention of comorbidities.

✦ Nurses can use counseling skills to assist families and individuals to cope with the stress of life challenges, powerlessness, and anticipatory and ambiguous losses that can accompany chronic illnesses at various life stages.

In 2004, about 133 million people or about half of all Americans lived with a chronic condition. As life expectancy continues to increase, it is predicted that by 2020 the number of persons living with a chronic illness will increase to 157 million, a number comprising all ages, races, and economic status (Partnership for Solutions, 2004). Seven of every 10 American deaths are caused by a chronic illness; this is more than 1.7 million people each year (Centers for Disease Control and Prevention [CDC], 2008). Chronic illnesses require complex care because many individuals have more than a single condition, which may require care from multiple physicians or specialists, a regimen of multiple prescription drugs, and care that would benefit from coordination across disciplines. The Institute of Medicine (2001) reports that the nation has a quality gap for several reasons: (1) increased medical care demands caused by rapid increases in chronic illness prevalence, and increased complexity of the underlying science and technology used for care; and (2) poorly organized health care systems and inadequate use of modern information technology to meet chronic illness demands. Greater focus on chronic conditions as a family's illness rather than a single person's illness could be an important way to consider economies of care and scalability of services.

Individuals and families can benefit from coordinated care that integrates health care services and relevant communication among the professionals providing care. Goals of coordinated care include improving health outcomes, identifying risks or problems early, avoiding crises, and assuring cost-effectiveness of service delivery. Persons experiencing even a single chronic condition may be given conflicting information, numerous diagnoses, or multiple medications by different professionals. Thus, poorly coordinated care has risks for preventable health complications, conflicts between professionals, increased stress for the individuals and their family, unnecessary hospitalizations, added expenses, and even death.

Chronic illness not only affects the lives of infants, children, adolescents, young adults, older adults, elderly, and the old-old, but also the physical, emotional, intellectual, social, and spiritual functioning of multiple family members. Wide variations exist in the ways chronic illness affects physical and mental health, employment, social life, and longevity. Chronic illness for an individual can entail single or multiple illnesses or conditions that last or are persistent over time. For example, a person that is newly diagnosed with type 2 diabetes may also have hypertension, hyperlipidemia, and neuropathy that are often linked with this diagnosis. The person could also have a condition that is unrelated, such as arthritis, asthma, or even Alzheimer disease as they age.

In fact, the term *chronos* is the root word for "chronic" and refers to time. When diagnosed with a chronic condition, it becomes necessary for individuals to learn to live and cope with the disease or disorder. The diagnosis of a chronic condition affects the family as a whole. Family members are challenged as they strive to assist a member diagnosed with a chronic condition to

stay healthy, prevent additional complications, incorporate changes in physical and mental status into the family's roles and functions, and manage any disabilities imposed.

Chronic illnesses can be categorized by their characteristics, including level of disability resulting from the condition, personal perception of disability, age of onset, stability (constant vs. relapsing vs. regression in symptoms), and impact on family functioning. For example, although some chronic conditions involve primary disabilities, such as those occurring from birth anomalies, other conditions, such as strokes, myocardial infarctions, secondary blindness, or kidney failure, are acquired disabilities resulting from life patterns or delayed or ineffective treatment of other conditions. The reaction and adaptation of the individual and family differs according to whether the disability is considered on-time and expected versus off-time and unexpected. Likewise, although some people with chronic conditions have lives fraught with pain, depression, and mental or physical difficulties, others experience satisfying lives with only minimal difficulties.

Differences in the ways families accommodate a chronic condition are influenced not only by the level of disability and associated symptoms, but also by the individual and family perception about the disability. Care needs can also differ depending on whether the symptoms are constant (e.g., those associated with cerebral palsy), episodic (e.g., those associated with migraine headaches), relapsing (e.g., those associated with sickle cell anemia), worsening or progressive (e.g., those associated with multiple sclerosis or certain types of cancer), or degenerative (e.g., those linked with Alzheimer disease and Rhett syndrome).

Regardless of the type of chronic illness experienced, family members are involved at several levels, depending on the age of the individual, the condition being cared for, previous family experiences, levels of expertise, unique relationships, and behavioral patterns. Over time, family is the biggest resource for care of individuals with chronic illnesses. Family members are the most enduring care providers, and offer the constancy and continuity of care needed. Professionals come and go, offering medical management, education, and counseling as needed, whereas family members provide ongoing and persistent care across time.

This chapter provides an integrative literature review primarily focused on diabetes and comparisons or explanations about ways this chronic disease affects families. Although many examples of other chronic conditions are presented throughout this chapter, discussions primarily focus on diabetes and ways to consider individual and family concerns when a single member has chronic illness as an exemplar of how nurses can assist families in the care of a chronic condition that is pervasive, and yet complications can be delayed or prevented, leading to improved quality of life for all family members. Two case studies are used in this chapter to depict concerns that families might encounter if they are at different life stages. Attempts are made to distinguish varied experiences that might occur in a family if a child has type 1 diabetes, as in the Yates Family, or an adult with type 2 diabetes, as in the Halloway Family. References to these case studies are made throughout this chapter.

Family Case Study

YATES FAMILY

Chloe Yates, age 13, was recently admitted to the pediatric intensive care unit with ketoacidosis, a complication of type 1 diabetes. On admission, her serum glucose level was 350 mg/dL, and she had passed out at school after vomiting and complaining of fatigue. Her glycosylated hemoglobin (HbA1c) was 11%, indicating poor metabolic control over the past 3 months.

Chloe's parents, Jack and Brenda, were surprised when they found out how poorly Chloe's metabolic control had been before her admission, because they feel their communication as a family is open and Chloe had been reporting that her glucose levels were "fine." Chloe is an honor-roll student at school, active in basketball and soccer, and well-liked by her peers.

The Yates family has recently experienced several stressors in addition to Chloe's hospitalization. Brenda's father, Henry, passed away 2 months ago after a long bout with Parkinson disease, and the family has moved to a new neighborhood and into a larger home. Fortunately, the children were able to remain in the same school district, and they can continue to receive their primary care in the clinic where their pediatric nurse practitioner has come to know the family over time.

Chloe was diagnosed with diabetes 2 years ago at the age of 11, and has been assuming more responsibility lately for monitoring her glucose levels and administering her insulin. At first, the family struggled to make changes to their routines and accommodate Chloe's dietary needs, and the frequent monitoring and management of her blood glucose levels. They have since been able to incorporate the management of her diabetes into the family's routines, and it seems less foreign to them now. They have made a point of eating at least one meal together as a family, which allows each family member to talk about their day. The family recently started "highlight/low light" time at dinner, during which each family member shares one high point and one low point about their day. Brenda recalls that lately, Chloe's highlights have been focused on her new friend at school, Brian. Her low lights have been focused on the "hassle" of checking her glucose and having to eat different food when she is out with friends.

Chloe's younger siblings, Leslie and Trevor, are staying with Jack's parents while Brenda and Jack prepare to take Chloe home from the hospital today. Leslie and Trevor have been asking about Chloe for several days, as they are worried about her "sugar." Leslie, age 11, has been feeling especially concerned about Chloe, because she and her sister have been arguing lately and Leslie feels responsible for Chloe's hospitalization. Trevor, age 4, has been asking if he can use Chloe's "finger pokers" and saying, "I have diabetes too!" Jack and Brenda think that he wants some of the special attention that his sister is getting at the hospital. They worry about being "spread too thin" as they try to attend to each child's needs while staying on top of Chloe's diabetes.

Chloe's parents are meeting with the nurse today in preparation for Chloe's discharge home. When the nurse asked whether they thought Chloe understood how to manage her diabetes, Jack said, "She not only understands, she could teach it! We just can't figure out why she had such a setback recently."

Family Case Study

HALLOWAY FAMILY

Sarah Halloway has recently been diagnosed with type 2 diabetes. For the last 2 years, each time she went to see Dr. Anderson, he warned, "Sarah, you have got to take better care of yourself. This continual weight gain and lack of physical activity is a problem, and you are putting yourself at risk for many chronic illnesses." Each time, she shrugged her shoulders and said, "I'm going to try harder." But at the next visit, she would not show improvement. About a year ago, Dr. Anderson told her, "You are borderline diabetic. You have gained fifty to sixty pounds of excess weight over the last four to five years; you must become more active and watch what you eat!"

On her last visit, Dr. Anderson warned, "Sarah, you are only thirty-eight years old; you are on your way to having diabetes. You have metabolic syndrome. You must change your habits if you want to live a long and healthy life." But Sarah continued her behavior patterns without making the needed lifestyle changes. Her husband and extended family members who live nearby have commented about the way she had become disinterested in things she once valued. She no longer seemed to enjoy being involved with family or friends. She often slept late and took long naps during the day. She dreaded going out in public. She had allowed the household to become disorganized as she allowed the wash to pile high and dirty dishes to clutter the kitchen. She never discussed these problems with her doctor but continued to take the same medicine he had prescribed for her nerves right after her mother had died.

At her last visit to Dr. Anderson she was really not surprised when he said, "Sarah, I have been telling you for years that you need to change your ways, and now you have type 2 diabetes. I want you to spend some time with our nurse educator before you leave today." Sarah spent about 30 minutes learning about her condition. She left the doctor's office armed with written materials about diet changes, medication prescriptions, a glucometer, and other tools for doing daily blood monitoring.

As she drove home, she thought about her condition. She was not prepared for the changes that needed to be made. In fact, she felt overwhelmed. Although she had had hypertension for years, she became especially frightened when she learned that diabetes also put her at greater risk for heart disease, stroke, kidney disease, and blindness. She also learned that the numbness and tingling in her feet and legs was called *neuropathy,* and if ignored, it could result in sores that healed slowly and could lead to an amputation.

On arriving home, Sarah began thinking about her family and how they would respond to her chronic illness. They were primarily meat and potato eaters! In fact, the preferred dinner meal was anything fried, plenty of biscuits, gravy over everything, and a luscious dessert. Fruits and green vegetables were not among the family favorites. Snacking was done regularly. Shopping habits meant the cupboards were usually full of cookies, chips, and prepared or microwaveable items.

Cooking family meals were linked with traditions Sarah cherished as she recalled growing up in a rural Eastern Kentucky home and community, a place some people called Appalachia. As an adult, she had not moved too far from the place where she was born. She still had many extended family members and friends living close by. Whereas regular family meals where everyone sat together to eat were important when she was a child, this rarely occurred with any regularity in her present household.

Family patterns were predominately sedentary, and she had little interest in a more active lifestyle. As Sarah thought about her family, she envisioned her two teenage sons, Harry, who is 17 years old, and Justin, who is 15, and their lively interest in football and basketball. Their interest was in watching it on television rather than playing it. Video games were the favorite pastime, with hours spent sitting almost glued to the couch, eyes fastened on the screen, and fingers diligently at work.

She had to admit that both boys were rather overweight, in fact, bordering on obese. Her husband, James, an independent truck driver for a local slag company, was up early every morning and arrived home tired most evenings. He thought that his work provided more than enough exercise. He lived a totally different lifestyle from his father, who had spent years working in the mines. James's larger pant size was indicative of his lifestyle. He had told stories to his sons about the work he did as a young teen in the family garden each spring and summer. Although their house was located on acreage large enough to have a nice family garden, it was not something they had considered.

James has been experiencing more stress than usual. He has become concerned about the impact the unstable economic market will have on the future of his job. He is afraid that they might also lose their home if he lost his job. The rising costs for transportation and food have already reduced the things his take-home pay will cover.

Sarah thought about her new diagnosis. Her mother was diagnosed with type 2 diabetes several years ago. Sarah recalled the problems her mother had with nerve damage and poor eyesight before she died. Sarah was full of uncertainty about the changes needed and fearful about what could happen if she did not heed Dr. Anderson's instructions. As she looked at the medications she had been taking for depression and hypertension, the new diabetes medication, the glucose monitor and all of the accessories that seemed to go with it, and the stack of written materials, she felt overwhelmed. Sarah realized that changes were needed, and that some changes would affect her entire family. As she thought about it all, she was left with an overwhelming feeling of uncertainty about what to do first and what the future might hold.

HISTORICAL PERSPECTIVES

Early in the 20th century, the nation's leading causes of death were tuberculosis, pneumonia, and influenza (Glasgow, Orleans, & Wagner, 2001). Dangerous work, poor dietary intake, contaminated water, inadequate sanitation, desperate living conditions, and lack of medical care often caused illness and death. Individual and population health greatly improved through the enactment of Title 42 of the U.S. Code, which was originally enacted in the early 1900s, but has been repeatedly amended over time. Several sections of this code provide permanent public health and welfare laws that protect the nation's residents against threatening health conditions (U.S. Code, 2007). In 1946, the passage of the Hill-Burton Act as Public Law 725 amended the Public Health Service Act and authorized state grants to survey, plan, and construct hospitals and public health centers (Schiller Institute, 2001). This act offered federal grants and guaranteed loans for the building and modernization of hospitals, and a total of $4.6 billion in grants and $1.5 billion in loans were given between the years 1946 and 1997, resulting in 6,800 health care facilities in more than 4,000 U.S. communities (Health Resources and Service Administration [HRSA], n.d.). This act required Hill-Burton hospitals to provide uncompensated services for 20 years after receiving funds, but Title XVI set the requirements to provide uncompensated services in perpetuity (HRSA, n.d.). More widely available medical care improved the health of individuals and society as a whole, and resulted in continued drops in communicable diseases. This trend, however, has been threatened today because of increasing numbers of families living in poverty and without stable health care, and decreased availability of access to uncompensated services.

Increased hospital and medical center care has shifted the primary focus of care delivery from care of acute conditions to care of acute complications of chronic diseases such as heart attacks and strokes, and the delivery of episodic care related to chronic illnesses. Although this trend has significantly reduced infectious diseases, the incidence of new diagnoses and new complications of chronic illnesses has continued to increase. This is partly due to our aging society, but it is also linked to treatment of illness conditions and complications as they occur rather than focusing on prevention of the occurrence or delay in the onset of the chronic conditions (e.g., heart disease, Alzheimer disease), or the prevention of preventable complications (e.g., kidney failure with diabetes). Many clinicians agree that much of the chronic-disease burden is preventable through management and modification of lifestyle behaviors (Glasgow et al., 2001). Another contributing factor to the increase in chronic illnesses is the growing concern about low health literacy, with many lacking access and understanding of wellness and healthy lifestyle behaviors (e.g., healthy nutrition, activity, stress management) that can prevent or delay illness onset, influencing the effectiveness of health care for many families.

Current Cost and Demographics

Chronic illness not only contributes to sickness, death, and disability, but it is widely prevalent and costly. *Chronic illness* is a term used to describe a health condition that lasts longer than 6 months, is not easily resolved, and is rarely cured by a surgical procedure or short-term medical therapy (Miller, 2000). According to the CDC (2008), the extended pain, suffering, and associated complications linked with diseases such as diabetes and arthritis often account for 7 of 10 U.S. deaths each year. The CDC (2008) notes that 133 million Americans live with chronic illness.

- Chronic diseases account for 70% of all deaths in the United States.
- Chronic diseases account for one-third of the years of potential life lost before age 65.
- The direct and indirect cost of diabetes is $174 billion a year.
- Each year, arthritis results in estimated medical care costs of nearly $81 billion, and estimated total costs (medical care and lost productivity) of $128 billion.
- The estimated direct and indirect costs associated with smoking exceed $193 billion annually.
- In 2008, the cost of heart disease and stroke in the United States is projected to be $448 billion.

- In 2000, the estimated total cost of obesity was nearly $117 billion.
- Cancer costs the nation an estimated $89 billion annually in direct medical costs.
- Nearly $98.6 billion is spent on dental services each year. Poor dental care is linked with an increased risk for chronic illness complications.

Prevention is certainly a concern when chronic illnesses are considered. Although not all chronic conditions are preventable, many are. For example, the CDC (2008) has identified several ways preventative financial investments can make important differences:

- For each $1 spent on water fluoridation, $38 is saved in dental restorative treatment costs.
- For each $1 spent on the Safer Choice Program (a school-based HIV, other sexually transmitted diseases, and pregnancy prevention program), about $2.65 is saved on medical and social costs.
- Every $1 spent on preconception care programs for women with diabetes, health costs can be reduced by up to $5.19, and prevent costly complications for mothers and babies.
- Implementing the Arthritis Self-Help Course among 10,000 individuals with arthritis will yield a net savings of more than $2.5 million whereas simultaneously reducing pain by 18% among participants.
- A mammogram every 2 years for women aged 50 to 69 costs about $9,000 per year of life saved, a cost that compares favorably with other widely used preventive services.

Each year in the United States, about 440,000 people die of a smoking-related illness; this results in 5.6 million years of potential life lost and $82 billion in lost productivity (Agency for Health Research and Quality, 2008). High utilization of health care services by those with chronic conditions accounts for 83% of health care spending, and two-thirds of all prescriptions filled (Partnership for Solutions, 2004). Numbers and costs will likely increase as society continues to age and numbers of those with chronic conditions grow.

Most agree that the toll of chronic disease on patients' families and society is enormous. A tudy conducted to quantify the costs of chronic disease, the potential effects on employers, the government, and the nation's economy found that the seven most common chronic diseases—cancer (broken into several types), diabetes, hypertension, stroke, heart disease, pulmonary conditions, and mental disorders—affect 133 million Americans (DeVol, 2008). These diseases have large-ticket economic costs of $1.3 trillion annually, and potential for lost work and productivity. Findings from the DeVol (2008) study also have the following indications:

- At the current rate, a 42% increase in cases of the 7 chronic diseases is predicted by 2023, with $4.2 trillion in treatment costs and lost economic output.
- Modest improvements in preventing and treating diseases could avoid 40 million cases of chronic disease by 2023, with the economic effect of chronic illness decreased by 27% or $1.1 trillion annually.
- Decreased obesity rates, a large risk factor linked with chronic illness, could result in productivity gains of $254 billion and avoid $60 billion in annual treatment expenditures.

Chronic illness is often linked to behavioral and environmental risk factors that could be effectively addressed through prevention programs. For example, the increasing rates of obesity, leading to several chronic complications, could be prevented with changes in dietary and exercise behaviors and changes in our environment that encourage exercise such as safe sidewalks.

Several reasons for the increase in prevalence of chronic conditions in children and adults should be noted. The percentage of preterm low-birth-weight (<2,500 g) infants born has steadily increased over the past few decades, and the number of multiple births has also increased (Perrin, Bloom, & Gortmaker, 2007). The result of preterm and low birth weight is a significant increase in the risk that a child will experience long-term disability. In addition, children who may once have died in infancy or childhood from conditions such as cystic fibrosis, Down syndrome, or spina bifida are now surviving well into adulthood. A child born with cystic fibrosis in the 1950s was not expected to live beyond 6 years, but a child born with cystic fibrosis today has a life expectancy of about 36 years; similarly, the life expectancy for a child born today with Down syndrome is 56 years (Lose & Robin, 2007). Some chronic conditions, such as autism, are being diagnosed more frequently, but this may not be entirely because of an increased prevalence of these conditions alone. Rather, the recognition and diagnosis of these conditions may be increasing, and individuals who may have gone undiagnosed in the past are now being identified and are able to receive services (National Center on Birth Defects and Developmental Disabilities, 2008). The three chronic conditions that affect the most children today at growing rates include obesity, asthma, and attention-deficit disorder, with most children continuing to have these disorders and related complications into adulthood (CDC, 2008).

As the population continues to age, the numbers of aging adults continue to increase. Chronic conditions can have a long-term and devastating impact on the lives of individuals and families in biological, psychosocial, and economic ways. Whereas children with special health care needs (SHCN) are likely to experience chronic conditions that are genetic or environmental in nature, many chronic illnesses experienced by adults are linked with lifestyle behaviors. Among children with SHCN, the most common conditions are obesity, asthma, allergies, learning disorders including attention-deficit disorders, and emotional problems (Child and Adolescent Health Measurement Initiative [CAHMI], 2008), and the most common chronic conditions in adulthood are related to cardiovascular disease and cancers (Martin et al., 2008). Increasing rates of childhood chronic conditions, particularly childhood obesity, suggest future increases in pulmonary, cardiovascular, and mental health burdens among adults as these children age (Perrin et al., 2007).

Other diseases such as arthritis, lupus, some cancers, and other mental health conditions such as autism are just a few of the other chronic conditions commonly experienced. Although some of these conditions may improve or disappear entirely with treatment and age, others can endure from childhood into adulthood and progress into secondary conditions. For example, conditions such as scoliosis, if treated early and appropriately, may improve as a child grows and ages. In contrast, hemochromatosis, a rare, chronic disease characterized by a lifelong excessive absorption of iron that accumulates in body organs and eventually causes inflammation, cirrhosis of the liver, liver cancer, heart failure, diabetes, impotence, arthritis, and other disorders (Cogswell et al., 2003), worsens over time. Likewise, Since 1996, as protease inhibitors have become more available, HIV has been recognized as a chronic illness, that continues to progress over time, eventually becoming fatal (Siegel & Lekas, 2002). Generally multiple chronic conditions occur more often with age, but 5% of children suffer from more than a single chronic condition. These children have more frequent activity limitations than children with a single chronic disorder and experience more days spent in bed and school absences (Partnership for Solutions, 2004). These early patterns affect these children well into adulthood with increased risk for physical and mental health and social disabilities.

Some people can manage their chronic illness without much difficulty, whereas others require a great amount of assistance. Many need little medical care, but others require extensive medical services that may include care from special health practitioners, regular treatments or testing, multiple medicines, or intense therapies. Life, as we imagine it, can be completely disrupted when confronting long-term or chronic illnesses that affect physical abilities, appearance, and independence. Diminished endurance capacities, continual discomfort in physical, emotional, and social realms, and financial problems are just a few of the challenges families face. New medical procedures, diagnostic tests, screening, and pharmaceuticals have improved health and the ability to live with chronic conditions and extended life span.

According to the Milken Institute's Center for Health Economics (DeVol, 2008), it is estimated that by 2014 the health care industry in the United States will be more than $3 trillion and account for 17% of the country's gross domestic product. Since the late 1980s, the percentage of the population diagnosed with diabetes and cardiovascular disease has grown dramatically, together with increased rates of stroke, pulmonary disease, and mental disorders (DeVol & Bedroussian, 2007). Chronically ill workers reduce the labor force because of absenteeism (i.e., more sick days than others) and constitute the part of the workforce that works inadequately but is present in spite of illness to avoid lost wages. This pattern of being at work but unproductive has become known as *presenteeism*.

In addition to health care in clinical settings, children with SHCN require illness management and health maintenance in the home. The increased time and care demands of SHCN make it difficult for family caregivers to be fully employed, and often lead to emotional stress and financial burdens. In the United States, 40% of families with children with SHCN (3,746,000 families in 2000) experienced financial burden related to their child's condition (Looman, O'Conner-Von, Ferski, & Hildenbrand, 2009). One in five families with a child with SHCN reported spending more than $1,000 on health care costs in the previous year for the care of their child (U.S. Department of Health and Human Services [DHHS], 2008).

Parents working in low-income jobs often do not receive health insurance benefits. These families typically earn too much money to qualify for public subsidies but not enough money to cover the health care expenses of raising a child with SHCN. Compared with children in higher-income households, children living in such "near-poor" families are more likely to have gaps in insurance coverage and more likely to be uninsured (Looman et al., 2009). Eleven percent of uninsured children did not receive needed family support services related to chronic illness care, compared with 7.7% of children with public insurance and 2.7% of privately insured children (U.S. DHHS, 2008). Families who lack health insurance are more likely to report that, although health and family support services are needed, they were not received.

Many individuals with chronic illnesses fear being unable to afford the medical care needed, a fear that is not unfounded as costs are up to five times higher for those with chronic illness regardless of the insurance type (Partnership for Solutions, 2004). Families often face economic challenges because of the needs of either a child or an adult with a chronic condition. For example, in diabetes management, although medical insurance may cover the costs of medications and supplies such as syringes and glucose testing strips, other health-promoting activities might require out-of-pocket expenses. A person with diabetes needs to eat a balanced diet, which requires the family to purchase foods high in nutritional value, food that can be far more expensive than unhealthful foods. In addition, if chronic illness care is not well coordinated with the multiple care providers, families might spend money for treatments that counteract one another or purchase medications that interact with one another and cause symptoms that are uncomfortable or life threatening. Families may also purchase over-the-counter medications or herbs that they believe will be helpful but have the potential for adverse interactions with prescribed medications. If a coordinated team does not assess the comprehensive care protocols during

chronic illness, it is possible to spend money unnecessarily and have untoward health problems or adverse interactions resulting from unmanaged regimens.

Economic costs for chronic illnesses such as diabetes are increasing for several reasons. For example, according to a study commissioned by the American Diabetes Association (2008), diabetes currently costs Americans $174 billion annually, a figure that has increased by 32% since 2002. Direct economic costs associated with diabetes have reached unprecedented levels with medical expenditures estimated to be $116 billion. A disproportionate percentage of these costs result from treatment and hospitalization of persons with diabetes-related complications. The study findings suggest that one of every five health care dollars is spent caring for someone diagnosed with diabetes. Financial costs for this disease are even greater when the family pays for additional health care needs, such as over-the-counter medication and medical supplies, additional visits to optometrists or dentists, health complications that occur before the diabetes is diagnosed, lost productivity at work for the individual and family members, and costs for informal caregiving. Because of continued emphasis on treatment of disease and related complications, rather than prevention, the cost of diabetes continues to climb.

The demographics of chronic illness are viewed by many as an epidemic in our country. Others refer to the increase as a cry for action. An optimistic scenario of increased weight reduction, healthy eating, a more active lifestyle, continued decrease in tobacco use, improved early detection, fewer invasive treatments, and quicker adoption of proved therapies could cut chronic illness treatment costs by $217 billion per year by 2023 (DeVol & Bedroussian, 2007), and change our profile from climbing rates of chronic illnesses and related complications to climbing health and preventive care.

THEORETICAL PERSPECTIVES TO UNDERSTANDING CHRONIC ILLNESS

A number of different theoretical perspectives are used to understand family nursing. This chapter utilizes three different theoretical perspectives: the

Chronic Care Model (CCM; Improving Chronic Illness Care, 2008), the Family Management Style Framework (Knafl & Deatrick, 1990, 2003), and the Family Health Model (FHM; Denham, 2003). These theoretical perspectives can assist nurses to understand family nursing, assessment, and intervention.

Chronic Health (or Care) Model

In the 1990s, the CCM was developed by Ed Wagner, MD, MPH, Director of the MacColl Institute for Healthcare Innovation, Group Health Cooperative of Puget Sound, and his colleagues from the Improving Chronic Illness Care program with support from the Robert Wood Johnson Foundation (Wagner, 1998; Wagner, Austin, Davis, Hindmarsh, Schaefer, & Bonomi, 2001). In this model, chronic illness is defined as any condition that requires ongoing adjustments by the affected person and interactions with the health care system. The model focuses on care system deficiencies that include things such as:

- Rushed practitioners not following established practice guidelines
- Lack of care coordination
- Lack of active follow-up to ensure the best outcomes
- Patients inadequately trained to manage their illnesses

The CCM calls for the transformation of health care from an essentially reactive system that responds when a person is sick to a proactive one that aims to keep persons healthy. It is viewed as a strategy that has been demonstrated to improve efforts by community health centers and health care teams to address diabetes and frailty in older persons. Initiatives based on this model aim to use best practices and innovative delivery systems to improve patient outcomes, make care delivery more efficient, improve access and timeliness of medical care, boost the usability of health care systems, lower costs, and reduce medical errors and inappropriate care (Wagner, Davis, Homer, Hagedorn, Austin, & Caplan, 2002).

Navigating the often confusing health care system can be extremely difficult for health care consumers. Some suggest a generalist model, or one that looks at chronic conditions as a whole, as the optimum approach to chronic care needs because many chronic illnesses have accompanying comorbidities and often occur simultaneously

(Grumbach, 2003). The reductionist perspective traditionally used for chronic conditions (e.g., diabetes, asthma, cardiovascular disease) ignores the overlap of needs that individuals and families incur. Seeking care from multiple specialists and health care practitioners also often means that care is parceled into complex and challenging clinical situations, rather than integrated into a coordinated whole. Chronic illness needs are often silent until symptoms become full-blown, and preventive care is frequently outside the scope of clinical medicine. Blueprints are needed to guide the redesign of medical and nursing care so that services provided assure high-quality and coordinated care for multiple needs. One of the main goals of the CCM is to redesign the model of health care to avoid this pattern through early prevention, early detection, and early treatment of individuals at risk for chronic conditions using a holistic and family approach to care.

The CCM provides an excellent tool for understanding ways the complex health care system addresses or fails to manage appropriately some of the most common health care problems. The CCM (Wagner, 1998; Wagner et al., 2001) implies that nurses will optimize the efficiency of the health care systems needed for care. Thus, a nurse interested in family-focused care might use case management as a way to address chronic care needs. In a condition such as diabetes, whether individuals receive care from a family physician, an endocrinologist, or other specialist, the individual outcomes must be focused on quality care, disease management, and family satisfaction. The CCM emphasizes that care is optimized through solving system management problems and not merely focused on the inadequacies of individuals or family members. Nurses who care for chronic disease prevention and management, conditions that usually span many years of medical management, must optimize the efficiencies and adequacies of the health care systems where they are employed. Education and appropriate referrals are two significant larger system concerns fundamental to adequate chronic disease management whether the client is a child or adult. Based on the CCM, improved disease management and preventive care outcomes depend on the community and health care system having collaborative interactions between informed active patients and a prepared proactive medical practice team (Glasgow et al., 2001).

Family Management Style Framework

The Family Management Style Framework was designed to study families who were managing chronic conditions. This framework was based on the identification of five categories of management styles (Knafl, Breitmayer, Gallo, & Zoeller, 1996), including thriving, accommodating, enduring, struggling, and floundering. The identification of these management styles has led to the connection between management styles and health outcomes. Thus, by identifying which style is predominant within the family, nursing interventions can be more accurately utilized to assist a family in changing to healthier patterns.

Understanding family's responses to childhood chronic illness provides ways to consider how effective interventions that meet individual and family demands might be constructed. Family typologies may be a useful way to understand how families cope and adapt when faced with illness. For example, Chesla (1991) has identified family patterns of engaged, conflicted, managed, and distanced family relationship styles when studying families who had a young adult with schizophrenia. Research findings suggest it may be useful to consider patterns and profiles of disease management, and consider a typology of family as balanced, traditional, disconnected, or emotionally strained when considering chronic care interventions (Fisher et al., 2000). This understanding led to Knafl and Deatrick's (1990) discussion of ways that family management style frameworks (FMSF) affect illness care by introducing a conceptual framework for understanding families' illness experiences. This conceptual framework leads to the study of family management, resulting in the description of five family management types (Knafl et al., 1996):

- Thriving
- Accommodating
- Enduring
- Struggling
- Floundering

After a comprehensive review of relevant literature about perceived influences on management, the original FMSF was modified (Knafl & Deatrick, 1990, 2003). The most recent revision includes three conceptual areas that are formed across perceptions and behaviors of multiple family members (Table 10-1). The ways parents perceive the child and the illness tend to be keys to the ways parents

TABLE 10-1

Concepts and Themes of Family Management Style Framework

CONCEPTS	THEMES
Definition of the situation	Child identity
	Illness view
	Management mindset
	Parental mutuality
Management behaviors	Parenting philosophy
	Management approach
Perceived consequences	Family focus
	Future expectation

attend to child capabilities or address their vulnerabilities as they manage a chronic situation. The perceived seriousness and uncertainty about the illness course and possible outcome(s) can influence the management mindset and the ease of which a treatment regimen is incorporated into family routines. The extent to which views about the chronic care situation are shared by multiple family members greatly affects how the disease is described and managed within a family household.

Parental management behaviors pertinent to a chronic illness are linked to their ability to establish consistent and effective treatment routines. Parents may not be prepared to handle the caregiving responsibilities (e.g., identify, access, or facilitate coordinated care resources) after early diagnosis of a chronic illness and often require some coaching (Sullivan-Bolyai, Knafl, Sadler, & Gilliss, 2004). Goals that entail regimented care without room for deviation or modification may result in care regimens quite different from ones that focus on disease control or normalcy of life. Stability in routines that allows for some form of equilibrium in daily life appears to be essential for optimal disease management over time and through life course changes. For example, if dietary changes are necessary because of a chronic illness, individuals must understand how personal food preferences and eating patterns previously practiced can be balanced with those of other family members and medical care needs. Although specific management or routine activities may vary, the presence of a predictable routine seems essential. Finally, the ways parents focus attention on a chronic illness is an important consideration.

Whether the illness is viewed as a central feature, an organizing family focus, or a life aspect that must be balanced with other life responsibilities and endeavors influences the family management style. When a disease has frequent exacerbations or a continual worsening progression, family management may be more stressful than if the disease is stable, has great predictability, or suggests a less fearful or frightening future.

The FMSF not only identifies cognitive and behavioral family aspects, but also points to factors that may be predictive of strength or problems (Knafl & Deatrick, 1990, 2003). Those using this model are urged to consider needs of individuals within the family, those of family members or member dyads, and the family as a whole. The FMSF has especially important implications for chronic care management in children. As the difficulties and trials of chronic illness care are encountered in family households, parents' management styles are extremely important. For example, the ways parents define the situation of a chronic illness will be closely linked to child identity, the ways the illness is viewed, whether parents are prepared to guide child management or whether they believe that they must do everything for the child, and the degree of parental agreement about the ways things should be done. All children with a chronic disease may not have two parents in the household; thus, external influences from other life partners, extended family members, or a parent who resides somewhere else but has a relationship with the child are areas that need to be assessed before plans for care management.

Family management style includes things such as parental philosophy and the usual ways they approach the child. If one set of parents leans toward encouraging child independence and another set of parents focuses on safety and protection, then the approaches they use to encourage the child's disease management may be quite different. In the former case, a child could have too much responsibility thrust on him or her too soon, whereas the latter case might mean that the child becomes overly dependent or even fearful of doing self-care. Nurses need to understand member dynamics and processes as they assess care needs and provide education and counseling. Using the FMSF, nurses would consider in their assessments and planned interventions the ways family members perceive the seriousness of the chronic condition, the ways family members identify with one another, and the perceived consequences of family management efforts.

Family Health Model

Nurses can use theory to provide a common language and foundation to understand abstract concepts and their connections. These connections between chronic illness and families are tied to ideas suggested by the FHM (Denham, 2003). This an ecological model that supplies a lens to consider the forces, processes, and experiences that influence the life course and health of interacting and developing persons. Nurses need to understand the infinite ways families and individual family members define themselves, as well as the ways family members interact and exchange information with larger societal systems and institutions, where the family household is situated. The FHM is used to identify connections among ideas relevant to chronic illness, and to assist the nurse to appreciate some ways a family and its members might be affected. In addition, this model encourages nurses to consider ecological factors such as community location and demographics, political milieu, and social environments that might influence responses to chronic illness, disease management, and result in disease outcomes.

Operational definitions can suggest ways to describe the complex relationships among the biophysical and holistic aspects of a chronic illness, and tie these to the contextual aspects of family, health, and family health. In the FHM (Denham, 2003), *health* is defined as an adaptive state experienced by household persons as they seek opportunities and wrestle with liabilities found within self, family, households, and diverse contexts throughout the life course. This definition provides a thoughtful way to consider nursing practice and appropriate family care when a member has a chronic illness. In chronic illness, health can be realized as personal abilities, and well-being is maximized. *Family health* suggests that member transactions occur through system and subsystems interactions, relationships, and processes that have the potential to maximize processes of becoming, enhance well-being, and capitalize on the household production of health. Families strive to achieve a state where members are content with themselves and one another. That is, family health includes the complex interactions of individuals, family subsystems, family, and the various contexts experienced over the life course. The household becomes the pivotal point for coping with health and family health needs.

Family health is depicted with contextual, functional, and structural dimensions (Fig. 10-1). The

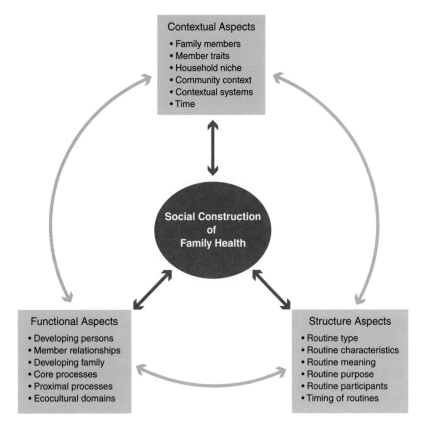

FIGURE 10-1 Contextual, functional, and structural aspects of family care.

contextual domain includes all of the environments where family members interact or have potential to be acted on, but also includes the characteristics or traits of the family (e.g., socioeconomic, educational attainment, extended kin relationships). The context is affected by the internal environments (i.e., member, family, and household context) and external environments (i.e., neighborhood, community, society, historical period, political context). An ecological model implies an understanding that nested domains challenge one's abilities to discern all of the interactions occurring over time, and the ways they overlap, intersect, and potentiate or negate important health factors. The *family household* is a key area of family context and refers to the physical structure(s), immediate surroundings, material goods, tangible and intangible family resources, and family interactions over the life course. The contextual domain pervades all family life aspects and effects personal interactions, values, attitudes, access to medical resources, availability of support systems, and health routines of individual members. For example, a family living in poverty or lacking adequate health care insurance may seek or obtain medical care quite differently from an affluent family with financial stability. A rural family with a long tradition of cultural behaviors linked with healing may minimize physical symptoms and be slower in seeking medical care than an urban family who has great confidence in the knowledge and services of health care professionals.

The *functional domain* refers to the individual and cooperative processes family members use to engage one another over the life course. This domain includes individual factors (e.g., values, perceptions, personality, coping, spirituality, motivation, roles), family process factors (e.g., cohesiveness, resilience, individuation, boundaries), and member processes (e.g., communication, coordination, caregiving, control). These dynamic factors have potential to mediate the work of individuals, family subsystems, and families as a whole as they seek to attain, sustain, maintain, and regain health. The core family processes of caregiving, celebration, change, communication, connectedness, and coordination describe concepts attuned to the family's functional domain, and are areas where nurses can collaborate with family members when chronic illness is a concern (Denham, 2003). When a family experiences chronic illness in one or more members, the functional capacities of the family and its members are tested. Individual and group strengths can be rallied to address pressing concerns, but in other families, something such as member conflict can become a threat to capacities for effective disease management.

The contextual and functional domains are the situational and behavioral antecedents that family members use to construct behavioral patterns linked with health outcomes. The *structural domain* is composed of six categories of family health routines (i.e., self-care, safety and precautions, mental health behaviors, family care, illness care, member care taking). These categories comprise complex habitual patterns that construct the lived health experience(s) of individuals and families (Denham, 2003). *Family health routines* are dynamic behavioral patterns with relative stability that can be recalled, described, and discussed from individual and family perspectives. Despite what might initially appear as random or chaotic health behavior patterns to an outsider, family members are cognizant of individual routines. Although routines have unique qualities and involve all household members, they often evolve over time as family maintains the integrity of routines viewed meaningful and adapts them to new life situations. Health routines tend toward steadfastness, but the diagnosis of a chronic condition that demands medical management and the availability of support or resources (i.e., contextual factors) can challenge prior routines that the family values. Families with effective modes of communication, abilities to share roles, and resilient personalities (i.e., functional domain) are likely to have greater capacities for deconstructing old routines and reconstructing new ones if a chronic condition becomes a family concern. Health routines have important implications for families when a member(s) has a chronic illness. Nurses can collaborate with family members to plan, implement, and evaluate coordinated care, and the process of deconstructing and reconstructing family routines.

When chronic illness is the concern, nurses can assist individuals and families to optimize resources to achieve health and well-being. *Well-being* is defined as a health state where opportunities are actualized, liabilities minimized, and contexts maximized. Well-being includes many dimensions (e.g., biophysical, psychological, emotional, social, spiritual, vocational) and is achieved through accomplishment of family goals (e.g., risk reduction, prevention, health maintenance, self-actualization). Nurses aim to provide holistic care that enhances well-being and partner with families to empower them when chronic illness is the concern. Nurses who provide *family-focused care* aid patients and families to achieve health goals. They also empower members to devise plans and identify ways to implement strategies, and also aid them to evaluate whether goals are met. Nursing encounters become a means to target the *household production of health,* or holistically address related or potentially related health attributes or threats. Thus, the *family is the unit of care* even when single patients with a chronic condition are encountered. In chronic illness, family-focused care assists family members to adapt, accommodate, and use household resources to achieve well-being for the entire family.

Family members are initially socialized about health by their families of origin, but over time, new information is gathered and some ideas, values, and behaviors are changed. Based on ideas described in the FHM (Denham, 2003), the functional domain suggests that both individuals and family members interact and respond to personal characteristic traits (e.g., worldview, religious perspectives, motivation, household factors), interaction with other household members (e.g., communication styles, problem-solving abilities, decision-making skills), and life approaches to tasks (e.g., collaborative, independent, demanding) relevant to chronic illness management. Functional perspectives give insight into ways families optimize health potentials and use resources to balance diverse and conflicting needs. As family members interact with one another and those outside the household, they translate health and illness information, experiences, and perceptions into socially constructed behavioral patterns. These patterns usually make sense to families but may need to be changed to manage a chronic illness effectively. Household members, through beliefs, values, attitudes, and abilities, can form supportive or threatening networks. Based on the FHM, nurses can use what are identified as core processes to consider family aspects relevant to chronic disease management and identify ways to empower individuals and families to meet care goals (Table 10-2).

TABLE 10-2

Core Family Processes and Chronic Illness

CORE PROCESSES	DEFINITION	AREAS OF CONCERN	
Caregiving	Concern generated from close intimate family relationships and member affections that result in watchful attention, thoughtfulness, and actions linked to members' developmental, health, and illness needs	Health maintenance Disease prevention Risk reduction Health promotion	Illness care Rehabilitation Acute episodic needs Chronic concerns
Cathexis	Emotional bonds between individuals and family that result in members' emotional and psychic energy investments into needs of the loved one	Attachment Commitment Affiliation Loss	Grief and mourning Normative processes Complicated processes
Celebration	Tangible forms of shared meanings that occur through family celebrations, family traditions, and leisure time that might be used to commemorate special times, days, and events; these times are often used to distinguish usual daily routines from special ones; they often occur across the life course and have special roles, responsibilities, and expectations	Culture Family fun Traditions Rituals	Religion Hobbies Shared activities
Change	A dynamic nonlinear process that demands an altered form, direction, and/or outcome of an expected identity, role, activity, or desired future	Control Meet expressed needs Meanings of change Contextual influences	Compare and contrast Similarities/differences Diversity
Communication	The primary ways children are socialized and family members interact over the life course about health beliefs, values, attitudes, and behaviors, and incorporate or apply health information and knowledge to illness and health concerns	Language Symbolic interactions Information access Coaching Cheerleading	Knowledge and skills Emotional needs Affective care Spiritual needs
Connectedness	The ways systems beyond the family household are linked with multiple family members through family, educational, cultural, spiritual, political, social, professional, legal, economic, or commercial interests	Partner relationships Kin networks Household labor Cooperation Member roles	Family rules Boundaries Tolerance for ambiguity Marginalization
Coordination	Cooperative sharing of resources, skills, abilities, and information within the family household, among members of extended kin networks, and larger contextual environments to optimize individual's health potentials, enhance the household production of health, maintain family integrity or wellness, and achieve family goals	Family tasks Problem solving Decision making Valuing Coping Resilience	Respect Reconciliation Forgiveness Cohesiveness System integrity Stress management

Source: Modified from Denham, S. A. (2003). *Family health: A framework for nursing.* Philadelphia: F.A. Davis, by permission.

Family Assessment

Many different factors influence the family response to chronic illness, and these are likely to vary from one family to another. The categories necessary to assess using the FHM (Denham, 2003) as a way to understand what happens when a member has a chronic illness may be contextual, functional, or structural in nature. Table 10-3 identifies a number of areas a family nurse might assess using this conceptual model. It is important to remember that nothing happens in isolation, and whenever a chronic illness occurs, it is always within the constraints of what else is occurring in the family at a particular point in time. For example, longstanding evidence exists that children from poorer, urban, minority households are at increased risk for morbidities associated with chronic health conditions because of the interaction between the context, function, and structure of these families resulting in insufficient support for the complex needs of chronic illness care (Fiese & Everhart, 2006).

A family that is already coping with multiple stressors such as a recent job loss, family disharmony, and death of a family member may or may not be more challenged as they live with a member who has a chronic illness than a family that appears to be problem free and has an abundance of resources. The level of dependence of the individual with the chronic illness (e.g., need for continuous assistance with activities of daily living such as feeding and toileting) may create far greater family challenges than when a person is more self-supporting and requires fewer family resources. The unique individual temperament of either the person with the chronic condition or family members, or both, can alter a family's coping capacities. Families address the balance between demands and resources differently, and these are areas where nurses can assess and consider interventions. An example of working with families to assess resources is the Yates family ecomap (Fig. 10-2).

Living with a chronic illness often requires a family to adapt to what is likely viewed as an undesirable situation while members find themselves needing to balance multiple resource demands. For some families, the absence of disease and the capacity to work may be essential to well-being, but for those living with chronic illness, well-being might be more closely linked with abilities for overcoming daily obstacles, resolving stresses, coping effectively, or family cohesiveness. Family factors will contribute to individual and family well-being, and may result in family beliefs that the illness situation is manageable. Activity limitation is often a challenge that accompanies chronic conditions and limits involvement in usual daily activities such as personal hygiene and walking unaided, and can affect school attendance or employment opportunities. Personal assistance is needed by many people living with a chronic condition. Although some require help from the beginning of life, others live in fear of the loss of independence and becoming a family burden. Caregivers often give many hours of uncompensated care for years to those living with long-term disabilities, care that would be extremely costly if it had to be purchased. Although many families manage well, others are continually threatened by the stress and demands commanded by a chronic illness. Family nurses are knowledgeable about family developmental alterations and sensitive

TABLE 10-3	
Assessment Using the Family Health Model	
CATEGORIES TO ASSESS	**SPECIFIC AREAS WITHIN EACH CATEGORY**
Contextual	▪ Developmental stage
	▪ Family traits
	▪ Availability of health insurance
	▪ Access to care
	▪ Demographics (age, education, sex, employment)
	▪ Social support
	▪ Culture and ethnicity
	▪ Political, historical, and environmental factors
Functional	▪ Stressors
	▪ Coping skills
	▪ Family roles
	▪ Member responsibilities
	▪ Communication patterns
Structural	▪ Illness characteristics
	▪ Family organization or chaos
	▪ Routines established
	▪ Ability and willingness to alter routines

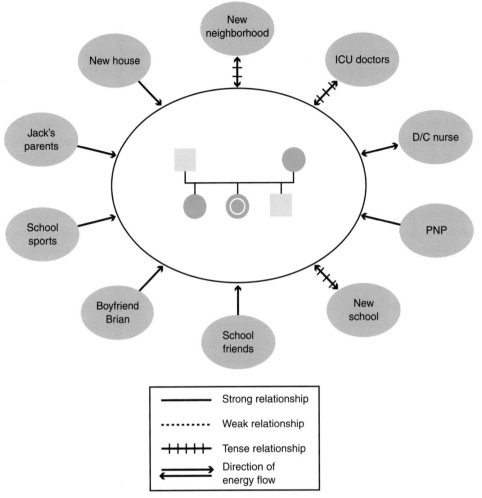

FIGURE 10-2 Yates family ecomap.

to members' expressed needs, as they aim to empower the household members to manage changes in chronic conditions over time.

Family Coping

Christopher Reeve, the actor who played Superman in four feature films, reminded us about the fragility of life and how quickly one can move from excellent health to life with a disability. In 1995, at the age of 42, he was transformed from an agile, able, and fit horseman to a man confined to a wheelchair and paralyzed from his neck down. This accident moved him from the image of a caped crusader who continuously championed good over evil, to a person with a disability who could not breathe on his own. His public face of coping presented a positive appearance of what persons with disabilities can accomplish. In an ABC television interview with Barbara Walters, Reeve said, "Let's look at the two choices I have. One is to vegetate and look out of my window and the other is to move forward. The second choice seems to be a whole lot more attractive" (Walters, 2004).

His valiant fight for those living with spinal cord injury, mobility impairment, and paralysis is characterized by the establishment of the Christopher and Dana Reeve Foundation Paralysis Resource Center (PRC), led by a group who aims to promote health and well-being of people living with disabilities. The public life of Christopher Reeve helped us to understand his deep-seated positive spirit and philosophy to live each day to the fullest. He gave a face and voice to neurologic conditions that were previously missing in the public consciousness (Reeve, 1999). His financial status and social clout provided him access to the best medical care, rigorous therapy, and support, things not usually available to many who cope with such a disability. Despite the numerous online photos and stories that chronicle his optimism and constructive activities, we know far less about the daily stresses, challenges, and difficulties that regularly pressed him and his family. Although his care was likely arduous and demanding, the resources accessible to him and his family were greater than those most Americans would have available. The FHM (Denham, 2003) can assist the nurse to understand the differences that one's contextual domain affords in a family's ability to cope with the stressors of chronic illness. Despite extensive and high-quality care, Christopher Reeve died of complications 9 years after his accident. Also, tragically, his wife, Dana, a nonsmoker, died 17 months later of lung cancer, a testament to the stress of caregiving, the strain of loss, and the possible effects of second-hand smoke exposure. Those living with a chronic illness are challenged in life as they are conflicted by stress, anxiety, and anger from the trials of daily tasks that others without such illnesses rarely consider. People living with a chronic disability are fatigued by the constant vigilance required to perform normal everyday activities of daily living. Family members are fatigued by the volume of help offered, the emotional strain that accompanies the daily hassles, and the relationship strain of constantly giving to another. Life with a chronic condition often entails a tentative life course that demands reliance on complicated and multisystem medical treatments. One person's chronic condition has great potential to impact the lives of many others. Management of these conditions involves the enlistment of a network of family, friends, health care professionals, and services. The odds of becoming a family caregiver to a family member with a chronic condition are continually increasing, and as more of the nation's population continues to age even greater risks will be experienced. The Chapter Web Sites section at the end of this chapter provides useful information about many concerns related to coping with chronic illness.

Caregiver Concerns

According to a recent (Gibson & Houser, 2007) report on caregiving, informal caregivers provided the nation's economy with an estimated economic value of about $350 billion in 2006 using conservative assumptions and estimates. Caregivers likely spend out-of-pocket costs ranging from $200 per month, or $2,400 per year, for those needing low-level care to $324 month per month, or $3,888 per year, or more for those with the greatest level of caregiving burden. Caregivers provide a variety of forms of care that range from the provision of highly skilled care to negotiation with health care providers and insurers for ways to help with daily activities that can have varied economic values per hour. This amount is greater than the $76.8 billion that was spent in 2005 for formal home care services (Georgetown University Health Policy Institute, 2007). In November 2006, about 30 to 38 million adult caregivers, 18 years or older, provided care to adults with limitations in activities of daily living for an average of 21 hours weekly, or 1,080 hours annually (Gibson & Houser, 2007). This is likely to be an underestimation, and the numbers will surely increase within the next decade as the baby boomers, those born in the era immediately following World War II, retire and age.

The cost of funding caregiver services and support is small compared with the value of their contributions. Several policy recommendations that can affect unpaid caregivers' services (Gibson & Houser, 2007) include:

- Implementing "family-friendly" workplace policies (e.g., flextime and telecommuting)
- Preserving and expanding the protections of the Family and Medical Leave Act
- Expanding funding for the National Family Caregiver Program
- Providing adequate funding for the Lifespan Respite Care Act
- Providing a tax credit for caregiving
- Permitting payment of family caregivers through consumer-directed models in publicly funded programs (e.g., Medicaid home, community-based services waivers)
- Assessing family caregivers' own needs through publicly funded home and community-based service programs and referral to supportive services

Implementing services that support caregivers is important for the continuance of informal caregivers and is an important investment in the nation's health.

Families have varied responses to living with chronic illness, and multiple factors can influence their actions. For example, the characteristics of the ill person (e.g., age, sex, developmental stage, care needs), those of the caregiver, as well as considerations for the types of additional demands and resources of the family influence coping capacities. Marital quality can be a source of stress or support with potential for a physical and a psychosocial impact on the well and the ill partner. A single parent as the sole caregiver, cohabitating relationships, or same-sex unions can each bring dimensions to the caregiving situation that require special understanding and support from nurses and other professional health care providers. Chronic illnesses force older persons to recognize potential loss of independence, income, and companionship as they deal with loss of place, things, family members, and friends. The availability or form of social support may vary widely in each of these family situations. The availability of an adequate job, income that provides financial security, or family beliefs, so that the illness situation is manageable financially, is something that can contribute to adaptive responses that enable the family to accommodate the life challenges faced. On the other hand, factors that contribute to the intensity of the stressful demands (e.g., insufficient or no health insurance, a high time demand that affects caregiver's sleep patterns, or beliefs that the illness situation is not manageable) can thwart a family's ability to meet the day-to-day demands of caregiving.

Family capacity to adapt successfully to evolving illness care demands can be quite different if the chronic illness is something such as Alzheimer disease where the individual needs can become more excessive as the condition worsens over time. In comparison, a chronic illness such as hypertension or arthritis may involve simply following a therapeutic self-management routine. A chronic illness such as asthma, sickle cell anemia, or diabetes can have times of great stability and be perceived as manageable, but may have periods of exacerbation that become life-threatening and require a great number of family resources. Caregiving is a dynamic process and is not consistently the same for caregivers. Although many families manage well, others may have more stressful demands than can be reasonably met with available resources. Nurses caring for families who have a member with a chronic illness need to understand the diversity of needs that may occur over time and be prepared to consider the unique ways these needs might be addressed.

Families and Children with Chronic Conditions

According to a recent survey entitled *National Survey of Children with Special Health Care Needs: Chart Book 2005–2006* (U.S. DHHS, 2008), one in five American households with children has at least one child with a chronic or disabling health condition. A child with a chronic physical, developmental, behavioral, or emotional condition who requires health and related services beyond that required by children generally is considered to have *special health care needs* (SHCN) (McPherson et al., 1998). By this definition, 10.2 million children (13.9%) in the United States from birth through 17 years of age have SHCN (U.S. DHHS, 2008). Children with SHCN have a wide range of conditions and risk factors that underlay many shared health conditions. Multiracial children (18%) have the greatest prevalence of SHCN, followed by non-Hispanic white (15.5%), non-Hispanic black (15%), American Indian/Alaska Native (14.5%), and Native Hawaiian/Pacific Islander children (11.5%) (U.S. DHHS, 2008). The prevalence rate of SHCN is lowest among Hispanic (8.3%) and Asian children (6.3%).

Children with SHCN are like typical children in many ways: they are actively growing and developing, enjoy playing and being with peers, and thrive in cohesive family environments. Children with chronic conditions, however, have limitations that affect daily lives and contribute to challenges unique from peers without chronic conditions. For example, 43% of children with SHCN have respiratory problems, 41% have learning problems, and 20% have trouble making or keeping friends (U.S. DHHS, 2008). In addition, 18% of children with SHCN have chronic pain and 12% have difficulty with self-care (U.S. DHHS, 2008). Many children have multiple functional difficulties that coexist, making daily life especially challenging.

Studies have shown that mothers of chronically ill children often have greater levels of distress than fathers, a concern thought to be related to the greater care demands placed on the mothers (Spilkin & Ballantyne, 2007). Twenty percent of families of children with SHCN report that they spend 2 to 7 hours a week providing health care for the child at home. Caring for the child at home is associated with a significant increase in the odds of having a family member reducing or quitting employment outside the home because of the child's health care needs (Looman et al., 2009). It is also not unusual for parents to differ in their perceptions about the impact of the chronically ill child on the family as a whole and on the marital relationship. Although mothers may find that caregiving demands influence their role performance, fathers may perceive the impact most in their expression of feelings and emotions (Rodrigues & Patterson, 2007). A study of 173 parent dyads of children with chronic conditions found mothers' marital satisfaction was influenced more than fathers' by perceptions about the effects of their child's condition on the family (Berge, Patterson, & Rueter, 2006). Parents' perceptions of the negative effects of the child's chronic condition were measured in terms of family social strain, role strain, and emotional strain. If parents differed in perceptions about the effects of the illness on the family or marital relationship, an increase in stress and frustration can result. Nurses can assist couples to recognize any differences in perception between parents, and facilitate discussions about the effects on roles and the benefits of sharing caregiving tasks (Berge et al., 2006; Spilkin & Ballantyne, 2007).

Family-centered or *family-focused care* are terms used interchangeably to consider approaches to the planning, delivery, and evaluation of health care that involves active participation between families and health care professionals. Family-focused care supports relationships that value and recognize the importance of family traditions, beliefs, and management styles as health care providers collaborate with family members in care management. When the general population of children with SHCN is considered, approximately 35% of them received care that lacked one or more of the essential components of family-centered care (U.S. DHHS, 2008). Table 10-4 provides an overview of the kinds of care that were lacking.

In general, families raising children with chronic illnesses face the joys and challenges that most typical families face, and are as unique and varied as families of typically developing children. These families want their children to be happy, have a high quality of life, and grow and develop into caring adults who can live independently and contribute to society. These families face additional stressors, and many researchers acknowledge that the children and parents in these families are at increased risk for stress-related health conditions and psychosocial problems (Barlow & Ellard, 2006; Berge, Patterson, & Rueter, 2006; McClellan & Cohen, 2007; Meltzer & Mindell, 2006; Mussatto, 2006). Box 10-1 provides a list of stressors likely to be experienced by

TABLE 10-4

Percentage of Children with Chronic Conditions Without Family-Centered Care

FAMILY-CENTERED CARE COMPONENT	PERCENTAGE
Health care provider does not usually spend enough time with the child	21.3
Health care provider does not usually provide enough information for the family	16.9
Health care provider does not usually make parent feel like a partner in the child's care	12.4
Health care provider is usually insensitive to the family's values and customs	11.1
Health care provider does not usually listen carefully to family's concern	11.2
Child does not have an interpreter when needed*	43.7

*This applies only to children who needed interpreter services (N=36,018).

Source: From U.S. Department of Health and Human Services, Health Resources and Services Administration, Maternal and Child Health Bureau. (2008). *The National Survey of Children with Special Health Care Needs Chartbook 2005–2006.* Rockville, MD: Author, by permission.

BOX 10-1

Potential Stressors When Raising a Child with Chronic Health Conditions

- Care regimen in meeting daily caregiving demands
- Grief, loss of anticipated child events or activities
- Financial and employment strains
- Uncertainty about future
- Access to specialty services
- Reallocation of family assets (e.g., emotional, time, financial)
- Recurrent crises and crisis management
- Foregone leisure time and social interactions
- Social isolation because of stigmatizing policies and practices
- Challenges in transporting disabled children (e.g., when architectural and other barriers restrict their inclusion)
- Physiological stress of caregiving

families with a chronically ill child. Despite the risks for problems, however, most children with chronic conditions and their families, including siblings, often demonstrate incredible resilience and capacity for finding positives amidst the challenges.

Given the marvels of modern medicine, children with chronic illnesses now live longer than ever before (Perrin et al., 2007), and this results in differing family demands as children with chronic illnesses live well into adulthood and later life. Although most young children with chronic conditions rely on and can count on their parents for supportive care, as these children age, their parents also age. For example, children with Down syndrome, cerebral palsy, or other genetic disorders may be dependent on siblings or other social agencies to care for them as their parents age or die, because these children now live well into their 40s or 50s (Lose & Robin, 2007). Mental illness such as schizophrenia may not manifest until the late teens or early 20s, and parents may not be able to provide necessary care at that time. Increased expenses for chronic care and aging parents who have their own health and financial issues can make the burdens of care exhaustive. Nurses who understand the complexities of chronic illness can begin to understand that the fragilities observed in a neonatal intensive care unit when a child is born prematurely with multiple SHCN continues to challenge individuals, families, medical care providers, and others across time.

Family Case Study

YATES FAMILY

The Yates family case study illustrates the multiple factors that face families who have a child with a chronic illness. This case study supports current literature and applies the theoretical concepts of normalization and resiliency, adolescent development and living with chronic illness, sibling reactions, family cohesion, relationships with health care providers, the transition issues between pediatric and adult care, and access to support systems and resources needed for optimal care across time.

The Yates family has three children, ages 13, 11, and 4 (Fig. 10-3). Chloe, the oldest child, has had diabetes for 2 years and has done well with parental guidance and self-management until recently. As a young teen, Chloe is moving into a new developmental stage, and her family is challenged as her disease management is threatened by interests and activities outside of the household. It is not unusual for families of children with SHCN to go through changes as children mature and encounter various life tasks. Family management style that might have been effective at an earlier point in life could prove to be less effective at a different developmental stage. Thus, nurses working with families with a child member who has a chronic condition must keep in mind that the support and guidance given should include these dynamic management needs.

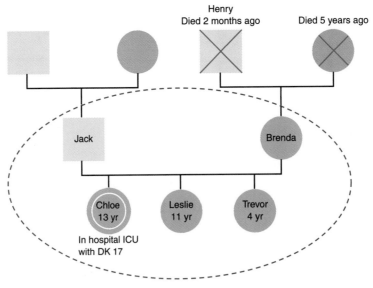

FIGURE 10-3 Yates family genogram.

SIBLINGS

In the Yates family case study, Leslie's and Trevor's reactions are typical for siblings of children with chronic conditions. Leslie, for example, feels responsible for Chloe's hospitalization, and has expressed possible guilt linked with recent arguments. Trevor's desire to have diabetes like his sister may represent his recognition that Chloe's diabetes is the source of much attention from their parents, attention that may be drawn away from him. Also, younger siblings often strive to model the behaviors of older siblings, including illness behaviors. Focus groups held with parents, siblings, and health care providers were conducted to develop a comprehensive list of psychosocial concerns specific to the experience of school-aged siblings (Strohm, 2001). Based on these conversations, seven issues were identified as significant feelings of siblings of children with chronic health care conditions (Strohm, 2001, p. 49):

- Feelings of guilt about having caused the illness or being spared the condition
- Pressure to be the "good" child and protect parents from further distress
- Feelings of resentment when their sibling with special needs receives more attention
- Feelings of loss and isolation
- Shame related to embarrassment about their sibling's appearance or behavior
- Guilt about their own abilities and success
- Frustration with increased responsibilities and caregiving demands

Other studies have been more positive in their focus, pointing out that siblings develop improved empathy, flexibility, pride in learning about and caring for a chronic illness, and understanding of differential treatment from parents based on ability and health. Siblings have been found to be more caring, mature, supportive, responsible, and independent than their peer counterparts who do not have siblings with chronic conditions (Barlow & Ellard, 2006). Other studies have found siblings to have high levels of empathy, compassion, patience, and sensitivity (Bellin & Kovacs, 2006). Siblings are interested in learning about diabetes and in being supportive of their ill brother or sister, and sometimes assume parental roles (Wennick & Hallstrom, 2007). Children who learn about their chronically ill sibling's illness and its mechanisms tend to feel more confident and competent in their ability to support their sibling (Lobato & Kao, 2005; Wennick & Hallstrom, 2007).

Families face the challenge of balancing the needs of the child with a chronic condition with those of the surrounding family, including siblings. In a study of parents and siblings of children with disabilities, Rabiee, Sloper, and Beresford (2005) have found that parents often could not give the time and attention siblings wanted because of the demands of caring for the child with a disability; this sometimes resulted in siblings resenting the child with disabilities. These researchers indicate that some parents rely on siblings to entertain or assist in the care of the child with disabilities, an action that puts additional stress on the other children. Chloe's parents have rearranged their lives to incorporate the management of her diabetes, but they also face the continued needs of their other children. Nurses working with the Yates family can facilitate the family's ability to balance the needs of their children by recognizing the ways Leslie's and Trevor's developmental needs influence their actions and assist the parents to consider the ways the psychosocial development of children at different ages will be attended to in the future (Bellin & Kovacs, 2006). Although siblings are likely to experience some distress when one has a chronic illness, some studies suggest that siblings of children with chronic conditions are rather resilient and have the potential for growth from their experiences in the context of a caring family (Bellin & Kovacs, 2006). The experience may catalyze siblings' abilities to tap into inner resources and develop empathy, compassion, patience, and sensitivity. Leslie and Trevor will benefit from age-appropriate, accurate information about Chloe's diabetes and from knowing that their responses are normal.

FAMILY FUNCTIONING

The Yates family demonstrates several examples of a cohesive family climate. For example, they value time together at mealtimes and encourage sharing of feelings. Studies have shown that high family cohesion is associated with adherence in children with diabetes. Cohesiveness allows for shared understanding, respect for differences of opinions, and an emotional investment in keeping the family together (Fiese & Everhart, 2006). The Family Management Style Framework could be useful here (Knafl & Deatrick, 1990, 2003). Chloe's parents have attempted to focus on the normal aspects of Chloe's early adolescence, and they see her as normal in many ways. For this reason, the Yates family might be considered accommodating. They have, up to this point, felt confident about Chloe's ability to manage her diabetes independently, but perhaps Chloe's transition into adolescence will require the family to reassess their assumptions. The Yates family has the resources and cohesiveness to negotiate the developmental changes that occur along the way.

Soon after the diagnosis of a chronic illness of a family member, caregivers must become proficient in many areas, including managing the illness, coordinating resources, maintaining the family unit, and caring for self (Sullivan-Bolyai et al., 2004). A multifaceted list of parent caregiving management responsibilities and associated activities to facilitate dialogue between health care providers and families of children with chronic conditions has been developed (Sullivan-Bolyai et al., 2004). These authors suggest that nurses assisting families who have children with SHCN can incorporate the following parental educational and counseling needs into the treatment plan:

- Monitoring conditions and behaviors
- Interpreting normal and expected behaviors from different and serious ones
- Provision of hands-on care
- Decision making
- Development of care routines
- Problem solving
- Teaching the child self-care management
- Teaching others about short-time care for the child

NORMALIZATION AND RESILIENCE

Normalization is a lens through which families of children with chronic conditions focus on normal aspects of their lives and de-emphasize those parts of life made more difficult by chronic conditions (Rehm & Bradley, 2005). Deatrick, Knafl, and Murphy-Moore (1999) identify five attributes of normalization for families of children with chronic conditions: (1) acknowledging the chronic condition and its potential to threaten their lifestyle, (2) adopting a normalcy lens to define the child and family, (3) engaging in parenting behaviors and routines that are consistent with a normalcy lens, (4) developing treatment regimens that are consistent with normalcy, and (5) interacting with others based on a view of

the child and family as normal (Deatrick et al., 1999). Although normalization is a useful conceptual and coping strategy for many families of children with chronic conditions, in families whose children have both complex physical and developmental disabilities, normalization as a goal may be neither possible nor helpful (Rehm & Bradley, 2005). When developmental delays compound the effects of a child's physical chronic conditions, a family's ability to organize and manage their daily lives is significantly affected. In this case, parents often recognize normal and positive aspects of their lives, whereas acknowledging the profound challenges that their families face, thus accepting a "new normal" (Rehm & Bradley, 2005). This capacity to normalize adversity and to define challenging experiences as manageable and surmountable fosters resilience in families, and nurses can use this knowledge to help families focus on the family's inherent strengths, resources, and functioning (Bellin & Kovacs, 2006).

It is important to realize that when a child or adult has a chronic illness, ideas about the process of normalization can vary. For example, giving injections to a child every day or sticking fingers to do blood screenings would not be viewed as normal, but in the Yates family, these things become part of normal daily processes. Yet, most of Chloe's day-to-day life, developmental needs, and experiences are similar to her peers. Likewise, although most of her parents' life is "normal," the frequency and type of doctor's appointments and communication with the school nurse become normal for this family. Social support depends on support for the developmental needs and typical challenges facing most families of 13-year-old children, and those that are normal for parents raising a child with diabetes.

CHANGE AND ADAPTATION

Adaptation of the family to the diagnosis of a child's chronic illness is a complex process that typically occurs in stages (McCubbin et al., 1996). Initially, families experience a period of adjustment, involving early responses and changes to cope with the stress of the diagnosis of chronic illness. Over time, most families progress to a state of long-term adaptation to the demands of the chronic illness suffered by their child, demonstrating the inherent resiliency of the human spirit (McCubbin et al., 1996). Examples of long-term adaptation may include tangible changes, such as moving to a home equipped to deal with mobility limitations or incorporating the administration of medications into daily routines (Mussatto, 2006).

The Yates family, although initially stressed by the demands of the diabetes management regimen, eventually found ways to incorporate Chloe's dietary requirements into family mealtime. They decided to have a weekly family meeting where all family members were encouraged to talk and share the strengths and stresses of their week. Nurses working with children and teens who are keenly aware of struggles around children's developmental stages can assist parents to identify what are normal or expected processes and things that are uniquely connected to the diabetes. Nurses can help families maintain stability by helping families with communication and relationships, and by encouraging a family routine of a weekly conference.

Adolescence is an exciting and challenging time for all families as they negotiate changes in roles, responsibilities, and relationships within and outside the family system. When a child has a chronic condition, this transitional time is especially challenging because the family must balance the adolescent's need for increased autonomy with the often complex self-care regimens of a chronic condition. Studies of adolescents consistently demonstrate a decline in self-care adherence as adolescents age and transition through puberty (Dashiff, Bartolucci, Wallander, & Abdullatif, 2005). This decline in self-care adherence can be considered a normal hurdle for families as they negotiate changes in responsibilities for a youth with chronic conditions, and nurses can support families by providing anticipatory guidance throughout a child's development.

In the case study, Chloe's parents were surprised to learn that her metabolic control is poor, because she previously managed to handle responsibilities linked with diabetes self-management with ease and skill. An early adolescent who has successfully managed diabetes may find it difficult to continue to manage the condition while simultaneously negotiating a move to social independence. Chloe's desire to fit in with her peers may be at odds with her need to check her blood glucose levels before meals, especially at school, and with her limitation on her diet, during social time with friends after school, at parties, and during weekend school events, such as a football game. Chloe's communication with her parents is particularly important at this transitional time. Parents are challenged to provide the adolescent with a level of autonomy that is developmentally appropriate whereas also monitoring abilities to adhere to complex medical regimens. Studies have shown that the more teens (particularly girls) perceive their mothers as controlling, the greater the effect on adherence (Fiese & Everhart, 2006). Nurses caring for Chloe could use the functional domain of the FHM (Denham, 2003) as the means to form a discussion with her parents about changes expected as children move through adolescence toward adulthood and consider ways this might affect the family as a whole.

It is possible that providers and parents may overestimate adolescents' desires for autonomy and confidentiality, especially of illness-related information (Britto et al., 2007). Also, adolescents, who tend to be more peer oriented, may wish to reduce the power differential between themselves and their care providers, and prefer that providers use direct communication styles. Adolescents with chronic illnesses may actually have fewer expectations for confidentiality and greater needs for parental involvement in care than healthy peers (Britto et al., 2007). Thus, nurses should not assume that all teens are seeking independence and autonomy just because they have reached the adolescent stage. In fact, nurses should consider the uniqueness of family situations before giving advice and avoid passing judgment. Nurses could use the FHM (Denham, 2003) and the Family Style Management Framework (Knafl & Deatrick, 1990, 2003) to conceptualize the forms and manner of care provided.

Although children may perform many disease management activities for many years, they might still need daily or intermittent reminders as adolescence nears. According to Schmidt (2007), families with an adolescent child with type 1 diabetes need to know that age-related challenges are likely to be encountered during the preteen and teen years (e.g., feeling angry or "different" from their friends), and families need to know that they can prepare for these transitions in the following ways:

- Finding opportunities for children or youths to interact with peers through attending diabetes camp, belonging to a support group, or interacting by phone or e-mail
- Obtaining information about gender differences in skill acquisition and adherence to diabetes management
- Setting realistic expectations for children's self-care

One of the ways the Yates family might prepare for their transition is through a family support group, where they can meet other families and discuss the age-related challenges of diabetes management in the teen years. Many cities offer support programs for families and peer support for siblings of youths with chronic conditions, such as Sibshops for Siblings of Children with Special Needs (http://www.siblingsupport.org).

TRANSITIONS

Transition is not an event, but rather a process that occurs over the lifetime. Successful change occurs when parents begin talking to youths early about adjustments that will be faced in the future. According to Blomquist (2006), this includes things such as:

- Including the children as soon as possible in medical care and upcoming transition issues
- Finding providers and insurance plans willing to take youths with particular diagnoses
- Planning ahead for insurance changes
- Allowing youths time alone with their health care provider during visits
- Helping youths learn to work with their health care providers

Families with a member who has a chronic illness will encounter many changes over time. Children and youths with chronic conditions and their families face several transitions at adulthood in the contexts of health care, education, and independent living. Finding a primary care provider who is a good "fit" for the family may be challenging. Families who establish trusting provider relationships often retain them for many years as the child grows and develops. When the child becomes a young adult, the transition from pediatric health care to adult health care can be a challenging period, especially as pediatric providers are reluctant to turn care over to a new provider after lifelong relationships have been established. Many pediatric providers and hospital units are unwilling or unable to take patients older than 18 years, and adult providers may have limited experience with conditions most common to a pediatric population. Individuals with conditions that once limited the life span, such as cystic fibrosis, are now living well into adulthood. The challenge for these individuals and families is finding providers who understand the condition and also provide adult care. The CCM (Wagner, 1998; Wagner et al.,

2001) may be helpful as the nurse considers ways to facilitate a family's transition to new providers.

Systems of Care for Children with Chronic Conditions

Often, bureaucracy and conditions in the health, education, and social services systems are sources of frustration for caregiving families. For example, many services are provided based on diagnosis or categorical determination of eligibility, so children need to fit certain categories to be eligible for services in acute care, community care, social services, or in the school system. Because clinics and subspecialists are in place to serve certain populations, children with uncommon diagnoses or multiple complex chronic conditions are at a disadvantage, and families must seek scarce resources and are forced to coordinate care from multiple specialists in multiple disciplines (Ray, 2003). Nurses working in medical care and community health settings can use the CCM to consider ways various providers and systems where they are employed can cooperate to provide coordinated care that provides what families need (Wagner, 1998; Wagner et al., 2001). Nurses who understand the complexity of care and chaos families experience as they cope with multiple care systems can assist them to move through the systems and obtain needed services.

When a child has a chronic illness, the family enters into a complex network of relationships with health care providers and other professionals in the care system. Families often feel as if they are thrown into these relationships (Dickinson, Smythe, & Spence, 2006). Nurses who provide family-focused care consider implications of dynamic care systems, refer the family to appropriate care centers, and evaluate the forms of care provided. Understanding the vulnerability of families in health care provider relationships helps nurses frame their family interactions in ways that create more horizontal than hierarchical relationships. Families are truly the "experts" when it comes to the day-to-day needs of children with chronic conditions, and they want professionals to recognize and respect this expertise. Parents and siblings of children with chronic conditions want professionals and community members to be informed about their child's diagnosis and the family implications. One parent described her frustration with staff poorly trained on sickle cell disease when she stated, "I knew we were in trouble when the nurse looked at me and said, 'so...how long has your daughter had sickle cell disease?' She did not even know that it was an inherited disease" (Mitchell, Lemanek, Palermo, Crosby, Nichols, & Powers, 2007). Through their multiple health care system encounters, parents of children with chronic health conditions tend to develop skills that aid them in the navigation of complex systems as they advocate for their child's needs (Mack, Co, Goldmann, Weeks, & Cleary, 2007). Frustration is experienced when parents encounter health care professionals who are insufficiently informed, lack knowledge about their child's condition, or who negate or discount their expertise in providing child care (Nuutila & Salantera, 2006).

SOCIAL SUPPORT

Social support is typically understood in terms of the *function* of relationships and can be categorized into four types of supportive behaviors: emotional, instrumental, informational, and appraisal (House, 1981). The family's capacity to mobilize social support to manage crisis periods and chronic stressors related to a child's health condition contribute to the well-being of all family members (Bellin & Kovacs, 2006). The need for support is typically greater among parents with special needs children than among families without a special needs child (Britner, Morog, Pianta, & Marvin, 2003). Table 10-5 provides examples of the four types of social support for families who have a member with a chronic health condition. The Chapter Web site section later in this chapter provides family caregiver resources.

Community contexts, such as the neighborhood, school, or church, support the child's development of positive values and foster strengths (Bellin & Kovacs, 2006). Social capital is a concept that can be useful in understanding the community context of health for children and families. Like social support, social capital is about resources that come

TABLE 10-5

Helpful Support for Families with a Chronically Ill Member

TYPE OF SUPPORT	DEFINITION	ACTIVITIES	EXAMPLE FROM CASE STUDIES
Emotional support	Provision of love, caring, sympathy, and other positive feelings	Listening; Offering commendations; Being present	The nurse working with the Yates family commends them by saying, "I am impressed by the commitment that your family has made to making life as 'normal' as possible for Chloe and her siblings."
Instrumental support	Tangible items, such as financial assistance, goods, or services	Assisting with household chores (e.g., laundry); Providing respite care; Providing transportation; Assisting with physical care	Jack's parents offer to take Chloe's siblings for a weekend, providing respite for the family and giving the siblings an opportunity to share time with their grandparents.
Informational support	Helpful advice, information, and suggestions	Sharing resources (i.e., books, Web sites, provider names); Educating family members on the health needs of the ill family member; Informational support groups	Sarah's brother David, who also has type 2 diabetes, recommends a Web site that provides healthy recipes for individuals with diabetes.
Appraisal support	Feedback given to individuals to assist them in self-evaluation or in appraising a situation	Reviewing daily logs; Sharing written feedback from providers (i.e., laboratory results)	The nutritionist provides appraisal support to Sarah during her regular appointments, offering feedback on how Sarah is doing with her lifestyle and dietary changes.

from relationships with other people and institutions. Social support is generally considered at the individual level, as there is a sender and a receiver of support. Social capital, in contrast, is generally considered at the level of relationships, and includes features of social life, such as norms, networks, and trust, that enable people to act together toward shared objectives (Putnam, 1996). Looman (2006) defines social capital in terms of investments in relationships that facilitate the exchange of resources. For families who have a chronically ill family member, social capital is especially relevant.

When an individual has a chronic illness, the members of the family (particularly caregivers) are required to engage with numerous professionals and institutions in the process of managing the condition and exchanging resources. The family benefits when a mutual investment exists in their relationships with nurses, physicians, teachers, other families, and even neighbors. For example, a parent might invest in her relationship with her child's teachers by providing them with information about her child's health condition, or by helping the teacher understand the child's unique learning style. The teacher, in return, might invest in his relationship with the child's family by scheduling additional parent-teacher conference sessions or by learning more about the child's specific health condition. The benefit of this investment in the family-school relationship, where the common goal is the success of the student, is an exchange of resources. The benefit of this investment may also reach to other students and families if this pattern of communication becomes a norm in the school, and if the general level of trust among parents and teachers increases. In this way, social capital facilitates the family's ability to acquire emotional, instrumental, informational, and appraisal support in many contexts.

In the Yates family, Jack and Brenda mobilized resources from extended family by having Jack's parents care for their two younger children while they prepare to take Chloe home from the hospital. Support from extended family members can be perceived as a double-edged sword, however, if obtaining that support is itself a source of stress (Brewer, Smith, Eatough, Stanley, Glendinning, & Quarrell, 2007). Nurses who understand the contextual domain and the nested interactions of complex systems described in the FHM (Denham, 2003) help families explore their options as resources from various care providers are sought. Assessment of resources and understanding what families have or lack can assist families to optimize their assets.

CURRENT RESEARCH ABOUT TYPE I DIABETES

Families of children with diabetes do not necessarily have poor family functioning, but in families where family functioning is poor, metabolic control is also likely to be poor, which seems to be particularly true for youths older than 12 years (Fiese & Everhart, 2006). In studies of families managing childhood diabetes, reports of a parent and child working together as a team around daily management tasks were associated with better adherence (Fiese & Everhart, 2006).

Mothers in families with children who have type 1 diabetes reported having less time to engage in activities with their children compared with mothers who do not have a child with diabetes (McClellan & Cohen, 2007). Parents of children with type 1 diabetes have also been identified as more likely to describe their families as less achievement oriented than families without children who have diabetes (McClellan & Cohen, 2007). Although nurses should be aware of the potential for family conflict around diabetes management, they should not assume that poor medical adherence is a product of the conflict observed, because conflict is a developmentally normal process in families with adolescents (Dashiff et al., 2005). It is important to keep in mind that conflict occurs in all families, regardless of the age of individual family members. What is essential is the way conflict is handled and resolved. Nurses can assist families by suggesting effective communication techniques and developmentally appropriate strategies to address problems and areas of conflict linked with healthy functioning and development. Studies of psychosocial well-being in families of children with chronic conditions too often focus on psychopathology and lack of adjustment, with less attention given to well-functioning and positive growth after childhood illness (Barlow & Ellard, 2006), an important area for future research. For example, more recent research on sibling relationships measures the positive attributes that occur in families with a child with a disability, instead of only pathologizing this experience (Barlow & Ellard, 2006; Bellin & Kovacs, 2006; Lobato & Kao, 2005; Wennick & Hallstrom, 2007).

Families and Adults with Chronic Conditions

The Halloway family provides a way for readers to consider the various ways a chronic illness of an adult household member might differ from a family with a child who has a chronic illness. Nevertheless, it is important for the reader to recognize that many family dimensions described in the discussion of the Yates family with a child who has type 1 diabetes would also be true with the Halloway family. Regardless of the member with chronic illness, family context, developmental stages of family members, and personal traits of individual members are likely to vary and result in different care needs.

The Halloway family is composed of James and Sarah and their two teenage sons. Although Sarah has a family history of diabetes, she has largely ignored her weight gain and the sedentary lifestyle she has adopted. The case study indicates that Sarah has been told recently that she has type 2 diabetes. When an adult is diagnosed with a chronic illness such as type 2 diabetes, she is confronted with the tasks aligned with making numerous lifestyle changes that also include and affect other household members. Adult family members may experience a chronic illness in ways quite different from the members of a family with a child either born with or developing a chronic illness in early childhood. If an adult member experiences a chronic illness, it is likely that he or she may need to cope with physiological, emotional, vocational, and social parameters linked with his or her illness. Marriage has been considered to have positive effects on couple relationships (Robles, & Kiecolt-Glaser, 2003; Tower, Kasl, & Darefsky, 2002), but more needs to be known about the effects of social contexts on marriage and the effects on chronic illness outcomes. In a chronic illness such as type 2 diabetes, family member support is extremely important to achieve self-management that results in tight diabetes control. Nurses and other health care professionals often fail to give the same forms of attention to family needs when an adult has a chronic illness diagnosis than might be provided to a family with a young child.

Diagnosis of the Condition

Diabetes affects nearly 24 million people in the United States, a disturbing increase of more than 3 million in approximately 2 years, according to new 2007 prevalence data estimates released by the CDC (2008). This means that nearly 8% of the U.S. population has diabetes. Therefore, when Sarah discovers that she is among that number of people who have the disease, she should not be entirely surprised given that she was aware of her family history of the disease and had been previously told by her physician that she was at risk for the condition. Keep in mind, however, that human nature allows for denial even in the face of evidence.

As Sarah and the Halloway family begin to face the changes implied by living with diabetes, they are likely to encounter concerns similar to those faced by other families. Therefore, knowing how family members share information and communicate news to one another could be important to nurses, as they assist individuals diagnosed with a chronic illness to identify how this new diagnosis and needed care routines will be conveyed to family members. Another nursing concern might be how well Sarah understands the information about diabetes management, the ways she plans to incorporate this new information into the family routines, and the level of comfort she feels with the skills needed. Knowing about these things and discussing them with Sarah before she leaves the doctor's office might help reduce some of the distress and confusion she may encounter when she is home and must face what living with this disease will mean for her family.

Often, family members are not knowledgeable about a new diagnosis and may underestimate or overestimate their knowledge about disease management. Sarah is from an Appalachian region; this means that she is likely to have family who wants to be supportive, but it is also possible that they may not have the newest information about diabetes management and may hold some myths to be true. Given that adults often see a health care provider alone, it is likely that, just like Sarah, they receive the first news or diagnosis without the support of a family member. Then, individuals must return home and inform their family about the diagnosis and interpret for them what this might mean. Individuals employed in nonmedical-related fields often have only limited understandings about medical conditions and may be hesitant to ask questions. Thus, it is a challenge when individuals begin telling their family about a newly diagnosed condition because they may fail to communicate adequately the important information or significance of therapeutic medical management. In addition, individuals may not explain ways that family members can provide needed support.

Nurses can use a theoretical model to consider ways to deliver nursing care. For example, both the FMSF (Knafl & Deatrick, 1990, 2003) and the FHM (Denham, 2003) can assist nurses to consider family communication patterns and ways to meet educational needs aligned with family households. Understanding the ways families define the situation (see Table 10-1) can assist nurses to understand what information to provide to the newly diagnosed adult. Nurses who understand about core family processes can suggest ways to help individuals with skills for unique family household concerns (see Table 10-2). Family theories are important tools for nurses as they assess, plan, implement, and evaluate family management of chronic illness.

Household Relationships in Diabetes Management

Sarah must share the information about her diagnosis with her family members, and together they will interpret what this disease and its care needs will mean to their household. Although she has the ultimate responsibility for her diabetes self-management, the disease will be managed within the family household and will require significant family cooperation. The need to balance the rigor of complex self-care behaviors autonomously and the need to care for others in a household is a struggle faced by many adults living with diabetes. Control mainly resides with the person with the chronic condition, but it is continuously influenced by routines and behaviors of others in the household, as well as those in the wider community (Denham, Manoogian, & Schuster, 2007). Thus, it is important to understand chronic illness as a family matter.

Sarah is faced with many concerns that have implications for herself and her family. She needs to follow a medical regimen, plan dietary changes that will affect her entire family, consider costs related to her disease management and balance these with other family needs, learn to do blood glucose management, observe and be conscious of risks for additional complications, and become more active. She already has hypertension, depression, and early stages of neuropathy. She should likely make an appointment with her ophthalmologist to get her eyes examined soon and be concerned about early

retinopathy damage that may have already occurred. Consideration of whether James's health insurance plan will cover this medical visit may well determine whether Sarah makes and keeps an appointment. Not only must she do these things, but she must do them now. In some families living in the Appalachian region, mothers may be more likely to attend to the health care needs of their family members and less likely to address their own needs (Denham, 1997). Thus, a nurse working with Sarah needs to be sensitive to the kinds of counsel that she might need as she takes on what likely seems to be an overwhelming task.

Sarah's entire household has adopted sedentary lifestyles, and now she realizes that she needs to make some changes. But she wonders how she will be able to motivate her husband, James, and sons, Harry and Justin, to join her in making changes. Growing adolescent boys always seem to be hungry, and suggesting smaller portion sizes, ceasing to purchase foods known to be less nutritious and high in fat, or suggesting turning off the television and video games may not be well received. James's concerns about his job and future employment are additional stressors linked to financial costs for disease management. How do the family economic resources get stretched to cover multiple member and household needs? As a nurse working with this family, what kinds of advice might you give? What kinds of education and support might be needed?

Diabetes Self-Management

Diabetes self-management is predominately behavioral and largely occurs outside health professionals' observation. Self-management calls for integration of standards and evidence of best practice into the lived experience of those with type 2 diabetes. Self-management involves active participation of the person with the disease, motivation to participate, and ability to incorporate new information into daily life. Diabetes educators and other health professionals are challenged to reframe their roles and practices in ways that empower individuals to meet stated concerns, clarify authentic priorities, and operate within the limits of patient resources (Anderson & Funnell, 2005). Too often, nurses ignore a family's economic constraints and fail to offer information about ways to address costs of health care services. Thus, with type 2 diabetes, it is essential to address the importance of adequate medical management that prevents comorbidities and unnecessary hospitalizations for hyperglycemia or other untoward events.

A large body of literature about self-efficacy has shown it to be an important factor linked with a willingness to participate in specific behavior; it has been negatively correlated to mood, anxiety, and feelings of helplessness. Persons with higher self-efficacy are more likely to engage in more challenging tasks, set higher goals, and achieve them (Bandura, 1977; Locke & Latham, 1990). The *Transtheoretical Model of Change* (Prochaska & DiClemente, 1983, 1984) has five stages: precontemplation, contemplation, preparation, action, and maintenance. Given that diabetes touches so many life areas, it is expected that individuals within a family may have different levels of self-efficacy and be at different levels of readiness for changes needed for diabetes self-management. Nurses who understand self-efficacy and readiness to change can use these concepts together with ideas about family health routines from the FHM (Denham, 2003) to empower individuals and family households. Specifically, a nurse can help Sarah and her family identify the ways they agree or differ in their willingness to make changes and assess their perceptions about unique abilities to make the changes. A nurse might identify that Harry and Justin are at different places in their personal willingness to alter lifestyle habits that might support their mother better. What might a nurse do to help the Halloway family identify Sarah's diabetes care needs and then incorporate these things into the existing or reconstructed daily family routines? How can the nurse assist Harry and Justin to identify ways their personal routines might need to be adjusted to support their mother and reduce their health risks?

Diabetes Comorbidities

Whether a person has type 1 or type 2 diabetes, they are at increased risk for additional disease-related complications or comorbid conditions. Sarah realizes that she has two coexisting chronic conditions (i.e., hypertension and depression) at the time of her diabetes diagnosis, and also becomes aware that the numbness that she has been experiencing is called *neuropathy* and may have serious future consequences. This case study does not provide enough information about the adequacy of her hypertension control or the length of time she has had the disorder. Neither does the case study tell us anything about her cholesterol level. Some critical information is portrayed, however: She is overweight, sedentary, and seems to consume a high-fat, high-calorie diet. Given the new diabetes diagnosis, a nurse might want to concentrate on aiming for tight glycemic management. Focusing on the management of her hypertension, if it is uncontrolled, may be a more immediate response for her overall health. Focusing on specific target goals is an excellent way to help Sarah make plans for lifestyle changes. Diabetes management, much like any other chronic disease management, can be overwhelming. How can a nurse assist Sarah and her family to prioritize their needs and at the same time make the changes that are absolutely essential as quickly as possible?

Depression is an additional comorbid condition for Sarah, which in her case, fortunately, had been diagnosed (American Diabetes Association, n.d.). The depression she experiences is likely to be an additional complicating factor in her daily outlook and energy levels. Although we can trust that Dr. Anderson is providing good medical management, it is possible that Sarah actually needs to see a specialist to assist her to get her depression under better control. A stigma is still linked with many forms of mental illness, including depression. Although Sarah is taking medication for the condition, she may be unwilling to discuss her concerns with others, admit she has any problems, or seek counseling if she thinks others will ridicule or think negatively about her. Relationships between diabetes and depression are still not completely understood, and the condition often goes undiagnosed and untreated. Thus, nurses working with clients with diabetes should be aware of the high risks for depression, assess whether the treatment received is adequate, and counsel about ways to manage and control the depression (Anderson, Freedland, Clouse, & Lustman, 2000). If the depression is not treated, it is likely that the diabetes will also be poorly managed. Research has also shown that depression, well-being, and psychosocial functioning are important quality-of-life indicators (de Groot et al., 2007). If Sarah has difficulty getting her blood glucose levels under control, then it is possible that her depression might worsen, which means that she might be even less likely to follow the needed routines for optimal self-management.

What interventions might nurses suggest as they work with Sarah and her family? How can a nurse assist Sarah to overcome the challenges she is apt to encounter as she copes with her multiple care needs? In what ways can the nurse provide family support that addresses the family members' concerns as they attempt to make needed lifestyle changes?

Current Research About Type 2 Diabetes

Research about type 2 diabetes is expanding to not only address adults, but also to consider the growing number of children and adolescents being diagnosed with the disease. Just over a decade ago, adolescents accounted for only about 3% of new-onset type 2 diabetes cases, but currently, 45% of adolescents diagnosed with new-onset diabetes are diagnosed with type 2 diabetes (Pinhas-Hamiel & Zeitler, 2005). Obesity has become increasingly recognized as a risk factor during adolescence, with costs likely exceeding $127 million for hospital costs for youths aged 6 to 17 years (Goran, Ball, & Cruz, 2008). A recent review of reports on acute and long-term comorbidities of youths with type 2 diabetes (Pinhaus-Hamiel & Zeitler, 2007) has indicated several critical concerns:

- Past research often has uncertain applicability because of small sample sizes, reports on only particular populations, broad variability in age range and duration of follow-up, and identification of many different comorbidities.
- We should recognize that obesity in all young people, regardless of whether they have been diagnosed with type 2 diabetes, is associated with risks for comorbidities.
- Occurrence of type 2 diabetes during youth or adolescence seems to place the individual at risk for morbidity and mortality during the most productive life years.
- Long-term data about potential benefits of early adjunctive treatments are scarce.

Studies about risks in children and youths will be important for establishing whether the pathophysiology, disease development, and premature cardiovascular disease are similar to adults, and whether treatments should be the same or different (Goran, Ball, & Cruz, 2008).

Research in all of these areas is important if we are to develop approaches to increase awareness and early medical management and initiation of adjunctive treatments. Still, the focus on medical management frequently underestimates the attention needed for prevention and lifestyle behaviors that occur within the family household and social context. For instance, behavioral factors such as tobacco use, heavy alcohol use, and obesity are prevalent concerns, have been linked with multiple chronic health conditions, and are closely connected to health care costs, disabilities, and mortality (Sturm, 2002). Some indications exist that obesity may be more closely related to chronic medical problems, quality of life, and health care or medication expenses than smoking or problem drinking (Sturm, 2002). Lifestyle behaviors occur within a family household where members often share common risks. Thus, parents who themselves are at risk for type 2 diabetes may have formed a family lifestyle that also puts their young children at risk for chronic health conditions. Use of the CCM (Glasgow et al., 2001) should enable nurses to see that interventions in the health care systems must be merged with those that occur at home and in the community. The FHM (Denham, 2003) can assist nurses to consider the many ways parents, family household, and larger social contexts are influencing lifestyle behaviors and health outcomes. Research is needed to understand these interactive processes and factors to develop family education pertinent to chronic illness that aids health promotion, disease prevention, and self-management of chronic illness.

Diabetes literature indicates much attention has been concentrated on improving diabetes self-management and self-efficacy; focus on the individual, however, has largely obscured the fact that families are and need to be involved (Fisher et al., 1998). Although thought is often focused on the family when the diagnosis is type 1 diabetes, far less attention is given to the needs of family when an adult is diagnosed with type 2 diabetes. In families with adult members who have type 2 diabetes, family health routines have been identified that correspond to the behavioral aspects of diabetes treatment and can serve as instrumental ways to consider self-management (Collier, 2007; Denham, Manoogian, & Schuster, 2007). A diabetes diagnosis affects previously constructed health routines; these old behaviors often need to be deconstructed and new ones formed in accord with unique family needs (Denham & Manoogian, unpublished). In diabetes self-management, differences in family members have implications for member support or threats to dietary and other care routines (Schuster, 2005).

Stimpson and Peek (2005) have studied the social concordance or social contextual factors that shape health in a shared living environment where one spouse has a chronic illness. In studying Mexican Americans, they found that a husband's risk for being diagnosed with hypertension, diabetes, arthritis, and cancer was significantly increased when the wife was diagnosed with the corresponding condition. Future research in this area needs to investigate the ways concordance operates, whether healthy individuals are more inclined to select healthier mates, or whether it is more of an effect caused by shared environmental stressors and risk factors or the ways mates influence one another. Research that provides nurses with evidence-based reports, best-practice guidelines, and standards of care that nurses can use to translate medical information into lifestyle routines by multiple-member households is needed to assist families with the many diverse types of chronic illnesses.

Summary of Family Nursing Intervention During Chronic Illness

Nurses' roles should be aimed primarily at assisting multiple family members to interact in ways that optimize each one's abilities and strengths. Although chronic illness care requires consideration of individual outcomes, this must be addressed within the family milieu to consider long-term caregiver needs and family outcomes. Across the life course, families use management styles, functional processes, and family health routines to address actual problems, minimize risks, and maximize potentials. Nurses who seek to empower and collaborate with families will most likely be most effective in meeting chronic care needs. Whether the chronic condition pertains to a child or an adult, at the time of diagnosis, nurses can use these ideas to discuss ways caregivers and nonafflicted members can integrate disease management routines into the family's daily life. These topics can be used as ways to support and acknowledge family caregivers' abilities and skills to learn to manage the illness proficiently.

Nurses assist families to find ways to balance illness needs by discussing areas such as family strengths, couple time, developmental milestones, sibling needs, economic restraints, and caregiver well-being. Adequacy of family communication and cooperation are areas for nurses to assess, make appropriate referrals, and evaluate over time.

In chronic illness care, nurses can provide family-focused care that assists family of origin and extended kin to obtain needed information, resources, education, counseling, or other needed support. (See the Chapter Web Site section later in this chapter for resources.) Family-focused care should address ways to prevent or reduce additional health risks, maintain optimal levels of wellness for all family members, develop therapeutic care management routines, set goals that enhance individual and family well-being and integrity, and enable members to accommodate unplanned changes. The FHM (Denham, 2003) suggests that families have *core processes* (i.e., caregiving, cathexis, celebration, change, communication, connectedness, coordination) or areas germane to ways families interact with one another. Nurses can use these ideas as targets when working with families who have a member with a chronic illness (see Table 10-3).

ILLNESS MANAGEMENT IN PRIMARY CARE

The CCM has implications for the development of truly collaborative interdisciplinary teams that use technologies and environments to support quality care (Grumbach, 2003). Unfortunately, although many programs are beginning to aim to use a CCM to focus on primary care, the emphasis is still too often on patient-centered rather than family-focused care. Using more global assessments of care needs, rather than merely using disease-specific foci, assists nurses to be more sensitive to family preferences and priorities. Consideration of family concerns such as quality of life, symptom management, and social needs at the beginning of care, rather than as outcomes, provides a more holistic approach to service delivery. Nurses that value the family's role in chronic illness management must advocate for care management that is inclusive of the breadth of family and meets the complex needs that occur outside the purview of medical professionals.

Families with chronic conditions, especially those whose conditions are complicated and require care from multiple specialists, often spend a great deal of time interfacing with the health care system for management of the condition and regular follow-up with specialists. For example, a family who has a child with Down syndrome may require regular visits for cardiac, ophthalmologic, developmental, and immunologic evaluations, physical and occupational therapy, and orthopedic assessments. In addition, parents typically spend a significant amount of time and energy advocating for their child within the school system, attending Individualized Educational Program (IEP) meetings, meeting with academic support professionals, and coping with worries about what is occurring when the child is out of sight.

In addition, children with chronic conditions still need well-child care similar to those without such an illness. Furthermore, they are susceptible to other infectious diseases or risks for injuries. It is important for children with chronic conditions to receive regular health maintenance visits with a primary care provider for anticipatory guidance, routine illness, and injury prevention discussions. Parents of children with chronic conditions expect to discuss illness concerns during the well-child care visit. Some providers may expect that care for chronic disease management will decrease opportunities for wellness discussion, but a study of primary care provision for children with SHCN demonstrated the opposite (Van Cleave, Heisler, Devries, Joiner, & Davis, 2007). For parents of children with SHCN and other parents, as more illness topics were discussed, more prevention topics were also discussed.

INFORMATION AND MUTUAL TRUST

Researchers who have interviewed parents of children with chronic conditions report some consistent expectations that parents have for their encounters with professionals. Especially important is parents' need for information and mutual trust (Nuutila & Salantera, 2006). Parents want information to be communicated clearly, honestly, respectfully, and with empathy. To be able to give advice and guidance applicable to the lives of a family, health professionals need to know about the family's everyday living and life conditions, and must recognize parents' abilities and skills in caring for their child (Nuutila & Salantera, 2006). Whether the chronically ill person is a child or an adult, family members require useful information that can be directly applied to real family needs. A trusting environment must be established where information can be exchanged easily, communication can be directed at meeting individual and family needs, and all perceive that they are treated with respect.

Families want information that will help them to care adequately for their child and anticipate the needs of their child into the future. Often, excellent informational resources are available but remain unknown to families because professionals assume that someone else has provided the family with the information (Ray, 2003). Parents' and others' needs for information and support change over time as they move through phases of the illness and the family life cycle (Nuutila & Salantera, 2006). At the time of diagnosis, parents want clear and consistent information, and possibly a more directive approach from the provider. For example, when a child with Down syndrome is born, the parents may want to know the immediate implications for the child's health and how that will affect their ability to care for the child at home. As the child grows older and the family gains experience in the care of the child, parents may want a less directive approach from the provider and more of a mutual exchange of information in a collaborative partnership (Nuutila & Salantera, 2006). The nurse who encounters this family at a 3-year well-child exam, for example, should acknowledge the parent's intimate understanding of the child, his or her reactions to the environment, and his or her unique needs during the clinical encounter. The most helpful advice from the nurse at this point is likely in the form of anticipatory guidance and planning for entry into the school system. However, nurses must recognize that individual and family needs will greatly differ for this same child as he or she becomes 16, 28, or 46 years of age, for example.

EMPOWERMENT

In chronic disease management, family-focused care needs to afford optimal clinical care services, and equip these individuals and their families with knowledge and tools to be effective self-managers (Wagner et al., 2001). Use of an empowerment model that includes several components (e.g., patient-centered care, problem-based, strength-based, evidence-based, culturally relevant) and uses an integrative process to respond to unique diabetes-related needs has been shown to be successful

(Tang, Funnell, & Anderson, 2006). Empowerment acknowledges that the patient is central to chronic care self-management. However, greater attention is still needed to the ways patient education and care can be reformed into family-focused care management. For example, when a child has diabetes, the education is aimed at the parents, considers the child's developmental abilities, and assists both in knowledge and skills for self-management. However, if an adult is diagnosed with type 2 diabetes, then although diabetes educators may be welcoming to additional family members, they are not considered necessary to the care and attention to empowering families. As nurses seek to empower families for chronic illness management, the CCM encourages flexibility, consideration of organizational characteristics, coordinated actions of multiple caregivers, use of evidence-based guidelines, identification of community resources, and education that builds confidence and skills in multiple family members (Wagner et al., 2001). More evidence about empowerment interventions is needed to show how they effectively address needs (Henshaw, 2006), but additional concerns are connected to the development and testing of effective chronic care family education models that empower individuals and family members to self-manage chronic conditions effectively.

ROUTINE INTERVENTIONS

Families typically vary in four systematic ways in their abilities to incorporate medical regimens into their daily routines, and these four R's of routine interventions are remediation, redefinition, realignment, and re-education (Fiese & Everhart, 2006). Remediation refers to a need to make slight alterations in daily routines to fit illness care into preexisting routines. For both the Yates and Halloway families, this might include changes in meal plans or timing of meals to incorporate dietary and insulin needs. Redefinition refers to a strategy whereby the emotional connections made during routine gatherings need to be redefined. For the Yates family, it is important for family members to consider the management of Chloe's diabetes an alteration, not an intrusion, in their daily lives. Chloe's recent poor metabolic control may represent her own perception that the management of her diabetes has taken over her life, especially with her peers. Realignment occurs when individuals within the family disagree

about the importance of different medical routines, and routines need to be realigned in the service of the child's health. The fourth form, re-education, is indicated when the family has little history or experience with routines and family life is substantially disorganized (Fiese & Everhart, 2006). These same ideas can also be used to consider changes and needs within the Halloway family.

Research about family health suggests that structural behaviors or family health routines are visible activities that family members can readily recall and discuss from multiple perspectives (Denham, 1997, 1999a, 1999b, 1999c). Although family members may report similarities in routines, unique variations are common. The nested family context is a powerful, persuasive, and motivating determinant that influences ways health information is incorporated into behaviors. Unique routine characteristics, rigidity and timing of activities, and member expectations vary across families and respond to different member beliefs, values, and perceived needs. One might expect that meaningful health information that fits with perceived family needs is most likely to be incorporated into behaviors that impact the management of a chronic condition. Thus, nursing assessment of chronic care management extends beyond the disease itself and is deeply entrenched in the ways a family functions and the life patterns they have previously established.

Family health routines include a number of categorically different foci. Self-care routines involve patterned behaviors related to usual activities of daily living. Safety and prevention routines are primarily concerned with health protection, disease prevention, prevention of unintended injury, and avoidance. However, a nurse assessing this routine area might also be interested in discerning less healthy habits and consider the impact of high-risk behaviors such as smoking, alcohol, and misuse of other substances on a chronic condition. Mental health routines are related to self-esteem, personal integrity, work and play, shared positive experiences, stress, self-efficacy, individuation, and family identity. Family-care routines are related to valued traditions, rituals, celebrations, vacations, and other events tied to making meaning and sharing enjoyable times. Illness-care routines are related to decisions about disease, illness, and chronic health care needs, and often determine when, where, and how members seek health care services and incorporate medical directives and health information into self-care routines. Family caregiving routines pertain to reciprocal member interactions believed to assist with health and illness care needs and support during times of crisis, loss, and death.

Families use these patterned behaviors or daily routines to arrange ordinary life and cope with health or illness events (Fiese & Wamboldt, 2000). These routines are embedded in the cultural and ecological context of families, and highlight ways to focus on family processes, individual, and family dynamics (Fiese, Tomcho, Douglas, Josephs, Poltrock, & Baker, 2002). Nurses aiming to provide education and counseling to individuals with a chronic illness need to understand the unique family routines of multiple household members and the ways chronic care management is going to alter patterns that are revered, cherished, and comfortable. Nurses who consider the four R's of routine intervention (Fiese & Everhart, 2006) in collaboration with families as assessments are completed, goals set, and outcomes measured increase the likelihood of achieving effective interventions that are sustainable over time.

SUMMARY

Family-focused care should not be considered optional when it comes to chronic illness. Chronic health conditions affect individuals and families differently than do acute conditions. Although the needs families experience may be similar initially, the duration of the illness alters the ways care is managed and perceived. The longevity, severity, and complexity of chronic care needs associated with chronic conditions have the potential to alter a desired or expected future into one that dramatically revolutionizes the lives of entire households. Financial costs and family resources are often highly taxed by years of debt and stress that would not be expected if a chronic condition had not occurred. Some children with SHCN and adults may require extraordinary adaptations by parents, siblings, and others that strain relationships. Although the chronic illnesses of children may be primarily genetic or environmental in nature, those of adults are often linked with lifestyle behaviors that might be prevented or delayed. Some conditions may worsen over time or require endless amounts of attention that can become especially burdensome as the child and

parent or caregiver ages, and either economic or family resources are exhausted. Family-focused care aimed at meeting needs of families who have a member or members with chronic illness requires nurses to have knowledge of many family dimensions and processes, and influences of other social contexts. To provide optimal nursing care related to chronic illness, nurses must be knowledgeable about individual and family developmental alterations, sensitive to their expressed needs, and willing to become collaborators that empower multiple household members to organize routines and manage resources for optimal disease management over time.

REFERENCES

Agency for Health Research and Quality. (AHRQ). (2008). *National Quality Measures Clearinghouse: Brief summary.* Retrieved July 12, 2008, from http://www.qualitymeasures.ahrq.gov/summary/summary.aspx?doc_id=12115

American Diabetes Association. (2008). Economic costs of diabetes in the U.S. in 2007. *Diabetes Care, 31*(3), 1–20.

American Diabetes Association. (n.d.). *Depression.* Retrieved June 29, 2008, from http://www.diabetes.org/type-2-diabetes/depression.jsp

Anderson, R. J., Freedland, K. E., Clouse, R. E., & Lustman, P. J. (2000). Prevalence of depression in adults with diabetes: A systematic review. *Diabetes, 49*(suppl 1), A64.

Anderson, R. M., & Funnell, M. M. (2005). Patient empowerment: Reflections on the challenge of fostering the adoption of a new paradigm. *Patient Education & Counseling, 57,* 153–157.

Bandura, A. (1977). Self-efficacy: Toward a unifying theory of behavioral change. *Psychological Review, 84,* 191–215.

Barlow, J. H., & Ellard, D. R. (2006). The psychosocial well-being of children with chronic disease, their parents and siblings: An overview of the research evidence base. *Child Care, Health & Development, 32*(1), 19–31.

Bellin, M. H., & Kovacs, P. (2006). Fostering resilience in siblings of youths with a chronic health condition: A review of the literature. *Health & Social Work, 31*(3), 209–216.

Berge, J. M., Patterson, J. M., & Rueter, M. (2006). Marital satisfaction and mental health of couples with children with chronic health conditions. *Families, Systems, & Health, 24*(3), 267–285.

Blomquist, K. B. (2006). Healthy and ready to work—Kentucky: Incorporating transition into a state program for children with special health care needs. *Pediatric Nursing, 32*(6), 515–528.

Brewer, H. M., Smith, J. A., Eatough, V., Stanley, C. A., Glendinning, N. W., & Quarrell, O. W. (2007). Caring for a child with Juvenile Huntington's Disease: Helpful and unhelpful support. *Journal of Child Health Care, 11*(1), 40–52.

Britner, P., Morog, M., Pianta, R., & Marvin, R. (2003). Stress and coping: A comparison of self-report measures of functioning in families of young children with cerebral palsy or no medical diagnosis. *Journal of Child and Family Studies, 12*(3), 335–348.

Britto, M. T., Slap, G. B., DeVellis, R. F., Hornung, R. W., Atherton, H. D., Knopf, J. M., et al. (2007). Specialists understanding of the health care preferences of chronically ill adolescents. *Journal of Adolescent Health, 40*(4), 334–341.

Centers for Disease Control and Prevention. (2008). Chronic disease overview. Retrieved April 14, 2008, from http://www.cdc.gov/nccdphp/overview.htm#2

Chesla, C. (1991). Parents' caring practices for the schizophrenic offspring. *Qualitative Health Research, 1*(4), 446–468.

Child and Adolescent Health Measurement Initiative (CAHMI). (2008). *2005/2006 national survey of children with special health care needs.* Retrieved July 14, 2008, from Data Resource Center for Child and Adolescent Health Web site: www.cshcndata.org

Cogswell, M. E., Gallagher, M. L., Steinberg, K. K., Caudill, S. P., Looker, A. C., Bowman, B. A., et al. (2003). HFE genotype and transferring saturation in the United States. *Genetics in Medicine, 5,* 304–310.

Collier, T. (2007). *Dietary routines and diabetes: Instrument development.* Unpublished master's thesis, Ohio University, College of Health and Human Services, Athens.

Dashiff, C., Bartolucci, A., Wallander, J., & Abdullatif, H. (2005). The relationship of family structure, maternal employment, and family conflict with self-care adherence of adolescents with type 1 diabetes. *Families, Systems, & Health, 23*(1), 66–70.

Deatrick, J. A., Knafl, K. A., & Murphy-Moore, C. (1999). Clarifying the concept of normalization. *Image: The Journal of Nursing Scholarship, 31*(3), 209–214.

de Groot, M., Doyle, T., Hockman, H., Wheeler, C., Pinkerman, B., Shubrook, J., et al. (2007). Depression among type 2 diabetes rural Appalachian clinic attendees. *Diabetes Care, 30,* 1602–1604.

Denham, S. A. (1997). *An ethnographic study of family health in Appalachian microsystems.* Unpublished doctoral dissertation, University of Alabama at Birmingham.

Denham, S. A. (1999a). The definition and practice of family health. *Journal of Family Nursing, 5*(2), 133–159.

Denham, S. A. (1999b). Family health: During and after death of a family member. *Journal of Family Nursing, 5*(2), 160–183.

Denham, S. A. (1999c). Family health in an economically disadvantaged population. *Journal of Family Nursing, 5*(2), 184–213.

Denham, S. A. (2003). *Family health: A framework for nursing.* Philadelphia: F.A. Davis.

Denham, S. A., & Manoogian, M. (unpublished). Patterns of support: Type 2 diabetes and older rural families.

Denham, S. A., Manoogian, M., & Schuster, L. (2007). Managing family support and dietary routines: Type 2 diabetes in rural Appalachian families. *Families, Systems, & Health, 25*(1), 36–52.

DeVol, R. (2008). Center for health economics. Retrieved June 28, 2008, from http://www.milkeninstitute.org/research/research.taf?cat=health

DeVol, R., & Bedroussian, A. (2007). *An unhealthy America: The economic burden of chronic disease charting a new course to save lives and increase productivity and economic growth.* Milken Institute. Retrieved June 28, 2008, from http://www.milkeninstitute.org/pdf/chronic_disease_report.pdf

Dickinson, A. R., Smythe, E., & Spence, D. (2006). Within the web: The family-practitioner relationship in the context of chronic childhood illness. *Journal of Child Health Care, 10*(4), 309–325.

Fiese, B. H., & Everhart, R. S. (2006). Medical adherence and childhood chronic illness: Family daily management skills and emotional climate as emerging contributors. *Current Opinion in Pediatrics, 18*(5), 551–557.

Fiese, B. H., & Wambolt, F. (2000). Family routines and asthma management: A proposal for family-based strategies to increase treatment adherence. *Families, Systems, & Health, 18,* 405–418.

Fiese, B. H., Tomcho, T. J., Douglas, M., Josephs, K., Poltrock, S., & Baker, T. (2002). A review of 50 years of research on naturally occurring family routines and rituals: Cause for celebration? *Journal of Family Psychology, 16,* 381–390.

Fisher, L., Chesla, C. A., Bartz, R. J., Gilliss, C., Skaff, M. A., Sabogal, F., et al. (1998). The family and type 2 diabetes: A framework for intervention. *Diabetes Educator, 24,* 599–607.

Fisher, L., Chesla, C., Skaff, M., Gilliss, C., Kanter, R., Lutz, C., et al. (2000). Disease management status: A typology of Latino and Euro-American patients with type 2 diabetes. *Behavioral Medicine, 26,* 53–65.

Georgetown University Health Policy Institute. (2007). *Long-term financing project: National spending for long term care.* Retrieved July 19, 2008, from http://ltc.georgetown.edu/pdfs/natspendfeb07.pdf

Gibson, M. J., & Houser, A. (2007). *AARP Policy Institute: Economic value of family caregivers brief.* Retrieved July 19, 2008, from http://www.nfcacares.org/pdfs/NewLookattheEconomicValueofFamilyCaregivingIssueBrief.pdf

Glasgow, R. E., Orleans, C. T., Wagner, E. H. (2001). Does the Chronic Care Model serve also as a template for improving prevention? *The Milbank Quarterly, 79*(4), 579–612.

Goran, M. I., Ball, G. D. C., & Cruz, M. L. (2008). Obesity and risk of type 2 diabetes and cardiovascular disease in children and adolescents. *Journal of Endocrinology & Metabolism, 88*(4), 1417–1427.

Grumbach, L. (2003). Chronic illness, comorbidities, and the need for medical generalism. *Annals of Family Medicine, 1*(1), 4–7.

Health Resources and Service Administration. (n.d.). *Hill-Burton free and reduced cost health care.* Retrieved June 24, 2008, from http://www.hrsa.gov/hillburton/

Henshaw, L (2006). Empowerment, diabetes and the National Service Framework: A systematic review. *Journal of Diabetes Nursing, 10*(4), 128, 130–135.

House, J. S. (1981). *Work stress and social support.* Reading, MA: Addison-Wesley.

Improving Chronic Illness Care. (2008). *The Chronic Care Model.* Retrieved June 24, 2008, from http://www.improvingchroniccare.org

Institute of Medicine. (2001). *Crossing the quality chasm: A new health system for the 21st century.* Washington, DC: National Academy Press.

Knafl, K., Breitmayer, B., Gallo, A., & Zoeller, L. (1996). Family response to childhood chronic illness: Description of management styles. *Journal of Pediatric Nursing, 11*(5), 315–326.

Knafl, K., & Deatrick, J. (1990). Family management style: Concept analysis and development. *Journal of Pediatric Nursing, 5*(1), 4–14.

Knafl, K., & Deatrick, J. (2003). Further refinement of the Family Management Style Framework. *Journal of Family Nursing, 9*(3), 232–256.

Kutner, M., Greenberg, E., Jin, Y., & Paulsen, C. (2006). *The health literacy of America's adults: Results from the 2003 National Assessment of Adult Literacy* (NCES 2006-483). Washington, DC: National Center for Education Statistics (NCES).

Libraries for the Future. (2006). *Health literacy basics.* Retrieved July 9, 2008, from http://www.lff.org/ffl/healthliteracy.rtf

Lobato, D. J., & Kao, B. T. (2005). Brief report: Family-based group intervention for young siblings of children with chronic illness and developmental disability. *Journal of Pediatric Psychology, 30,* 678–682.

Locke, E. A., & Latham, G. P. (1990). *A theory of goal setting and task performance.* Englewood Cliffs, NJ: Prentice Hall.

Looman, W. S. (2006). Development and testing of the Social Capital Scale for families of children with chronic conditions. *Research in Nursing & Health, 29*(4), 325–336.

Looman, W. S., O'Conner-Von, S. K., Ferski, G. J., & Hildenbrand, D. A. (2009). Financial and employment problems in families of children with special health care needs: Implications for research and practice. *Journal of Pediatric Health Care, 23*(2), 117–125.

Lose, E. J., & Robin, N. H. (2007). Caring for adults with pediatric genetic diseases: A growing need. *Current Opinion in Pediatrics, 19*(6), 611–612.

Mack, J. W., Co, J. P., Goldmann, D. A., Weeks, J. C., & Cleary, P. D. (2007). Quality of health care for children: Role of health and chronic illness in inpatient care experiences. *Archives of Pediatrics & Adolescent Medicine, 161*(9), 828–834.

Martin, J. A., Kung, H., Matthews, T. J., Hoyert, D. L., Strobino, B. G., Guyer, B., & Sutton, S. R. (2008). Annual summary of vital statistics: 2006. *Pediatrics, 121,* 788–801.

McClellan, C. B., & Cohen, L. L. (2007). Family functioning in children with chronic illness compared with healthy controls: A critical review. *Journal of Pediatrics, 150*(3), 221–223.

McCubbin, H. I., Thompson, A. I., & McCubbin, M. A. (1996). Resiliency in families: A conceptual model of family adjustment and adaptation in response to stress and crisis. In H. I. McCubbin, A. I. Thompson, & M. A. McCubbin (Eds.), *Family assessment: Resiliency, coping and adaptation—inventories for research and practice* (pp. 1–64). Madison: University of Wisconsin Publishers.

McPherson, M., Arango, P., Fox, H., Lauver, C., McManus, M., Newacheck, P., et al. (1998). A new definition of children with special health care needs. *Pediatrics, 102*(1), 137–140.

Meltzer, L. J., & Mindell, J. A. (2006). Impact of a child's chronic illness on maternal sleep and daytime functioning. *Archives of Internal Medicine, 166*(16), 1749–1755.

Miller, J. F. (2000). Client power resources. In J. F. Miller (Ed.), *Coping with chronic illness* (pp. 3–19). Philadelphia: F.A. Davis.

Mitchell, M. J., Lemanek, K., Palermo, T. M., Crosby, L. E., Nichols, A., & Powers, S. W. (2007). Parent perspectives on pain management, coping, and family functioning in pediatric sickle cell disease. *Clinical Pediatrics, 46*(4), 311–319.

Mussatto, K. (2006). Adaptation of the child and family to life with a chronic illness. *Cardiology in the Young, 16*(suppl 3), 110–116.

National Center on Birth Defects and Developmental Disabilities. (2008). *Autism information center.* Retrieved July 14, 2008, from http://www.cdc.gov/ncbddd/autism/faq_prevalence.htm#whatisprevalence

Nuutila, L., & Salantera, S. (2006). Children with a long-term illness: Parents' experiences of care. *Journal of Pediatric Nursing, 21*(2), 153–160.

Partnership for Solutions. (2004). *Chronic conditions: Making the case for ongoing care.* Retrieved June 24, 2008, from Robert Wood Johnson Web site: http://www.rwjf.org/pr/product.jsp?id=14685

Perrin, J. M., Bloom, S. R., & Gortmaker, S. L. (2007). The increase of childhood chronic conditions in the United States. *JAMA, 297,* 2755–2759.

Pinhas-Hamiel, O., & Zeitler, P. (2005). The global spread of type 2 diabetes mellitus in children and adolescents. *Journal of Pediatrics, 146,* 693–700.

Prochaska, J. O., & DiClemente, C. C. (1983). Stages and processes of self-change of smoking: Toward an integrative model of change. *Journal of Consulting and Clinical Psychology, 51,* 390–395.

Prochaska, J. O., & DiClemente, C. C. (1984). *The transtheoretical approach: Crossing traditional boundaries of change.* Homewood, IL: Irwin.

Putnam, R. (1996). Who killed civic America? *The American Prospect, 4*(13), 11–18.

Rabiee, P., Sloper, P., & Beresford, B. (2005). Desired outcomes for children and young people with complex health care needs, and children who do not use speech for communication. *Health & Social Care in the Community, 13*(5), 478–487.

Ray, L. D. (2003). The social and political conditions that shape special-needs parenting. *Journal of Family Nursing, 9*(3), 281–304.

Reeve, C. (1999). *Still me.* New York: Ballantine Books.

Rehm, R. S., & Bradley, J. F. (2005). Normalization in families raising a child who is medically fragile/technology dependent and developmentally delayed. *Qualitative Health Research, 15*(6), 807–820.

Robles, T. F., & Kiecolt-Glaser, J. K. (2003). The physiology of marriage: Pathways to health. *Physiological Behavior, 70,* 409–416.

Rodrigues, N., & Patterson, J. M. (2007). Impact of severity of a child's chronic condition on the functioning of two-parent families. *Journal of Pediatric Psychology, 32*(4), 417–426.

Schiller Institute. (2001). The Hill-Burton Act. Retrieved June 24, 2008, from http://www.schillerinstitute.org/health/hill_burton.html#anchor

Schmidt, C. (2007). Self-care in children with type 1 diabetes: A survey of mothers. *MCN, American Journal of Maternal Child Nursing, 32*(4), 223–229.

Schuster, L. (2005). Family support in dietary routines in Appalachians with type 2 diabetes. Unpublished master's thesis, Ohio University, Athens.

Siegel, K., & Lekas, H. (2002). AIDS as a chronic illness: Psychosocial implications. *AIDS Supplement, 16,* S69–S76.

Spilkin, A., & Ballantyne, A. (2007). Behavior in children with a chronic illness: A descriptive study of child characteristics, family adjustment, and school issues in children with cystinosis. *Families, Systems, & Health, 25*(1), 68–84.

Stimpson, J. P., & Peek, M. K. (2005). Concordance of chronic conditions in older Mexican American couples. *Preventing Chronic Illness, 2*(3), 1–7.

Strohm, K. (2001). Sibling project. *Youth Studies Australia, 20*(4), 48–53.

Sturm, R. (2002). The effects of obesity, smoking, and drinking on medical problems and costs. *Health Affairs, 21*(2), 245–253.

Sullivan-Bolyai, S., Knafl, K. A., Sadler, L., & Gilliss, C. L. (2004). Family matters. Great expectations: A position description for parents as caregivers: Part II. *Pediatric Nursing, 30*(1), 52–56.

Tang, T. S., Funnell, M. M., & Anderson, R. M. (2006). Group education strategies for diabetes self-management. *Diabetes Spectrum, 19*(2), 99–105.

Tower, R. B., Kasl, S. V., & Darefsky, A. S. (2002). Types of marital closeness and mortality risk in older couples. *Psychosomatic Medicine, 64*, 644–659.

U.S. Code. (2007). *Title 42: The public and health law.* Retrieved June 3, 2008, from http://www.access.gpo.gov/uscode/title42/title42.html

U.S. Department of Health and Human Services, Health Resources and Services Administration, Maternal and Child Health Bureau. (2008). *The National Survey of Children with Special Health Care Needs Chartbook 2005–2006.* Rockville, MD: Author.

Van Cleave, J., Heisler, M., Devries, J. M., Joiner, T. A., & Davis, M. M. (2007). Discussion of illness during well-child care visits with parents of children with and without special health care needs. *Archives of Pediatrics & Adolescent Medicine, 161*(12), 1170–1175.

Wagner, E. H. (1998). Chronic disease management: What will it take to improve care for chronic illness? *Effective Clinical Practice, 1*, 2–4.

Wagner, E. H., Austin, B. T., Davis, C., Hindmarsh, M., Schaefer, J., & Bonomi, A. (2001). Improving chronic illness care: Translating evidence into action. *Health Affairs, 20*, 64–78.

Wagner, E. H., Davis, C., Homer, C. J., Hagedorn, S. D., Austin, B., & Caplan, A. (2002). *Accelerating change today: Curing the system: Stories of change in chronic illness care.* The National Coalition of Health Care, the Institute for Health care Improvement. Retrieved July 15, 2008, from http://www.improvingchroniccare.org/downloads/act_report_may_2002_curing_the_system.pdf

Walters, B. (2004). Barbara Walters's Last Interview with Christopher Reeves. Retrieved on May 9, 2009, from http://abcnews.go.com/2020/ABCNEWSSpecial/story?id=124364&page=1

Wennick, A., & Hallstrom, I. (2007). Families' lived experience one year after a child was diagnosed with type 1 diabetes. *Journal of Advanced Nursing, 60*, 299–307.

CHAPTER WEB SITES

Chronic Illness

- *Centers for Disease Control and Prevention: National Center on Birth Defects and Developmental Disabilities:* http://www. cdc.gov/ncbddd
This Web site offers information about prevention, causes of birth defects and developmental disabilities, ways to help children develop and reach their full potential, and ways to promote health and well-being among people with disabilities of all ages.
- *Centers for Disease Control and Prevention: National Center for Chronic Disease Prevention and Health Promotion:* http:// www.cdc.gov/nccdphp

This site provides access to many resources relevant to chronic conditions.
- *Center for Health Care Strategies (CHCS):* http://www.chcs.org
This nonprofit health policy resource center is dedicated to improving the quality and cost effectiveness of health care services for low-income populations and people with chronic illnesses and disabilities.
- *Christopher and Dana Reeve Foundation Paralysis Resource Center:* http://www.paralysis.org/site/c.erJMJUOxFmH/b.1169107/k.BE3A/Home.htm
This site offers information and resources for those with spinal cord injury, mobility impairment, and paralysis.
- *Chronic Conditions: Making the Case for Ongoing Care (2004):* http://www.rwjf.org/pr
This chart book provides an overview of chronic health conditions in the United States and the impact of these conditions on individuals, their caregivers, and the U.S. health care system.
- *Conill Institute for Chronic Illness:* http://www.conillinst.org
This nonprofit organization develops educational programs to help patients, families, care partners, and employers deal effectively with chronic illness and disability.
- *CSHCN Screener:* http://www.cahmi.org
The CSHCN Screener is a five-item survey tool that uses noncondition-specific, consequence-based criteria to identify children with special health care needs. It is available at no charge with supporting materials, scoring programs, and technical documentation. English- and Spanish-language versions of the CSHCN Screener, as well as adolescent and adult self-report versions, are also available.
- *CureResearch.com:* http://www.cureresearch.com/index.htm
This Web site is maintained by an independent technology company that claims not to be affiliated with a medical or drug organization and suggests that the information offered is factual and unbiased.
- *Data Resource Center for Child and Adolescent Health:* http://www.childhealthdata.org
This site enables individuals to search and compare national, state, or regional results on key health outcomes based on the 2005–2006 National Survey of Children with Special Health Care Needs. It includes results for survey sections on Family-Centered Care and Impact on Families.
- *Family History Resources and Tools:* http://www.cdc.gov/genomics/public/famhist.htm
In 1997, the Centers for Disease Control and Prevention (CDC) established the Office of Genetics and Disease Prevention, which has been named the National Office of Public Health Genomics (NOPHG) since 2006. This office aims to use genomic knowledge to improve the lives and health of all people. This site provides many tools for working with families as you consider ways to use their family history to promote health.
- *HealingWell.com:* http://www.healingwell.com/pages
HealingWell.com is a community and information resource for patients, caregivers, and families coping with diseases, disorders, and chronic illnesses. They offer health resources, interactive tools, and community support to enable individuals to take control of chronic illness.
- *Improving Chronic Illness Care:* http://www.improvingchroniccare.org
This site provides information about the Chronic Care Model, a model that originated from a synthesis of the literature by the

MacColl Institute for Healthcare Innovation in the 1990s and has been supported by the Robert Wood Johnson Foundation.

- *MedlinePlus: Coping with Chronic Illness:* http://www.nlm.nih.gov/medlineplus/copingwithchronicillness.html
This site provides a number of resources relevant to living with chronic illness.
- *Science Daily: Chronic Illness News:* http://www.sciencedaily.com/news/health_medicine/chronic_illness/
This site is an excellent place to find recent and archived news pertaining to chronic illness conditions, together with videos, images, and book information.
- *The Sibling Support Project:* http://www.siblingsupport.org
This project is a national effort dedicated to the lifelong concerns of brothers and sisters of people who have special health, developmental, or mental health concerns.
- *Transition Timeline for Children and Adolescents with Special Health Care Needs:* http://depts.washington.edu/healthtr/Timeline/timeline.htm
Developed by the Adolescent Health Transition Project, the timeline can be printed as a handout or wall chart, and provides ideas to help children and youth to achieve independence in their own health care and in other areas of life as they grow. Forms for children and adolescents with developmental disabilities or delays, or both, or chronic illnesses or physical disabilities, or both, are available in English, Spanish, Russian, Chinese, and Vietnamese.
- *Who Cares: Chronic Illness in America (PBS):* http://www.pbs.org/inthebalance/archives/whocares
This 2001 television program explored the many problems linked with chronic illness played out in homes and health care centers across the nation. Multiple resources linked with this presentation are located at this site.

Family Caregiver Resources

- *Family Caregiving 101:* http://www.familycaregiving101.org
The site is designed for families and individuals to provide assistance, answers, new ideas, and helpful advice.
- *Family Caregiver Alliance:*
http://www.caregiver.org/caregiver/jsp/home.jsp
This was the first community-based nonprofit organization in the country to address the needs of families and friends who provide long-term care at home. The group offers programs

at national, state, and local levels to support and sustain caregivers.

- *National Alliance for Caregivers:* http://www.caregiving.org
This is a nonprofit coalition of national organizations that focus on issues of family caregiving. Alliance members include grassroots organizations, professional associations, service organizations, disease-specific organizations, a government agency, and corporations. The alliance was created to conduct research, do policy analysis, develop national programs, increase public awareness of family caregiving issues, work to strengthen state and local caregiving coalitions, and represent the U.S. caregiving community internationally.
- *National Family Caregivers Association:* http://www.nfcacares.org
This organization provides education, reports, and support to empower and speak for the needs of the millions of Americans who care for loved ones with a chronic illness or disability or the frailties of old age. Check out the *National Family Caregiver Story*, a collection of stories about caregivers' experiences.

Additional Health Literacy Information

- *American Medical Association Foundation: Health Literacy:* http://kb.ncchca.org/article.aspx?id=10157&cNode=8M6C6P
This site provides information about toolkits, professional, and patient education tools pertaining to health literacy.
- *Clear Communication: An NIH Health Literacy Initiative:* http://www.nih.gov/icd/od/ocpl/resources/clearcommunication/healthliteracy.htm
This site provides relevant research and resources about health literacy.
- *Health Resources and Service Administration (HRSA): Health Literacy:* http://www.hrsa.gov/healthliteracy
HRSA provides information for health care providers about health literacy including a training program that can be accessed at this site.
- *National Assessment of Adult Literacy:* http://nces.ed.gov/naal
This site provides information about adult literacy and links to the 2006 *NAAL Health Literacy Report*.
- *Pfizer Clear Health Communication Initiative:* http://www.pfizerhealthliteracy.org
This site provides resources for researchers, health professionals, public health workers, and others.

CHAPTER 11

Families in Palliative and End-of-Life Care

Rose Steele, PhD, RN

Carole Robinson, PhD, RN

Lissi Hansen, PhD, RN

Kimberly A. Widger, PhD(c), RN

CRITICAL CONCEPTS

+ Palliative care is both a philosophy and a type of care.

+ Palliative care involves a focus on quality of life, or living well, for all family members when they are dealing with a life-limiting illness. It can start long before end-of-life, as early as at the diagnosis of a life-limiting illness.

+ The principles of palliative care also are applicable in a sudden, acute event, such as an accident, suicide, or myocardial infarction, though the context is different because there is a shorter time span in which to work with a family.

+ Interdisciplinary teamwork is essential in palliative and end-of-life care.

+ Illness is a family affair.

+ People who have advanced, life-limiting illnesses worry about being a burden on their families and about the consequences of their death on their families. Family members worry about burdening their ill member. Everyone involved is often afraid. This fear can lead to communication problems, isolation, and lack of support within the family.

+ Perceived barriers to nurses providing quality end-of-life care may be ameliorated when the nurse assumes a palliative care perspective.

+ Nurses need strong patient and family assessment skills to provide optimal palliative and end-of-life care.

+ Skilled nursing interventions and relationships between nurses and families are crucial in effecting positive outcomes in palliative and end-of-life care.

(continued)

✦ End-of-life decision making is a process that involves all relevant family members identified by the family and evolves over time.

✦ A "good" death is one that happens in alignment with patient and family preferences.

Nurses encounter families who are facing end-of-life issues in virtually all settings of practice. From newborns to seniors in their 90s and older, people die and their families are affected by the experience. Nurses are in an ideal position to influence a family's experience, either positively or negatively. Ideally, nurses facilitate a positive experience for families, one that will bring them comfort as they recall what it was like when their loved one died. Unfortunately, not all families have a positive experience, and it is often because health care providers do not know how to work effectively with families at this challenging time (Andershed, 2006). Yet, palliative and end-of-life nursing can be extremely rewarding and professionally fulfilling. It offers an opportunity for personal growth in patients, families, and health care providers; interactions among all concerned are especially meaningful (Webster & Kristjanson, 2002). This chapter details the key issues to consider in providing care, as well as families' most important concerns and needs when a family member is dying. It also presents some concrete strategies to assist nurses in providing optimal care to families with a member who is at the end of life.

PALLIATIVE AND END-OF-LIFE CARE

Palliative care and end-of-life care are not synonymous terms. End-of-life care focuses on the immediate period around death, whereas palliative care can last for many months, even years (especially in children), and can coexist with active treatments (World Health Organization [WHO], 2006). Palliative care focuses on improving the quality of life of patients and their families facing problems associated with life-limiting illness. Palliative care helps them live well by preventing and relieving suffering through early identification, and excellent assessment and treatment of pain and other physical, psychosocial, or spiritual symptoms (WHO, 2006). Through a team approach, palliative care offers a support system to help patients live as actively as possible, and to help families cope during the patient's illness and their own bereavement. Life is affirmed and dying is regarded as a normal process (WHO, 2006).

Although focus on the family as a unit is a key principle in palliative care, support of individual family members and the family as a whole is the particular focus of care when a child is the patient, because a child is dependent on the family. The age range of patients receiving pediatric palliative care, typically 0 to 19 years of age, requires that children's developmental, social, educational, recreational, and relational needs be considered. The developmental stages of families must also be considered, regardless of the patient's age.

Palliative care in adults developed primarily around care for patients with cancer. Still, patients and their families have similar needs for information, care, and support in a wide variety of chronic illnesses, including heart disease (Barnes et al., 2006; Horne & Payne, 2004), muscular dystrophy (Dawson & Kristjanson, 2003), motor neurone disease (Dawson & Kristjanson, 2003; Hughes, Sinha, Higginson, Down, & Leigh, 2005), dementia (Caron, Griffith, & Arcand, 2005), Parkinson disease (Goy, Carter, & Ganzini, 2007), and neurodegenerative diseases (Kristjanson, Aoun, & Oldham, 2006), as well as when patients are "simply" of an advanced age (Forbes Thompson & Gessert, 2005).

Palliative care is about creating and maintaining quality of life from diagnosis of life-limiting illness through bereavement. The approaches encompassed by palliative care can be used in any setting with any family, regardless of how long a person has to live or how sudden the death is. Communication about transition from curative to palliative intent is crucial and requires discussion about how to shift the primary focus to quality of life rather than prolonging life. When a sudden or traumatic event occurs, there is little time to hold such discussions. But when someone has a protracted illness, this discussion can be introduced gradually and over time.

Unfortunately, in many clinical settings, palliative care is raised only in the last few days of life, even when death has been anticipated. The introduction of palliative care is particularly challenging for health care providers when patients suffer from illnesses that are difficult to prognosticate, such as advanced lung, heart, and liver disease (Fox, Landrum-McNiff, Zhong, Dawson, Wu, & Lynn, 1999). Regardless of when the conversation occurs, it needs to take place to ensure that patients, family members, and health care providers are aligned in their goals for care (Thompson, McClement, & Daeninck, 2006). A need exists to determine what quality of life means for the patient and family; it will be unique in each situation and should tailor care to each particular family. Key to supporting families is the ability of nurses to identify and respond to the needs of all family members (Heyland, Dodek, et al., 2006; Teno, 1999), because it determines the quality of care provided. Quality of care, in turn, is important because of its links to the long-term health of family members.

Death occurs in many settings, from various causes, and across the life span. Some differences can be expected in families' experiences depending on the context, for example:

- Where the death takes place (e.g., home vs. intensive care unit [ICU])
- The cause of death (e.g., natural progression of a chronic illness vs. an unexpected, acute event)
- The dying trajectory (e.g., over a period of years vs. sudden)
- The age of the family member who is dying (e.g., a 3-year-old child vs. an 85-year-old person)
- The cultural and spiritual backgrounds of families (e.g., white vs. Chinese; religious faith vs. no faith)

However, the principles of palliative care should be consistent and can be enacted by health care professionals regardless of the different contexts. Use of these principles contributes to quality end-of-life care (see Box 11-1).

> ### BOX 11-1
> ### Palliative Care Principles
>
> - Patient and family are cared for as a unit.
> - Attention is paid to physical, psychological, social, and spiritual needs and concerns.
> - Education and support of patient and family are crucial.
> - Interdisciplinary approach is required.
> - Care extends across settings.
> - Bereavement support must be provided.

Identifying Relevant Literature

The amount of research about the provision of end-of-life care to adults is growing. Research in pediatric end-of-life care is much more limited, but many of the reported issues for families are similar across the life span. An electronic search of the Cumulative Index to Nursing & Allied Health Literature (CINAHL) database from 2002 until spring 2008 uncovered more than 1,500 articles that reported on some aspect of patient or family perceptions of the palliative, end-of-life, or bereavement care provided to the family by health professionals. However, there were only 161 research studies.

The studies included exploration of patient and family concerns and needs in relation to different diseases (cancer being the most common) and causes of death (sudden deaths, deaths after illness), different care settings (long-term care, acute hospital care, critical care, home, and hospice), different ages (pediatric to elderly patients), different countries, and different cultures. Often, great variation existed in beliefs and needs within a given cultural or other type of group, as well as within individual families (Aspinal, Hughes, Dunckley, & Addington Hall, 2006; Heyland, Dodek, et al., 2006; Mularski, Curtis, Osborne, Engelberg, & Ganzini, 2004; Torke, Garas, Sexson, & Branch, 2005). Therefore, one cannot determine from the literature what the exact needs of, for example, family members of an elderly African American person living with Alzheimer disease in a long-term care setting will be. But the literature does highlight the key issues to consider in providing palliative and end-of-life care, important areas to assess for any family facing an end-of-life experience, and interventions that may be helpful for many families or that can be adjusted to fit with a particular family's assessed needs. The literature found through this search forms the evidence base for the remainder of this chapter.

KEY ISSUES IN PALLIATIVE AND END-OF-LIFE CARE

Personal Assumptions and Biases about People and Death and Dying

As a nurse, you need to be aware of the assumptions and stereotypes that you hold, and you need to recognize each person as being valuable in his or her own right. Valuing patients and their families as human beings and as capable people is a prerequisite and a corequisite for nursing care that fully involves families. Unless you have respect for the inherent worth of others, you will find it difficult, if not impossible, to provide successful and adequate end-of-life care to your patients and their families. Valuing appreciates the possibility that every human being has the potential for actualization or optimal development (Davies & Oberle, 1990).

To be effective in providing optimal palliative and end-of-life care, nurses also need to be aware of their own assumptions and biases about death and dying. As a nurse, you need to explore your own beliefs, attitudes, and personal and professional experiences to understand how they may influence your attitudes toward death, dying, and bereavement. It is neither possible nor wise to separate the "nurse as person" from the "nurse as professional," because if your personal reactions are ignored, then you are less able to focus on meeting the needs of patients and their families (Davies & Oberle, 1990). Many nurses do not know how to deal with dying and death. They are afraid, nervous, or anxious when faced with a dying patient and grieving family. But other nurses experience great satisfaction when working with dying patients. They have become comfortable with death, not simply through caring for many dying patients, but through reflecting on their experiences with those patients and in their personal lives, on the meaning of life and death, and on their own behavior. They are able, therefore, to provide not only competent physical care, but also a welcome presence to those who are dying and their families.

As a novice nurse, you can build on your own strengths and learn ways to become comfortable with death and dying. You must think not only about what death means for your patients and their families, but what life and death mean to you personally. Reflecting on your beliefs about life and death will help clarify your understanding of and appreciation for the human condition. This reflection will form the foundation for the inner strength that will enable you to provide optimal end-of-life care (Davies & Oberle, 1990). When you are ready, you may want to further your education in caregiving at life's end through one of the many available resources, such as workshops, books, and conferences. Gaining knowledge through formal education can help improve your comfort with caregiving (Kwak, Salmon, Acquaviva, Brandt, & Egan, 2007).

Cultural and Spiritual Backgrounds

An underlying principle in palliative care is respect for persons. Implementing the palliative care philosophy means that you must understand diversity and be able to deal with issues that arise when caring for people with varied backgrounds (Davies & Oberle, 1990). The cultural and spiritual backgrounds of families with whom you work need to be taken into account. Cultural beliefs, as well as spirituality, spiritual beliefs, or faith, may be important in how some patients and families cope (Aspinal et al., 2006; Ferrell, Ervin, Smith, Marek, & Melancon, 2002; Perreault, Fothergill Bourbonnais, & Fiset, 2004; Robinson, Thiel, Backus, & Meyer, 2006; Sharman, Meert, & Sarnaik, 2005; Torke et al., 2005). Spiritual well-being may be associated with quality of life to the same degree as physical well-being (Brady, Peterman, Fitchett, Mo, & Cella, 1999). Although across cultures different needs may exist, there is likely more similarity than differences among cultures in terms of basic human needs for connections with others, physical care, dignity, and support (Diver, Molassiotis, & Weeks, 2003). It also is important to recognize your own cultural background and how it might influence your practice, as well as your expectations of others. The cultural and spiritual implications discussed elsewhere in this text also are relevant to quality end-of-life care.

Interdisciplinary Versus Multidisciplinary Teams and Role in End-of-Life Care

Although the focus of this chapter is on the role of the nurse, provision of care through an interdisciplinary team approach is one of the principles of palliative care. Team members need to work toward a common vision, and the underlying definitions and principles of palliative care guide team members toward a clearly defined vision. Despite sharing common goals, however, each member will still bring different ideas and skills to the team; the challenge is how to make best use of each person's attributes while ensuring that the team is effective in providing benefit to patients and families. It is critical to remember that the patient and family are not only at the center of the team, they are team members (Oliver, Porock, Demiris, & Courtney, 2005). For nurses, being an effective team player often means that they share information and consult with other team members, mediate on behalf of patients and families when necessary, and act as a liaison between various members, institutions, and programs. Knowledge about group dynamics is invaluable in learning how to become a successful team member. Everyone also needs to know and accept that each member of the team is unique and valuable, and good communication skills are crucial so that supportive rather than defensive communication can be fostered. A lack of communication among health professionals is common and frustrating for families because they then receive conflicting information or need to repeat information and relay decisions that have been made already (Antle, Barrera, Beaune, D'Agostino, & Good, 2005; Hammes, Klevan, Kempf, & Williams, 2005; Hudson, 2006; Macdonald et al., 2005; Perreault et al., 2004; Widger & Picot, 2008; Wiegand, 2006).

In health care settings, traditional roles and expectations among the professions involved in providing care can raise barriers to integrated and effective teams. Traditional medical services have been based on a multidisciplinary model that has tended to hinder the development of an effective team because a *multidisciplinary* team is composed of individuals from different disciplinary backgrounds who work with the same patient and family, but who may develop individual goals and work relatively independently. In contrast, the *interdisciplinary* team approach focuses on collaboratively working with a patient/family to develop and achieve common goals. The level of collaboration permits role maximization and sharing or overlap in achieving the common goals.

One of the clear differences between these two approaches is the enactment of professional roles within a team; because of the interdisciplinary approach, palliative care is often noted for blurring of these roles. Families receiving end-of-life care will benefit from an interdisciplinary approach because they are both central to the care and members of the collaborative team. Thus, the focus can be on promoting quality of life as determined by the family (see Box 11-2).

BOX 11-2
Interdisciplinary Versus Multidisciplinary Teams

Multidisciplinary Team	Interdisciplinary Team
▪ Medical treatment model	▪ Holistic, "patient-centered" approach to care
▪ Fragmented approach to care	▪ Group control
▪ Centralized control	▪ Facilitative team leader
▪ Autocratic team leader	▪ Decision making by consensus
▪ Decision making by team leader	▪ Leadership by team members
▪ Vertical communication between disciplines	▪ Horizontal communication between disciplines
▪ Treatment geared toward *intra*disciplinary goals	▪ Treatment geared toward *inter*disciplinary goals
▪ Separate goals among disciplines	▪ Common goals among disciplines
▪ Discipline goals basis of plan	▪ Patient goals basis of care plan
▪ Families are peripheral	▪ Families are integral
▪ Meetings/rounds involve individual discipline reporting	▪ Meetings/rounds involve group problem solving and decision making

Illness Is a Family Affair

Evidence from the literature is clear that families play an important role in end-of-life care (Andershed, 2006). Life-threatening illness is often referred to by family members as "our" illness (Ferrell et al., 2002). When the ill person is having a "good" day, so is the caregiver (Stajduhar, Martin, Barwick, & Fyles, 2008). If the ill person is in emotional or physical pain, the suffering of the caregiver dramatically increases (Brajtman, 2005). Parents suffer by watching their child suffer (Sharman et al., 2005). Similarly, parents' needs are met when the child's needs are met (James & Johnson, 1997). Siblings too may suffer if parents are too focused on the ill child to meet sibling needs (de Cinque, Monterosso, Dadd, Sidhu, Macpherson, & Aoun, 2006; Horsley & Patterson, 2006). Likewise, children suffer when they see their parents suffer. Therefore, interventions directed at one family member can also be supportive to other family members. Family members feel supported when they believe that professionals have the best interests of their loved one at heart; therefore, nurses who practice from a family perspective at the end of life need to ensure that the patient is well cared for.

In contrast, patients are often most concerned about the well-being of their family members in terms of caregiving burden and their ability to cope after the death (Aspinal et al., 2006; Fitzsimons et al., 2007; Jo, Brazil, Lohfeld, & Willison, 2007; Kristjanson, Aoun, & Yates, 2006; Perreault et al., 2004). Even ill children may make decisions based on what they believe is best for their family rather than what they particularly want (Hinds et al., 2005). Patients do not want to become a burden to their families (Fitzsimons et al., 2007; Heyland, Dodek, et al., 2006; Heyland et al., 2005). If patients know that their family is well supported, it may reduce their own suffering.

Issues for Family Members

Family members may experience emotional (e.g., fear, helplessness), physical (e.g., fatigue, insomnia), psychological (e.g., anxiety, depression), and financial distress when a family member is dying (Andershed, 2006). Uncertainty and loss of control also can affect family members negatively. In addition, general physical health and quality of life often suffers when a loved one is dying. When a child dies, from any cause, mothers in particular have a greater risk for psychiatric hospitalization and death from suicide or accidents shortly after their child's death, compared with those who have not experienced a child's death (Li, Precht, Mortensen, & Olsen, 2003; Li, Laursen, Precht, Olsen, & Mortensen, 2005; Qin & Mortensen, 2003). Bereaved mothers also have a greater risk for death from cancer and cardiovascular disease long after their child has died (Li, Johansen, Hansen, & Olsen, 2002; Li et al., 2003, 2005). Family members may experience issues regardless of whether their relative is mostly at home (Andershed, 2006) or in an institutional setting (Abma, 2005). They often have increased responsibilities and may view the situation as burdensome (Andershed, 2006). Yet, family caregivers are often more concerned about the care of the dying person than about their own health. They may keep their own concerns to themselves so as not to burden the patient (Fridriksdottir, Sigurdardottir, & Gunnarsdottir, 2006; Perreault et al., 2004; Proot, AbuSaad, Crebolder, Goldsteen, Luker, & Widdershoven, 2003; Riley & Fenton, 2007). Caregiver burdens include ill health (e.g., depression, back pain, shingles, difficulty sleeping, and preexisting chronic illnesses), conflicting family responsibilities (e.g., caring for the ill parent or spouse plus their own children), little time to meet their own needs, fear, anxiety, insecurity, financial concerns, loss of physical closeness with a spouse, and lack of support from other family members and health professionals (Ferrell et al., 2002; Hudson, 2004; Jo et al., 2007; Osse, Vernooij Dassen, Schade, & Grol, 2006; Perreault et al., 2004; Proot et al., 2003; Riley & Fenton, 2007; Sherwood, Given, Doorenbos, & Given, 2004; Wollin, Yates, & Kristjanson, 2006). The work of caregiving can be both physically and mentally exhausting (Riley & Fenton, 2007; Sherwood et al., 2004). There also may be an ambivalent sense of waiting for the person to die but not wanting the patient to die (Riley & Fenton, 2007).

Although patients may want to remain at home, family members often have to assume extra responsibilities, such as administering medications, which can lead to a great deal of anxiety and fear about giving too much, too little, or giving the medication at the wrong time (Kazanowski, 2005). Further, when patients choose a home death—perhaps to increase their quality of life through greater normalcy; increased contact with family, friends, and pets; and the familiar, comfortable surroundings

(Tang, 2003)—this location may not be the caregiver's first choice. For some families, a home death brings additional burdens, worry, and responsibility, and the home becomes more like an institution (Brazil, Howell, Bedard, Krueger, & Heidebrecht, 2005; Milberg, Strang, Carlsson, & Borjesson, 2003). Decisions related to care location and use of palliative surgery or other interventions must be viewed as a family event because the course chosen has a profound impact on the well-being of both the patient and the family (Borneman et al., 2003; Stajduhar, 2003; Tang, Liu, Lai, & McCorkle, 2005).

Family members may not be available or able to give care at home, patients and family members may perceive that hospitals or hospices are able to provide a higher quality of end-of-life care than can be given at home, or the patient and family may feel a close connection to the health care providers in the institution (Tang et al., 2005). Some family members may experience profound guilt if they are not able to provide end-of-life care at home. Health care professionals can alleviate some of this guilt if they alert patients and families early on that plans for location of care may need to change as time goes on to ensure provision of the best possible care (Stajduhar, 2003).

Family caregivers may be vulnerable to burnout if they are not able to cope with the caregiving requirements (Proot et al., 2003). The burden may be increased by the physical and emotional demands of the patient, reduced opportunities for the caregiver to participate in usual activities, and feelings of fear, insecurity, and loneliness (Proot et al., 2003). Caregiver strain also may increase when patients need more assistance with activities of daily living or have greater levels of psychological and existential distress. Differences may exist in needs based on age and sex, with younger caregivers having more concerns about finances, and maintaining social activities and relationships. Female caregivers may have more difficulties with their own health (lack of sleep and muscle pain), with transportation, coordinating care, and feeling underappreciated (Osse et al., 2006). Strain may be reduced when families are more accepting of the patient's illness, and feel more capable in their ability to provide and manage the patient's end-of-life care (Redinbaugh, Baum, Tarbell, & Arnold, 2003). Facilitating hope for a longer life or for a peaceful death, having positive feeling about the care they are able to provide, receiving adequate information, and having emotional and instrumental support also may reduce the burden (Proot et al., 2003).

On the other hand, some people report positive aspects of caregiving, such as feelings of satisfaction, learning more about themselves, and being able to show their love for their family member (Andershed, 2006). Some family members may view care provision as an opportunity and a privilege (Hudson, 2004, 2006; Jo et al., 2007; Kazanowski, 2005; Sherwood et al., 2004). Positive aspects include greater appreciation for life, greater purpose and meaning to life, increased closeness and intimacy, newfound personal strength and ability, and the opportunity to share special time together (Ferrell et al., 2002; Hudson, 2004, 2006; Jo et al., 2007; Riley & Fenton, 2007; Sherwood et al., 2004). Hudson (2004, 2006) suggests a link between the caregiver's ability to see the positives in the situation, and both better coping and less traumatic grief. In parents of children dying of a neurodegenerative disease, increased spirituality (Steele, 2005a), personal growth (Steele 2005a; Steele & Davies, 2006), and an increased appreciation of life have been noted (Steele, 2005a, 2005b; Steele & Davies, 2006). It is important, therefore, to uncover the positive aspects and help families recognize the value in what they are doing because it may contribute to their overall well-being and may enhance their experience. Further, quality of care has also been shown to increase length of survival for caregivers of adults (Christakis & Iwashyna, 2003), and some researchers have found links between parents' satisfaction with care, or assessment of care quality, and their coping ability or emotional state in the years after the child's death (Kreicbergs, Valdimarsdottir, Onelov, Bjork, Steineck, & Henter, 2005; Meert, Thurston, & Sarnaik, 2000; Seecharan, Andresen, Norris, & Toce, 2004; Surkan et al., 2006). Nurses are in an excellent position to identify, prevent, and alleviate many of the negative aspects of providing end-of-life care, as well as to identify and foster a family's strengths. Thus, nurses can have a significant, life-long effect on well-being of family members.

Bereavement

One of the principles of palliative care is that care continues after the death and into bereavement. The need for follow-up with the family after the death by involved health professionals is considered by many families to be a crucial component of end-of-life care, but unfortunately one that is often missing

(Cherlin, Schulman Green, McCorkle, Johnson Hurzeler, & Bradley, 2004; D'Agostino, Berlin-Romalis, Jovcevska, & Barrera, 2008; de Jong-Berg & Kane, 2006; Kreicbergs et al., 2005; Macdonald et al., 2005; Meyer, Ritholz, Burns, & Truog, 2006; Widger & Picot, 2008; Wisten & Zingmark, 2007; Woodgate, 2006). Families sometimes feel abandoned after the death, which adds to the grief they experience (D'Agostino et al., 2008; de Cinque et al., 2006; Heller & Solomon, 2005; Meert et al., 2007; Widger & Picot, 2008). Bereavement care is important because family caregivers may experience negative effects, such as feelings of loneliness, sadness, and physical exhaustion caused by difficulty sleeping, as well as the aftermath of the demands of caregiving. These feelings may be juxtaposed with feelings of relief that the patient's suffering ended and that everything possible was done to keep the patient comfortable (Hudson, 2006; Sherwood et al., 2004; Wollin et al., 2006). After the death, some caregivers may feel "lost" because they now have "free" hours that had been previously devoted to caregiving (Sherwood et al., 2004). Support for families after the death may help prevent or alleviate prolonged suffering.

Barriers to Optimal End-of-Life Nursing Care

Although effective palliative and end-of-life care is desirable and possible, some barriers may have a negative effect on quality of care. The major barrier to optimal end-of-life care for patients and their families relates to the limited formal education and training nurses have received. In the past, little attention has been given to end-of-life and palliative care in nursing curricula, and this is true of other health professionals as well. Although this is changing somewhat, it still exists. Other barriers, such as the work environment, delayed referral to hospice and palliative care services, a lack of availability of ethics consultations, and lack of 24/7 access to care at home also play a role. In many cases, the program set up and lines of communication do not allow for families to be included to the extent they could and should be. Uncertainties about prognosis and differences in treatment goals between family members and professionals, as well as communication issues, also have been reported as barriers in pediatric palliative care (Davies et al., 2008). Although work needs to be done to remove these barriers, it is possible

for nurses to practice high standards within constraining contexts.

One other barrier that can be more challenging to deal with is the moral distress that can arise for nurses who practice in intensive care units (ICUs) when they provide end-of-life care to patients and their families (Elpern, Covert, & Kleinpell, 2005). Moral distress may be experienced by nurses when vulnerable patients receive advanced medical treatments that the nurses believe to be both inappropriate and contributing to patients' suffering. This moral distress can affect critical care nurses' job satisfaction, physical and psychological well-being, self-image, spirituality, and decisions about their own health. Such distress may lead to burnout, job dissatisfaction, and leaving the work environment (Elpern et al., 2005; Meltzer & Huckabay, 2004).

FAMILY NURSING PRACTICE ASSESSMENT AND INTERVENTION

Nurses must possess strong patient and family assessment skills if they are going to provide optimal care (e.g., excellent pain and symptom management, psychosocial support), because the most appropriate interventions can be designed and implemented only once a family's needs and goals have been assessed accurately. Assessment should be ongoing and sequential, building on what is known about the family and shaping interventions to meet the family's changing needs and preferences throughout the palliative process.

This section is organized around interventions that may be helpful to families. But you must never forget that each family is unique. Your assessment will help you determine what a specific family needs, and you can then tailor your approach in consultation with the family. Although your practice should be evidence based, do not try to apply theory and research uncritically. What works for one family may not be right for another. You must not lose sight of the need to assess and critically analyze each situation on its own merits, rather than simply treating all families as if they are the same. Because we can never know whether an intervention will be useful to a particular family, interventions should always be offered tentatively and then evaluated from the family perspective. Assessment and intervention are, therefore, intertwined and are discussed together in the following sections.

The interventions discussed are supported by research. They also have been used successfully in the authors' clinical practices. They are guidelines and practical suggestions about how you might approach a family, and how you might support and guide a family at the end of a family member's life. But it is not possible to cover every potential scenario in end-of-life care; therefore, the focus is on discussing the main concepts that you need to be aware of for end-of-life care. Most deaths you will encounter when providing end-of-life care occur as the result of chronic disease rather than an acute event. Therefore, these situations are the focus of the remaining discussion and the case study.

Connections Between Families and Nurses

The relationships or connections that families develop with health care professionals have a significant effect on how families will manage end-of-life events and their sequelae. In your nursing education so far, you may have learned about the characteristics of a "helping relationship" between nurses and families, but in practice, nurses often speak of their "connections" with families rather than their "relationships." Whether nurses are working in home, hospice, long-term care, or hospital settings (including general medical and surgical units, outpatient departments, ICUs, and emergency departments), the presence of a mutual, trusting relationship is foundational to all the assessment and intervention that nurses have to work with the family to ensure optimal care is provided.

Families typically are not used to talking about death and dying; therefore, it is often an unfamiliar pattern of communication for many people (Andershed, 2006). Thus, the relationship between families and nurses is crucial in providing a safe environment for families who often need guidance and support. Nurses need to understand the conditions that are necessary for establishing and maintaining connections, and they have to build trust by providing open and honest communication, demonstrating commitment and a caring attitude to the family, and being reliable and accessible (Aspinal et al., 2006; Heyland, Dodek, et al., 2006; Kristjanson, Aoun, & Oldham, 2006; Milberg et al., 2003; Mok, Chan, Chan, & Yeung, 2002; Mok & Chiu, 2004; Shiozaki, Morita, Hirai, Sakaguchi, Tsuneto,

& Shima, 2005; Torke et al., 2005). Simple acts of addressing all family members by name, smiling, making eye contact, showing emotion, and physical contact with a hand on the shoulder can foster connections between family members and the health professional (Heller & Solomon, 2005; Macdonald et al., 2005; Pector, 2004a; Sharman et al., 2005). Patients and families also appreciate when a nurse is able to anticipate and respond to needs without being asked, because it demonstrates how well the nurse knows the patient and family (Mok & Chiu, 2004). Identifying and understanding possible needs and issues is important because families may not know what they need or what might be possible (Pector, 2004b; Rini & Loriz, 2007; Selman et al., 2007).

It is the professional's responsibility to develop a trusting relationship with families and to provide an environment of openness where families feel comfortable asking questions. As a nurse, you must cultivate relationships with families. You must show families through your attitude and behaviors that you not only have the knowledge to assist them, but that you are willing and able to be there for them. Although some families will need your assistance more than others, it is important to recognize that the sense of security and trust families experience in relationships with health care professionals can add to and strengthen a family's resources (Andershed, 2006). Nurses need to be respectful, open, collaborative, willing to listen, trustworthy, inquisitive, reliable, accessible, compassionate, and nonjudgmental (accept family's differences). In addition, a nurse's competence must be above reproach—excellent pain and symptom management, and empathy in all interactions with both patient and family. When nurses are competent at completing tasks but are unable or unwilling to imagine what it is like for the patient and family, the connection is usually weak and is less satisfying for the patient and family. Box 11-3 provides some questions to help you open up communication and learn about family members' perspectives as you build your relationship with a family.

Making a connection does not necessarily happen instantly, nor does it have to take a lot of time. Sometimes you will feel a connection exists between you and a family; other times, you may have to make an extra effort to get to know the family and to establish a relationship. You might feel as if you have to "prove" yourself to the family or overcome your own negative reaction to a particular family or

BOX 11-3

Key Questions to Ask Families to Open up Communication and Obtain Family Members' Perspectives

Ideally, questions to open up communication and obtain family members' perspectives should be asked with all involved family members present including the patient; however, knowing that family members do not want to burden their ill member with their emotions and concerns, you may find that some of these questions need to be asked of family members alone. You will need to tailor questions depending on where the ill family member is in the palliative care experience. Also, decisions about how and what information is shared, with whom, and how decisions are made, as well as how family members are involved in care, are ultimately those of the patient (if an adult).

Start by saying, "I'd like to understand what it has been like for your family to live with [illness]." Then use the following key questions to open up communication and obtain family members' perspectives:

- What is your understanding of what is happening with [ill family member]?
- What experience do you have as a family in dealing with serious health problems? With death and dying?
- If you were to think ahead a bit, how do you see things going in [the next few days, the next few weeks, the next few months (use the timeframe that is most appropriate)]?
- How are you hoping this will go?
- What is most important for me to know about your family?
- What are you most concerned or worried about?
- When you think about your loved one getting really sick, what fears or worries do you have?
- I've found that many families caring for someone with this condition think about the possibility of their loved one dying. They have questions about this. Do you have questions?
- Who is suffering most?
- How do they show their suffering?
- How are you managing?
- I understand that different family members will have different talents: How do you most want to be involved?
- How can I be most helpful to you at this time?
- How does your family like to talk about challenging things?
- How have you been talking about the situation you find yourselves in? Who has been involved?
- Is there anyone involved who is important and who I haven't met?
- How are important decisions made in your family? How would you like important decision making to go now?
- Families often find it helpful to talk about the care they want at end of life. Have you been able to have a conversation about this? I wonder if I might be able to help you start this conversation.
- Do you have any cultural beliefs, rituals, or traditions around illness and end of life that I should be aware of?
- What have you found most helpful or useful to you as a family at this time?
- What do you most need to manage well?
- What has not been helpful?
- What sustains you in challenging times?
- What is going well?
- What do you most want to be doing at this time? What brings you joy (or helps you get out of bed in the morning)?
- If your loved one were to die tonight, is there anything you have not said or done that you would regret? If so, how can I help you do or say what you need to do? (Ask this of the patient as well, i.e., If you were die suddenly, is there anything you would regret not doing or saying?)
- In families, often many things are happening apart from the illness that we do not know about. Is there anything going on that is adding to what you are already coping with?

family member. Nevertheless, it is important to make an effort to establish connections with each family member, to get to know each on an individual and personal level. Making a connection with family members helps you discover what is meaningful to them, builds a bridge between you as human beings, and crosses the gap that often exists between professionals and family members. Getting to know each family member demonstrates respect for the patient's and family members' individuality, dignity, needs, and feelings (Aspinal et al., 2006; Kristjanson, Aoun, & Oldham, 2006; Riley & Fenton, 2007; Shiozaki et al., 2005). Further, it acknowledges differences within the family. Simply giving undivided attention by taking time to listen to the family's needs and worries is a demonstration of respect, and the importance of the person and the relationship (Aspinal et al., 2006; Dwyer, Nordenfelt, & Ternestedt, 2008; Milberg et al., 2003; Mok & Chiu, 2004).

Understanding the family's situation apart from the illness is important (Contro, Larson, Scofield, Sourkes, & Cohen, 2002, 2004; Maynard, Rennie, Shirtliffe, & Vickers, 2005; Steele, 2002; Steele & Davis, 2006; Surkan et al., 2006; Tomlinson et al., 2006). Connecting means acquiring knowledge of the patients and family as people with personal histories, hopes, and dreams rather than as objects of biomedical science. Having this knowledge and understanding allows you to see their perspective, and appreciate the creativity and ingenuity of their efforts. Connecting allows you to apply your general scientific knowledge in ways that are best for the individual patients and their families, given their specific background, needs, and ways of being in the world. Connecting is a two-way process where both the nurse and the patients and family get to know one another at a personal level and begin to establish trust. With trust comes a greater sense of comfort and ease for patients, and an increased ability for nurses to offer effective interventions and to act as advocates (Davies & Oberle, 1990). But communication and interpersonal skills can facilitate or hinder connecting with patients and families, and nurses need to be aware of how their personal styles of interaction and communication can make, sustain, and break connections.

Unfortunately, all too often, families report a lack of support and connection that contribute to negative experiences (Andershed, 2006). When families sense a lack of respect and sincerity from many

professionals, they are affected negatively. Even single incidents related to lack of communication and interpersonal skills on the part of health professionals can contribute to intense emotional distress long after the event (Contro et al., 2002, 2004; Meert et al., 2007; Pector, 2004a; Rini & Loriz, 2007; Surkan et al., 2006; Widger & Picot, 2008).

Sometimes nurses worry about saying the wrong thing, or they do not understand the need to listen carefully and to reassure patients and families. Humor may be one way to facilitate a connection with families, but it is important first to assess receptivity to humor (Dean & Gregory, 2005). Generally, when families use humor, it is fine to enter into the humor with them, but it may be more difficult for the nurse to initiate humor. The use of humor can provide respite from thinking about the illness, relieve tension, and demonstrate value for the patient and family members as people. Some strategies that nurses can use to make a connection between themselves and patients and families are provided in Box 11-4.

SPECIAL CONSIDERATIONS: CONNECTING IN THE INTENSIVE CARE UNIT AND EMERGENCY DEPARTMENT. In critical care areas, nurses may be less apt to support patients and their families psychologically (Nordgren & Olsson, 2004; Price, 2004) because they give more attention to managing the patient's physical symptoms systematically and efficiently. Families may not be attended to as nurses deal with the acuity of evolving situations. Yet, we know that family members of patients in ICUs often experience anxiety and depression (Pochard et al., 2001). Furthermore, insufficient information and death in the ICU have been associated with posttraumatic stress disorder in families of ICU patients (Azoulay et al., 2005). Therefore, it is necessary to offer psychological support, such as ongoing assessment of and information for families of patients who are cared for and who may ultimately die in ICUs (White & Luce, 2004).

Whether during a sudden or traumatic event that necessitates admission to the emergency department or the quickly shifting situations in ICU, nurses need to remember that despite and amidst the technology are real people who need connections. You may need to take a breath and step back so you can focus on the "bigger picture" before you are able to help the family, but it is critical that someone takes time for them. All of the ways that you can connect

BOX 11-4

Suggestions About How to Establish and Sustain Connections with Families

- Patients and families need to know who you are; when you meet a patient and family for the first time, make them feel welcome, introduce yourself by name, then find out who they are and learn about them as people as well. Ask them how they would like to be called (e.g., by full name or first name).
- Begin any interaction by clarifying your role and telling the patient and family about your "professional" self so you establish your credentials. For example, "Hello, Mr. Li. My name is Rose Steele. I'm a third-year Student Nurse. Sandyha Singh, who is the Registered Nurse supervising me, and I are taking care of your wife today. I'm working until 3.30 p.m. today and also will be here tomorrow, so I'll be her nurse then too. I have worked on this unit for the past three weeks, so I am pretty familiar with all the routines, but I'm really interested in finding out how we can fit in with what you and Mrs. Li want."
- The best approach is not "This is how we do it here," but rather "How do you like to do this?" and "How can we find a way to do that in this context?"
- Ensure a comfortable physical environment; let patients and families know the routines and how they can get help as needed, to provide a sense of familiarity and help you begin to make the connection.
- Privacy is often an issue and is critical to some of the sensitive discussions that occur in palliative and end-of-life care. Try to find a private location before broaching sensitive issues.
- Describe who other team members are and what their roles are so families understand the context. Family members often do not know who to ask for what.
- Attend to the patient's and family's immediate state of well-being; it is impossible to connect with someone when you have not attended to their basic needs first; if a patient is lying in a wet bed or is in pain, family members will not be open to a "connecting" conversation with the nurse.
- Be sensitive to an individual's particular characteristics such as cultural or gender differences; making eye contact is a useful strategy for connecting in many cases, but a First Nations person may be uncomfortable with direct eye contact. Touch is often welcome but is not universally experienced as supportive.
- Do not let your observations of particular characteristics limit your perception by stereotyping the person; be aware of your own assumptions and biases, guarding against "operationalizing" your biases—for example, do not assume that an elderly person is deaf.
- Be sensitive to a person's way of being. Some people are outgoing and talkative; others are more withdrawn. Humor may be appropriate for some people or situations, but not for others. Responding to people in ways that match their style enhances their comfort level. Another useful habit is to use the family's language. If you need to use medical terms, then be sure to explain them.
- Not all people will want the same level of connection; you need to respect where the person is coming from and not try to force a deeper relationship.
- Patients and families differ in their expectations of what health care workers should provide; some only want information, some expect only physical care, and still others expect more of a supportive relationship. The key here is in asking for expectations. This does not mean that you can meet the expectations and you may want to preface the request with a statement such as this: "To be most helpful to you, I need to know what you would like. I may not be able to do things exactly as you prefer, but we can work together to get as close as possible."
- Many times you will find that when you simply meet the patient's and family's expectations without imposing your own, further opportunities for connecting may evolve.
- Once the connection has been made, you have to work at sustaining it.
- Sustaining the connection allows you to learn even more about the patient and family so you can continually adapt your care according to their needs; it is also a way of demonstrating your trustworthiness as the patient and family get to know and trust you. When you are well connected, you are more likely to offer useful interventions that the family will accept.
- Ways of sustaining the connection include giving of self, spending time with the patient and family, and being available. Sometimes the only thing we can do is to stay with patients and families as a witness to their suffering.

> ### BOX 11-4
> ### Suggestions About How to Establish and Sustain Connections with Families—cont'd
>
> ▨ Making and sustaining the connection is a two-way process that has to do with sharing parts of yourself with patients and families as you seek a common bond. It does not mean that you uncritically relate your entire life history, but that you feel comfortable in talking about pieces of your personal life.
> ▨ Sustaining the connection requires that you spend time with patients and their families.
> ▨ Continuity of care, such as having the same nurse be in contact with the same patient over some period of time, is important. It is critical that team members effectively communicate with one another to support continuity of care.
> ▨ It is not just the quantity but also the quality of time that makes the difference.
> ▨ The "best" nurses are those who give the impression of "having all the time in the world," even when they are really busy. One way of doing this is to come into the room and sit or stand by the bedside, even if only briefly.
> ▨ Taking the time to "be there" for patients and families instead of being in a rush maintains the connection. This requires you to be mindful and to let go momentarily of all the demands that compete for your attention.
> ▨ Even when you are not actually with patients and families, it is important that they feel as if you will be available when they need you; simple things such as saying hello and good-bye at the beginning and end of shifts, and also at break times help them know your availability.
> ▨ Informing patients and families so they know what to expect and keeping your word, such as being there when you say you will be, also sustain the connection.
> ▨ Instead of having your routine set for the day, adapt your routine to what the patient and family needs at the time.
> ▨ Be flexible because you are always working under constraints; share these constraints with patients and families, and tell them if you need to change the plan you have made with them.
> ▨ Changing plans often requires the support of colleagues who can take over for you or help out as needed.

with families can still work in ICU and emergency department settings, but you need to create some space for the family to ensure the connections and communication can happen. If family members are in the room, then you need to talk with them, explain what is happening, and be available to answer their questions. If they are waiting outside, ensure they have somewhere comfortable and private to sit, and provide frequent updates about their loved one. If you yourself are too busy with urgent care for the patient, make sure that someone is designated to care for the family and to keep them involved as much as they want to be.

Relieving the Patient's Suffering

For many nurses, the concrete actions involved in technical skills and nursing tasks, such as giving medications and changing intravenous infusions, are viewed as the most important clinical components of professional practice. Less tangible aspects, such as

helping patients and their families manage emotions, are frequently undervalued in nursing practice. Relieving symptoms and making patients comfortable are crucial to good end-of-life care, because unless patients are physically comfortable, they may be unable to attend to other issues in their lives, and their quality of life may be compromised. Nurses need to understand the variety of symptoms common to patients at the end of life, and gain the knowledge needed for anticipating, recognizing, assessing, preventing, and managing symptoms with both traditional and complementary therapies. You also need to develop strategies for promoting comfort and quality of life for patients and their families and then analyze the effectiveness of these strategies when implemented in nursing care.

Support for the dying family member must go beyond relief of physical symptoms. Psychosocial and spiritual suffering also need to be attended to and are no less important than physical discomfort. It is imperative in family care at the end of life to attend to all aspects of the patient's needs, in part because of the effect it has on family (Brajtman, 2003). Unless families believe you are taking good care of their loved one, you will not be able to begin to meet the family's other needs.

Relieving suffering includes improving quality of life, but no single definition exists for the most important factors for a good quality of life (Johansson, Axelsson, & Danielson, 2006; Norris, Merriman, Curtis, Asp, Tuholske, & Byock, 2007). Individual needs must be assessed. For example, Norris and colleagues (2007) found that higher patient quality of life ratings were associated with playing music that was meaningful to the patient, attending a place of worship, having a familiar health care team available at all times (for patients at home), and having individual preferences respected. Other components contributing to better quality of life include valuing everyday things, maintaining a positive attitude, having symptoms relieved, feeling in control, and feeling connected to and needed by family, friends, and health professionals (Aspinal et al., 2006; Johansson et al., 2006).

Empowering Families

Family palliative and end-of-life care is a strength-based approach. It is about building and nurturing family strengths to ensure that quality of life, as defined by the family, can be achieved as closely as possible. Rather than solely focusing on deficits or areas that the nurse perceives as problematic, end-of-life care should emphasize empowering families to manage this challenging time in their own unique way by noticing and growing strengths, whereas at the same time effectively addressing problems. Families appreciate recognition for their competencies and caring; therefore, nurses should make a point of commending family strengths (Houger Limacher & Wright, 2003; Mok et al., 2002; Wright & Leahey, 2005), especially in the presence of the ill person. Caregivers may be better able to cope with caregiving when the ill person recognizes and appreciates their role (Stajduhar et al., 2008), so nurses can role model this appreciation by commending the work of the caregiver in the presence of the ill person. This can be done by making specific observations of patterns of family strengths that occur across time (Wright & Leahey, 2005). Similarly, parents appreciate recognition of their parenting role and skills. Nurses' commendations may help to strengthen

parental relationships with their child and their view of their role (Antle et al., 2005; Steele, 2002).

Empowering is also about making patients and families aware of options and constraints about clinical care so they can make choices that are most appropriate for them. For example, families may be unaware of the possibility of having death occur outside the hospital or at home when life support is discontinued, yet that may be a support for some families (Pector, 2004b).

Empowering patients and families also involves helping them to do what they themselves want and need to do, rather than professionals taking over and doing it for them. For example, although it may appear quicker and easier for the nurse to assist a patient out of bed, it may be important that the patient moves by him or herself. All of the empowering strategies require good communication skills, and nurses must understand various strategies for empowering patients and families. The focus should be on maximizing the patient's and family's capacity to use their own resources to meet their needs and respecting their ability to do so. Nurses empower patients and families by creating an environment in which their strengths and abilities are recognized, by encouraging them to consider various options, by assisting them in fulfilling their needs and desires through the provision of information and resources, and by supporting their choices. Therefore, it is important to assess the capacity of patients and families to do for themselves, and then find ways of supporting them when hopes and expectations exceed capacity. For example, sometimes a person's capacity is diminished because of fatigue, severe pain, or other sources of distress that may be physical or emotional in nature. If a patient or family member is limited in their capacity to do things for themselves, the nurse often needs to "do for" them instead. When a nurse acts in such situations, the patient and family often feel more comfortable again, and are able to regain control and reclaim their sense of competency, so "doing for" complements empowering (Davies & Oberle, 1990). Careful assessment of the situation is central to knowing when to act on behalf of patients and families, and when to encourage them to manage themselves, because if you "do for" patients and families when they can care for themselves, then you may diminish their sense of competency and disempower them.

Balancing Hope and Preparation

A fair amount of ambiguity always exists when working with families at end of life, regardless of whether the situation is acute or chronic. Nurses need to become comfortable with the inherent uncertainty and help families live well within an uncertain context. One common ambiguity is around prognostic uncertainty. Given that we cannot predict when death will occur, families need to be encouraged to attend to what they view as important and to take advantage of the moment. When a patient or family member asks, "How long?" you might reply by asking, "What would you be doing differently now if you knew that the time was very short?" In response to their answer, you might suggest that they do whatever "it" is, and if they get to do "it" again next week or next month or even next year, then that would be a bonus.

For some families and in some cultures, a need is present to keep fighting for every chance at life, hoping for a miracle, until the last possible moment even when they may know this is unrealistic (Kirk, Kirk, & Kristjanson, 2004; Shiozaki et al., 2005; Torke et al., 2005). As a nurse, you need to find the balance between supporting families in their hopes and still being comfortable talking about death and preparing the patient and family for what is to come, including advance care planning (Davies & Connaughty, 2002; Hsiao, Evan, & Zeltzer, 2007; Rini & Loriz, 2007; Robinson et al., 2006; Shiozaki et al., 2005; Steele, 2005a). Therefore, when preparing the family for what is to come, the information must be provided in a sensitive manner that still acknowledges hope (Kirk et al., 2004; Shiozaki et al., 2005). One way of doing this is to use a hypothetical question (Wright & Leahey, 2005), such as "If things don't go as we hope, what is most important for you to have happen?"

Providing Information

Families often have a need for information, but it is not always easy to obtain because professionals may not be open to sharing. Family members often do not know what questions to ask, yet lack of knowledge and feeling uninformed can leave people isolated, frustrated, and distressed (Andershed, 2006). Some families want a great deal of detailed information, whereas others feel overwhelmed and

find that it interferes with their ability to live as normal a life as possible. Therefore, ongoing assessment of how much and what types of information families want is important (Maynard et al., 2005; Pector, 2004a; Steele, 2005a, 2005b). This assessment also needs to include how much information should be offered directly to the patient, especially a child (Hays et al., 2006; Hsiao et al., 2007; Mack et al., 2005). A wide variation can exist in the ages some parents feel are too young to include, ranging from 4 months to 13 years, and the age at which other parents feel the child is old enough to be included, ranging from 2 to 25 years (Mack et al., 2005). Even when the patient is an adult, some families may believe that not all information should be shared with the patient (Royak Schaler, Gadalla, Lemkau, Ross, Alexander, & Scott, 2006). It can be a delicate balance to comply with legal requirements within your geographical jurisdiction, yet not alienate family members. As a nurse, you need to be aware of your legal responsibilities and ensure that you do not withhold information inappropriately. You also must convey your responsibilities to the family and initiate an open dialogue about the importance of communication.

There may be little sharing of information, concerns, wishes, and needs among family members as they each do not want to upset the other (Fridriksdottir et al., 2006; Perreault et al., 2004; Proot et al., 2003; Riley & Fenton, 2007). Keep in mind, however, that this conspiracy of silence as family members try to "protect" one another may lead to increased fears and anxiety in all family members (Riley & Fenton, 2007; Selman et al., 2007), and can result in silence and isolation. Family members' wishes about what information should be shared with the patient may need to be negotiated, especially if there are differing opinions.

When patients and family members are empowered with the amount of information they want, it results in more effective partnerships with professionals. Nurses are in a key position to act as liaison between the professional team members and the family. Patients and families should be encouraged to ask questions, and these questions should be answered with full explanations and support. Nurses are an important source of information about a wide range of issues as patients and their families cope with the end-of-life experience. Nurses also need to provide education and preparation that will support families to do their job (i.e., caregiving); at the same time, nurses must facilitate "normal" roles within a family, for example, as a parent or as an adult caregiver. Beginning nurses are sometimes reluctant to invite questions from families because an expectation exists that you will have an answer. Simply knowing the questions is valuable information, and many times the questions do not have answers. As a novice, you may not know the answer, and that is all right. If possible, however, you can show your trustworthiness by seeking the information and providing it in a timely fashion.

Families need to have honest and understandable information about a variety of areas, including the patient's condition, the illness trajectory, symptoms to expect and treatment options, how to provide physical care, what to expect (including signs of impending death, which allow family members the opportunity to say final good-byes), ways of coping (including helping families become aware of possible strategies such as respite and mental pauses), the dying process, how to access additional support, what aids (e.g., wheelchairs, beds, lifts) may be helpful and where to get them, and the care system in which this all occurs (Andershed, 2006; Aspinal et al., 2006; Fridriksdottir et al., 2006; Heyland et al., 2005; Hudson, 2006; Kreicbergs, Lannen, Onelov, & Wolfe, 2007; Kristjanson, Aoun, & Yates, 2006; Mok et al., 2002; Osse et al., 2006; Proot et al., 2003; Sherwood et al., 2004; Shiozaki et al., 2005; Wollin et al., 2006).

The way in which information is shared is as important as the content of the information. Critical components of the process of sharing information include timing, pacing, and both verbal and nonverbal conveyance of respect, empathy, and compassion (Kirk et al., 2004). The timing and pacing, in particular, are important to allow families to absorb the reality of the situation and to make informed decisions (Meert et al., 2007). Do not rush families to make decisions, and give information as early as possible to allow for ongoing discussions and decision making with a clearer mind rather than waiting for a crisis that may be fraught with emotion (Hammes et al., 2005; Macdonald, Liben, & Cohen, 2006; Sharman et al., 2005).

Through learning about other families' experiences, patients and family members can better understand their own experience, so nurses can share insights gained from other families both from practice and research. For example, "Other families

have told me that talking about what their child's death might be like was one of the hardest things they ever had to do, but once they knew there was a plan in place for how to handle the possible symptoms or issues that may happen, they were able to stop worrying about all the 'what-ifs' and just focus on having the best time possible with their child." Having information enables patients and families to collaborate with health care providers from an informed position, and is required for making decisions and planning for the future.

Facilitating Choices

Families may be facing their first experience with death and dying, and they often depend on nurses to help them in their process. Families may not know what they need or what might be possible (Selman et al., 2007); they may expect health professionals to bring up issues when appropriate—that is, the family members may feel it is not their place to raise issues first. It is important to assess and respect the patient's and family's desired level of involvement in discussions about end of life and in decision making. Some patients and families may want full responsibility for decisions, some may want to be involved but not make final decisions, some may want the physician to take the initiative and make all decisions (Milberg et al., 2003; Selman et al., 2007; Shiozaki et al., 2005), and some patients want their family members to make decisions (Torke et al., 2005). The involvement of family members in decision making can have a life-long effect on the well-being of family members (Christakis & Iwashyna, 2003; Kreicbergs et al., 2005; Meert et al, 2000; Seecharan et al., 2004; Surkan et al., 2006; Tilden, Tolle, Nelson, & Fields, 2001). Nurses, therefore, must foster good communication to ensure that the patient's and family's needs and wishes are understood and supported within a caring relationship that is built on partnership between professionals and families. Many times health care providers block families from participating because they feel they know what is best or because they are trying to protect families. But effective end-of-life care is not possible unless open and mutual communication occurs between families and professionals, and families participate in shared decision making to the extent they desire.

Some parents feel that making decisions for the child is inherently a parental role, but not all want to have complete responsibility for final decisions (Brinchmann, Forde, & Nortvedt, 2002; Brosig, Pierucci, Kupst, & Leuthner, 2007; Contro et al., 2002, 2004; Hays et al., 2006; Meyer, Burns, Griffith, & Truog, 2002; Meyer et al., 2006; Pector, 2004b; Sharman et al., 2005). Again, assessment of parents' preferences about decision making is important. Regardless of their actual role in the decision-making process, parents want to be recognized as the experts on their child and as the central, consistent figures in their child's life. As such, they want health professionals to seek out and respect their knowledge, opinions, observations, and concerns about their child (Brinchmann et al., 2002; Hsiao et al., 2007; Meyer et al., 2006; Steele, 2002, 2005a; Widger & Picot, 2008; Woodgate, 2006).

At the end of life, patients may be unable to participate in making decisions about their care, leaving family members to make decisions based on their understanding of what the patient would want if they were able to participate. This process of surrogate decision making can be a very demanding one for families (Meeker, 2004). Nurses can facilitate the process and empower both patients and families by encouraging them to talk about end-of-life issues and preferences long before they are faced with the situation and by initiating discussions about surrogate decision making, including the legalities of representation. Written advance directives also can be helpful to family members, particularly in reminding them of their loved one's wishes when there may be differences in what each thought would be best. Less than 30% of adults have an advance directive, and even for those adults who do have them, they may not be available when needed or be specific enough (Dunn, Tolle, Moss, & Black, 2007).

We are coming to understand that advance care planning is a process that is best initiated early in the illness experience and revisited as the illness progresses because preferences can change over time. These types of conversations are difficult to have among family members, and families may appreciate your assistance to initiate and facilitate the conversation. In addition, when faced with actually making decisions, family members often appreciate acknowledgment of the difficulty of their role, and your attentive, respectful support throughout the process will be very helpful (Meeker, 2004).

A sudden or traumatic death leaves little time for families to come to terms with the situation.

Further, the nature of a frequently chaotic environment may contribute to a lack of communication between professionals and families. It is important that the information given to families include the big picture; otherwise, families often receive different pieces of information from each health professional and may have trouble putting it all together to understand that it actually means the patient is dying. This may be more of an issue in situations when there is a sudden illness or injury because the family has little experience and may be unprepared for what is happening (Meert, Thurston, & Briller, 2005; Rini & Loriz, 2007; Wiegand, 2006).

Lack of early information about the possibility of death makes it difficult for family members to come to terms with decisions such as the withdrawal of life-sustaining therapy or the use of cardiopulmonary resuscitation (Counsell, 2002; Heyland, Frank, et al., 2006; Norton, Tilden, Tolle, Nelson, & Eggman, 2003). Families faced with these types of decisions usually place great value on open, honest, and timely information, but they also need to be listened to rather than just spoken to (Heyland, Rocker, O'Callaghan, Dodek, & Cook, 2003; McDonagh et al., 2004; Norton et al., 2003). Moreover, it is crucial to prepare the family for what to expect when life-sustaining therapy is withdrawn. For example, families need to be aware that death may occur very quickly, or may take hours or days (Wiegand, 2006). When decisions are made, such as withdrawal of life-sustaining therapy, any delays past the agreed-on time for implementing the decision may greatly increase the family's anxiety (Wiegand, 2006).

Nurses need to recognize the individual's and family's rights and abilities to make their own decisions and then make an effort to find out what is important to them. You should focus on what patients and families *can* do, rather than on what they cannot. As a nurse, you can reinforce those aspects of the self that remain intact, and assist patients and families to recognize their own strengths and abilities. Once you identify and build on individual and family strengths, you can smooth the way for patients and families to meet their own needs. Nurses can work with patients and families by making suggestions, providing options, and planning strategies that will allow them to achieve their goals. Your professional knowledge may be invaluable in guiding families to consider options and possible routes of actions that they would not have thought of without your input. Furthermore, you may have a clearer sense of the consequences of certain choices, which again is extremely valuable information.

Facilitating choices also means identifying and accepting a patient's and family's limitations, and finding ways to work with them so they achieve an outcome that is both positive and satisfactory to them. For example, you can suggest new activities that are appropriate for the patient's current capabilities. It is important that relationships remain mutual and reciprocal, and patients in particular need to experience their positive contribution to their family members. Thus, as patients get sicker, their contribution will look different and may focus on such things as words of wisdom. Sometimes you will need to be creative in finding ways to empower patients and families. You might find that your abilities are stretched as you try to accommodate them, especially within the constraints of your clinical setting, so do not be afraid to talk with your clinical facilitator or other staff members about your struggles. They can be great resources for you. At the same time, you might have some innovative ideas to share that they will find useful in their practice.

Offering Resources

One nurse cannot be all things to every patient and family. It is important to be aware of other team members, such as spiritual or pastoral care providers (Wall, Engelberg, Gries, Glavan, & Curtis, 2007), social workers, and others who may be available to provide support to the family. Furthermore, the nurse should be knowledgeable about hospital- and community-based services, such as hospice, that may be available to support families both before and after the death (Casarett, Crowley, Stevenson, Xie, & Teno, 2005). You should offer these other resources and services to families, but each family must decide what will actually be helpful for them. For some families, using inpatient respite services during the last year of life may help relieve their burden if only for short time, whereas other caregivers may experience feelings of guilt and increased stress caused by worrying about the quality of care provided (Skilbeck, Payne, Ingleton, Nolan, Carey, & Hanson, 2005). Caregivers may be supported in their role simply by knowing there are other resources and support readily available,

even if they do not make use of them (Stajduhar et al., 2008).

Encouraging Patients and Families

Patients and family members often seek approval and encouragement from professionals as they make decisions about how to meet their needs. Encouraging is an important strategy in empowering patients and families to do for themselves. It means verbally and nonverbally supporting patients and families in their choices, providing reinforcement for each individual's ideas, and demonstrating your agreement to find ways to facilitate their choices. Encouraging does not necessarily mean that you *agree* with the choice, merely that you support the patient or family member in finding ways to enact the choice. Encouraging allows families to figure out ways to do what is important for them. As a nurse, you can encourage families to include their cultural and religious practices as part of their palliative care experience. You need to be aware of those traditions that are important to families during the dying process, such as specific rituals at the time of death. Taking the time to discuss such issues before the patient's death and exploring ways to support their choice will empower patients and families.

It can sometimes be too easy to think that you know what is "best" for patients and their families. As a caring professional, you have their best interests at heart and you want to protect them as much as possible. Yet, if you value each person as a worthwhile individual who has the right and ability to make his or her own choices and decisions, then you may find that the patient's and family's wants conflict with what you believe is "best" based on your professional experience and knowledge. Times like these can cause you moral distress as you struggle with supporting the patient, yet remaining "true" to the knowledge you have. Your negotiation skills may be severely tested in such situations, and sometimes you will be tempted to override a patient's wishes. Some nurses describe their bottom line as "ensuring patient safety," and unless the patient's physical safety is compromised, they will support the patient's choice, even when they disagree with it. Honoring patient and family member preferences does not mean abandoning your professional expertise. Sharing your knowledge and perspective contributes to fully informed decision making.

Managing Negative Feelings

End-of-life care is not all encouragement and positive feelings. Many patients and family members also have negative feelings that influence their experiences. Talking with patients and families about those negative feelings gives them permission to have, experience, and deal with them. For many people, negative feelings, such as guilt or anger, are suppressed or internalized. Others openly express their anger but displace it onto someone else, often the nurse or other family members. The ability to diffuse a situation effectively requires nurses to learn how to accept someone else's negative feelings in an open and nondefensive manner. It means not taking their words as a personal attack, but realizing that patients and family members simply need a safe outlet for their frustrations and negative feelings. Your role is to listen in an accepting way and allow them to ventilate. It can be hard to face an angry tirade, but most people will calm down once they have said what they need to say, and they realize that you value their feelings even if they are negative ones. Questions that are often useful include "How can I help?" or "What needs to be different?"

Sometimes, however, people will remain angry or guilty despite your best efforts. Diffusing will not always be as successful as you would like. Some people are so angry about what is happening to their loved one and their family that they cannot move to any other emotional state. You will need to accept that this is their reality and find ways to work with them. This is often a time when nurses need the support of colleagues, and a team approach may help to lessen the effects of working with these patients and families (Namasivayam, Orb, & O'Connor, 2005).

Facilitating Healing Between Family Members

Negative feelings and misunderstandings can cause or expand rifts in families. If a nurse can facilitate healing between family members that unifies the family, then the family can function as a team and members are able to move through the dying process. You can help mend relationships by interpreting family members' behaviors to one another and helping them to see each other's point of view. Sometimes an outsider can bring clarity to a situation that is impossible when you are enmeshed

in it. Be careful, though, that you do not try to "fix broken families." Many families that you might think are dysfunctional do not see themselves as having difficulties or needing to change. They will not invite you to fix them and, indeed, may find your concern about the family intrusive. Furthermore, relationships develop over many years, and your interventions will occur in a relatively short period. Do not expect a huge change in family dynamics during the time you know a family, unless the family wants to change and makes an effort to do so. Sometimes all you can do is acknowledge to yourself that certain things cannot be fixed and your presence is all you have to offer. Levels of family functioning will need to be attended to carefully as you work with a family, and the expectations that a family will pull together to cope with the process of dying may be unrealistic. Noticing the family members' love for the ill member and acknowledging their mutual desire for the best for their ill member (even though there may be quite different ideas about what is best) is sometimes helpful.

Family Conferences

Family meetings with health professionals are beneficial to ensure consistency in everyone's understanding of the situation and the expected course for the illness (Wiegand, 2006). They enable patients, family members, and professionals to meet together to discuss any issue, but they are not family therapy (Fineberg, 2005). Nurses are ideal partners to lead these end-of-life family conferences. In all settings, you can assist families in preparing for the meetings by helping them to write down questions that they want to raise at the meeting, informing the family about what to expect during the conference, and discussing what the patient values in life, the patient's and the family members' spiritual and religious needs, and what the patient may want if he or she is unable to participate in the conference (Curtis, Patrick, Shannon, Treece, Engelberg, & Rubenfeld, 2001). It is helpful to begin by eliciting the family's understanding of the situation before moving to the health professionals' perspectives. Furthermore, it is to be expected that different family members and professionals will have different ideas, so it is useful to request different perspectives. Afterward, you can talk with the family about how the conference went, what the changes in the patient's plan of care are and what they mean, and how the family feels about the conference and changed plan of care (Curtis et al., 2001). You also should talk with the family about the decisions that were made and then support them in these decisions.

More than one meeting is likely necessary as the patient's condition changes or if the family needs time to think or further discuss issues before decisions are made (Wiegand, 2006). The proportion of time the family spends talking during these conferences is more important than the total length of the conference in increasing family satisfaction and decreasing conflict between families and health professionals (McDonagh et al., 2004). Yet, on average, typical family conferences involve the health professional speaking for 70% of the time and listening for only 30% of the time (McDonagh et al., 2004). You need to pay careful attention to ensuring that families do the majority of talking during family conferences. In addition, be mindful of the power of your nonverbal communication, as it is often our main method of communication, particularly when the topics are emotional.

Finding Meaning

When recovery is impossible, nurses must consider their role in helping patients and families find meaning in the experience as they care for and assist families. Patients and families often struggle to understand why the patient is dying. They try to give the experience some meaning, and they search for ways to make the patient's life and inevitable death worthwhile. Much of their search for meaning will involve examining relationships within the family, and some people will be more successful at finding meaning than others.

As a nurse, you can assist in this process of finding meaning by truly listening and hearing what family members have to say. Engaging in relationship and dialogue will be empowering and can help families create meaning even in a difficult situation (Abma, 2005). But there are many different ways of finding meaning, and not all individuals will overtly search for meaning. As a nurse, you will accompany people as they try to make sense of their situation. You cannot find meaning for someone else, however. Each individual will seek his own meaning in his own unique way. Some may be very articulate about their philosophical and spiritual beliefs. Others may talk about these issues in more concrete terms, perhaps rarely having articulated their thoughts and feelings. Still others may "talk" through their actions. Finding meaning gives strength to people, and therefore, you will find that it is empowering for families. Nurses who examine the concepts of meaning of illness and dying with patients may gain a deepened understanding of the patients' experiences, which may lead to changes and improvements in the way care is provided (Gauthier, 2002). You might begin this examination by asking the patient: "Can you tell me what it is like to be at this point in your life?"

Care at the Time of Death

A "good death" may contribute to family members feeling more at peace with the death (Mok et al., 2002), and also having a sense of satisfaction and accomplishment (Perreault et al., 2004). Parents often believe that their child's peaceful death means that they made the right choices and that they did all that they could for their child (Davies et al., 1998; Hinds et al., 2000; Vickers & Carlisle, 2000). Thus, facilitating a good death is an imperative for nurses. What constitutes a good death, however, is not well understood. From observations of patients, family members, and health care providers, six major components of a good death have been identified: pain and symptom management, clear decision making, preparation for death, completion, contributing to others, and affirmation of the whole person (Steinhauser, Clipp, McNeilly, Christakis, McIntyre, & Tulsky, 2000). A bad death has been defined by a "lack of opportunity to plan ahead, arrange personal affairs, decrease family burden, or say good-bye" (Steinhauser et al., 2000, p. 829).

In the context of a palliative care approach, the language of care, quality of life, relief of suffering, and the principles of palliative care become important in helping families attain a "good death." When a cure is not possible, families often react to the news with a blanket statement: "We want everything done." But that may not be what they mean literally. Rather, they want a "good death," but families may believe that if they agree to palliative care, then care, as well as treatment, will be withheld, and they will be abandoned because death is the expected outcome (Gillis, 2008). Clear discussions are needed about the continued provision of active care with a shift in emphasis to quality of life instead of prolongation of life. Such discussions will ensure families that, indeed, everything is being done and they are not being abandoned.

No matter the setting, family members are often afraid of the actual death event and have little or no understanding of what dying entails. You will find that sometimes the greatest gift you can give families as they prepare for the death is helping them release the dying person, to forgive themselves and their loved one so he or she can die in peace (Cooke, 1992). Nurses can help alleviate families' fears by finding out what they know and what they need. You can then prepare families for the death and help them to recognize the signs of imminent death so they are aware of what will likely happen when the signs appear (see Box 11-5). This preparation may be even more crucial for families in the home, who may be alone at the time. It also is important in the ICU and emergency department to tailor your information to the situation, for example, the effects drugs and machines (e.g., ventilator) might have on what signs are even possible around imminent death in these settings. For example, a patient's breathing will not change if they are on a ventilator.

BOX 11-5
Signs of Imminent Death

- Decline in physical capabilities
- Decreased alertness and social interaction
- Decreased intake of food and fluids
- Difficulty swallowing medications, food, and fluids
- Visual and auditory hallucinations
- Confusion, restlessness, agitation
- Physical changes as death nears include the following:
  - Circulation gradually shuts down; hands and feet feel cool, and a patchy, purplish color called *mottling* appears on the skin; heart speeds up, but also weakens, so pulse is rapid and can be hard to feel.
  - Bowel movements and urine production decrease as less food and fluid is taken in; may be no urine output in last day or two of life; constipation is not usually an issue to be managed in the last week of life; loss of bladder or bowel control can be managed with frequent skin care and the use of adult incontinence products, or even a urinary catheter if needed.
  - Changes in breathing often provide clues about how close someone is to death. As the automatic centers in the brain take over the regulation of breathing, changes generally occur in the following ways:
    - The rate of breathing: tends to be more rapid
    - The pattern or regularity in breathing: becomes very regular, almost mechanical
    - How deep the breaths are (may be shallow, deep, or normal): tends to become more shallow; may have periods of apnea where breathing pauses for a while; when the pauses in breathing appear, a noticeable pattern often develops: clusters of fairly rapid breathing that start with shallow breaths that become deeper and deeper, and then fade off, becoming shallower and shallower; may be 5 to 10 breaths in each cluster, and each cluster is separated by a pause that may last a few seconds or perhaps up to 30 seconds; called the Cheyne–Stokes pattern of breathing and is occasionally seen in healthy elderly people as well, especially during sleep
    - The kinds of muscles used in breathing: may start to use the neck muscles and the shoulders, but though it may look as if the person is struggling, unless they are agitated, it is simply "automatic pilot"
    - The amount of mucus or secretions that build up because the person is unable to cough: can be noisy (rattling or gurgling) and sometimes upsets people at the bedside even though is unlikely to be distressing to the person who is usually unconscious; some people call it the "death rattle," and it can be treated by medication to dry up the secretions; because the term *death rattle* may cause strong emotional reactions, the term *respiratory congestion* is now recommended
    - The pattern of breathing in the final minutes or perhaps hours of life: the breathing takes on an irregular pattern in which there is a breath, then a pause, then another breath or two, then another pause, and so forth. There may be periods of 15 to 30 seconds or so between final breaths.
    - After the last breath: very slight motions of breathing may happen irregularly for a few minutes after the final breath; these are reflex actions and are not signs of distress

Generally, an illness begins to weaken the body when a person is nearing death. Some health conditions affect vital body systems, such as the brain and nervous system, lungs, heart and blood vessels, or the digestive system, including the liver and bowels. As illnesses progress, the body becomes unable to use the nutrients in food, resulting in weight loss and a decline in appetite, energy, and strength. More time is spent resting, and in the final few days before death, people usually sleep most of the time. If families are aware of this natural progression, then they may be less distressed, for example, when their loved one stops eating. One sign of imminent death, terminal restlessness, can be distressing for family members to watch (Brajtman, 2003). Sedation at the end of life may be necessary to control severe symptoms such as terminal restlessness. Box 11-5 lists signs of imminent death that should be shared with families.

Communication and relationships continue to be important as death approaches (Munn & Zimmerman, 2006). Nurses can encourage family members to continue talking to their loved ones even if they are nonresponsive, because they may still be able to hear (Brajtman, 2005). You can model this type of interaction by continuing to speak to the patient and treating him or her with dignity throughout the dying process. You can also demonstrate respect for the family and their intimate knowledge of the patient by seeking their advice on things that were soothing or calming to the patient in the past, such as particular music, foot rubs and back rubs, or a particular way of arranging the pillows, then following these suggestions or encouraging the family to do so (Brajtman, 2005).

Many family members want to be present when their loved one is imminently dying; it is often important that they have an opportunity to say good-bye (Andershed, 2006). Thus, you need to be aware ahead of time about a family's wishes and ensure that they are called if there is a change in the patient's condition so they can be present at the time of death if that is what they want. The days, hours, and minutes leading up to a child's death are often seen by parents as their last opportunity to be a "good parent" to the child. Their ability to be physically present, emotionally supportive, and an effective advocate for their child is often key to viewing themselves as good parents in the years after their child's death (Meert et al., 2005; Rini & Loriz,

2007; Sharman et al., 2005; Woodgate, 2006). "Normal" parent activities such as bathing, feeding, or holding the child, even in the midst of technology that is being used to support the child's life, allow parents to develop or continue their bond with their child and sometimes to be able to say good-bye to their child (Brosig et al., 2007; Meert et al., 2005; Meyer et al., 2006; Pector, 2004a, 2004b; Rini & Loriz, 2007; Robinson et al., 2006; Sharman et al., 2005; Steele, Davies, Collins, & Cook, 2005). As a nurse, therefore, you need to facilitate parents' wishes at this time and provide an environment that allows for parents to fulfil their parental role. We cannot know when a patient will die, and despite our best efforts, sometimes this happens when family members are not present. When family members wish to be present, it is important to talk about the possibility that this may not happen. Sometimes the patient dies when the family member has nodded off to sleep or stepped out of the room for a cup of tea. It is often helpful for family members to know of this possibility.

Bereavement Care

Once the patient dies, the work of the nurse does not end (O'Connor, Peters, Lee, & Webster, 2005). A lot of family members may be present for the death, all of whom may need support, advice, information, and time to begin the grieving and healing process. Family members may wish to stay by the bedside and say whatever words seem appropriate. For some cultures, rituals may need to be conducted (O'Connor et al., 2005). Some families may want active involvement in caring for the patient's body or at least to know the body will be cared for in a respectful manner (Pector, 2004a; Widger & Picot, 2008). There is no harm in touching the person's body, and there should be no rush to move the person until everyone has had a chance to say their final good-byes.

Family members who were not present for the death may need to be contacted and may wish to see the patient before he or she is taken to the morgue or a funeral home. As a nurse, you can encourage the family to be together if they wish and to take as much time as needed after the death. Your presence as family members express their emotions may help them to create meaningful final memories and begin to process their experience (Hannan & Gibson, 2005; Macnab, Northway, Ryall, Scott, & Straw, 2003; Meert et al., 2005; Pector, 2004a; Rini & Loriz, 2007; Steele et al., 2005; Wisten & Zingmark, 2007). You may need to contact pastoral care or other professionals to assist in supporting the family. Some families will appreciate your assistance with or information on arranging funerals (de Jong-Berg & Kane, 2006; Macnab et al., 2003; Pector, 2004a; Rini & Loriz, 2007).

Particularly when the patient who has died is a child, families may appreciate you giving them a collection of mementos such as pictures, locks of hair, and handprints or footprints (de Jong-Berg & Kane, 2006; Macnab et al., 2003; Meert et al., 2005; Pector, 2004b; Rini & Loriz, 2007; Widger & Picot, 2008). Some families later regret not taking mementos (de Jong-Berg & Kane, 2006), but others may be distressed if you take mementos, especially pictures, against their wishes (Skene, 1998); therefore, determining what each family wants and needs requires sensitivity and a careful approach.

In some cases, autopsy and organ or tissue donation may be possible. Nurses and other health professionals sometimes view such discussions as an intrusion, and thus because of their own discomfort, they do not approach families. Parents may have lingering regrets, however, if they miss an opportunity to help another child or to receive answers to some questions about their own child's death (Macdonald et al., 2006; Widger & Picot, 2008). Therefore, you should not be afraid to initiate these conversations should they be indicated, or at least ensure that someone initiates them. It is also important to make sure that when autopsies are done, families are given the results in a timely and compassionate manner (Macdonald et al., 2006; Meert et al., 2007; Rini & Loriz, 2007; Wisten & Zingmark, 2007). Families may want to meet with health professionals to discuss autopsy results, clarify the events leading to and the circumstances of the death, and be reassured that everything possible was done and the right decisions were made (Kreicbergs et al., 2005; Macdonald et al., 2006; Pector, 2004a; Wisten & Zingmark, 2007; Woodgate, 2006).

It was previously thought that healing meant a person got over their loss and severed ties with the deceased. It is now known that one does not "get over" the loss of a loved one; rather, families will forever have links with the person who has died (Moules, Simonson, Fleiszer, Prins, & Rev Bob, 2007; Moules, Simonson, Prins, Angus, & Bell, 2004). As a nurse, you can do much to facilitate a healthy start to their grieving journey and to help them find meaning in death. Your actions at the actual death event are critical. Family members vividly remember the moment of their loved one's death. They often remember who was present, what was said, what was done that was helpful, and what was not so helpful. Many remember that it was the nurse who was with them at the moment of death, or that the nurse was the first to respond to the family's call about a change in their loved one's condition. More often than not, families clearly recall the nurse's words and actions. What you do for and with family members at the time of their loved one's death can have a profound and long-lasting impact on them. It is important to remember that, although the death may be one of many for the nurse, it may be the first and only for the family; therefore, a person's death should never be treated as "just a job" on the part of the nurse (Shiozaki et al., 2005). Be cognizant too that clichés such as "this was meant to be," "he or she is in a better place," or referring to the deceased person as an angel may make families feel that you are minimizing the impact of the death on the family (Pector, 2004a, 2004b). Simple expressions, such as "I am sorry your husband is dying" (Tilden, Tolle, Garland, & Nelson, 1995, p. 637), are more often appreciated.

Nurses should have an understanding of loss, know how to support families in grief, and be able to provide quality bereavement care. Beginning nurses often worry about showing emotion, such as crying, in the presence of family members. Family members are often deeply touched when they see a nurse's genuine emotional response, but it is critical that the family not be put in the position of caring for the nurse.

Provision of bereavement care by the nurse offers the opportunity for continued contact with the family and signifies the importance of the family to the nurse (Davies, Collins, Steele, Cook, Distler, & Brenner, 2007; de Cinque et al., 2006; de Jong-Berg & Kane, 2006; Kreicbergs et al., 2005; Macdonald et al., 2005; Meert et al., 2007; Rodger, Sherwood, O'Connor, & Leslie, 2007). Follow-up activities that many families appreciate include calls, cards, attendance at the funeral, and offers to make referrals to additional sources of support as needed (Cherlin et al., 2004). Written information on practical issues and what to do next may be helpful (D'Agostino et al., 2008; de Cinque et al., 2006; Rini & Loriz, 2007; Rodger et al., 2007). Families may also appreciate written information about grief or other sources of support (D'Agostino et al., 2008; de Cinque et al., 2006; de Jong-Berg & Kane, 2006; Pector, 2004a; Rini & Loriz, 2007), as well as information to share with extended family and friends on how to offer effective support. Depending on the setting, bereavement care may continue for a period of time in the community. Sometimes health care professionals call or send a card to families on the first anniversary of the patient's death, especially if it was a child who died. This simple contact acknowledges that the grieving process takes time and can make families feel really cared for, once again highlighting the importance of the patient and family to the professional.

Special Situations

Some situations that can be challenging for nurses to consider, such as how to respond when a child wants to visit a dying family member in the ICU or when a parent wants to observe resuscitation attempts, and how to help families when caring for a family member at home, deserve additional attention.

FACILITATING CONNECTIONS FOR CHILDREN WHEN A FAMILY MEMBER IS CRITICALLY ILL. When a family member is critically ill, families and professionals may have a concern about the importance and impact of bringing children to visit, whether at home, in the ICU, or in any other setting. Yet, these visits may reduce feelings of separation, guilt, abandonment, fear, loneliness, and worry for the child (Nolbris & Hellstrom, 2005; Vint, 2005). Children can generally decide for themselves if they do wish to visit. Those younger than 10 visiting a relative may be most interested in the equipment, whereas older children may spend more time focused on the person they are visiting (Knutsson & Bergbom, 2007). The visit can also benefit the patient by acting as a diversion, offering hope, and bringing a sense of normality (Vint, 2005). Thus, nurses should offer families the option of bringing children in to visit loved ones. You can assist families to prepare children beforehand about what they

will see and what to expect; you also can be present during the visit to support family members in answering questions and to make the child feel welcome and an important part of the family (Knutsson & Bergbom, 2007; Nolbris & Hellstrom, 2005; Vint, 2005). If the child chooses not to visit, you can still assist in maintaining connections between the child and the ill family member through facilitating cards, calls, and frequent updates about how the patient is doing.

WHEN DEATH IS SUDDEN OR TRAUMATIC. Sudden life-threatening events bring the possibility of administering cardiopulmonary resuscitation. Although some debate exists regarding the presence of family members during attempts at resuscitation, many settings do allow for it. Parents in particular may voice a strong belief that it is their right to be present during these events (McGahey Oakland, Lieder, Young, & Jefferson, 2007; Meert et al., 2005; Rini & Loriz, 2007; Wisten & Zingmark, 2007), because they believe that their presence is a source of strength and support for the child, and being present offers the opportunity to see for themselves that everything possible was done to assist their child. Families need frequent updates if they choose not to be present and must be given information about what is happening if they are present (McGahey Oakland et al., 2007).

DYING AT HOME. Families need professional support, particularly in the area of symptom control, to make a home death "happen" (Brazil et al., 2005). Caring for a dying family member at home can be extremely demanding work—physically, emotionally, psychologically, and spiritually. The primary caregivers require support and resources to be successful. First and foremost, the family and the nurse need to discuss the dying process, existing resources, and present and future needs. Then together they can develop a plan that anticipates changes. For example, symptom crises, such as escalating pain, need to be anticipated and addressed in advance. When the family is committed to supporting death at home, it can be devastating when a symptom crisis results in death in the middle of a busy emergency department. Box 11-6 provides some practical suggestions about what you need to consider and perhaps facilitate when someone is dying at home.

BOX 11-6

Practical Considerations When Someone Is Dying at Home

- Involvement of expert resources such as hospice and an interdisciplinary team including volunteers
- Advance care planning including the presence of a "Do Not Resuscitate" order if necessary
- Equipment such as a hospital bed and commode
- Identification of willing informal support persons (friends, church, extended family)
- Development of a list of things that willing people can do, for example, a calendar for preparation of meals, house cleaning, someone to visit so the caregiver can get out for a walk
- Respite for the caregiver(s), which may be planned hospice admissions or the overnight placement of a paid professional
- Financial implications and available support, for example, compassionate benefits program
- Symptom management plan, including anticipating changes such as inability to swallow and the need for parenteral medications
- Contact numbers of resources
- Discussion of unfinished business to enable a peaceful death
- Discussion of alternatives should dying and death at home become impossible for any reason

Jones Family Case Study

The Jones family was introduced in Chapter 3 and is reintroduced here to demonstrate working with a family at the end of life. Please return to Chapter 3 and reacquaint yourself with the family and the Jones Family Genogram in Figure 11-1. You will remember that Linda, the mother in the family, had been living with multiple sclerosis (MS) for 13 years. Early in the illness, Linda experienced relapses where her symptoms worsened, but these were followed by periods of remission where she recovered back to "normal." But since Travis's birth, her relapses had become more frequent, and although her symptoms sometimes improved a little, her condition was steadily getting worse.

Before Linda's discharge from the hospital where she had been treated with antibiotics for pneumonia after aspiration, the primary nurse, Catherine, initiated a family meeting with Linda, Robert, and Linda's physician. Catherine had noticed Robert's fatigue and repeated questions about whether Linda was really ready to come home. Catherine had also noticed Linda's reluctance to take medications (particularly for pain), her determination to walk with her cane despite serious unsteadiness, and the deepening silence between the husband and wife.

Catherine began the conversation by asking Linda and Robert about their understanding of the MS at this point. Linda quickly responded, saying that the pneumonia was really an unusual "one-time" problem, and although it had set her back, it would not be long before she was back on her feet. Robert worried out loud that it seemed things were getting progressively worse. He was concerned about how Linda would manage at home alone in the mornings and with Travis in the afternoon when he returned from preschool. Noticing the difference in perspective, Catherine acknowledged she could see how there might be differences because MS is, indeed, a "tricky" illness that is difficult to predict. She asked Linda and Robert to think back to how things were a year ago and to what had happened over the last year. Both noticed that the hospitalizations had become more frequent, the recoveries were more difficult, and overall, Linda was not doing as well. The physician, Dr. Brooks, who had been listening quietly, remarked that, although MS was often an unpredictable disease, it seemed that Linda's MS had changed into a different kind of illness than it had been at first. He agreed that now the MS was more steadily progressing, and that it seemed things were getting worse more quickly. Linda said she could see this but kept hoping that the situation would turn around.

Catherine then asked what the family's goals for care were. Linda was quick to answer, "Remission—I want full remission." Robert was slower to reply. He said, "I am so tired, and it hurts me so much to see you suffer. I want you to be comfortable, to be free of pain, to enjoy the kids rather than snapping at them...." Linda said, "I'm just trying so hard to get back to normal. I always thought that a wheelchair would be the end for me. And I'm just so tired." Catherine acknowledged that MS often creates profound tiredness in many family members and wondered which of the children might be most affected. Both Linda and Robert agreed that, of the children, Katie was suffering the most from tiredness. She picked up a lot of the pieces of Linda's work in the home, beginning supper preparations and looking after Travis. Often she would be up late at night working on homework, but her grades had been slipping and she had

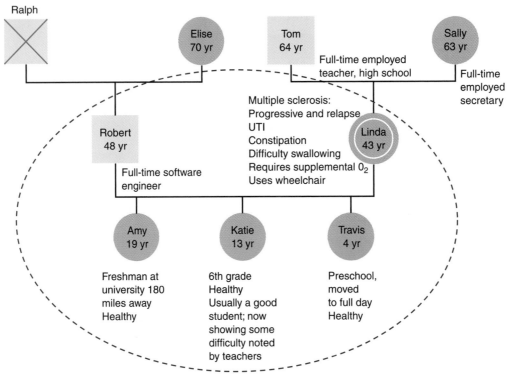

FIGURE 11-1 Jones family genogram.

been crying more. Linda worried that Amy was also tired as she spent a great deal of time driving home on weekends to care for the family.

Dr. Brooks interjected at this point saying that their primary goal for care during this hospitalization had been to cure the pneumonia. He noted that, although they were successful, they had not been able to assist Linda toward a remission. He remarked that with the change in the MS, it seemed that the hope for remission might not be possible. He then asked, "If things continue the way they are going, where do you think you will be in six months?" Linda began to cry and said she was thinking she might not be alive. The pneumonia scared her, and she was frightened about aspirating again, so she had been decreasing what she ate and drank. Robert was worried about how he could continue to work full time supporting the family and also care for Linda at home, especially as it seemed there was so little he did that was "right" for Linda.

Catherine replied that the "new" MS was clearly creating challenges for the family and wondered if it was time to shift the focus of care more toward comfort and quality of life for all family members, whereas at the same time working to prevent problems such as aspiration. She

explained that as illness gets more demanding, additional supports are needed. She also explained that as illness gets intrusive, attention needs to be paid to what is most important to living well for all family members. Linda was getting tired at this point and having a lot of difficulty holding her head up, so Catherine asked if she could schedule another meeting. Robert and Linda readily agreed, saying they knew they needed to talk about these things but just did not know how. Catherine asked them to do some homework: to each identify their biggest concern, as well as what was most important to living well at this time. They were asked to find this out from the children, too, and a meeting was scheduled for the next day. Dr. Brooks let them know that he wanted to speak with them about Linda's preferences for care should she have another experience with pneumonia.

The next day, Linda, Robert, Catherine, and Dr. Brooks all met again. Linda began the conversation, saying she had done a great deal of soul searching and was most worried about suffering from unmanageable pain and being a burden to her family. She was wondering if perhaps she should not go home but should be admitted into a care facility. Robert was most worried about burning out and not being able to support

Linda and the children as he wanted. They had had a three-way conversation with each of the children last evening. Amy was most worried that her mother was going to die, and she let her parents know that she was planning on leaving university to move back home. Katie was most troubled by her lack of friends as her friends were no longer including her in their activities. Travis missed his mother, and wanted her to be able to read stories to him and play with him more.

The things that were most important to Linda's quality of life were reducing her pain, having Amy continue at university, being more involved in Katie's and Travis's everyday lives, being able to attend a service at her church on a weekly basis, and reconnecting with Robert. She said her greatest hope was to be at home as long as possible. Robert wanted to be able to sleep, to go to work without constantly worrying about Linda, and to reconnect to Linda. He too wanted her at home as long as possible. Both Linda and Robert agreed that for them to live well, they needed more help in their home. Options were discussed, including the possibility of Elise (Robert's mother) moving in to be of assistance and preplanned, short stays in hospice for respite. Linda did not want Elise doing her personal care, so again, options were discussed. Dr. Brooks and the family developed a systematic plan for pain management. During the assessment process, he learned that Linda was refusing her medications because she was concerned they were contributing to her irritability with Robert and the children. He was able to reassure her that this was not the case; in fact, her unmanaged pain was more likely a major negative influence. They devised a plan for long-acting pain medication so that Robert would be able to sleep through the night. A dietician was consulted regarding ways to manage swallowing problems, and a home assessment by the team physiotherapist was scheduled so that Linda's mobility could be safely maximized.

Both Catherine and Dr. Brooks commended Linda and Robert on the deep love they saw between the couple and how effective they were at problem solving, systematically working their issues through until achieving a mutually satisfying outcome.

Finally, Dr. Brooks raised the topic of what Linda's preferences for care would be if she should experience development of pneumonia again. He explained that this was a real possibility because Linda's respiratory muscles were weakening. Dr. Brooks understood that both Linda and Robert wanted her home as long as possible, so he was curious about whether she would

want to come to the hospital to be treated with intravenous antibiotics as she had during this hospitalization. Linda stated this would be her preference, especially if she was likely to be able to go home again after the treatment. Dr. Brooks explained that as her muscles become weaker, she might need the assistance of a breathing machine (ventilator) to give the antibiotics time to work against the infection, and asked whether she would want that. Linda was not sure what her preference would be in this situation, but she was very clear that she did not want to be "kept alive on a machine." She and Robert wanted more time to discuss this question, and they wanted to consult with their pastor, so they agreed to continue the conversation at the next doctor's appointment. Robert and Linda agreed to visit the local hospice to explore respite opportunities, as well as end-of-life care, should staying at home prove too difficult.

Three weeks later at the scheduled appointment with Dr. Brooks, Linda let him know that many things were going better with Elise in the house and home visits from Catherine, as well as a personal care aide. Amy had agreed to stay in college with the promise from her parents that she would be told immediately if Linda's health changed. All family members were feeling less tired. Linda stated that she was not ready to leave Robert and the children, but was in a dilemma about the use of a ventilator if she experienced development of pneumonia. She continued to worry that she might be kept alive on the machine, and to her that would not be living. Dr. Brooks explained that, if necessary, one possibility was a time-limited trial of a ventilator to determine whether the antibiotics would work. Both Linda and Robert agreed. This was a difficult discussion, and Linda expressed distress about her loss of independence and her deep sorrow about the possibility of leaving her children. She admitted to swinging between despair and anger, and that both made it hard for her to enjoy her days. This was new information to Robert, who had noticed her struggling but thought things would work out over time. Through assessment, it became apparent that Linda was experiencing depression. She agreed to try an antidepressant medication and to join a local MS support group.

EIGHT MONTHS LATER

Linda experienced fever, congestion, and shortness of breath after aspiration. Antibiotics were initiated, and symptom management was maximized to relieve pain, breathlessness, fever, and constipation. Linda occasionally had periods of acute shortness of breath where she worried that she might not be able to take her next breath. The fear served to make the breathlessness worse, so the visiting nurse showed both Linda and the family how to slow and deepen breathing by consciously breathing together. Dr. Brooks made a home visit and asked Linda about admission to hospital. When he could not assure her that she would get off the ventilator, Linda declined, saying she wanted to stay with her family. Robert agreed. A family meeting with Catherine and Dr. Brooks was held at Linda's bedside to discuss what the family would experience if the pneumonia progressed. A family ecomap was developed (Figure 11-2) and support services were increased with more frequent visits from the nurse, care aide, and friends (particularly from Linda's support group). A move to hospice was discussed, but all agreed that home was the best

place for Linda, and that death at home was their preference.

Linda engaged in one-on-one time with each of her children. They talked about their best memories together, what they most loved about each other, and their hopes and dreams for the future as the children grow up. Robert participated by videotaping the conversations. Each child was given a journal, and together with Linda they drew pictures, wrote notes, and gathered mementos to capture these conversations. She organized gifts for their birthdays and for Christmas in the upcoming year. It was not that she knew she was dying, but she had been encouraged to plan for the worst and hope for the best, to do the things that needed doing. The family had received the same encouragement so they had all been able to have special time with Linda over the last few months. Linda died surrounded by her family.

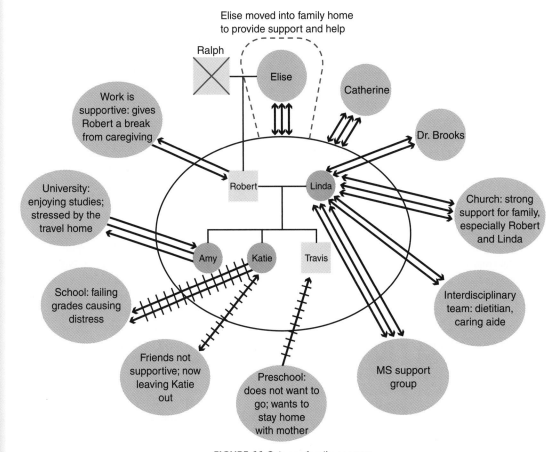

FIGURE 11-2 Jones family ecomap.

SIX WEEKS LATER

Catherine visited the family 6 weeks after Linda's death and found them managing well. Pictures of Linda were everywhere. Elise continued to live with the family, and they thought this was the best plan for the time being. Robert had taken some time off work to be with the children after Linda's death, but shortly afterward all went back to work and school. Amy still came home on some weekends. Robert, Amy, and Katie talked of their sense of having done the very best they could to honor Linda's preferences. They took comfort in the fact that she died at home. They had marked the 1-month anniversary of Linda's death with a visit to her grave site, taking flowers and a picture Travis had drawn of his mother. Family members drew support from different sources: each other, friends, their pastor, and some of the people from the MS support group who continued to visit. The children continued to read and reread the letters Linda had written; for Travis this was part of his bedtime ritual. They were sad, and some days were better than others; they had a sense that the weight of their grief was lifting.

SUMMARY

Nurses are in a unique position to help families manage their lives when a loved one has a terminal illness or faces an acute or sudden death. Providing palliative and end-of-life nursing care as you accompany a family during this intense period is a privilege that should not be taken lightly. The importance of the nurse-family relationship in effecting positive outcomes cannot be overstated; this relationship can make the difference between a family who has good memories about their loved one's death and a family who experiences prolonged suffering because of a negative experience. Open and trusting communication, physical, psychological, and spiritual support, and respect for the families' right to make their own decisions, as well as support to facilitate these decisions, are essential components of quality palliative and end-of-life care. It is a privilege to have the unique opportunity to form close relationships with the dying person and their family, to make a difference at this time in the family's life, and to learn from the people we nurse (Cooke, 1992). How often do nurses really have an opportunity to engage with patients and their families in such a powerful way?

REFERENCES

Abma, T. A. (2005). Struggling with the fragility of life: A relational-narrative approach to ethics in palliative nursing. *Nursing Ethics, 12*(4), 337–348.

Andershed, B. (2006). Relatives in end-of-life care. Part 1: A systematic review of the literature the five past years, January 1999–February 2004. *Journal of Clinical Nursing, 15*, 1158–1169.

Antle, B. J., Barrera, M., Beaune, L., D'Agostino, N., & Good, B. (2005, Fall). Paediatric palliative care: What do parents want? *Rehab and Community Care Medicine*, 24–26.

Aspinal, F., Hughes, R., Dunckley, M., & Addington Hall, J. (2006). What is important to measure in the last months and weeks of life? A modified nominal group study. *International Journal of Nursing Studies, 43*(4), 393–403.

Azoulay, E., Pochard, F., Kentish-Barnes, N., Chevret, S., Aboab, J., Adrie, C., et al. (2005). Risk of post-traumatic stress symptoms in family members of intensive care unit patients. *American Journal of Respiratory and Critical Care Medicine, 171*(9), 987–994.

Barnes, S., Gott, M., Payne, S., Parker, C., Seamark, D., Gariballa, S., et al. (2006). Characteristics and views of family carers of older people with heart failure. *International Journal of Palliative Nursing, 12*(8), 380–389.

Borneman, T., Chu, D. Z., Wagman, L., Ferrell, B., Juarez, G., McCahill, L. E., et al. (2003). Concerns of family caregivers of patients with cancer facing palliative surgery for advanced malignancies. *Oncology Nursing Forum, 30*(6), 997–1005.

Brady, M. J., Peterman, A. H., Fitchett, G., Mo, M., & Cella, A. (1999). A case for including spirituality in quality of life measurement in oncology. *Psycho-Oncology, 8*, 417–428.

Brajtman, S. (2003). The impact on the family of terminal restlessness and its management. *Palliative Medicine, 17*(5), 454–460.

Brajtman, S. (2005). Helping the family through the experience of terminal restlessness. *Journal of Hospice and Palliative Nursing, 7*(2), 73–81.

Brazil, K., Howell, D., Bedard, M., Krueger, P., & Heidebrecht, C. (2005). Preferences for place of care and place of death among informal caregivers of the terminally ill. *Palliative Medicine, 19*(6), 492–499.

Brinchmann, B. S., Forde, R., & Nortvedt, P. (2002). What matters to the parents? A qualitative study of parents' experiences with life-and-death decisions concerning their premature infants. *Nursing Ethics, 9*(4), 388–404.

Brosig, C. L., Pierucci, R. L., Kupst, M. J., & Leuthner, S. R. (2007). Infant end-of-life care: The parents' perspective. *Journal of Perinatology, 27*, 510–516.

Caron, C. D., Griffith, J., & Arcand, M. (2005). End-of-life decision making in dementia: The perspective of family caregivers. *Dementia, 4*(1), 113–136.

Casarett, D., Crowley, R., Stevenson, C., Xie, S., & Teno, J. (2005). Making difficult decisions about hospice enrollment: What do patients and families want to know? *Journal of the American Geriatrics Society, 53*(2), 249–254.

Cherlin, E., Schulman Green, D., McCorkle, R., Johnson Hurzeler, R., & Bradley, E. (2004). Family perceptions of clinicians' outstanding practices in end-of-life care. *Journal of Palliative Care, 20*(2), 113–116.

Christakis, N. A., & Iwashyna, T. J. (2003). The health impact of health care on families: A matched cohort study of hospice use by decedents and mortality outcomes in surviving, widowed spouses. *Social Science & Medicine, 57*, 465–475.

Contro, N., Larson, J., Scofield, S., Sourkes, B., & Cohen, H. (2002). Family perspectives on the quality of pediatric palliative care. *Archives of Pediatrics & Adolescent Medicine, 156*(1), 14–19.

Contro, N. A., Larson, J., Scofield, S., Sourkes, B., & Cohen, H. J. (2004). Hospital staff and family perspectives regarding quality of pediatric palliative care. *Pediatrics, 114*(5), 1248–1252.

Cooke, M. A. (1992). The challenge of hospice nursing in the 90's. *American Journal of Hospice & Palliative Care, 9*(1), 34–37.

Counsell, C. (2002). Exploring family needs during withdrawal of life support in critically ill patients. *Critical Care Nursing Clinics of North America, 14*(2), 187–191.

Curtis, J. R., Patrick, D. L., Shannon, S. E., Treece, P. D., Engelberg, R. A., & Rubenfeld, G. D. (2001). The family conference as a focus to improve communication about end-of-life care in the intensive care unit: Opportunities for improvement. *Critical Care Medicine, 29*(2 suppl), N26–N33.

D'Agostino, N. M., Berlin-Romalis, D., Jovcevska, V., & Barrera, M. (2008). Bereaved parents' perspectives on their needs. *Palliative and Supportive Care, 6*(1), 33–41.

Davies, B., Collins, J., Steele, R., Cook, K., Distler, V., & Brenner, A. (2007). Parents' and children's perspectives of a children's hospice bereavement program. *Journal of Palliative Care, 23*(1), 14–23.

Davies, B., & Connaughty, S. (2002). Pediatric end-of-life care: Lessons learned from parents. *Journal of Nursing Administration, 32*(1), 5–6.

Davies, B., Deveau, E., deVeber, B., Howell, D., Martinson, I., Papadatou, D., et al. (1998). Experiences of mothers in five countries whose child died of cancer. *Cancer Nursing, 21*(5), 301–311.

Davies, B., & Oberle, K. (1990). Dimensions of the supportive role of the nurse in palliative care. *Oncology Nursing Forum, 17*(1), 87–94.

Davies, B., Sehring, S. A., Partridge, J. C., Cooper, B. A., Hughes, A., Philp, J. C., et al. (2008). Barriers to palliative care for children: Perceptions of pediatric health care providers. *Pediatrics, 121*(2), 282–288.

Dawson, S., & Kristjanson, L. J. (2003). Mapping the journey: Family carers' perceptions of issues related to end-stage care of individuals with muscular dystrophy or motor neurone disease. *Journal of Palliative Care, 19*(1), 36–42.

Dean, R. A., & Gregory, D. M. (2005). More than trivial: Strategies for using humor in palliative care. *Cancer Nursing, 28*(4), 292–300.

De Cinque, N., Monterosso, L., Dadd, G., Sidhu, R., Macpherson, R., & Aoun, S. (2006). Bereavement support for families following the death of a child from cancer: Experience of bereaved parents. *Journal of Psychosocial Oncology, 24*(2), 65–83.

De Jong-Berg, M. A., & Kane, L. (2006). Bereavement care for families. Part 2: Evaluation of a paediatric follow-up programme. *International Journal of Palliative Nursing, 12*(10), 484–494.

Diver, F., Molassiotis, A., & Weeks, L. (2003). The palliative care needs of ethnic minority patients attending a day-care centre: A qualitative study. *International Journal of Palliative Nursing, 9*(9), 389–396.

Dunn, P. M., Tolle, S. W., Moss, A. H., & Black, J. S. (2007). The POLST paradigm: Respecting the wishes of patients and families. *Annals of Long-Term Care, 15*(9), 33–40.

Dwyer, L., Nordenfelt, L., & Ternestedt, B. (2008). Three nursing home residents speak about meaning at the end of life. *Nursing Ethics, 15*(1), 97–109.

Elpern, E. H., Covert, B., & Kleinpell, R. (2005). Moral distress of staff nurses in a medical intensive care unit. *American Journal of Critical Care, 14*(6), 523–530.

Ferrell, B., Ervin, K., Smith, S., Marek, T., & Melancon, C. (2002). Family perspectives of ovarian cancer. *Cancer Practice: A Multidisciplinary Journal of Cancer Care, 10*(6), 269–276.

Fineberg, I. C. (2005). Preparing professionals for family conferences in palliative care: Evaluation results of an interdisciplinary approach. *Journal of Palliative Medicine, 8*(4), 857–866.

Fitzsimons, D., Mullan, D., Wilson, J. S., Conway, B., Corcoran, B., Dempster, M., et al. (2007). The challenge of patients' unmet palliative care needs in the final stages of chronic illness. *Palliative Medicine, 21*(4), 313–322.

Forbes Thompson, S., & Gessert, C. E. (2005). End of life in nursing homes: Connections between structure, process, and outcomes. *Journal of Palliative Medicine, 8*(3), 545–555.

Fox, E., Landrum-McNiff, K., Zhong, Z., Dawson, N. V., Wu, A. W., & Lynn, J. (1999). Evaluation of prognostic criteria for determining hospice eligibility in patients with advanced lung, heart, or liver disease. *Journal of the American Medical Association, 282*(17), 1638–1645.

Fridriksdottir, N., Sigurdardottir, V., & Gunnarsdottir, S. (2006). Important needs of families in acute and palliative care settings assessed with the family inventory of needs. *Palliative Medicine, 20*(4), 425–432.

Gauthier, D. M. (2002). The meaning of healing near the end of life. *Journal of Hospice and Palliative Nursing, 4*(4), 220–227.

Gillis, J. (2008). "We want everything done." *Archives of Disease in Childhood, 93*(3), 192–193.

Goy, E. R., Carter, J. H., & Ganzini, L. (2007). Parkinson disease at the end of life: Caregiver perspectives. *Neurology, 69*(6), 611–612.

Hammes, B. J., Klevan, J., Kempf, M., & Williams, M. S. (2005). Pediatric advance care planning. *Journal of Palliative Medicine, 8*(4), 766–773.

Hannan, J., & Gibson, F. (2005). Advanced cancer in children: How parents decide on final place of care for their dying child. *International Journal of Palliative Nursing, 11*(6), 284–291.

Hays, R. M., Valentine, J., Haynes, G., Geyer, J. R., Villareale, N., McKinstry, B., et al. (2006). The Seattle pediatric palliative care project: Effects on family satisfaction and health-related quality of life. *Journal of Palliative Medicine, 9*(3), 716–728.

Heller, K. S., & Solomon, M. Z. (2005). Continuity of care and caring: What matters to parents of children with life-threatening conditions. *Journal of Pediatric Nursing, 20*(5), 335–346.

Heyland, D. K., Dodek, P., Rocker, G., Groll, D., Gafni, A., Pichora, D., et al. (2006). What matters most in end-of-life care: Perceptions of seriously ill patients and their family members. *Canadian Medical Association Journal, 174*(5), 627–633.

Heyland, D. K., Frank, C., Groll, D., Pichora, D., Dodek, P., Rocker, G., et al. (2006). Understanding cardiopulmonary resuscitation decision making: Perspectives of seriously ill hospitalized patients and family members. *Chest, 130*(2), 419–428.

Heyland, D. K., Groll, D., Rocker, G., Dodek, P., Gafni, A., Tranmer, J., et al. (2005). End-of-life care in acute care hospitals in Canada: A quality finish? *Journal of Palliative Care, 21*(3), 142–150.

Heyland, D. K., Rocker, G. M., O'Callaghan, C. J., Dodek, P. M., & Cook, D. J. (2003). Ethics in cardiopulmonary medicine. Dying in the ICU: Perspectives of family members. *Chest, 124*(1), 392–397.

Hinds, P. S., Drew, D., Oakes, L. L., Fouladi, M., Spunt, S. L., Church, C., et al. (2005). End-of-life care preferences of pediatric patients with cancer. *Journal of Clinical Oncology, 23*(36), 9146–9154.

Hinds, P. S., Oakes, L., Quargnenti, A., Furman, W., Bowman, L., Gilger, E., et al. (2000). An international feasibility study of parental decision making in pediatric oncology. *Oncology Nursing Forum, 27*(8), 1233–1243.

Horne, G., & Payne, S. (2004). Removing the boundaries: Palliative care for patients with heart failure. *Palliative Medicine, 18*(4), 291–296.

Horsley, H., & Patterson, T. (2006). The effects of a parent guidance intervention on communication among adolescents who have experienced the sudden death of a sibling. *The American Journal of Family Therapy, 34*, 119–137.

Houger Limacher, L., & Wright, L. M. (2003). Commendations: Listening to the silent side of a family intervention. *Journal of Family Nursing, 9*(2), 130–135.

Hsiao, J. L., Evan, E. E., & Zeltzer, L. K. (2007). Parent and child perspectives on physician communication in pediatric palliative care. *Palliative & Supportive Care, 5*(4), 355–365.

Hudson, P. (2004). Positive aspects and challenges associated with caring for a dying relative at home. *International Journal of Palliative Nursing, 10*(2), 58–60, 62–64.

Hudson, P. (2006). How well do family caregivers cope after caring for a relative with advanced disease and how can health professionals enhance their support? *Journal of Palliative Medicine, 9*(3), 694–703.

Hughes, R. A., Sinha, A., Higginson, I., Down, K., & Leigh, P. N. (2005). Living with motor neurone disease: Lives, experiences of services and suggestions for change. *Health and Social Care in the Community, 13*(1), 64–74.

James, L., & Johnson, B. (1997). The needs of parents of pediatric oncology patients during the palliative care phase. *Journal of Pediatric Oncology Nursing, 14*(2), 83–95.

Jo, S., Brazil, K., Lohfeld, L., & Willison, K. (2007). Caregiving at the end of life: Perspectives from spousal caregivers and care recipients. *Palliative & Supportive Care, 5*(1), 11–17.

Johansson, C. M., Axelsson, B., & Danielson, E. (2006). Living with incurable cancer at the end of life—Patients' perceptions on quality of life. *Cancer Nursing, 29*(5), 391–399.

Kazanowski, M. (2005). Family caregivers' medication management of symptoms in patients with cancer near death. *Journal of Hospice and Palliative Nursing, 7*(3), 174–181.

Kirk, P., Kirk, I., & Kristjanson, L. J. (2004). What do patients receiving palliative care for cancer and their families want to be told? A Canadian and Australian qualitative study. *British Medical Journal, 328*(7452), 1343–1347.

Knutsson, S. E., & Bergbom, I. L. (2007). Custodians' viewpoints and experiences from their child's visit to an ill or injured nearest being cared for at an adult intensive care unit. *Journal of Clinical Nursing, 16*(2), 362–371.

Kreicbergs, U. C., Lannen, P., Onelov, E., & Wolfe, J. (2007). Parental grief after losing a child to cancer: Impact of professional and social support on long-term outcomes. *Journal of Clinical Oncology, 25*(22), 3307–3312.

Kreicbergs, U., Valdimarsdottir, U., Onelov, E., Bjork, O., Steineck, G., & Henter, J. I. (2005). Care-related distress: A nationwide study of parents who lost their child to cancer. *Journal of Clinical Oncology, 23*(36), 9162–9171.

Kristjanson, L. J., Aoun, S. M., & Oldham, L. (2006). Palliative care and support for people with neurodegenerative conditions and their carers. *International Journal of Palliative Nursing, 12*(8), 368–377.

Kristjanson, L. J., Aoun, S.M., & Yates, P. (2006). Are supportive services meeting the needs of Australians with neurodegenerative conditions and their families? *Journal of Palliative Care, 22*(3), 151–157.

Kwak, J., Salmon, J. R., Acquaviva, K. D., Brandt, K., & Egan, K. A. (2007). Benefits of training family caregivers on experiences of closure during end-of-life care. *Journal of Pain and Symptom Management, 33*(4), 434–445.

Li, J., Johansen, C., Hansen, D., & Olsen, J. (2002). Cancer incidence in parents who lost a child: A nationwide study in Denmark. *Cancer, 95*(10), 2237–2242.

Li, J., Laursen, T. M., Precht, D. H., Olsen, J., & Mortensen, P. B. (2005). Hospitalization for mental illness among parents after the death of a child. *New England Journal of Medicine, 352*(12), 1190–1196.

Li, J., Precht, D. H., Mortensen, P. B., & Olsen J. (2003). Mortality in parents after death of a child in Denmark: A nationwide follow-up study. *Lancet, 361*(9355), 363–367.

Macdonald, M. E., Liben, S., Carnevale, F. A., Rennick, J. E., Wolf, S. L., Meloche, D., et al. (2005). Parental perspectives on hospital staff members' acts of kindness and commemoration after a child's death. *Pediatrics, 116*(4), 884–890.

Macdonald, M. E., Liben, S., & Cohen, S. R. (2006). Truth and consequences: Parental perspectives on autopsy after the death of a child. *Pediatric Intensive Care Nursing, 7*(1), 6–15.

Mack, J. W., Hilden, J. M., Watterson, J., Moore, C., Turner, B., Grier, H. E., et al. (2005). Parent and physician perspectives on quality of care at the end of life in children with cancer. *Journal of Clinical Oncology, 23*(36), 9155–9161.

Macnab, A., Northway, T., Ryall, K., Scott, D., & Straw, G. (2003). Death and bereavement in a paediatric intensive care unit: Parental perception of staff support. *Paediatrics & Child Health, 8*(6), 357–362.

Maynard, L., Rennie, T., Shirtliffe, J., & Vickers, D. (2005). Seeking and using families' views to shape children's hospice services. *International Journal of Palliative Nursing, 11*(12), 624–630.

McDonagh, J. R., Elliott, T. R., Engelberg, R. A., Treece, P. D., Shannon, S. E., Rubenfeld, G. D., et al. (2004). Family satisfaction with family conferences about end-of-life care in the intensive care unit: Increased proportion of family speech is associated with increased satisfaction. *Critical Care Medicine, 32*(7), 1484–1488.

McGahey Oakland, P. R., Lieder, H. S., Young, A., & Jefferson, L. S. (2007). Family experiences during resuscitation at a children's hospital emergency department. *Journal of Pediatric Health Care, 21*(4), 217–225.

Meeker, J. (2004). A voice for the dying. *Clinical Nursing Research, 13*(4), 326–342.

Meert, K. L., Eggly, S., Pollack, M., Anand, K. J., Zimmerman, J., Carcillo, J., et al. (2007). Parents' perspectives regarding a physician-parent conference after their child's death in the pediatric intensive care unit. *Journal of Pediatrics, 151*(1), 50–55, 55.e1–55.e2.

Meert, K. L., Thurston, C. S., & Briller, S. H. (2005). The spiritual needs of parents at the time of their child's death in the pediatric intensive care unit and during bereavement: A qualitative study article. *Pediatric Critical Care Medicine, 6*(4), 420–427.

Meert, K. L., Thurston, C. S., & Sarnaik, A. P. (2000). End-of-life decision-making and satisfaction with care: Parental perspectives. *Pediatric Critical Care Medicine, 1*(2), 179–185.

Meltzer, L. S., & Huckabay, L. M. (2004). Critical care nurses' perceptions of futile care and its effect on burnout. *American Journal of Critical Care, 13*(3), 202–208.

Meyer, E. C., Burns, J. P., Griffith, J. L., & Truog, R. D. (2002). Parental perspectives on end-of-life care in the pediatric intensive care unit. *Critical Care Medicine, 30*(1), 226–231.

Meyer, E. C., Ritholz, M. D., Burns, J. P., & Truog, R. (2006). Improving the quality of end-of-life care in the pediatric intensive care unit: Parents' priorities and recommendations. *Pediatrics, 117*(3), 649–657.

Milberg, A., Strang, P., Carlsson, M., & Borjesson, S. (2003). Advanced palliative home care: Next-of-kin's perspective. *Journal of Palliative Medicine, 6*(5), 749–756.

Mok, E., Chan, F., Chan, V., & Yeung, E. (2002). Perception of empowerment by family caregivers of patients with a terminal illness in Hong Kong. *International Journal of Palliative Nursing, 8*(3), 137–145.

Mok, E., & Chiu, P. C. (2004). Nurse-patient relationships in palliative care. *Journal of Advanced Nursing, 48*(5), 475–483.

Moules, N. J., Simonson, K., Fleiszer, A. R., Prins, M., & Rev Bob, G. (2007). The soul of sorrow work: Grief and therapeutic interventions with families. *Journal of Family Nursing, 13*(1), 117–141.

Moules, N. J., Simonson, K., Prins, M., Angus, P., & Bell, J. M. (2004). Making room for grief: Walking backwards and living forward. *Nursing Inquiry, 11*(2), 99–107.

Mularski, R., Curtis, J. R., Osborne, M., Engelberg, R. A., & Ganzini, L. (2004). Agreement among family members in their assessment of the quality of dying and death. *Journal of Pain and Symptom Management, 28*(4), 306–315.

Munn, J. C., & Zimmerman, S. (2006). A good death for residents of long-term care: Family members speak. *Journal of Social Work in End-of-Life & Palliative Care, 2*(3), 45–59.

Namasivayam, P., Orb, A., & O'Connor, M. (2005). The challenges of caring for families of the terminally ill: Nurses' lived experience. *Contemporary Nurse, 19*(1-2), 169–180.

Nolbris, M., & Hellstrom, A. (2005). Siblings' needs and issues when a brother or sister dies of cancer. *Journal of Pediatric Oncology Nursing, 22*(4), 227–233.

Nordgren, L., & Olsson, H. (2004). Palliative care in a coronary care unit: A qualitative study of physicians' and nurses' perceptions. *Journal of Clinical Nursing, 13*(2), 185–193.

Norris, K., Merriman, M. P., Curtis, J. R., Asp, C., Tuholske, L., & Byock, I. R. (2007). Next of kin perspectives on the experience of end-of-life care in a community setting. *Journal of Palliative Medicine, 10*(5), 1101–1115.

Norton, S. A., Tilden, V. P., Tolle, S. W., Nelson, C. A., & Eggman, S. T. (2003). Life support withdrawal: Communication and conflict. *American Journal of Critical Care, 12*(6), 548–555.

O'Connor, M., Peters, L., Lee, S., & Webster, C. (2005). Palliative care work, between death and discharge. *Journal of Palliative Care, 21*(2), 97–102.

Oliver, D., Porock, D., Demiris, G., & Courtney, K. (2005). Patient and family involvement in hospice interdisciplinary teams. *Journal of Palliative Care, 21*(4), 270–276.

Osse, B. H., Vernooij Dassen, M. J., Schade, E., & Grol, R. P. (2006). Problems experienced by the informal caregivers of cancer patients and their needs for support. *Cancer Nursing, 29*(5), 378–390.

Pector, E. A. (2004a). How bereaved multiple-birth parents cope with hospitalization, homecoming, disposition for deceased, and attachment to survivors. *Journal of Perinatology, 24,* 714–772.

Pector, E. A. (2004b). Views of bereaved multiple-birth parents on life support decisions, the dying process, and discussions surrounding death. *Journal of Perinatology, 24,* 4–10.

Perreault, A., Fothergill Bourbonnais, F., & Fiset, V. (2004). The experience of family members caring for a dying loved one. *International Journal of Palliative Nursing, 10*(3), 133–143.

Pochard, F., Azoulay, E., Chevret, S., Lemaire, F., Hubert, P., Canoui, P., et al. (2001). Symptoms of anxiety and depression in family members of intensive care unit patients: Ethical hypothesis regarding decision-making capacity. *Critical Care Medicine, 29*(10), 1893–1897.

Price, A. M. (2004). Intensive care nurses' experiences of assessing and dealing with patients' psychological needs. *Nursing in Critical Care, 9*(3), 134–142.

Proot, I. M., AbuSaad, H. H., Crebolder, H. F., Goldsteen, M., Luker, K. A., & Widdershoven, G. A. (2003). Vulnerability of family caregivers in terminal palliative care at home; balancing between burden and capacity. *Scandinavian Journal of Caring Sciences, 17*(2), 113–121.

Qin, P., & Mortensen, P. B. (2003). The impact of parental status on the risk of completed suicide. *Archives of General Psychiatry, 60*(8), 797–802.

Redinbaugh, E. M., Baum, A., Tarbell, S., & Arnold, R. (2003). End-of-life caregiving: What helps family caregivers cope? *Journal of Palliative Medicine, 6*(6), 901–909.

Riley, J., & Fenton, G. (2007). A terminal diagnosis: The carers' perspective. *CPR, 7*(2), 86–91.

Rini, A., & Loriz, L. (2007). Anticipatory mourning in parents with a child who dies while hospitalized. *Journal of Pediatric Nursing, 22*(4), 272–282.

Robinson, M. R., Thiel, M. M., Backus, M. M., & Meyer, E. C. (2006). Matters of spirituality at the end of life in the pediatric intensive care unit. *Pediatrics, 118*(3), e719–e729.

Rodger, M. L., Sherwood, P., O'Connor, M., & Leslie, G. (2007). Living beyond the unanticipated sudden death of a partner: A phenomenological study. *Omega: Journal of Death and Dying, 54*(2), 107–133.

Royak Schaler, R., Gadalla, S. M., Lemkau, J. P., Ross, D. D., Alexander, C., & Scott, D. (2006). Journal club. Family perspectives on communication with healthcare providers during end-of-life cancer care. *Oncology Nursing Forum, 33*(4), 753–760.

Seecharan, G. A., Andresen, E. M., Norris, K., & Toce, S. S. (2004). Parents' assessment of quality of care and grief following a child's death. *Archives of Pediatrics & Adolescent Medicine, 158,* 515–520.

Selman, L., Harding, R., Beynon, T., Hodson, F., Coady, E., Hazeldine, C., et al. (2007). Improving end-of-life care for patients with chronic heart failure: "Let's hope it'll get better, when I know in my heart of hearts it won't." *Heart, 93*(8), 963–967.

Sharman, M., Meert, K. L., & Sarnaik, A. P. (2005). What influences parents' decisions to limit or withdraw life support? *Pediatric Critical Care Medicine, 6*(5), 513–518.

Sherwood, P. R., Given, B., Doorenbos, A. Z., & Given, C. W. (2004). Forgotten voices: Lessons from bereaved caregivers of persons with a brain tumour...including commentary by Krishnasamy M. *International Journal of Palliative Nursing, 10*(2), 67–75.

Shiozaki, M., Morita, T., Hirai, K., Sakaguchi, Y., Tsuneto, S., & Shima, Y. (2005). Why are bereaved family members dissatisfied with specialised inpatient palliative care service? A nationwide qualitative study. *Palliative Medicine, 19*(4), 319–327.

Skene, C. (1998). Individualised bereavement care. *Paediatric Nursing, 10*(10), 13–16.

Skilbeck, J. K., Payne, S. A., Ingleton, M. C., Nolan, M., Carey, I., & Hanson, A. (2005). An exploration of family carers' experience of respite services in one specialist palliative care unit. *Palliative Medicine, 19*(8), 610–618.

Stajduhar, K. I. (2003). Examining the perspectives of family members involved in the delivery of palliative care at home. *Journal of Palliative Care, 19*(1), 27–35.

Stajduhar, K. I., Martin, W. L., Barwich, D., & Fyles, G. (2008). Factors influencing family caregivers' ability to cope with providing end-of-life cancer care at home. *Cancer Nursing, 31*(1), 77–85.

Steele, R. (2002). Experiences of families in which a child has a prolonged terminal illness: Modifying factors. *International Journal of Palliative Nursing, 8*(9), 418–434.

Steele, R. (2005a). Navigating uncharted territory: Experiences of families when a child is dying. *Journal of Palliative Care, 21*(1), 35–43.

Steele, R. (2005b). Strategies used by families to navigate uncharted territory when a child is dying. *Journal of Palliative Care, 21*(2), 103–110.

Steele, R., & Davies, B. (2006). Impact on parents when a child has a progressive, life-threatening illness. *International Journal of Palliative Nursing, 12*(12), 576–585.

Steele, R., Davies, B., Collins, J. B., & Cook, K. (2005). End-of-life care in a children's hospice program. *Journal of Palliative Care, 21*(1), 5–11.

Steinhauser, K. E., Clipp, E. C., McNeilly, M., Christakis, N. A., McIntyre, L. M., & Tulsky, J. A. (2000). In search of a good death: Observations of patients, families, and providers. *Annals of Internal Medicine, 132*(10), 825–832.

Surkan, P. J., Kreicbergs, U., Valdimarsdottir, U., Nyberg, U., Onelov, E., Dickman, P. W., et al. (2006). Perceptions of inadequate health care and feelings of guilt in parents after the death of a child to a malignancy: A population-based long-term follow-up. *Journal of Palliative Medicine, 9*(2), 317–331.

Tang, S. T. (2003). When death is imminent: Where terminally ill patients with cancer prefer to die and why. *Cancer Nursing, 26*(3), 245–251.

Tang, S. T., Liu, T., Lai, M., & McCorkle, R. (2005). Discrepancy in the preferences of place of death between terminally ill cancer patients and their primary family caregivers in Taiwan. *Social Science & Medicine, 61*(7), 1560–1566.

Teno, J. (1999). Putting patient and family voice back into measuring quality care for the dying. *The Hospice Journal, 14*(3/4), 167–176.

Thompson, G. N., McClement, S. E., & Daeninck, P. J. (2006). "Changing lanes": Facilitating the transition from curative to palliative care. *Journal of Palliative Care, 22*(2), 91–98.

Tilden, V. P., Tolle, S. W., Garland, M. J., & Nelson, C. A. (1995). Decisions about life-sustaining treatment. *Archives of Internal Medicine, 155*(6), 633–638.

Tilden, V. P., Tolle, S. W., Nelson, C. A., & Fields, J. (2001). Family decision-making to withdraw life-sustaining treatments from hospitalized patients. *Nursing Research, 50*(2), 105–115.

Tomlinson, D., Capra, M., Gammon, J., Volpe, J., Barrera, M., Hinds, P. S., et al. (2006). Parental decision making in pediatric cancer end-of-life care: Using focus group methodology as a prephase to seek participant design input. *European Journal of Oncology Nursing, 10*(3), 198–206.

Torke, A. M., Garas, N. S., Sexson, W., & Branch, W. T., Jr. (2005). Medical care at the end of life: Views of African American patients in an urban hospital. *Journal of Palliative Medicine, 8*(3), 593–602.

Vickers, J. L., & Carlisle, C. (2000). Choices and control: Parental experiences in pediatric terminal home care. *Journal of Pediatric Oncology Nursing, 17*(1), 12–21.

Vint, P. E. (2005). An exploration of the support available to children who may wish to visit a critically adult [sic] in ITU. *Intensive & Critical Care Nursing, 21*(3), 149–159.

Wall, R. J., Engelberg, R. A., Gries, C. J., Glavan, B., & Curtis, J. R. (2007). Spiritual care of families in the intensive care unit. *Critical Care Medicine, 35*(4), 1084–1090.

Webster, J., & Kristjanson, L. (2002). "But isn't it depressing?" The vitality of palliative care. *Journal of Palliative Care, 18*(1), 15–24.

White, D. B., & Luce, J. M. (2004). Palliative care in the intensive care unit: Barriers, advances, and unmet needs. *Critical Care Clinics, 20*(3), 329–343.

Widger, K., & Picot, C. (2008). Parents' perceptions of the quality of pediatric and perinatal end-of-life care. *Pediatric Nursing, 34*(1), 53–58.

Wiegand, D. L. (2006). Withdrawal of life-sustaining therapy after sudden, unexpected life-threatening illness or injury: Interactions between patients' families, healthcare providers, and the healthcare system. *American Journal of Critical Care, 15*(2), 178–187.

Wisten, A., & Zingmark, K. (2007). Supportive needs of parents confronted with sudden cardiac death: A qualitative study. *Resuscitation, 74*(1), 68–74.

Wollin, J. A., Yates, P. M., & Kristjanson, L. J. (2006). Supportive and palliative care needs identified by multiple sclerosis patients and their families. *International Journal of Palliative Nursing, 12*(1), 20–26.

Woodgate, R. L. (2006). Living in a world without closure: Reality for parents who have experienced the death of a child. *Journal of Palliative Care, 22*(2), 75–82.

World Health Organization. (2006). *WHO definition of palliative care.* Retrieved May 30, 2008, from http://www.who.int/cancer/palliative/definition/en/

Wright, L. M., & Leahey, M. (2005). *Nurses and families: A guide to family assessment and intervention* (4th ed.). Philadelphia: F.A. Davis.

CHAPTER WEB SITES

- *American Academy of Hospice and Palliative Medicine:* http://www.aahpm.org/
- *American Association of Colleges of Nursing End-of-Life Nursing Education Consortium (ELNEC) Project:* http://www.aacn.nche.edu/elnec/
- *The American Geriatrics Society:* http://www.americangeriatrics.org/
- *The Association for Children's Palliative Care:* http://www.act.org.uk
- *Association for Death Education and Counseling:* http://www.adec.org/
- *Canadian Hospice Palliative Care Association:* http://www.chpca.net
- *Canadian Organization for Rare Disorders:* http://www.cord.ca/
- *Canadian Network of Palliative Care for Children:* http://cnpcc.ca/
- *Canadian Virtual Hospice:* http://www.virtualhospice.ca
- *The Compassionate Friends of Canada resource Links:* http://www.tcfcanada.net/links/index.htm
- *Education on Palliative and End-of-Life Care EPEC Project:* http://www.epec.net/
- *End of Life/Palliative Education Resource Center:* http://www.eperc.mcw.edu/
- *European Organization for Rare Diseases:* http://www.eurordis.org
- *GriefNet.org:* http://griefnet.org/
- *Hospice and Palliative Nurses Association:* http://www.hpna.org/
- *Institute of Medicine of the National Academies:* http://www.iom.edu/
- *National Hospice and Palliative Care Association:* http://www.nhpco.org
- *National Organization for Rare Disorders:* http://www.rarediseases.org
- *Promoting Excellence in End-of-Life Care (tools):* http://www.promotingexcellence.org
- *World Health Organization:* http://www.who.int/cancer/palliative/definition/en/

3

Nursing Care of Families in Clinical Areas

CHAPTER 12

Family Nursing with Childbearing Families

Linda Veltri, MSN, RN

- ✦ Childbearing family nursing is not synonymous with obstetrical nursing, which considers the woman as the client and context for care. In contrast, childbearing family nursing considers the family as client, the family as context for the care of its members, or both. Childbearing family nursing primarily focuses on health and wellness rather than on procedures and medical treatment.

- ✦ Nurses must understand and utilize multiple theories to plan and guide nursing care for childbearing families.

- ✦ Nurses need to be aware of stressors childbearing families encounter before, during, and after reproductive events so they can anticipate, identify, and respond to needs appropriately.

- ✦ Nursing care for adoptive families should be provided in a manner similar to that which is provided to biological families.

- ✦ Nurses caring for childbearing families experiencing infertility must consider, understand, and address the emotional and physical needs.

- ✦ Understanding the many ways families experience loss allows nurses to advocate for practices that best facilitate childbearing as a transitional event in the life of the family.

- ✦ When a mother or a newborn has serious threats to health, family nurses act to maintain and promote family relationships.

- ✦ Understanding the effect a new baby has on all family members allows nurses to work to help parents develop realistic expectations about themselves, each other, and their children, as well as to identify appropriate support and resources.

- ✦ Postpartum depression (PPD) is treatable and recoverable. Therefore, family nurses must work diligently to identify and refer women for appropriate treatment *early* to reduce the effects of maternal depression on the woman and her family.

- ✦ Family nurses can be leaders in practice, policy development, and research related to childbearing families.

*B*efore the onset of professional nursing in North America during the late 19th century, caregivers for childbearing families were women. Female family members, in-laws, neighbors, friends, and midwives came to the home to encourage, support, and nurture a woman during and after childbirth (Mander, 2004). These women caregivers maintained family functions of the household, tended to new babies and mothers' other children, and provided postpartum physical care. During these years, the father's role in childbirth was limited to announcing labor had begun and seeking assistance from other women (Mander, 2004). The practice of excluding male individuals, as well as other family members, from the childbirth experience continued through the 1970s primarily because of concerns they would be carriers of infection into the perinatal setting.

Beginning in the late 1960s, families became increasingly knowledgeable about childbearing and desirous of a more satisfying birth experience. As a result, families began to question hospital routines and policies that required strict adherence to newborn feeding and sleeping schedules and that kept fathers out of the delivery room and parents separated from their newborns. Informed families then lobbied for changes in childbearing practices in light of available research that provided evidence for not separating mothers and babies immediately after delivery, as well as other hallmark findings demonstrating improved parent-child attachment with immediate and frequent contact between mothers and fathers with their newborns (de Chateau, 1976, 1977; Klaus, Jerauld, Kreger, McAlpine, Steffa, & Kennel, 1972; Martell, 2006).

In time, nurses, hospitals, and other health care providers for women began to recognize the effect reproductive events have on all family members, as well as the influence of the family on the parents and infants. This recognition has resulted in inclusion of family concepts into care. With the trend for increased family education about reproductive events, increased responsibility for family members to plan for care of the infant during pregnancy and delivery, and shorter hospital stays after birth, postpartum care is becoming family based and is occurring at home with nursing guidance, rather than medically based in a hospital. This shift in focus from the individual to consideration and inclusion of the family in the care from preconception to the postpartum period is known as *childbearing family nursing*. The historical perspective is outlined in Box 12-1.

BOX 12-1
Historical Perspective of Childbearing Family Nursing

HISTORICAL PERSPECTIVE
Late 1800s: Industrialization
- Families moved to more urban areas; household size and functions diminished.
- Traditional networks of women were not always available, and mothers needed to replace care previously carried out in the home.
- Childbearing still occurred at home for many middle-class families (Leavitt, 1986; Wertz & Wertz, 1989).

First Third of the 20th Century
- The hospital became the place for labor, birth, and early postpartum recovery for middle-class families.
- Many immigrant and working-class urban families continued to have newborns at home with their traditional care providers.
- An impetus to the development of public health nursing was concern for the health of urban mothers and babies.
- Realizing that the health needs of all the family members were intertwined, early public health nurses considered families, not individuals, as their clients.

1930s Through the "Baby Boom" of the 1950s
- With the dramatic shift of births to hospitals, family involvement with childbearing diminished (Leavitt, 1986).
- Concerns about infection control contributed to separation of family members.
- Family members were forbidden to be with women in the hospital.

Continued

BOX 12-1
Historical Perspective of Childbearing Family Nursing—cont'd

- Babies were segregated into nurseries and brought out to their mothers only for brief feeding sessions.
- Nurses focused on the smooth operation of postpartum wards and nurseries through the use of routine and orderliness.
- Despite these inflexible conditions, families tolerated them because they believed that hospital births were safer for mothers and newborns.

1960s to 1970s
- Some women and a few physicians began to question the need for heavy sedation and analgesia for childbearing, and embraced natural childbirth.
- A feature of natural childbirth was the close relationship between the laboring woman and a supportive person serving as a coach, and in North America, husbands assumed this supportive role (Wertz & Wertz, 1989).
- Expectant parents actively sought out physicians and hospitals that would best meet their expectations for father involvement, and the control over childbearing began to shift from health care professionals to families.
- Some nurses were skeptical about the changes families demanded, but others were enthusiastic about increased family participation.
- Many hospital-based maternity nurses began to consider themselves to be mother-baby nurses rather than nursery or postpartum nurses, and labor and delivery nurses often collaborated with family members in helping women cope with the discomforts of labor.

1980s to the Present
- Klaus and Kennel's research (1976) served as the impetus for the growth of family-centered care (American College of Obstetricians and Gynecologists and the Interprofessional Task Force on Health Care of Women and Children, 1978).
- Today, promotion of family contact is becoming the hallmark of childbearing care.
- Many hospitals have renamed their obstetrical services, using names such as Family Birth Center to convey the importance of family members in childbearing health care even though obstetrical care is becoming more dependent on technology.

Notably, the practice of childbearing family nursing is not synonymous with obstetrical nursing, which considers the woman as the client and context for care. Childbearing family nursing, by contrast, considers the family as client, the family as context for the care of its members, or both primarily. Additionally it is a health and wellness, rather than an illness model of care.

Family nursing with childbearing families covers the period before conception, pregnancy, labor, birth, and the postpartum period. Childbearing family nursing traditionally begins when families are considering whether to start having children and continues until parents have achieved a degree of relative comfort in their roles as parents of infants and have ceased the addition of new children to their families. Often, childbearing family nursing expands to include the periods between pregnancies and other aspects of reproduction such as family planning, sexuality, adoption, foster care, and parenting grandchildren. Decisions and changes surrounding childbearing vary for families according to their cultural and psychological needs; therefore, the beginning and end points of the reproductive periods may be different for each family.

At any one time in the reproductive cycle, family members may have related but different health needs pertaining to the same family health concern. Therefore, childbearing family nursing practice utilizes the family nursing process of assessment, diagnosis, planning, implementation, and evaluation to orient knowledge and direct care activities to the entire childbearing family, thus bringing the focus of childbearing family nurses on family relationships and the health of all family members. Nurses involved with childbearing families use family concepts and theories as part of developing the plan of nursing care. Theoretical perspectives that guide nursing practice with childbearing families are presented in this chapter, followed by an exploration of family nursing with childbearing families before conception through the postpartum period. This chapter concludes with implications for nursing practice, research, and policy. A case study showing family stresses with the birth of a preterm infant is at the end of the chapter.

THEORY-GUIDED, EVIDENCE-BASED CHILDBEARING NURSING

Application of theory to family health situations during childbearing can guide family nurses in making more complete assessments and planning interventions congruent with the predictable events during childbearing. Several of the theories discussed in Chapter 3 contribute to nurses' understanding of how families grow, develop, function, and change during childbearing. Two of these theories, Family Systems Theory and Family Developmental and Life Cycle Theory, are especially applicable to childbearing families. A brief summary of these theories and their application to childbearing families follows.

Family Systems Theory

Becoming parents or adding a child brings stress to a family by challenging family stability, not only for the nuclear and extended family systems, but also for the individual members and subsystems of the family. As new subsystems are created or modified by pregnancy and childbirth, a sense of disequilibrium exists until a family adapts to its new member and re-achieves stability. For example, changes in the husband-wife subsystem occur as a response to development of the new parent-child subsystems.

Imbalance, or disequilibrium, occurs while adjustments are still needed and new roles are being learned. Families with greater flexibility in role expectations and behaviors tend to experience these periods of disequilibrium with less discomfort. The greater the range or number of coping strategies available to the family, the greater the ability to engage in various family roles, and the more effective the family's response will be to both internal strains and external stress associated with childbearing. External stresses such as outside employment and child care concerns may be important in predicting disequilibrium in pregnant women, and nurses should assess the effect of stress on family stability.

Family Systems Theory is especially effective for use by childbearing family nurses. A family, while in a state of change and readjustment tends to have more permeable boundaries or is more open to the outside environment because the family needs resources beyond itself. Consequently, the family is apt to be engaged in more interactions with systems outside the family and may become more receptive to interventions such as health teaching than they would be at other times in the family life cycle (Martell, 2005). This openness of family boundaries allows nurses more access to the family for health promotion.

On the other hand, family nurses should be aware of very closed or enmeshed families who may have nonpermeable boundaries and reject outside influences, including nursing care. Families can become closed because they interpret the outside environment and systems as hostile, threatening, or difficult to cope with. These families are challenging for nurses because they are less readily accessible or responsive to family nurses.

Family Developmental and Life Cycle Theory

Family Developmental and Life Cycle Theory describes a process of developing over time that is predictable, and yet individual, based on unique life circumstances and family interactions. Although the life cycle of most individual families around the world follows a universal sequence of family development, it is important for childbearing family nurses to recognize that wide variations exist in the timing and sequencing of family life cycle phases (Berk, 2007; Carter & McGoldrick, 2005; Duvall, 1977). Many present-day childbearing families do not fit precisely into the classic sequence and timing of family developmental stages and tasks originally described by Duvall and Miller (1985) because they are constructed differently than the traditional nuclear family that was common after World War II. For example, families might be blended with one or both partners having children from previous relationships; parents also may be cohabitating, unmarried, single, of the same sex, or have children born later in life (Berk, 2007; Pillitteri, 2003).

Despite how diverse the family is today, Family Developmental and Life Cycle Theory remains helpful to guide the practice of family nurses because it addresses the patterns of adaptation to parenthood that are typical for many families. This theory also has relevance for family nurses regardless of how families are structured because the essential tasks all families must perform to survive as a healthy unit are generally present to some extent in all families (Pillitteri, 2003). The Sanders family case study at the end of this chapter addresses families and how roles are changed with the birth of a preterm child.

According to Family Developmental and Life Cycle Theory, changes occur in stages during which there is upheaval while adjustments are being made. What occurs during these stages is generally referred to as developmental tasks. The Childbearing Family with Infants stage is defined as the period from the beginning of the first pregnancy until the oldest child reaches 18 months of age. During this stage, childbearing families have nine specific tasks to accomplish to grow and achieve family well-being. The nine tasks for childbearing families and nursing interventions are explained in the following subsections.

TASK ONE: ARRANGING SPACE (TERRITORY) FOR A CHILD

Arranging space (territory) involves families making space preparations for their infants. Families accommodate newborns by moving to a new residence during pregnancy or the first year after birth, or by modifying their living quarters and furnishings. Families may delay or avoid space preparations for a new baby for several reasons. For example, busy families, those who fear or have experienced prior fetal loss, and families involved with adoption or foster placement may delay or avoid space preparations. For some groups, preparation for a baby's material needs during pregnancy is not acceptable; it may mean bad luck or misfortune for the baby (Lewis, 2003). The lack of space preparation may also result from the parents not having accepted the reality of the coming baby, inadequate or unsafe housing, or homelessness. In addition, adolescent parents may not make space arrangements because of denial of the pregnancy or fear about repercussions from their families if pregnancy is revealed.

Family Nursing Interventions

- Inquire about the living space, material, and physical preparation all families have made for the baby.
- Inquire about the families' thoughts, values, beliefs, and possible fears about making preparations for the anticipated arrival of the baby.
- Assist families to explore and manage their fear about survival of the baby and then mobilize resources to help them cope so that family development can continue.
- Assist adolescents to find ways to communicate with their families and make plans for the future of the infant and the adolescent parents.
- Refer families who are homeless or live in inadequate or unsafe housing to appropriate resources for obtaining safer housing.

TASK TWO: FINANCING CHILDBEARING AND CHILDREARING

Childbearing results in additional expenses and lower family income. Most employed women will miss some employment and forego possible career advancement during childbearing. Men are more likely to take on additional paid work, leaving them less time for family matters, which may be a source of more anxiety and stress for the family (Martell, 2005; Mennino & Brayfield, 2002). Families may fall back onto savings, increase their debt, or alter their lifestyles to match changing levels of income. Financial stresses can be even harder for mothers without partners or for women who provide most of the income for their families. Adolescent mothers are especially prone to financial difficulties because childbearing may disrupt their education, which increases their risk for future poverty because they may not be able to obtain jobs that pay well enough to support a family. Health care surrounding childbirth can add another layer of financial stress on a family. Health care providers may not be able to accept patients who are not privately insured, insured by federal or state programs, or cannot pay out of pocket for obstetrical services.

Family Nursing Interventions

- Assist families to find needed resources, such as nutrition programs and prenatal clinics, that fit with the financial resources of the family.

- Provide families with information and resources that will help them choose safe and appropriate child care.
- Identify associated barriers to prenatal care, such as lack of transportation and child care, hours of service that conflict with family employment, and difficulty obtaining or using health care benefits.

TASK THREE: ASSUMING MUTUAL RESPONSIBILITY FOR CHILD CARE AND NURTURING

The care and nurturing of infants bring sleep disruptions, demands on time and energy, additional household tasks, and personal discomfort for caretakers. The affectionate bonds (or attachment) that develop between parents and their children may be one of the driving forces for engaging in infant care and nurturing even under difficult circumstances.

Family Nursing Interventions

- Educate parents about the realities of parenting, such as interrupted sleep and a change in how time is spent.
- Teach a family to alternate who responds to the baby's needs, including feeding, changing, and comforting.
- Assist parents to develop new skills in care giving and ways of interacting with their babies.
- Observe for signs of attachment by listening to what parents say about their babies and observing parent behaviors (see Box 12-2, which outlines parental behaviors that facilitate attachment).
- Refer families who do not demonstrate nurturing behaviors to other professionals who can provide more intensive intervention.

TASK FOUR: FACILITATING ROLE LEARNING OF FAMILY MEMBERS

Learning roles is particularly important for childbearing families. For many couples, taking on the role of parents is a dramatic shift in their lives. Difficulty with adaptation to parenthood may be related to the stress of learning new roles. Role learning involves expectations about the role, developing the ability to assume the role, and taking on the role.

BOX 12-2
Parental Behaviors that Facilitate Attachment

Arranges self or the newborn so as to have face-to-face and eye-to-eye contact with infant

Directs attention to the infant; maintains contact with infant physically and emotionally

Identifies infant as a separate, unique individual with independent needs

Identifies characteristics of family members in infant

Names infant; calls infant by name

Smiles, coos, talks to, or sings to infant

Verbalizes pride in the infant

Responds to sounds made by the infant, such as crying, sneezing, or grunting

Assigns meaning to the infant's actions; interprets infant needs sensitively

Has a positive view of infant's behaviors and appearance

Source: Davidson, M. R., London, M. L., & Ladewig, P. A. (2008). *Olds' maternal-newborn nursing and women's health across the lifespan* (8th ed.). Upper Saddle River, NJ: Pearson Prentice Hall; Lowdermilk, D. L., & Perry, S. E. (2004). *Martenity and women's health care* (8th ed.). St. Louis, MO: Mosby; and Schenk, L. K., Kelley, J. H., & Schenk, M. P. (2005). Models of maternal-infant attachment: A role for nurses. *Pediatric Nursing, 31*(6), 514–517, by permission.

Family Nursing Interventions

- Assist and encourage pregnant couples to explore their attitudes and expectations about the role of their partners.
- Encourage contact with others who are in the process of taking on the parenting role, especially if the parents are isolated, adolescent, or culturally diverse and living apart from traditional networks.
- Encourage expectant women to bring their partners into the experience by sharing their physical sensations and emotions of being pregnant.
- Provide opportunities for fathers and other partners to become skilled infant caregivers.

TASK FIVE: ADJUSTING TO CHANGED COMMUNICATION PATTERNS

Communication patterns change in order for the family to accommodate newborn and young children. As parents and infants learn to interpret and respond to each other's communication cues, they develop effective, reciprocal communication patterns. Infant cues may be so subtle, however, that parents may not be sensitive to cues until nurses point them out (Martell, 2005; Schiffman, Omar, & McKelvey, 2003). For example, many babies respond to being held by cuddling and nuzzling, but others respond by back arching and stiffening. Parents may interpret the latter as rejecting and unloving responses, and these negative interpretations may adversely affect the parent-infant relationship.

Communication between parents also changes with the transition to parenthood. During the years of childbearing, many men and women devote considerable time to career development. The time demands of work may affect a couple's relationship. While taking on the everyday aspects of rearing children, parents often do not give their couple relationship the attention needed to sustain it (Martell, 2005).

Family Nursing Interventions
- Educate parents about different infant temperaments so they are able to interpret their baby's unique style of communication.
- Encourage parents to talk to and engage in eye contact with the baby.
- Incorporate couple communication into care and education of expectant parents.
- Promote effective couple communication by encouraging the partners to listen to each other actively, using "I" phrases instead of blaming the other.
- Encourage couples to set aside a regular time to talk and enjoy each other as loving partners.

TASK SIX: PLANNING FOR SUBSEQUENT CHILDREN

After the birth, some parents will have definite, mutually agreed-on plans for additional children, whereas others will have decided against future children or will be ambivalent about family plans. Families who have definite plans primarily need information about family planning options so that they can carry out their plans.

Family Nursing Interventions
- Consider a family's cultural and religious background, and identify the power structure and locus of decision making in the family when discussing reproductive matters.
- Provide current, evidenced-based information about family planning options.

- Refer to a nurse genetic specialist for assessment and counseling when appropriate.

TASK SEVEN: REALIGNING INTERGENERATIONAL PATTERNS

The first baby adds a new generation in the family lineage that carries the family into the future. Expectant parents change from being children of their parents to becoming parents themselves. Childbearing may signify the onset of being an adult for adolescent parents and some cultural groups. Childbearing changes relationships within extended families as parents' siblings become aunts and uncles, children from previous relationships become stepsiblings, and their own parents become grandparents.

Family Nursing Interventions
- Assist new parents to seek support from friends, family members, organized parent groups, and work colleagues as a way to cope with the demands of parenting.
- Work with families to develop strategies that maintain their couple activities, adult interests, and friendships.
- Facilitate partner discussions about perceptions of extended family involvement in care of the new child.

TASK EIGHT: MAINTAINING FAMILY MEMBERS' MOTIVATION AND MORALE

After the initial excitement surrounding the arrival of a new baby, families must learn to adjust to and cope with the new demands that caring for the baby will have on their time, energy, sexual relationship, and personal resources. Many new moms experience postpartum fatigue, which is a feeling of exhaustion and decreased ability to engage in physical and mental work (Davidson, London, & Ladewig, 2008). Women may be fatigued for months from the blood loss associated with birth, breast-feeding, sleep difficulties, depression, the demands of multiple roles, or returning to work outside the home, all of which are compounded by the demands of infant care (Davidson, London, & Ladewig, 2008; Martell, 2005; Troy, 2003). In addition, a relationship exists between maternal fatigue and postpartum depression (PPD), both of which affect family processes (Davidson, London, & Ladewig, 2008).

In the months following childbirth, families must be realistic about infant sleep patterns and crying behaviors, the potential to experience loneliness, and changes in their sexual relationship. For example, many young families experience loneliness in the postpartum period because they live in communities far from their extended families. Some families have recently moved into a new neighborhood and may not have established friendships or a sense of community. Many ethnically diverse groups had special support and recognition of the postpartum period in their countries of origin, but in North America, replacements may not exist for traditional postpartum care (Martell, 2005).

Family Nursing Interventions
- Inform family members about ways to promote comfort, rest, and sleep, which will make it easier for them to cope with fatigue.
  - Promote parental rest while a baby needs nighttime feedings by encouraging parents to alternate who responds to the baby.
- Teach parents ways to cope with a crying infant, which will boost family morale, increase confidence, and allow family members to get additional sleep.
- Provide information on ways parents can reduce isolation and loneliness by seeking support from friends, family members, organized parent groups, and work colleagues.
- Encourage parents to articulate their needs and to find help in ways that support their self-esteem as new parents.
- Counsel couples about changes in sexuality after birth and help them develop mutually satisfying sexual expression.
- Help families to develop strategies that maintain their couple activities, adult interests, and friendships.

TASK NINE: ESTABLISHING FAMILY RITUALS AND ROUTINES

Rituals develop as children come into a family, and these rituals become a source of comfort, as well as part of the uniqueness and identity of a family (Fomby, 2004). The predictability of rituals helps babies develop trust. Family rituals include bedtime and bathing routines, baby's special possessions such as a treasured blanket, and nicknames for body functions. For some families, rituals have special cultural meanings that nurses should respect. When families are disrupted or separated during childbearing, nurses can help them deal with stress by encouraging them to carry out their usual routines and established rituals related to their babies and other children.

Family Nursing Interventions
- Determine the special cultural meaning each ritual has for the family and respect those meanings.
- Encourage families to carry out their usual routines and established rituals related to their babies and other children.
- Facilitate couple discussion of bedtime and bathing routines, a baby's special possessions such as a treasured blanket, nicknames, language for body functions, and welcoming rituals such as announcements, baptisms, circumcision, or other celebrations.

FAMILY TRANSITIONS

Transition, a major concept of Family Developmental Theory, is similar to change theory. Inherent in transition from one developmental stage to the next is a period of upheaval as the family moves from one state to another. Historically, "transition to parenthood" was thought by early family researchers to be a crisis (LeMasters, 1957; Steffensmeier, 1982). The notion of transition to parenthood as a crisis is now being abandoned. More recent work focuses on the transition processes associated with change in families. In a more contemporary approach, transition to parenthood has been defined as a long-term process that results in qualitative reorganization of both inner life and external behavior (Carter & McGoldrick, 2005).

Nurse researchers have focused on transition to motherhood. Even though other family members experience the transition when a newborn joins the family, concepts related to motherhood give nurses insight into family transition. For example, Nelson (2003) describes the primary process of transition as "engagement," or opening one's self to the opportunity to grow and be transformed. Opening of self relates to making a commitment to mothering, experiencing the presence of a child, and caring for the child. The notion of family transition gives foundation to nursing interventions that promote parenting because opening of self involves the real experience of being with and caring for the child. Nurses who understand the stressors that families experience as they transition from one state to another can use this theoretical concept to realize that a mother may be frustrated over not being able to cope in her old ways.

Just as no one theory covers all aspects of nursing, no single theory will work for every situation involving childbearing families. Therefore, nurses must understand and utilize multiple theories to plan and guide nursing care for childbearing families. Major concepts from Family Systems Theory and Family Developmental and Life Cycle Theory help nurses organize assessments and manage the predictable and unpredictable experiences childbearing families encounter.

CHILDBEARING FAMILY STRESSORS

Childbearing family nursing begins when a couple anticipates and plans for pregnancy, has already conceived, or may be planning to adopt a child. Reproductive life planning is an emotional task all types of families, such as the traditional nuclear, blended, gay or lesbian, and adoptive families, as well as other heterosexual couples who cohabitate, must negotiate (Pillitteri, 2003). Any pregnancy-related event such as infertility, adoption, pregnancy loss, or even an unplanned pregnancy may be enough to disrupt the delicately formed bonds of the family in this stage. Nurses need to be aware of problems childbearing families might encounter before, during, and after reproductive events so that they can anticipate, identify, and respond to needs appropriately.

Infertility

Men and women perceive fertility to be a sign of competence as reproductive human beings. Therefore, the experience of infertility can be a life crisis that disrupts a couple's marital or sexual relationship, or both. Infertility is of concern to childbearing family nurses, especially in cultures where the expectation of motherhood is strong (Day, 2005; Sherrod, 2006). Infertility or the inability to conceive after 12 or more months of unprotected, regular intercourse is a common stress-producing event

that 8% to 15% of couples experience during their reproductive lives (Day, 2005; Sherrod, 2004).

Nurses should anticipate that infertile couples will experience several different physical, emotional, and psychological symptoms. Couples dealing with infertility struggle between feelings of hope and hopelessness, report feelings of being on a roller-coaster ride, feel a sense of despair, and feel that time is running out (Day, 2005; Sherrod, 2004). Problems with infertility change a couple's social relationships and support, which results in increased levels of depression and psychological distress (see Table 12-1).

Men and women respond to infertility in very different ways. Sherrod (2006) reports that women coping with infertility have greater anxiety, impaired self-esteem, depression, and hostility than men. Women want to spend time talking about their infertility experience, whereas men report that talking about it only increases their anxiety. As a result, men dealing with infertility tend to talk, communicate, and listen less. In addition, men coping with infertility tend to disguise their feelings to protect themselves, their partners, or both (Sherrod, 2006).

Testing and treatment for infertility is expensive, painful, time consuming, and inconvenient. It can lead to a loss of spontaneity and privacy in sexual activities, which only compounds the stress and strain couples are experiencing. Although every test or

TABLE 12-1
Common Symptoms and Stressors Infertile Couples May Experience
▪ Irritability
▪ Insomnia
▪ Tension
▪ Depression
▪ Increased anxiety
▪ Anger toward each other, God, friends and other fertile women
▪ Feel rejected, alienated, stigmatized, isolated and estranged

Source: From Sherrod, R. A. (2004). Understanding the emotional aspects of infertility. Implications for nursing practice. *Journal of Psychosocial Nursing, 42*(3), 42–47; and Day, R. D. (2005). Relationship stress in couples. In P. C. McKenry & S. J. Price (Eds.), *Families and Changes: Coping with stressful events and transition* (3rd ed., pp. 332–353). Thousand Oaks, CA: Sage, by permission.

treatment is another painful reminder of the inability to reproduce, it is nurses' lack of knowledge and understanding of the emotional aspects of infertility that frustrates infertile couples. As a result, couples interpret nursing care to be insensitive when it primarily focuses on the physiologic rather than emotional aspects of infertility (Sherrod, 2004). Therefore, it is vital that nurses caring for childbearing families experiencing infertility understand, consider, and address the emotional and physical needs of couples undergoing treatment for infertility. Families experiencing the crisis of infertility are in as much need of an empathetic ear as they are in need of accurate, evidence-based information about testing and treatment options. See Table 12-2 for specific nursing interventions to help couples deal with infertility.

Adoption

Today, children are being adopted by many different family types, such as nuclear, single-parent, gay, or lesbian families (Pillitteri, 2003). Adoption is also considered an alternative for resolving infertility. Nevertheless, nurses must not assume it to be an appropriate or best solution for every infertile couple (London, Ladewig, Ball, & Bindler, 2007; Sherrod, 2004), just as they must not assume that every couple who has adopted has done so because of infertility. Once families decide to adopt a child, they may

pursue several routes such as international adoption (also known as intercountry), or private domestic adoption. In the United States, domestic adoption can be a difficult, lengthy, bureaucratic, and costly process taking anywhere from 12 months to 5 or 6 years (Fontenot, 2007; London et al., 2007; Pillitteri, 2003). The laws favoring birth mothers also complicate domestic adoption. This long waiting period and fear of the court system has resulted in many families turning to international/intercountry adoptions, which can provide a child in a much shorter amount of time. It is estimated that more than 20,000 children are adopted into Western countries every year, with most being children of color adopted by white parents, known as transracial (or cross-cultural) adoption (Rykkje, 2007). One drawback to an international adoption is that little to no information about the child's birth parents' background or prenatal health care may be available to the adopting family. The lack of birth history places families at risk for adopting a child who may have experienced a significant number of threats to normal brain and behavioral development, which can contribute to future struggles as families cope with the consequences of these problems (Gunnar & Pollak, 2007). Table 12-3 lists other issues and challenges related to international and transracial adoption.

Private adoption is a third alternative for families considering adoption. Private adoptions can range from being strictly anonymous to very open, where the adopting couple and birth mother get to know each other extremely well. Often, the Internet is a place where women wanting to place babies for adoption and families seeking to adopt connect. Regardless of how families connect or interact with the birth mother, it is paramount that families pursuing private adoption retain professional legal advice and counsel to ensure that everyone involved understands the legal ramifications and to work out all aspects related to the adoption before the baby's birth. Nurses should be aware that when a private adoption has been negotiated, one of the important points is whether the adopting family will be present at the child's birth. Nurses must also be prepared and ready to intervene should a birth mother reverse her decision to give the baby up for adoption (Pillitteri, 2003).

Adoption is just one of the many ways women may become mothers. Although adoptive mothers/ families may not experience the physical context of

---

TABLE 12-2

Nursing Interventions that are Helpful to Couples Dealing with Infertility

- Avoid assigning blame to one partner or the other.
- Facilitate communication between couples in order to give men in particular the opportunity to acknowledge and express their feelings and process their response to the infertility experience.
- Provide information related to cost and insurance coverage for treatment.
- Suggest appropriate stress relieving activities.
- Refer to support groups and/or other professionals for counseling.

Source: From Sherrod, R. A. (2004). Understanding the emotional aspects of infertility. Implications for nursing practice. *Journal of Psychosocial Nursing, 42*(3), 42–47; and Sherrod, R. A. (2006). Male infertility: The element of disguise. *Journal of Psychosocial Nursing, 44*(10), 31–37.

TABLE 12-3

International and Transracial Adoption: Issues and Challenges

Issues and Challenges to Families Before International and Transracial Adoption

▨ Ability to travel on short notice to pick up a child

▨ Changing political conditions may stop the adoption process at any time

▨ Ways family will maintain the adopted child's natural heritage

▨ Ways family will deal with racial and other types of prejudice

Issues and Challenges to Families After International Adoption

▨ Limited postadoption resources such as pediatricians trained in international adoption or international adoption clinics for families seeking help for a child's developmental and behavioral problems

▨ Child's emotional and developmental issues can be exhausting and financially tax the family

Issues and Challenges to Families After Transracial Adoption

▨ Need to redefine the family as multiracial and multiethnic when white families adopt non-white children

▨ Extra attention and comments about the child's looks from strangers in public places

▨ Neighbors, family members, and others may express prejudice toward the child

Source: Gunnar, M., & Pollak, S. D. (2007). Supporting parents so that they can support their internationally adopted children: The larger challenge lurking behind the fatality statistics. *Child Maltreatment, 12*(4), 381–382; Pillitteri, A. (2003). *Maternal and child health nursing* (4th ed.). Philadelphia: Lippincott Williams & Wilkins; and Rykkje, L. (2007). Intercountry adoption and nursing care. *Scandinavian Journal of Caring Sciences, 21*(4), 507–514, by permission.

(Hockenberry, Wilson, Winkelstein, & Kline, 2006; Rykkje, 2007). Therefore, nurses caring for women in the preadoptive and early postadoptive period must recognize and provide care in a manner similar to that provided to biological mothers during the prenatal and postpartum periods (Fontenot, 2007). See Table 12-4 for appropriate nursing interventions when caring for adoptive families.

Perinatal Loss

Loss of a child during pregnancy, after birth, or in the early postpartum period is one of the hardest losses for a family. The loss may be anticipated and voluntary, such as with abortion or relinquishing parental rights for adoption, or unanticipated, such as death or loss of custody to the state. An adoptive family may lose their intended child if a birth mother changes her mind about giving a baby up for adoption. Perinatal loss is not an uncommon event, with 25% to 50% of pregnancies ending before 20 weeks' gestation, stillbirth occurring in 7 fetuses per 1,200 live births, and 16 in 1,000 pregnancies ending with death of an infant after

TABLE 12-4

Nurse Interventions for Adoptive Families

▨ Encourage families to seek help from adoption experts and agencies

▨ Refer families to adoption specialists such as social workers and counselors

▨ Recommend families speak with and secure pediatric providers during the preadoptive process

▨ Recommend adoptive parents attend parenting classes and include them in prenatal and infant care classes

▨ Incorporate adoptive sensitive material into classes and other educational resources

▨ Keep lines of communication open between nurses and adoptive families as a way to alleviate fears about being judged or undermined

▨ Address other siblings' response to the adopted child because a biological child's feelings of inferiority or superiority to an adopted child can interfere with relationships within the family

Source: From Fontenot, H. (2007). Transition and adaptation to adoptive motherhood. *Journal of Obstetrics, Gynecologic and Neonatal Nursing, 36*(2), 175–182; and Pillitteri, A. (2003). *Maternal and child health nursing* (4th ed.). Philadelphia: Lippincott Williams & Wilkins, by permission.

pregnancy, nurses should be aware that adoptive mothers and families will have many of the same feelings and fears as biological families (Fontenot, 2007). All parents react to the strong intense feelings and emotions, ranging from happiness to distress, at the first moments they meet their child, regardless of the way in which a family is formed. Even though the child is not biological or the parental relationship may not be established immediately at birth, bonding can be just as strong and immediate for adoptive parents and children birth (Callister, 2006). These sobering statistics serve to alert nurses about the prevalence of pregnancy loss, as well as point out the need for ongoing nursing assessment and intervention related to potential, previous, or current loss when caring for families during the childbearing family with infants stage. Table 12-5 lists other types of perinatal loss that families may experience.

Loss of a child is a unique and profound experience for parents. When parents lose a child, they lose a part of their hoped-for identity as a parent, as well as all hopes and dreams held for the child they anticipated and loved (Callister, 2006; O'Leary & Thorwick, 2006). Despite the intense effect pregnancy loss has on the family, it is often only minimally recognized or acknowledged by society. Societal invisibility of infant loss contributes to parental frustration, especially when they are denied time to mourn or asked why they are not yet over their loss (Callister, 2006; Chichester, 2005). One mother put it this way when describing her loss experience during the second trimester of pregnancy: "When I lost my baby there was no memorial service, no outpouring of sympathy, no evidence that I gave birth and lost a baby" (Callister, 2006, p. 228).

Nurses providing care to childbearing families should anticipate that each family member will experience loss differently. For example, mothers are more apt to grieve visibly by emotional expression, sharing of feelings, and participation in grief support groups. Fathers, in contrast, tend to feel a sense of loneliness and isolation and have feelings of helplessness rather than control. Fathers, who see their role as primarily supportive, may hold back their own feelings to conform to societal and culture pressure to be the strong one (Callister, 2006; O'Leary & Thorwick, 2006; Robson, 2002). Siblings may describe their grief experience as "hurting inside" as a way to express feelings of sadness, frustration, loneliness, fear, and anger (Davies, 2006). Likewise, grandparents experience their own grief and pain at the loss of their grandchild, and the pain of seeing their own children suffer (Lemon, 2002).

Considering the effect of perinatal loss on all family members, nurses must work to support and strengthen the familial bond in the face of such loss (Callister, 2006). Often, losing a child is a young couple's first experience with death, grief, and sorrow, which can lead to a reliance on nurses and other health care providers for support and knowledge (Callister, 2006; Chichester, 2005). Nurses can support families' experience of perinatal loss by being present, expressing emotions, gathering memorabilia, and helping the family make meaning of the experience (Callister, 2006). Referral to support groups may be helpful depending on the needs of the grieving couple or family (Callister, 2006). Compassionate Friends is one of many groups to which nurses might refer grieving parents, siblings, and grandparents for support.

Culture influences how families respond to perinatal loss. Therefore, it is essential for nurses to understand several different culturally diverse practices and rituals associated with loss, as well as provide culturally competent care. Nurses demonstrate cultural sensitivity when they validate what families perceive to be the "right way" to grieve (Callister, 2006; Chichester, 2005). Table 12-6 lists cultural perinatal loss practices and rituals of select cultural groups.

TABLE 12-5

Types of Perinatal Loss Families May Experience

- Miscarriage
- Elective abortion
- Ectopic pregnancy
- Selective reduction after in vitro implantation of multiple fertilized eggs
- Stillbirth
- Death of a child after a live birth
- Recurrent pregnancy loss
- Loss of a perfect child because of anomalies or malformations
- Death of a twin during pregnancy, labor, birth, or after birth
- Termination of pregnancy for identified fetal anomalies, which is increasing because of technologic advances in prenatal diagnosis of such anomalies

Source: From Callister, L. C. (2006). Perinatal loss: A family perspective. *Journal of Perinatal Neonatal Nursing, 20*(3), 227–234; and Robson, F. (2002). Yes! A chance to tell my side of the story: A case study of a male partner of a woman undergoing termination of pregnancy for fetal abnormality. *Journal of Health Psychology, 7*(2), 183–193, by permission.

TABLE 12-6

Perinatal Loss Cultural Practices and Rituals

- Jewish families may request to remain with the body at all times out of respect. Newborns are named and circumcised at burial so they can be included in family records.

- Muslim babies born after more than 4 months' gestation are to be named, bathed, wrapped in a seamless white sheet, and buried within 24 hours. Bodies are buried intact, so taking locks of hair is not permitted.

- Puerto Rican families may call on faith healers and spiritualists to assist the baby on their journey into the next life.

- Roma (gypsy) families want to avoid any association between death and bad luck/impurity (mahrime), so they may leave the hospital suddenly and shift responsibility for burial to the hospital.

- American Indians/Alaskan Natives may request to remain with the baby until death to pray and perform a ritual.

Source: From Callister, L. C. (2006). Perinatal loss: A family perspective. *Journal of Perinatal Neonatal Nursing, 20*(3), 227–234; Chichester, M. (2005). Multicultural issues in perinatal loss. *Lifelines, 9*(4), 314–320; Palacios, J., Butterfly, R., & Strickland, C. J. (2005). American Indians/Alaskan Natives. In J. G. Lipson & S. L. Dibble (Eds.), *Cultural and clinical care* (pp. 27–41). San Francisco: The Regents University of California; and Sutherland, A. H. (2005). Roma (Gypsies). In J. G. Lipson & S. L. Dibble (Eds.), *Cultural and clinical care* (pp. 404–414). San Francisco: The Regents University of California.

Pregnancy After Perinatal Loss

Women may not perceive pregnancy as normal after experiencing perinatal loss but rather may be plagued with a sense of anxiety, insecurity, ambivalence, doubt, and concern that another loss may occur (Callister, 2006; Davidson et al., 2008). Fathers also may shut down their feelings when pregnancy occurs after loss because of unresolved feelings related to prior pregnancy loss. They may even be too frightened to share or be conscious of their feelings. Nurses caring for childbearing families during pregnancy after perinatal loss are in a prime position to help mothers and fathers open doors of communication that may have been closed because of fear. One strategy nurses could use to encourage communication is to ask fathers "How are you

doing?" in front of the mothers, which provides an opportunity to share what they are feeling (Davidson et al., 2008; O'Leary & Thorwick, 2006).

THREATS TO HEALTH DURING CHILDBEARING

For the majority of families, childbearing is a physically healthy experience. For some families, health during childbearing is threatened, and the childbearing experience becomes an illness experience. In such cases, concern for the physical health of the mother and the fetus tends to outweigh other aspects of pregnancy, and rather than eagerly anticipating the birth and baby, family members experience fear and apprehension. Moreover, the family's functioning and developmental tasks are disrupted as the family focuses its attention on the health of the mother and survival of the fetus or baby. Childbearing nurses must be aware that families with threats to health have additional needs for maintaining and preserving family health.

Acute and Chronic Illness During Childbearing

This chapter defines "acute" as health threats that come on suddenly and may have life-threatening implications. Examples of acute health threats childbearing families may encounter are fetal distress during labor and pulmonary embolism for postpartum women. In contrast, "chronic" defines conditions that occur during pregnancy that persist, linger, need control, or have no cure, and which require careful monitoring and treatment to avoid becoming an acute threat to maternal or infant health. Pregnancy-induced hypertension, gestational and preexisting diabetes, and PPD are some examples of chronic health threats. Some threats to health during childbearing vacillate between acute and chronic. For example, preterm labor can be an acute health threat that results in a preterm birth. If preterm labor contractions are suppressed, it becomes a "chronic" health threat, requiring adherence to prescribed regimens to keep contractions from reoccurring.

Effect of Threats to Health on Childbearing Families

Chronic threats to childbearing health are disruptive to childbearing families. Knowledge of the family as a dynamic system explains why the effects of these chronic conditions extend to the entire family and result in the upset of family functioning, development, and structure that keep the family system stable (Maloni, Brezinski-Tomasi, & Johnson, 2001). When childbearing health is threatened, all family members experience stress as families strive to regain balance. For example, three sources of stress that alter family processes when the mother or infant experiences a chronic health threat are: (1) assuming household tasks, (2) managing changes in income and resources, and (3) facing uncertainty and separation.

ASSUMPTIONS OF HOUSEHOLD TASKS

When women experience chronic threats to childbearing health, other members of the family must assume responsibility for household tasks and functioning, regardless of whether the condition is managed at the hospital or at home. Assumption of household tasks by others creates family stress, as each participant must take on household and other tasks so the expectant mother or infant, or both, can follow prescribed regimens (Bomar, 2004). Shifting these tasks may be stressful and affect the family's functioning (Bomar, 2004). Expectant fathers especially may find that all their time and energy are consumed by employment and household management, tasks that previously were shared or done solely by their partners. Children's lives change when mothers have to limit activities. Toddlers do not understand why their mothers cannot pick them up or run after them. The resulting frustration for children can manifest itself in behavioral changes, such as tantrums and regression in developmental tasks such as toilet training.

MANAGING CHANGES IN INCOME AND RESOURCES

An at-risk pregnancy is stressful in terms of the family's financial and other resources. Changes in the family's income, financial stability, and resources occur because one or both parents have to take time away from paid employment at a time when they are coping with increased medical and personal expenses (Maloni et al., 2001). For example, if a mother is placed on bed rest because of risk for premature labor, she may miss time away from paid employment, which may result in loss of income. At the same time, medical expenses may increase because of the need for increased care, including possible neonatal intensive care and maintaining multiple health care provider visits or hospital stays, as can personal expenses associated with the cost of specialized diets, medications, and hiring personnel to assist with household tasks. For families already in debt, threats to health serve to increase the burden of debt.

Although assets such as energy and social networks cannot be measured as easily as money, family nurses are in a position to help families consider and manage changes in their nonmonetary resources. Some of the nonmonetary changes that family nurses should anticipate families will encounter include the need for others outside of the nuclear family to assume various household tasks such as meal preparation, laundry, and cleaning; that all families may not have social networks or extended families in the immediate vicinity; that changes in employment may cause separation from persons and activities that were stimulating; and that isolation, regardless of the cause, can increase a family's burden.

FACING UNCERTAINTY AND SEPARATION OR LOSS

The unpredictable nature of high-risk childbearing makes planning for the future difficult for childbearing families because it leaves them facing uncertainty and possible separation. For example, expectant parents, especially employed women, face uncertainty with pending preterm birth because they may not be able to determine accurately when to begin and end parental leave because of the need to cope with sudden hospitalization. Separation can occur when mothers are suddenly hospitalized or when families living in remote rural areas are transferred to a distant perinatal center for days or weeks. When families are separated, it becomes difficult for them to maintain and develop family relationships. Separation from the family and concerns about family status are two of the greatest stressors women hospitalized for chronic threats to childbearing health experience (Maloni, Margevicius, & Damato, 2006). In addition, small children experience extreme anxiety over the sudden departure of their mother, especially if they are unprepared or unable to comprehend what is happening to their mother and the new baby.

Even if the logistical problems related to separation are solved and a family can be together, coping with basic tasks of living is challenging in new settings. For instance, a family may not know where to stay, how to find reasonably priced meals, how to obtain transportation, or where to park a car. Table 12-7 presents nursing interventions related to childbearing families who are experiencing chronic threats to health.

TABLE 12-7

Family Nursing Interventions for Childbearing Families who are Experiencing Chronic Threats to Health

Assuming Household Tasks
- Help families find ways to streamline and prioritize household tasks to reduce stress and increase adherence to medical regimens.
- Assist adults to list household management tasks and determine who does what when so that the family can be more efficient and effective in managing these tasks.
- Educate families about the impact of parents' health difficulties on children.
- Provide practical, age-appropriate suggestions for managing children such as hiring a teenager after school for active play with young children.
- Encourage parents to provide ways for young children to have some quiet one-on-one time with their mothers as a way to reduce stress for both mothers and children.

Managing Changes in Income and Resources
- Refer to an appropriate counselor who can assist the family explore ways to manage financial problems.
- Assist families to identify others outside of the nuclear family who can assume various household tasks such as meal preparation, laundry, and cleaning.
- Help families identify and use resources, such as home-health agencies and parents' groups in the community, that will assist with household management.
- Encourage families with necessary resources to use a computer to connect with each other, friends, coworkers, and other at-risk families to prevent or decrease feelings of isolation.
- Direct families to appropriate Internet sites such as the ones listed in the Selected Resources section at the end of this chapter.

Facing Uncertainty and Separation and Loss: Nursing Interventions
- Acknowledge the difficulties of uncertainties associated with difficult perinatal situations.
- Be honest and informative about the condition and prognosis of both the mother and fetus.
- Use terms understood by all family members to provide accurate and thorough explanations tailored to families' anxiety levels.
- Assist families to cope with basic tasks of living in high-tech settings such as the neonatal intensive care unit.
- Investigate and reduce the barriers families encounter at the distant perinatal center, such as lack of transportation, other responsibilities, employment, and the threatening environment of the setting.
- Provide families with information on where to stay, how to find reasonably priced meals, how to obtain transportation, or where to park a car.
- Encourage use of electronic communication, such as e-mail, which facilitates contact between family members and health care professionals.
- Encourage calling families about their members' progress and sending photographs as a way to help families cope with uncertainty and enhance relationships of physically separated family members.
- Encourage family members to participate in care of their infants to promote development of parenting skills.

Source: From Martell, L. (2005). Family nursing with childbearing families. In S. M. H. Hanson, V. Gedaly-Duff, & J. R. Kaakinen (Eds.), *Family health care nursing: Theory, practice & research* (3rd ed., pp. 291–323). Philadelphia: F.A. Davis.

FAMILY NURSING OF POSTPARTUM FAMILIES

All family members experience household upheaval during the first few days and weeks a newborn is in the home. Throughout the childbearing cycle, nurses assist families to understand and respond to the effect of a new baby on the family. Assisting parents to be realistic in their expectations about themselves, each other, and their children helps them to plan ahead by identifying appropriate support and resources. This section discusses appropriate nursing assessments and interventions family nurses should incorporate into practice when caring for families during the postpartum period.

Feeding Management

Success in feeding their babies induces feelings of competency in mothers. A family's comfort with its infant feeding method is as crucial for physical, emotional, and social well-being of the infant as the food itself. Regardless of the parents' choice of feeding method, nurses' instructions need to emphasize the development of relationships between infant and parent through feeding. Being held during feeding enhances social development whether a baby is being breast-fed or bottle-fed. Parents should take the time during feedings to enjoy interacting with their babies. When the infant is adopted, social interaction with feeding is a special opportunity for developing attachment.

Even though the act of breast-feeding is a strictly female function, fathers need not be excluded from the feeding experience. Nurses can promote paternal-infant attachment by encouraging fathers to be involved with feeding. For example, the father can burp the baby during or after feedings, as well as hold and comfort the infant once feeding has been completed. Another way to involve fathers is to have them give the breast-fed baby an occasional bottle of expressed breast milk once breast-feeding is well established (Davidson et al., 2008). Early involvement of fathers in feeding offers an excellent opportunity for family nurses to observe interactions between parent and infant for signs of positive attachment behaviors (Lowdermilk & Perry, 2004). It is also beneficial later when infants are being weaned from the breast or mothers are preparing to return to employment.

Attachment

Positive parent-infant attachment must take place to foster optimal growth and development of infants, as well as to encourage the parent-infant love relationship. The attachment process requires early involvement and physical contact between parents and their infant for a strong link to develop (Schenk et al., 2005). Extreme stress, health risk factors, and illness can interfere with the physical contact and early parent-infant involvement needed for the development of attachment. Stressful conditions that pull parents' energies and attention away from their newborns can be detrimental to attachment.

Nurses should be alert for families who are likely to have difficulty with attachment, especially if family history indicates a parent has suffered abuse, neglect, and abandonment during childhood. In addition, nurses may identify families at risk for poor attachment through listening to what parents say about their babies and observing parent behaviors. Families at risk for poor attachment may have misconceptions about infant behavior such as believing that infants cry just to annoy their parents. Hence, family nurses must address verbal expressions of dissatisfaction with the infant, comparison of the infant with disliked family members, failure to respond to the infant's crying, lack of spontaneity in touching the infant, and stiffness or discomfort in holding the infant after the first week. Although isolated incidences of these behaviors are probably not detrimental to attachment, persistent trends and patterns could be an indicator of future relationship difficulties.

Another signal of attachment difficulty is inconsistent maternal behaviors, such as a mother who exhibits intense concern at times interspersed with apathy at other times without any predictable cause or pattern. Therefore, an important step when assessing attachment behaviors is to evaluate whether the parent-infant relationship is progressing positively, and the enjoyment and love of children grow over time. If the parents' enjoyment of the baby as a unique individual and commitment to the baby are not progressing, the nurse needs to help the family to understand what attachment is, and to identify factors that might be interfering with attachment to their infant. For example, mothers struggling with PPD need treatment for their depression before they can address attachment to the infant. Childbearing family nurses may need to refer families who do not demonstrate nurturing behaviors to other professionals such as social workers, psychotherapists, and developmental specialists who can provide more intensive interventions that will help parents care for and nurture their children.

Siblings

No matter what age siblings are, the addition of a new baby affects the position, role, and power of older children, thereby creating stress for both parents and children. Teaching parents to emphasize the positive aspects of adding a family member helps them focus on sibling "relationships" rather than "rivalry." Parents need help to address *all* of the children's needs, not just those of the new baby. Parents may be concerned whether they have "enough" energy, time, and love for additional children. Practical ideas for time and task management can alleviate some of their concerns, as well as helping parents delegate nonparenting tasks such as housecleaning and meal preparation to friends and relatives when possible.

Postpartum Depression

The period after childbirth can be a stressful time for women because of their need to face the new tasks of the maternal role. Changes in relationships, economic demands, and social support also take place during this time and can result in postpartum stress (Hung, 2005). PPD has been described as "a dangerous thief that robs women of precious time together with their infants that they had been dreaming of throughout pregnancy" (Beck, 2001, p. 275). Although the "baby blues" are a predictable and temporary mood shift that occurs during the first 2 weeks after childbirth, symptoms of stress that take hold and persist during the first year are of concern to family nurses because they can adversely affect maternal health and the ability of mothers to function in their new role (Blass, 2005; Hung, 2005). Ten percent to 15% of all postpartum mothers and 48% of postpartum adolescent mothers will experience a major depressive disorder known as PPD after the birth or adoption of a baby (Driscoll, 2006). The effects of maternal depression are not limited to the mother herself but spread to family, friends, and coworkers alike (Grantmakers in Health, 2004). Left unidentified and untreated, PPD leads to serious consequences for families, such as maternal suicide, poor attachment to the infant, altered family dynamics, and lowered cognitive development in children. Considering these consequences, it becomes imperative that family nurses immediately identify and appropriately refer women experiencing PPD so that early treatment can begin (Driscoll, 2006). Box 12-3 lists signs of PPD.

Usually women do not volunteer information about their depression. Therefore, nursing assessment during the postpartum period must be aimed at determining a woman's moods, sleep, appetite, energy, fatigue level, and ability to concentrate. Childbearing family nurses might consider incorporating

---

BOX 12-3
Signs of Postpartum Depression

Sadness
Frequent crying
Insomnia or excessive sleeping
Lack of interest or pleasure in usual activities, including sexual relations
Difficulties thinking, concentrating, or making decisions
Lack of concern about personal appearance
Feelings of worthlessness
Fatigue or loss of energy
Depressed mood
Thoughts of death: suicidal ideation without a plan; suicide plan or attempt

Source: Davidson, M. R., London, M. L., & Ladewig, P. A. (2008). *Olds' maternal-newborn nursing and women's health across the lifespan* (8th ed.). Upper Saddle River, NJ: Pearson Prentice Hall; and Driscoll, J. W. (2006). Postpartum depression: How nurses can identify and care for women grappling with this disorder. *Lifelines, 10*(5), 399–409.

the two-question screening measure that Jesse and Graham (2005) developed as a rapid way to begin the identification of women at risk for PPD. Use of this scale simply involves nurses asking women two questions: "Are you sad or depressed?" and "Have you experienced a loss in pleasurable activities?" Nurses would recommend that women who answer yes to both of these questions be referred to a mental health provider (Driscoll, 2006). Family nurses might also consider using one of many readily available and easy-to-use depression scales such the Postpartum Depression Predictor Inventory (PDPI-Revised) or the Edinburgh Postnatal Depression Scale as a routine assessment screening tool for PPD (Davidson et al., 2008). In particular, the Edinburgh Postnatal Depression Scale has been found to be valid for several cultures, translated into several different languages, and has been used with men (Driscoll, 2006; Eberhard-Gran et al., 2001; Goodman, 2004). Regardless of which screening tool is used to identify women at risk for PPD, childbearing family nurses have a professional responsibility to assess for the disorder, recommend women be referred for treatment, and provide self-care strategies and support to the woman and her family (Driscoll, 2006).

Although much attention has been given to maternal PPD, shifting gender roles and paternal involvement in child care requires adjustments for men, which puts them at risk for experiencing depression after the birth of a child, especially if the mother is depressed. This makes sense to the nurses who understand Family Systems Theory because anything that affects one family member directly or indirectly affects other family members. Viewed from this theoretical perspective, it is easy to see how maternal or paternal depression affects all family members and relationships within the family, and results in serious implications for family health and well-being. Therefore, family nurses must recognize PPD in fathers just as in mothers because when both parents are depressed, the risk to infants and children increases (Goodman, 2004). As with mothers, recommendation of a referral for fathers to mental health care providers should be made in an effort to initiate early treatment and reduce negative effects on the family system (Goodman, 2004). Table 12-8 lists additional nursing interventions for PPD.

TABLE 12-8

Nursing Interventions for Postpartum Depression

- Help women differentiate between myths of the mother role, which imply at 6 weeks after birth women are ready to resume all their previous activities, versus the reality of motherhood where prepregnancy clothes do not fit, infants periodically become demanding malcontents, and houses are messy because family members are too exhausted to clean.

- Encourage women with postpartum depression to share feelings as they grieve the loss of who they were and begin to build on who they are becoming.

- Encourage women to seek help with symptoms of anxiety, anger, obsessive thinking, fear, guilt, and/or suicidal thoughts.

- Assist women to recreate, restructure, and integrate changes that new motherhood brings into their daily lives.

- Develop standard protocols for screening of men whose partners are depressed after childbirth.

Source: From Driscoll, J. W. (2006). Postpartum depression: How nurses can identify and care for women grappling with this disorder. *Lifelines, 10*(5), 399–409; Goodman, J. H. (2004). Paternal postpartum depression, its relationship to maternal postpartum depression, and implications for family health. *Journal of Advanced Nursing, 45*(10), 26–35; and Martell, L. K. (2005). Family nursing with childbearing families. In S. M. H. Hanson, V. Gedaly-Duff, & J. R. Kaakinen (Eds.), *Family health care nursing: Theory, practice and care* (3rd ed., pp. 267–289). Philadelphia: F.A. Davis, by permission.

IMPLICATIONS FOR FAMILY NURSING PRACTICE

The concerns of childbearing family nursing go beyond care of the individual family. Nurses are participants in guiding nursing practice, developing and using research, and setting and implementing policy.

Practice

Family-centered care is an approach to care that "recognizes the strengths and needs of patients and families and the essential roles that family members play in the promotion of health and the management of illness" (Roudebush, Kaufman, Johnson, Abraham, & Clayton, 2006, p. 202). Family-centered maternity care encourages mothers and families to assume active roles in caregiving and decision making, places an emphasis on education and preparation for childbirth, encourages family presence during labor and birth, focuses on enhancing and supporting the normal birth and screens, and intervenes when deviations from normal birth occur (Roudebush et al., 2006). Nurses may find barriers in their practice settings that interfere with promoting family development. For example, lack of privacy, complex machinery, and location of a neonatal intensive care unit may stifle interaction between family members and newborns. To some nurses, "mother/baby" means that the family members will assume all the care for the baby with nurses periodically "checking in" and renewing baby care supplies. In such situations, families feel ignored or burdened with too much independence (Martell, 2001, 2003). Some suggestions for making family-centered care a reality include identifying physical, psychological, and nursing staff requirements for family-centered care; developing a clear vision of family-centered care units; and involving nurses in the planning and implementation of change (Martell, 2003). In settings other than hospitals, changing the focus of care from individuals to families is the most important step in promoting family care. In-home care will be more effective when it includes family members in care.

Research

Technologic advances such as gene therapy in human reproduction are rapidly increasing and becoming more commonplace. (See Chapter 8 for a more detailed discussion on genomics and family nursing.) The scientific knowledge about the effect of these technologies on families still needs investigation. Because nurses focus on the full range of human experiences, the nursing profession has an opportunity to be the leader in launching such studies. Areas for study include the most effective ways to counsel or interact with clients about infertility, genetic counseling, in vitro surgeries, and other medical advances.

Childbearing families represent the increasing diversity of families. The content of this chapter is partially based on study of two-parent, middle-class, North American families. Research on the childbearing experience of ethnic and blended families is

increasing, but more is needed on the full range of present-day families. In addition to studying various family cultures and types, it is critical to advance the studies relative to multiple births. Another aspect that needs study is how alternative families adjust to miscarriages, stillbirths, and infertility issues. Adoption issues for the childbearing family and how men cope with prenatal loss and early infancy are two other issues in need of further study.

Research on family nursing interventions and outcomes for childbearing families needs support to develop evidence-based nursing practice. Evaluation of the effectiveness of family nursing interventions is especially critical when health care costs are under close scrutiny.

Policy

Much of Chapter 5 addresses important issues for childbearing families. The legal definitions of family, official recognition of the diversity of families, access to health care, alternatives to traditional childbearing such as cross-cultural adoption, and growing needs of poverty-stricken families are just a few of the policy areas vital to childbearing family nursing.

Nurses need to be aware of the effect of legislation on childbearing families. One example is family leave for childbirth, which can profoundly affect the health and development of childbearing families. The Family and Medical Leave Act entitles family members to take *unpaid* time away from employment without penalizing them, to care for a family member, such as a newborn, with health care needs. Unfortunately, many families cannot take advantage of the benefits of this act because it applies only to certain size businesses, and employers are not obligated to pay on-leave employees. Unlike the citizens of many developed nations, parents in the United States are not entitled to government benefits for childbearing except for tax deductions and other incentives. Many European countries, by contrast, offer paid paternity leave.

All types of policies affect family nursing every day. Hospitals often have policies that form barriers to family welfare and relationships, which should be of concern to family nurses considering how varied the family of today is. For example, increasing numbers of nontraditional families, such as lesbian couples, are having children through donor insemination or adoption (Roberts, 2006). However, policies that guide perinatal practices from the visual images hanging on the wall to if or how well partners are welcomed in prenatal groups, the delivery room or other hospital environments may be a barrier to these particular families' welfare and relationships (Goldberg, 2005; Roberts, 2006). In these situations, family nurses have an obligation to speak out on behalf of families. Often, nurses think of policies as entities beyond their control. In actuality, nurses have a voice and power in forming and changing policies. Beginning steps include close scrutiny of their practice settings for issues related to the welfare of families and their members.

Family Case Study

THE SANDERS: A FAMILY WITH A PRETERM BIRTH

Tom and Mary Sanders have been married to each other for 6 years. Tom, age 28, and Mary, age 24, have one child named Jenny, who was born at full term 2 years ago. Mary did not experience any health problems with this first pregnancy. At that time, the Sanders lived in a large city in the western part of the United States, near their parents, siblings, and childhood friends. Two years later, the Sanders moved to a small town 500 miles away from their friends and families to find better professional opportunities for Tom, a software engineer, and more affordable housing. A month after the move, they discovered that Mary was about 3 months pregnant. Even though it would strain family finances, Mary decided to postpone seeking employment as a secretary until after the birth and to concentrate instead on fixing up the older two-story house they had bought.

Unexpectedly, Mary had health problems with this pregnancy. At 27 weeks' gestation, her obstetrician diagnosed gestational diabetes, which required Mary to modify her diet to keep her blood glucose under control. At 29 weeks, she began to have preterm labor. To stop the contractions, her physician insisted that Mary stay on bed rest around the clock except for a very brief daily shower and use of the bathroom. Tom had to take over meal preparation, house cleaning, and caring for Jenny. He arranged the living room so Mary could lie on the couch and Jenny could play near her mother while he was at work. Because he had not yet accrued vacation or sick time, Tom could not take off time from his job to help Mary and take care of Jenny without sacrificing pay.

Mary found it difficult to follow her diet and stay on bed rest. She was frustrated because she had to stop her house renovation, and Tom's cooking and housecleaning were not up to her standards. She was tempted to run the vacuum cleaner, wash dishes, and eat sweets while Tom was at work. The medication to suppress contractions made her so anxious and tremulous that she could not amuse herself with crafts, sewing, or puzzles. She was lonely for her mother and friends, who were 500 miles away; she longed for companionship but found herself complaining and nagging Tom when he was home. Jenny frequently had tantrums because she could not play outside with her mother and began to have lapses in toilet training.

At 32 weeks of pregnancy, Mary's membranes ruptured; her physician sent her to a perinatal center 100 miles away from Mary's home because it had better facilities to care for preterm babies. Jenny went with her parents to the perinatal center to wait until one of her grandmothers could come and take care of her. Jason was born 28 hours after the Sanders arrived at the perinatal center hospital. (Figure 12-1 presents a Sanders family genogram.)

Mary was discharged from the perinatal center within 24 hours after Jason's birth. At home, she felt extremely weak and was overwhelmed by household tasks and caring for Jenny. She was disappointed that she was unable to breast-feed the baby. Two weeks later, she was weeping frequently, felt very sad, had no appetite, and had difficulty sleeping. Being with their new son was difficult because each visit required a 200-mile round-trip, Tom had a full-time job, and Mary cared for Jenny during the day. Jason, the new baby, remained at the perinatal center in the special care nursery until he was mature and stable enough to go home 4 weeks later. At her 6-week postpartum checkup, Mary told the office nurse that she did not enjoy caring for her new baby and she had difficulty with her sleep. Figure 12-2 presents the Sanders family ecomap and how the nurse mobilized resources to help this family.

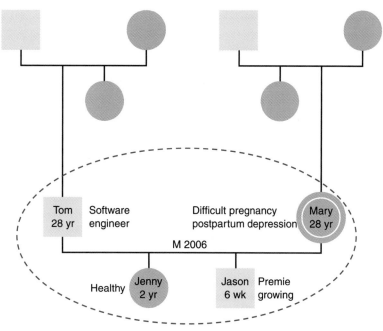

FIGURE 12-1 Sanders family genogram.

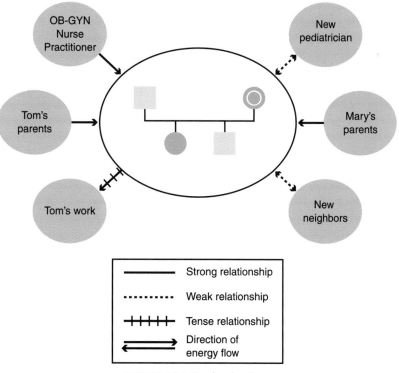

FIGURE 12-2 Sanders family ecomap.

SUMMARY

Childbearing family nursing focuses on family relationships and the health of all members of the childbearing family even during times of extreme threats to maternal health. Several different theories are available to nurses encountering families during childbearing, which can help guide their assessment of, plan of care, and interventions for the family. Nurses are also in a position to have a powerful influence on the ways in which family centered care is practiced and on the development of family friendly policies at both the federal and practice setting level. In addition nurses can contribute to the knowledge base of childbearing families through design and implementation of research aimed at understanding their unique experiences.

- While giving direct physical care, teaching patients, or performing other traditional modes of maternity nursing, family nurses focus on family relationships and health of all members of the childbearing family.
- Several theories are helpful to guide nurses' understanding of childbearing families and to structure nursing care, particularly Family Systems Theory and Family Developmental Theory.
- Even in extreme threats to health, family nurses do not ignore the whole of the family.
- Nurses have a powerful influence on family practice, policy, and research for childbearing families.

REFERENCES

American College of Obstetricians and Gynecologists (ACOG) and the Interprofessional Task Force on Health Care of Women and Children. (1978). *Joint statement on the development of family centered maternity/newborn care in hospitals.* Chicago: ACOG.

Beck, C. T. (2001). Predictors of postpartum depression: An update. *Nursing Research, 50*(5), 275–285.

Berk, L. (2007). *Development through the lifespan* (4th ed.). Boston: Allyn and Bacon.

Blass, D. (2005). *Riding the emotional roller coaster.* Washington, DC: American College of Obstetricians and Gynecologists.

Bomar, P. (Ed.). (2004). *Promoting health in families: Applying family research and theory in nursing practice* (2nd ed.). Philadelphia: Saunders.

Callister, L. C. (2006). Perinatal loss: A family perspective. *Journal of Perinatal Neonatal Nursing, 20*(3), 227–234.

Carter, B., & McGoldrick, M. (2005). *The expanded family life cycle: Individual, family and social perspectives* (3rd ed.). New York: Allyn & Bacon, Pearson Education Company.

Chichester, M. (2005). Multicultural issues in perinatal loss. *Lifelines, 9*(4), 314–320.

Davidson, M. R., London, M. L., & Ladewig, P. A. (2008). *Olds' maternal-newborn nursing and women's health across the lifespan* (8th ed.). Upper Saddle River, NJ: Pearson Prentice Hall.

Davies, B. (2006, January/February/March). Sibling grief throughout childhood. *The Forum.* Retrieved May 5, 2008, from Association for Death Education and Counseling: http://www.adec.org/coping/PDF/Sibling%20Grief.pdf

Day, R. D. (2005). Relationship stress in couples. In P. C. McKenry & S. J. Price (Eds.), *Families and Changes: Coping with stressful events and transition* (3rd ed., pp. 332–353). Thousand Oaks, CA: Sage.

de Chateau, P. (1976). Influence of early contact on maternal and infant behavior in primiparae. *Birth Family Journal, 6,* 149–155.

de Chateau, P. (1977). Importance of the neonatal period for the development of synchrony in the mother-infant dyad. *Birth Family Journal, 4*(1), 10–22.

Driscoll, J. W. (2006). Postpartum depression: How nurses can identify and care for women grappling with this disorder. *Lifelines, 10*(5), 399–409.

Duval, E. M. (1977). *Marriage and family development* (5th ed.). Philadelphia: J.B. Lippincott.

Duvall, E. M., & Miller, B. C. (1985). *Marriage and family development* (6th ed.). New York: Harper & Row.

Eberhard-Gran, M., Eskild, A., Tambs, K., Opjordsmoen, S., & Samuelsen, S. O. (2001). Review of validation studies of the Edinburgh Postnatal Depression Scale. *Acta Psychiatrica Scandinavica, 104*(4), 243–249.

Fomby, B. W. (2004). Family routines, rituals, recreation and rules. In P. Bomar (Ed.), *Promoting health in families: Applying family research and theory in nursing practice.* (2nd ed.). Philadelphia: Saunders.

Fontenot, H. (2007). Transition and adaptation to adoptive motherhood. *Journal of Obstetrics, Gynecologic and Neonatal Nursing, 36*(2), 175–182.

Goldberg, L. (2005). Understanding lesbian experience: What perinatal nurses should know to promote women's health. *AWHONN Lifelines, 9*(6), 463–467.

Goodman, J. H. (2004). Paternal postpartum depression, its relationship to maternal postpartum depression, and implications for family health. *Journal of Advanced Nursing, 45*(10), 26–35.

Grantmakers in Health. (2004). *Fact sheet. Addressing maternal depression.* Washington, DC: Grantmakers in Health.

Gunnar, M., & Pollak, S. D. (2007). Supporting parents so that they can support their internationally adopted children: The larger challenge lurking behind the fatality statistics. *Child Maltreatment, 12*(4), 381–382.

Hockenberry, M. I., Wilson, D., Winkelstein, M. L., & Kline, N. E. (2006). *Wong's nursing care of infants and children* (7th ed.). St. Louis, MO: Mosby.

Hung, C. H., (2005). Women's postpartum stress, social support and healthk status. *Western Journal of Nursing Research, 27*(2), 148–159.

Jesse, D. E., & Graham, M. (2005). Are you often sad and depressed? Brief measures to identify women at risk for depression in pregnancy. *American Journal of Maternal Child Nursing, 30*(1), 40–45.

Klaus, M. K., Jerauld, R., Kreger, N. C., McAlpine, W., Steffa, M., & Kennel, J. M. (1972). Maternal attachment: Importance of the first postpartum days. *New England Journal of Medicine, 286*(9), 460–463.

Klaus, M. H., & Kennel, J. H. (1976). Maternal-infant bonding. St. Louis, MO: Mosby.

Leavitt, J. W. (1986). *Brought to bed: Childbearing in America 1750-1950*. New York: Oxford University Press.

LeMasters, E. E. (1957). Parenthood as crisis. *Marriage and the Family, 31*, 352–355.

Lemon, B. S. (2002). Experiencing grandparent grief: A piece of my heart died twice. *AWHONN Lifelines, 6*(5), 470–472.

London, M. L., Ladewig, P. W., Ball, J. W., & Bindler, R. C. (2007). *Maternal and child nursing care* (2nd ed.). Upper Saddle River, NJ: Pearson.

Lowdermilk, D. L., & Perry, S. E. (2004). *Maternity and women's health care* (8th ed.). St. Louis, MO: Mosby.

Maloni, J. A., Brezinski-Tomasi, J. E., & Johnson, L. A. (2001). Antepartum bed rest: Effect upon the family. *Journal of Obstetric, Gynecologic, and Neonatal Nursing, 30*(2), 165–172.

Maloni, J. A., Margevicius, S. P., & Damato, E. G. (2006). Multiple gestation: Side effects of antepartum bed rest. *Biological Research for Nursing, 8*(2), 115–128.

Mander, R. (2004). *Men and maternity*. New York: Routledge.

Martell, L. K. (2001). Heading toward the new normal: A contemporary postpartum experience. *Journal of Obstetric, Gynecologic, and Neonatal Nursing, 30*(5), 65–72.

Martell, L. K. (2003). Postpartum women's perceptions of the hospital environment. *Journal of Obstetric, Gynecologic, and Neonatal Nursing, 32*(4), 478–485.

Martell, L. K. (2005). Family nursing with childbearing families. In S. M. Hanson, V. Gedaly-Duff, & J. R. Kaakinen (Eds.), *Family health care nursing: Theory, practice and care* (3rd ed., pp. 267–289). Philadelphia: F.A. Davis.

Martell, L. K. (2006). From innovation to common practice: Perinatal nursing pre-1970 to 2005. *Journal of Perinatal and Neonatal Nursing, 20*(1), 8–16.

Mennino, S. F., & Brayfield, A. (2002). Job-family trade-offs: The multidimensional effects of gender. *Work and Occupations, 29*(2), 226–256.

Murray, T. R. (1992). *Comparing theories of child development*. Belmont, CA: Wadsworth.

Nelson, A. M. (2003). Transition to motherhood. *Journal of Obstetric, Gynecologic, and Neonatal Nursing, 32*(4), 465–477.

O'Leary, J., & Thorwick, C. (2006). Fathers' perspective during pregnancy, post perinatal loss. *Journal of Obstetrics, Gynecology and Neonatal Nursing, 35*(1), 78–86.

Palacios, J., Butterfly, R., & Strickland, C. J. (2005). American Indians/Alaskan Natives. In J. G. Lipson & S. L. Dibble (Eds.), *Cultural and clinical care* (pp. 27–41). San Francisco: The Regents University of California.

Pillitteri, A. (2003). *Maternal and child health nursing* (4th ed.). Philadelphia: Lippincott Williams & Wilkins.

Prugh, D. (1983). *The psychological aspects of pediatrics*. Philadelphia: Lea & Febiger.

Roberts, S. J. (2006). Healthcare recommendations for lesbian women. *Journal of Obstetrics, Gynecology and Neonatal Nursing, 35*(5), 583–591.

Robson, F. (2002). Yes! A chance to tell my side of the story: A case study of a male partner of a woman undergoing termination of pregnancy for foetal abnormality. *Journal of Health Psychology, 7*(2), 183–193.

Roudebush, J. R., Kaufman, J., Johnson, B. H., Abraham, M. R., & Clayton, S. P. (2006). Patient and family-centered perinatal care: Partnerships with childbearing women and families. *The Journal of Perinatal and Neonatal Nursing, 20*(3), 201–209.

Rykkje, L. (2007). Intercountry adoption and nursing care. *Scandinavian Journal of Caring Sciences, 21*(4), 507–514.

Schenk, L. K., Kelley, J. H., & Schenk, M. P. (2005). Models of maternal-infant attachment: A role for nurses. *Pediatric Nursing, 31*(6), 514–517.

Schiffman, R. F., Omar, M. A., & McKelvey, L. M. (2003). Mother-infant interaction in low-income families. *MCN: The American Journal of Maternal/Child Nursing, 28*(4), 246–251.

Sherrod, R. A. (2004). Understanding the emotional aspects of infertility. Implications for nursing practice. *Journal of Psychosocial Nursing, 42*(3), 42–47.

Sherrod, R. A. (2006). Male infertility: The element of disguise. *Journal of Psychosocial Nursing, 44*(10), 31–37.

Steffensmeier, T. H. (1982). A role model of the transition to parenthood. *Journal of Marriage and the Family, 44*(2), 319–334.

Sutherland, A. H. (2005). Roma (Gypsies). In J. G. Lipson & S. L. Dibble (Eds.), *Cultural and clinical care* (pp. 404–414). San Francisco: The Regents University of California.

Troy, N. W. (2003). Is the significance of postpartum fatigue being overlooked in the lives of women? *MCN: The American Journal of Maternal/Child Nursing, 28*(4), 252–257.

Wertz, R. W., & Wertz, D. C. (1989). *Lying-in: A history of childbirth in America*. New Haven, CT: Yale University Press.

SELECTED RESOURCES

Organizations

- *The Association of Women's Health, Obstetric, and Neonatal Nurses (AWHONN):* http://www.awhonn.org
- *Depression After Delivery, Inc.:* http://www.depressionafterdelivery.com
- *The Compassionate Friends, Inc.:* www.compassionatefriends.org
- *International Childbirth Education Association (ICEA):* http://www.icea.org
- *The International Lactation Consultant Association (ILCA):* http://www.ilca.org
- *La Leche League International:* http://www.lalecheleague.org
- *National Council on Family Relations (NCFR):* http://www.ncfr.org
- *NCAST-AVENEW:* University of Washington: http://www.ncast.org

Journals

- Birth
- Family Relations
- Journal of Obstetric, Gynecologic, and Neonatal Nursing (JOGNN)
- Journal of Perinatal and Neonatal Nursing
- Nursing for Women's Health (formally AWHONN Lifelines)
- MCN The American Journal of Maternal Child Nursing

CHAPTER 13

Family Child Health Nursing

Vivian Gedaly-Duff, DNSc, RN

Ann Nielsen, MN, RN

Marsha L. Heims, EdD, RN

Mary Frances D. Pate, DSN, RN

CRITICAL CONCEPTS

✦ Family child health nurses focus on the relationship between family life and children's health and illness, and they assist families and family members to achieve well-being.

✦ Through family-centered care, family child health nurses enhance family life and the development of family members to their fullest potential.

✦ The family child health concepts incorporate relevant components of family life and interaction, family development and transitions, and family health and illness, and help nurses to take a comprehensive and collaborative approach to families.

✦ The family child health concepts enable nurses to screen for potentially harmful situations, instruct families about health issues, and help families cope with acute illness, chronic illness, and life-threatening conditions.

A major task of families is to nurture children to become healthy, responsible, and creative adults who can develop meaningful relationships across the life span. An important task of all parents is to keep children healthy and care for them during illness. Yet, most mothers and fathers have little formal education for health care of children. In fact, most parents learn the role "on the job," relying on memories of their childhood experiences in their families of origin to help them.

Family nurses help families promote health, prevent disease, and cope with illness. The importance of family life for children's health and illness care is often invisible, because families' everyday routines are commonplace and lie below the level of awareness. Family life influences many aspects of children's health, however, including the promotion of health and the experience of illness in children. Likewise, family life is influenced by the children's health and illness.

Families are groups with unique characteristics, including specific family memories and intergenerational relationships, family structure and membership, family rules and routines, family aspirations and achievements, and ethnic or cultural patterns (Burr, Herrin, Beutler, & Leigh, 1988). Family changes in structure and function interact with and are influenced by these family characteristics. Healthy outcomes for children (e.g., tripling their birth weight by 1 year of age, or successfully completing high school) are partially attributable to the intangible, invisible daily interactions among family members. Nurses, in partnership with families, examine how the characteristics of families influence health.

Family child health nursing entails applying nursing actions that consider the relationship between family tasks and health care, and their effects on family well-being and children's health. Nurses care for children within the context of their family, and they care for children by treating the family as a whole. In both approaches, families affect their children's health, whereas children's health affects their families. Nurses care for children in a variety of clinical settings and care situations.

This chapter provides a brief history of family-centered care of children and then presents foundational concepts that will be used to guide nursing practice with families with children. The chapter goes on to describe nursing care of well children and families in community settings with an emphasis on health promotion. It discusses nursing care of children with chronic illness and their families and nursing care of children and families in acute care settings. A case study is used to illustrate application of the family-centered care. Finally, the chapter discusses implications for practice, research, education, and policy.

FAMILY-CENTERED CARE

Family-centered care is a system-wide approach to child health care. It is based on the assumption that families are their children's primary source of nurturance during childhood. "Family-centered care" has emerged in response to increasing family responsibilities for health care. The principles of family-centered care include: (1) recognizing families as "the constants" in children's lives while the personnel in the health care system fluctuate; (2) openly sharing information about alternative treatments, ethical concerns, and uncertainties about health care treatments; (3) forming partnerships between families and health professionals to decide what is important for families; (4) respecting the racial, ethnic, cultural, and socioeconomic diversity of families and their ways of coping; and (5) supporting and strengthening families' abilities to grow and develop (Lewandowski & Tesler, 2003) (see Box 13-1). For example, families who live with the everyday routine of a child's chronic disease not only know the disease, drugs, and other medical treatments, but they also know the responses of the child and family members to these factors (Gedaly-Duff, Stoeger, & Shelton, 2000).

Families acknowledge the uncertainty that surrounds their child's disease, but they want to be informed partners of the health team decision making and valued collaborators in the care of their child (Griffin, 2003). In societies that respect diverse opinions, a health team that includes the family is preferable to a hierarchical team with physicians at the top, nurses in between, and families at the bottom. Family-centered care attends to the importance of families in health care.

Although family-centered care is recognized as being key in the care of children, the term itself is not consistently defined (Shields, Pratt, & Hunter, 2006), nor is family-centered care consistently practiced (Corlett & Twycross, 2006; Power & Franck, 2008). Conflicting assumptions have been made between nurses and parents about the degree of parent participation during hospitalization, ranging from expecting parents to do all the feeding and bathing of their children to doing technical procedures and giving medicines (Kirk, 2001). Rather than a direct discussion about what caregiving parents wanted and could do, nurses and parents indirectly worked out their roles during their interactions surrounding the care of the child (Corlett & Twycross, 2006). In an integrative review of 11 qualitative studies about family-centered care, Shields and colleagues (2006) found that care was a negotiation between families and staff. Some parents felt imposed on when nurses made the assumption that they would do their children's basic care while in the hospital without discussing it with them first (Shields et al., 2006). Kirk (2001) reports that parental skills to negotiate with health professionals began after discharge, after the parents had gained experience caring for their child and interacting with professionals in the hospital.

BOX 13-1
Elements of Family-Centered Care

Elements	Definition
1. The family is at the center	The family is the constant in the child's life.
2. Family-professional collaboration	Collaboration includes the care of the individual child, program development, policy formation at all levels of care—hospital, home, and community.
3. Family-professional communication	Information exchange is complete, unbiased, and occurs in a supportive manner at all times.
4. Cultural diversity of families	Honors diversity (ethnic, racial, spiritual, social, economic, educational, and geographic), strengths, and individuality within and across all families.
5. Coping differences and support	Recognizes and respects family coping, supporting families with developmental, educational, emotional, spiritual, environmental, and financial resources to meet diverse needs.
6. Family-centered peer support	Families are encouraged to network and support each other.
7. Specialized service and support systems	Support systems for children with special health and developmental needs in the hospital, home, and community are accessible, flexible, and comprehensive.
8. Holistic perspective of family-centered care	Families are viewed as families, and children are viewed as children, recognizing their strengths, concerns, emotions, and aspirations beyond their specific health needs.

Source: From Lewandowski, L., & Tesler, M. (Eds.). (2003). *Family-centered care: Putting it into action. The SPN/ANA guide to family-centered care.* Washington, DC: Society of Pediatric Nursest/American Nurses Association, by permission.

CONCEPTS OF FAMILY CHILD HEALTH NURSING

Several foundational concepts guide nursing care of families with children. These are family development or career, individual development, and transitions (e.g., developmental, situational, and health/illness). Development theories assume that families and individuals change over time. Not only do families experience the various developmental stages of each member, but they also progress through a series of family developmental stages. Nurses, by comparing their observations of particular families with expected family and individual developmental stages, can plan appropriate care. See Box 13-2 for definitions of family career, individual development, and health and illness.

Family Career

Family career is the dynamic process of change that occurs during the life span of the unique group called the *family*. Family career incorporates stages, tasks, and transitions. Family career is similar to family development theory in that it takes into account family tasks and raising children. Whereas Family Developmental Theory views the family in standard sequential steps progressing from the birth of the first child to raising and launching children to experiencing the death of a parent figure in old age (Duvall & Miller, 1985), *family career* takes into account the diverse experiences of American families (Aldous, 1996). The family career includes both the expected developmental changes of the family life cycle and the unexpected changes of situational crises such as divorce, remarriage, adoption, and death.

BOX 13-2
Definitions of Family Career, Individual Development, and Patterns of Health/Disease/Illness

Term	Definition
Family career	The dynamic process of change that occurs during the life span of the unique group called the *family*. Whereas family development views the family in standard sequential steps or stages, family career takes into account the diverse experiences of American families that do not occur in anticipated stages.
Individual development	Physical and maturational change of the individual over time. Some theories perceive change as stages, and others are interactional change.
Health and illness	Health is behavior that promotes optimal dimensions of well-being. Family and individual health is multidimensional; therefore, a family or a member can have a disease and be "healthy" in another dimension of health.
	Illness is family and individual activities that manage a disease that may be acute (time limited), chronic (live with over time), or terminal (palliative/end of life).
	Families and their members experience dimensions of health while managing illness among members.

The notion of family career involves the many paths that families can take during their life span. Changes do not necessarily occur in a linear fashion. For example, Family Developmental Theory assumes that families raising more than one child have already experienced the stage of birthing and resulting family development tasks. Family career, similar to family life course theory, takes into account the possibility that a person without children may marry a partner who already has adolescent children resulting in the experience of parenthood, starting at adolescence. This new parent does not build on parenting based on parenthood of young children. This helps explain interactions of many types of families in which the adults are married, cohabiting, single, divorced, remarried, or homosexual. Family career is a useful concept because it reminds us that families are dynamic. Nurses working with childrearing families need to know that family careers are inclusive of family development stages, transitions, and diversity, because these dynamics affect family health.

Family Stages

Duvall's eight stages of family development, based on the oldest child, describe expected changes in families who are raising children (Duvall & Miller, 1985). According to Duvall, family careers start with marriage without children, then proceeds to childbearing, preschool children, school children, adolescents, the launching of young adults (i.e., first child gone to last child leaving home), middle age of parents (i.e., empty nest to retirement), and aging of family members (i.e., retirement to death of both parents). Knowledge of *family stages* helps nurses anticipate the reorganization necessary to accommodate the expected growth and development of family members. For example, families with school-aged children expect children to be able to take care for their own hygiene, whereas families with infants expect to do all the hygiene care. Likewise, family activities shift with the developmental needs of the individual family members. Families with preschoolers may enjoy a day at the playground, whereas families with adolescents would likely not choose this outing.

Family Tasks

Across all family stages, basic *family functions and tasks* are essential to survival and continuity (Duvall & Miller, 1985): (1) to secure shelter, food, and clothing; (2) to develop emotionally healthy individuals who can manage crises and experience nonmonetary achievement; (3) to assure each individual's socialization in school, work, spiritual, and community life; (4) to contribute to the next generation, by giving birth, adopting a child, or fostercaring for a child; and (5) to promote the health of family members and care for them during illness. The aim of nurses is to help families develop appropriate ways to carry out the tasks necessary to prevent or handle illness and disease, and to promote health.

Transitions

Transitions are central to nursing practice because they have profound health-related effects on families and family members (Meleis, Sawyer, Im, Hilfinger Messias, & Schumacher, 2000). They can be developmental, situational, or health and illness. *Family transitions* are events that signal a reorganization of family roles and tasks. *Developmental transitions* are predictable changes that occur in an expected timeline congruent with movement through the eight family stages (e.g., the addition of a family member by birth). Because they are typical and expected, developmental transitions are also called *normative transitions*. Thus, family members expect and learn to interact differently as children grow. Sometimes families may not make the transition to an expected family stage. For example, families with children who have disabilities and are not capable of independent living have difficulty launching their children because of lack of residential living facilities and caregivers.

Situational transitions include changes in personal relationships, roles and status, the environment, physical and mental capabilities, and the loss of possessions (Rankin, 1989; Rankin & Weekes, 2000). Situational transitions are also called *nonnormative transitions*. Not all families experience each situational transition. Furthermore, they can occur irrespective of time. For example, changes occur in personal relationships when a stepchild is integrated into the family group when one becomes a new stepparent after divorce and remarriage.

Changes in role and status happen when an only child becomes a sibling after the family adopts another child. Changes in the familiar environment occur when working parents move to a new job, and family members adjust to a new house, school, friends, and community. Even greater changes occur when families immigrate to a new country, learn a new language and a new culture, and perhaps have to work at a lower-status job. Changes in physical and mental capabilities (e.g., an illness that incapacitates a working parent) may shift caregiving activities to other members of the family (Meleis et al., 2000). A natural disaster can destroy family possessions and heirlooms, resulting in stress, fear, a sense of loss, and problems with family members' ways of being and interacting (Schumacher & Meleis, 1994). See Chapter 18 for nursing care of families during disaster and war. *Health-illness transitions* are changes in the meaning and behavior of families as they experience an illness over time. Even though there are different diseases and conditions, the illness experience follows a pattern of prediagnosis signs and symptoms, crisis of diagnosis, daily management of the condition called the "long haul," and resolved or terminal phase (Rolland, 2005). Knowing the trajectory of a condition helps nurses and families recognize transition points and learn new ways of coping. For example, a family who has learned to manage its child's asthma experience hospitalization when the child's asthma symptoms are complicated by an upper respiratory illness and become too severe. The family will need to reorganize itself to deal with the child's hospitalization and quite possibly learn to implement different asthma management approaches after hospitalization.

Transition events, either developmental (normative) or situational (non-normative), are signals to nurses that families may be at risk for health problems. Families develop ways of keeping their children safe. These work until the children grow and develop new abilities. A developmental example is an infant who is crawling and may be placed in a playpen to decrease the risk for harm while the parent is temporarily busy. When an infant transitions from crawling to pulling up to standing and walking, the family needs to modify the environment by removing things from low tables and covering electric plugs because young children explore the floor environment by touching things with their fingers and mouth. A situational example is a married family transitioning to a divorced family. Parents will need to think about new routines for caring for the children. In a two-parent family, one parent may have gotten breakfast ready whereas the other got the child dressed. Now one parent will be doing both. An example of a health and illness transition would be when a child is diagnosed with type 1 diabetes mellitus. The family will need to make major changes in family tasks to accommodate the nutrition and medication needs of one member. Nurses, by assessing families for anticipated changes related to family and child developmental transitions, as well as situational and health-illness transitions, can help families plan for changes.

It is important to consider the *individual development* of all the family members in nursing care of families with children. Child-raising families are complex groups of adults and children at different stages of development. Some family developmental stages are specific to the growth of individual members and the differing needs of maturing human beings. A schematic overview of human development highlights the stages of individual experiences over time (Table 13-1). Adult landmarks are included because adult developmental needs may complement or conflict with their children's developmental needs.

When nurses review with families the individual family member's developmental stages that are occurring concurrently among children and adults, they validate the complexity of family interactions. Through this review process, nurses can assist families to accommodate to children's and adults' changing needs, abilities, and thought processes across time. Table 13-1 presents three dimensions of individual development: social-emotional, cognitive, and physical. The table is meant to be a guide and is not all-inclusive. Some items may not be representative of all cultures or socioeconomic status. The table contains the following eight columns:

- Column 1, developmental period and age, shows orienting timelines. The period identifies eight stages from infancy through late adulthood, and the age is divided into chronologic years from birth through 18 years, plus the adult years beyond.
- Column 2, social-emotional stages, represents Erikson's perspective, which views social-emotional development across the eight stages of human life (Erikson, 1973), and significant relations, which shows how the world of

individuals expands as they move beyond their immediate families.
- Column 3, stage-sensitive family developmental tasks, provides the orientation of families as they raise and launch children (Duvall & Miller, 1985).
- Column 4, values orientation, reflects moral development from undifferentiated to complex stages (Bukatko & Daehler, 2004; Kohlberg, 1984). Individual family members have their own values, but their values also relate to the values of their family and community.
- Column 5 shows the cognitive stages of development (Bukatko & Daehler, 2004; Piaget & Inhelder, 1969).
- Column 6, the developmental landmarks, shows milestones that families use to measure their children's progress.
- Column 7, physical maturation, shows bodily changes as children grow.
- Column 8 lists the developmental steps that individuals experience.

Nurses can use this table to identify expected developmental progression and potential areas of concern for families.

CARE OF CHILDREN AND FAMILIES IN THE COMMUNITY

Families are the context for health promotion and illness care for all family members, including children. Family behaviors and practices affect health. This includes traditional health practices around food, eating, and types of food served at meals; physical activity and rest; use of alcohol and other substances; and providing care and connection for their members (Novilla, Barnes, De La Cruz, Williams, & Rogers, 2006). Christensen (2004) concludes that the role of families in health promotion of children goes beyond protecting their health, well-being, and development, and decreasing risk behavior, to teaching children to be "health-promoting actors" by encouraging their active participation in health care, and by providing information and having them make their own healthy life choices. The family, of course, is linked to the larger environment, with dynamic interaction with it. See Chapter 3 for a discussion on the bioecological theory.

TABLE 13-1

Social-Emotional, Cognitive, and Physical Dimensions of Individual Development

PERIOD	SOCIAL-EMOTIONAL STAGES/ SIGNIFICANT RELATIONSHIPS	STAGE-SENSITIVE FAMILY DEVELOPMENT TASKS	VALUES ORIENTATION
Infancy: birth to 1 year of age	Trust vs. mistrust (I am what I am given.) Primary parent	Having, adjusting to, and encouraging the development of infants Establishing a satisfying home for both parents and infant(s) Establishing well-child health care	Undifferentiated
Toddlerhood: 1–3 years old	Autonomy vs. shame or doubt (I am what I "will.") Parental persons	Parenting role development: learning to parent toddler; developing approaches to discipline; understanding child's increasing autonomy Family planning Providing safe environment Maintaining well-child health care	Punishment and obedience

COGNITIVE STAGES OF DEVELOPMENT	DEVELOPMENTAL LANDMARKS	PHYSICAL MATURATION	DEVELOPMENTAL STEPS
Sensory-Motor ages: birth to 2 years Infants move from neonatal reflex level of complete self world undifferentiation to relatively coherent organization of sensory-motor actions; they learn that certain actions have specific effects on the environment	Gazes at complete patterns Social smile (2 months) 180-degree visual pursuit (2 months) Rolls over (5 months) Ranking grasp (7 months) Crude purposeful release (9 months) Inferior pincer grasp Walks unassisted (10–14 months)	*Rapid (Skeletal)* Transitory reflexes present (3 months) (i.e., Moro, sucking, grasp, tonic neck reflex) Muscle constitutes 25% of total body weight Birth weight doubles (6 months) Eruption of deciduous central incisors (5–10 months) Birth weight triples (1 year) Anterior fontanel closes (10–14 months) Transitory reflexes disappear (10 months) Eruption of deciduous first molars (11–18 months)	Anticipation of feeding Symbiosis (4–18 months) Stranger anxiety (6–10 months) Separation anxiety (8–24 months) Self-feeding
Recognition of the constancy of external objects and primitive internal representation of the world begins; uses memory to act; can solve basic problems	Words: 3–4 (13 months) Builds tower of 2 cubes (15 months) Scribbles with crayon (18 months) Words: 10 (18 months) Builds tower of 5–6 cubes (21 months) Uses 3-word sentences (24 months) Names 6 body parts (30 months) Uses appropriate personal pronouns, i.e., I, you, me (30 months) Rides tricycle (36 months) Copies circle (36 months) Matches 4 colors (36 months) Talks to self and others (42 months) Takes turns (42 months)	Babinski reflex extinguished (18 months) Bowel and bladder nerves myelinated (18 months) Increase in lymphoid tissue Weight gain 2 kg per year (12–36 months)	Oppositional behavior Messiness Exploratory behavior Parallel play Pleasure in looking at or being looked at Beginning self-concept Orderliness Curiosity

Continued

TABLE 13-1

Social-Emotional, Cognitive, and Physical Dimensions of Individual Development—cont'd

PERIOD	SOCIAL-EMOTIONAL STAGES/ SIGNIFICANT RELATIONSHIPS	STAGE-SENSITIVE FAMILY DEVELOPMENT TASKS	VALUES ORIENTATION
Preschool age: 3–5 years old	Initiative vs. guilt (I am what I imagine I can be.) Basic family	Adapting to the critical needs and interests of preschool children in stimulating, growth-promoting ways; monitoring child development; seeking developmental screening as needed Coping with energy depletion and lack of privacy as parents; socializing children; providing safe environment/accident prevention; maintaining a couple relationship; fostering sibling relationships	Punishment and obedience moves to meeting own needs and doing for others if that person will do something for the child
School age: 6–12 years old	Industry vs. inferiority (I am what I learn.) Neighborhood and school	Fitting into the community of school-age families in constructive ways; letting child go, as they become increasingly independent Encouraging child's education achievement; balancing parental needs with children's needs	Moves from instrumental exchange: "If you scratch my back, I'll scratch yours" into wanting to follow rules to be "good"; then to rule orientation for maintenance of social order
Adolescence: 13–20 years	Identity vs. role confusion (I know who I am.) Peer in-groups and out-groups Adult models of leadership	Balancing freedom with responsibility as teenagers mature and emancipate themselves Maintaining communication with teen Establishing postparental interests and careers as growing parents	Increasing internalization of ethical standards; can use to make decisions

COGNITIVE STAGES OF DEVELOPMENT	DEVELOPMENTAL LANDMARKS	PHYSICAL MATURATION	DEVELOPMENTAL STEPS
Preoperational Thought (Prelogical): ages 2–7 Begins to use symbols; thinking tends to be egocentric and intuitive; conclusions are based on what they feel or what they would like to believe	Uses 4-word sentences (48 months) Copies cross (48 months) Throws ball overhand (48 months) Copies square (54 months) Copies triangle (60 months) Prints name Rides two-wheel bike	Weight gain 2 kg per year (4–6 years) Eruption of permanent teeth (5.5–8 years) Body image solidifying	Cooperative play Fantasy play Imaginary companions Masturbation Task completion Rivalry with parents of same sex Games and rules Problem solving Achievement Voluntary hygiene Competes with partners Hobbies Ritualistic play Rational attitudes about food Companionship (same sex) Invests in community leaders, teachers, impersonal ideals
Concrete Operational Thought: ages 7-12 Conceptual organization increasingly stable; children begin to seem rational and well-organized; increasingly systematic in approach to the world; weight and volume are now viewed as constant, despite changes in shape and size	As child moves through stage, copies diamond; knows simple opposite analogies; names days of the week; repeats 5 digits forward; defines "brave" and "nonsense"; knows seasons of the year; is able to rhyme words; repeats 5 digits in reverse; understands pity, grief, surprise; knows where sun sets; can define "nitrogen" and "microscope"	Weight gain 2–4 kg per year (7–11 years) Uterus begins to grow Budding of nipples in girls Increased vascularity of penis and scrotum Pubic hair appears in girls Menarche (9–16 years)	Task completion Rivalry with parents of the same sex Games and rules Problem solving Achievement Voluntary hygiene Competes with partners Has hobbies Ritualistic play Rational attitudes about food Values companionship Invest in community leaders, teachers, impersonal ideals
Formal Operational Thought Abstract thought and awareness of the world of possibility develop; adolescents use deductive reasoning and can evaluate the logic and quality of their own thinking; increased abstract power allows them to work with laws and principles	Knows why oil floats on water Can divide 72 by 4 without pencil or paper Understands "belfry" and "espionage" Can repeat six digits forward and five digits in reverse	*Spurt (Skeletal)* Girls 1.5 years ahead of boys Pubic hair appears in boys Rapid growth of testes and penis Axillary hair starts to grow Down on upper lip appears Voice changes Mature spermatozoa (11–17 years) Acne may appear	"Revolt" Loosens tie to family Cliques Responsible independence Work habits solidifying Heterosexual interests Recreational activities

Continued

TABLE 13-1

Social-Emotional, Cognitive, and Physical Dimensions of Individual Development—cont'd

PERIOD	SOCIAL-EMOTIONAL STAGES/ SIGNIFICANT RELATIONSHIPS	STAGE-SENSITIVE FAMILY DEVELOPMENT TASKS	VALUES ORIENTATION
Early adulthood	Intimacy vs. isolation Partners in friendship, sex, completion	Releasing young adults into work, military service, college, marriage, and so on with appropriate rituals and assistance Maintaining a supportive home base	Principled social contract
Middle adulthood	Generativity vs. self-absorption or stagnation Divided labor and shared household	Refocusing on the marriage relationship Maintaining kin ties with older and younger generations	Self-actualization: doing what one is capable of
Late adulthood	Integrity vs. despair, disgust "Humankind" "My kind"	Coping with bereavement and living alone Closing the family home in adapting to aging Adjusting to retirement	Universal ethical principles

Adapted from Prugh, D. (1983). *The psychological aspects of pediatrics*. Philadelphia: Lea & Febiger; Murray, T. R. (1992). *Comparing theories of child development* (pp. 166–167, 501). Belmont, CA: Wadsworth; Duvall, E. M., & Miller, B. C. (1985). *Marriage and family development* (6th ed., p. 62), New York: Harper and Collins; and London, M., Wieland, P., Ladewig, J., & Bindler, R. (2006). *Maternal & child nursing care* (2nd ed.). Upper Saddle River, NJ: Prentice Hall.

In well-child care, families are considered the care environment for their children. Proposed outcomes of current well-child care focus on family functioning and capacity. Specific outcomes include: (1) parents are knowledgeable about their children's physical health status and needs; (2) parents feel valued and supported as their children's primary caregivers, and function in partnership with their children's health care providers; (3) maternal depression, family violence, and family substance abuse are detected and referral initiated; (4) parents understand and are able to fully use well-child care services; (5) parents understand and can implement developmental monitoring, stimulation, and regulation such as reading regularly to their children; (6) parents are skilled in anticipating and meeting their children's developmental needs; and (7) they have access to consistent sources of emotional support and are linked to appropriate community services (Schor, 2007). In promotion of child and family well-being, nurses support families in care of their children using various skills and interventions.

Communication with Families

A foundation of nursing care of families with children is therapeutic communication with family groups. One important feature is including all the family members in a discussion or interaction (Wright & Leahey, 1999). A nurse may talk directly to the parents because they are the anchors and are often the decision makers in the child-raising family. In initial communication, Cooklin (2001) recommends that each member be asked to introduce herself or himself, beginning with the parent or adults of the family, and proceeding with each family member in order of age from oldest to youngest. North American children are often valued as autonomous beings. Research supports that children want to be consulted about decisions concerning their health care and want their opinions to be respected (Coyne, 2006). Assurance that children have a "real voice" is fostered by inviting them to speak, conveying that their opinion really matters, and demonstrating genuine interest in their point of view. Because the role of children in

COGNITIVE STAGES OF DEVELOPMENT	DEVELOPMENTAL LANDMARKS	PHYSICAL MATURATION	DEVELOPMENTAL STEPS
		Cessation of skeletal growth	Preparation for occupational choice
		Involution of lymphoid tissue	Occupational commitment
		Muscle constitutes 43% total body weight	Elaboration of recreational outlets
		Permanent teeth calcified	Marriage readiness
		Eruption of permanent third molars (17–30 years)	Parenthood readiness

social situations is influenced by family culture, it is important to confirm that the children feel that they have permission not to answer questions, and that the parents will allow the children to participate freely in the discussion (Cooklin, 2001).

Another important feature of communication with families is consideration of developmental appropriateness of communication style, content of message, and vocabulary for each family member, and adjusting communication accordingly (Barnes, Kroll, Lee, Burke, Jones, & Stein, 2002; Cooklin, 2001; McKinney, James, Murray, & Ashwill, 2005). Engaging children in a casual conversation initiates a beginning relationship. Coyne's study (2006) finds that children wanted to "chat" with the nurse, to know a little about the nurse as a person, and wanted the nurse to know about them. Instead of starting the conversation about why they are in the hospital or at the clinic, children wanted to start the conversation with questions they were familiar with and were used to answering, such as their age, grade, and where they live. Asking children what they are good at, followed by asking about personal experiences, can enhance the start of a therapeutic relationship. Playfulness may assist in establishing communication with children. Children's temperament influences how they engage with new experiences and new people. A quiet, shy child, for example, often wants to watch and see what others are doing before being willing to interact with new people. Instead of asking questions, a nurse may elicit more conversation by inviting the shy child to color together and chat during an activity instead of putting the focus on what the child is saying. "Draw and tell" helps nurses learn what children are thinking (Driessnack, 2005). Asking children to draw their family and tell the nurse about the picture starts a meaningful conversation. As a child becomes more comfortable with the nurse, the nurse can ask the child to draw the clinic or hospital and tell about the picture. Another strategy to use with children is play.

Similar to drawing, playing a developmentally appropriate game with children helps them to relax and share their thoughts and feelings. Cognitively, children developmentally move from concrete to abstract thought. Careful explanation of abstract concepts using real objects is especially important when working with children younger than middle-school age. If explaining surgery, children will understand more if shown what the incision and bandage will look like by showing a doll or stuffed animal with a drawn incision and bandage on the appropriate body part (Li & Lopez, 2008) (see Box 13-4 for an example). It is important to validate or confirm with all family members that the message conveyed is understood, and that medical words are explained fully. Use of clichés and euphemisms, such as "this won't hurt" or "it will be over before you know it," are rarely appropriate when communicating with children and adolescents. See Chapter 4 for a discussion about family health literacy. Developing a therapeutic relationship with parents and other adults in the family is important. Parents have reported establishment of a rapport when health care providers showed an interest in their child, knew their child's and their family's needs, as well as included them in taking care of the child (Espezel & Canam, 2003). A significant family nursing intervention is identifying and commending on the strengths observed in the family and individual members (Wright & Leahy, 1999). This strategy, when used with contextual sensitivity, builds trust in the nurse-family relationship. Families begin to view themselves in a new way based on the nursing observation, and may be more receptive to new ideas and teaching offered by nurses (Limacher & Wright, 2006).

Supporting Development of Parenting Skills and Family Functioning

Providing support for the development of parenting skills is an important nursing intervention. Beginning at birth, children have a need for warm, affectionate relationships with parents. One of the earliest parenting skills found to establish healthy caregiving behavior is a parent's responsiveness to the infant's cues. Responsiveness is noticing and interpreting the infant's cues, then acting promptly in response to those cues. For example, if an infant looks away from a parent, a responsive parent will decrease stimulation until the infant turns back and reestablishes eye contact. An integrative research review about responsive parenting concluded that, in developed countries, maternal responsiveness in early childhood was positively correlated with increased intelligence quotient, whereas unresponsiveness was associated with lower intelligence quotients and greater childhood behavior problems. In developing countries, maternal responsiveness was associated with increased IQ, as well as increased survival and growth, which is thought to be related to improved nutrition (Eshel, Daelmans, de Mello, & Martines, 2006).

After the infancy period, parents begin to develop a "style" of nurturing and caring for their children. The parenting style of either two-parent or one-parent families influences outcomes in children including health, academic achievement, and social development (Baumrind, 1991, 2005; Richaud de Minzi, 2006). An *authoritative* parenting style is distinguished by reciprocity, mutual understanding, shared decision making, and flexibility (Sorkhabi, 2005). Although parents using this style convey clear expectations and "demands" of their children, those expectations take into consideration their children's developmental level, and parents provide rationales for and support to meet those demands, as well as warmth in their relationship with the children (Baumrind, 2005). This parenting style promotes feelings of competence. The ultimate goal is to promote self-control and autonomy in children. Parenting styles influence health, providing the ongoing message that the children have some control over good health and healthy lifestyle choices (Luther, 2007).

Authoritarian parenting style, in contrast, is an inflexible and unilateral style in which parents have clear expectations and demands of their children but insist on compliance with the parental perception of what is best for their children with limited explanation and rationale or acceptance of their children's perceptions (Sorkhabi, 2005). The authoritarian style promotes the belief that children cannot control their own behavior and cannot contribute to decisions about their own health care (Luther, 2007).

The *permissive* parenting style allows children to pursue self-determined goals with little guidance from the parents. Parents using this style tend to ignore behavior problems and may not provide the organizational support needed to assist children in reaching goals (Sorkhabi, 2005). Children raised in the permissive style are less assertive and achievement oriented, and more likely to develop ineffective and possibly dangerous coping strategies, such as using drugs, compared with the other two styles (Baumrind, 1991).

Rejecting or neglecting parenting style, in which there are limited expectations and responsiveness, and a punitive or negative reaction to parent-child interaction, as well as lack of parental involvement with the children, is associated with generally poorer outcomes than all of the other styles (Baumrind, 1991). The findings regarding parenting style and childhood outcomes are similar across cultures and geographic locations. One review, for example, concludes that, in collectivist or interdependent cultures, authoritarian and authoritative styles had similar outcomes as found in individualist cultures (Sorkhabi, 2005). Nurses can teach about parenting styles and help parents adopt authoritative parenting strategies when doing health promotion and illness care with child-raising families. In two-parent families, each parent may have a different style. Using reflection with parents can help them recognize their differences that can lead to a conversation about how they want to parent, which can lead to supporting each other so that they parent as a unit.

Parental behavior has been associated with parents' abilities to understand new and complex knowledge. Bond and Burns (2006) have found that mothers who conceptualized knowledge in concrete and absolute terms were more likely to use authoritarian parenting strategies. Mothers who thought about knowledge as more complex and viewed child development as less categorical and considered diverse perspectives were more likely to use authoritative approaches. These mothers talked with their children and explained the reasons for their "demands." Nursing interventions that use reflective strategies, group narrative, and collaborative problem solving support parents' insights about the advantages of diverse types of knowledge (Bond & Burns, 2006). Because parents' understanding of parenting styles and roles and child development vary, it is important for nurses to explore parent beliefs to tailor health-promotion activities to specific families.

Another important variable that influences childhood outcomes, including health, is parents' use of developmentally appropriate discipline (Bright Futures, 2002). Although teaching, engaging in pleasurable experiences, guiding, and supporting children should fill the majority of time parents spend nurturing their children, parents often struggle with discipline. Exploring parental approaches to discipline is an important part of family health promotion. For example, a temper tantrum in a 2-year-old child might be perceived by a parent as being stubborn rather than the toddler's increasing autonomy and struggle to communicate needs and emotions. A teenager demonstrating typical adolescent behavior, such as complaining that the school-night curfew is too early, may be perceived as being disrespectful of parental values. The parent may not understand that the adolescent is practicing a self-identity that is separate from family. Helping parents recognize what is normal or typical childhood behavior helps parents interpret some of their children's actions as developmental changes rather than undesirable behaviors.

Other family characteristics associated with well-child health outcomes are parent engagement, closeness, communication, and healthy role modeling. These positive qualities have correlated with increased adolescent social competence, health-promoting behaviors, and self-esteem, as well as less externalizing (e.g., aggression and anger) and internalizing behaviors (e.g., depression). Conversely, family aggression and parental aggravation were associated with less social competence, less health-promoting behavior, and lower self-esteem scores (Youngblade, Theokas, Schulenberg, Curry, Huang, & Novak, 2007). Children's readiness for school was related to identifying and supporting parental strengths, promoting strong parent-child relationships, teaching parents about child development, and involving parents in activities that encourage learning (Zigler, Pfannenstiel, & Seitz, 2008).

Nursing interventions for family-focused well-child care include identification of teachable moments to discuss child development, exploring parental feelings, modeling positive interactions with children, and reframing parents' negative attributions about their children's behavior. For example, a nurse may reflect that a child's temper tantrum may be a sign of independence and the need to communicate new thoughts and feelings without the language to do so, rather than a deliberate behavior to embarrass or disobey the parent. The positive health outcomes from parents learning more appropriate parenting include using less physical and harsh discipline approaches, increasing use of safety strategies such as placing newborns on their backs to sleep, increasing likelihood that children will have up-to-date vaccines, and increasing family time spent in pleasurable interactions and experiences. Nursing actions to reduce negative outcomes in child-raising families are to identify parental risk factors associated with abuse/neglect such as depression, family violence, drug and alcohol use, and cigarette smoking (Zuckerman, Parker, Kaplan-Sanoff, Augustyn, & Barth, 2004).

UNDERSTANDING AND WORKING WITH FAMILY ROUTINES

Establishing daily routines and family rituals is an important health-promotion strategy. These predictable patterns influence the physical, mental, and social health of children, as well as the health of the family itself (Denham, 2002). Nurses help families integrate physical, social-emotional, and cognitive health promotion into family routines, and in doing so, they also affirm positive patterns of health or provide alternative ones (Greening, Stoppelbein, Konishi, Jordan, & Moll, 2007). Discussing or observing family routines and rituals has the potential, in a nonthreatening way, to gain entrée and understand family dynamics to a greater depth (Denham, 2003). Routines are important to all families in all settings. For instance, predictable and familiar routines were used by parents in homeless shelters to preserve family bonds and their connection with their community (Schultz-Krohn, 2004). Conversely, because routines and rituals have great meaning and stability for families, it is important to recognize that they are potential threats and barriers when implementing new prevention or treatment interventions (Segal, 2004). A nursing action is to remind families that it is not unusual to relapse into old behaviors, and that nurses can provide ongoing support that changes as families remake their routines and rituals to improve their health. See Chapter 9 for a more detailed discussion about nursing interventions and family routines.

CHILD CARE, AFTER-SCHOOL ACTIVITIES, AND CHILDREN'S HEALTH PROMOTION

Child-raising families nurture children through partnerships with child care providers, teachers, and other adults within the community. Families sometimes experience conflict between family goals and the needs of individual family members, such as the parents' need to work and their children's need for care and nurturing. Parents work hard to try to balance these conflicts. Often, balancing these types of conflicts in a successful way is critical to family and child health. An important feature of American family life today is that a large percentage of households have a parent or both parents working outside the home. In 1970, 29% of women with children younger than 6 years were in the labor force; by 1990, that figure was 52% (Bianchi, 1995). By 2005, that figure increased to 62.5%. Fifty-nine percent of mothers with children younger than 3 years were in the labor force (Mosisa & Hipple, 2006). Although the workforce participation of mothers who have college educations has declined slightly, the workforce participation rate of mothers who have dropped out of high school has increased dramatically from 1994, likely because of welfare reform during the 1990s (Mosisa & Hipple, 2006). Care for children while mothers are at work is divided among fathers, grandparents, other relatives, friends, neighbors, other nonpaid care, lay professional care (e.g., nannies and unlicensed providers), licensed home care providers, or licensed and certified center care providers. In 2005, 30% of the 11.3 million children younger than 5 years whose mothers were employed were cared for by a grandparent during their mother's working hours. A slightly greater percentage was cared for in a home-based or center-based child care facility or preschool. Fathers cared for 25% of children, whereas 3% were cared for by siblings and 8% by other relatives during mothers' working hours (U.S. Census Bureau, 2008).

Working parents of infants must decide whether and when to place their infants in child care. Working parents of school-aged children and adolescents must decide whether the children can be at home without adult supervision during the after-school period before parents return home from work. In both situations, the family task is to provide economic resources for shelter and food, as well as meet their children's need for a safe, developmentally appropriate environment. Families settle these conflicts differently. Nurses can help families resolve the issues through anticipatory guidance that involves providing information about what to expect in various situations, how to choose quality and affordable care, discussing the pros and cons of different types of care and duration of care, and exploring how to cope with unwanted developmental and life changes in family members (Limbo, Petersen, & Pridham, 2003).

Protection against injuries and infections is a key issue when selecting child care and after-school programs. Nurses can provide families with a series of questions to help them check safety and access how a facility will handle their children's illnesses. For example, asking to be shown the indoor and outdoor activity areas can provide information about the safety for active children. Care settings should have functioning toilets and wash sinks that children can reach. Observing whether care providers wash their hands is important. Encourage parents to review the policy for children who arrive ill or develop an illness during their stay at the center. Do guidelines exist about what illnesses cannot be cared for at the setting, when children can return to child care after an illness, and the availability of a health care professional for consultation when children become ill while at child care? Does a policy exist for administering prescribed medications (e.g., children with asthma or diabetes)? Parents need information about what foods are served, how they are prepared, and how mealtimes are managed at the child care setting.

Besides health and safety concerns, parents should be encouraged to evaluate the quality of early childhood education and support for their children. For example, multiple studies have documented the importance of education and training of early childhood teachers; developmentally appropriate environments, activities, and equipment; and a recommended safe and effective teacher. Child ratio, culturally appropriate learning strategies, family involvement, and nurturing and caring interactions between the teacher and the children are important considerations (for a full review of research on child outcomes related to quality indicators for early childhood education and care, access the National Association of Education for Young Children Web site at www.NAEYC.org). In spite of the research evidence shared with families, most families are forced to choose child care based on cost rather than quality. Families composed of minority groups and families with children with disabilities require special consideration when choosing child care and after-school options (U.S. Census Bureau, 2008).

School-aged children often attend before- and after-school care programs. Some children care for themselves, and that number increases with the age of the child. Six percent of children aged 5 to 11 years care for themselves and 33% of children aged 12 to 14 years regularly care for themselves (U.S. Census Bureau, 2008). Nurses, parents, teachers,

governmental agencies, and other invested community members must work together to develop before- and after-school programs at schools, homework telephone services with teachers and teachers' aides during the school year, and community center programs during the summer months, holidays, and other events when school is not in session and parents continue to work. Nurses can help families review the types of child care and after-school options available, select compatible philosophies for health promotion, and examine the site for health protection features. They can also participate on community boards that advocate for and regulate these facilities. It is important that families whose children care for themselves understand safety measures, such as having a contact person the child can call in an emergency, concealing the house key during the school day so that it is not readily apparent that the child will be going home alone, setting rules about safety such as cooking and use of the stove, setting clear rules about allowance of friends in the house when parents are not present, and setting safe, developmentally appropriate rules for screen time (e.g., television, video games, and computer) when parents are not present. Nurses can educate parents on the risks of children being alone at home during afternoon and early evening hours, including loneliness, increased fears, increased criminal activity, and increased adolescent sexual activity and teen pregnancy during these hours unsupervised by adults.

GRANDPARENTING AND HEALTH PROMOTION

Although grandparenting is not fully acknowledged as a way to promote health in children, grandparents influence the values that parents bring to their parenting, because parenting values are derived in part from families of origin. During illness, a grandparent may serve as a valued backup, watchdog, safety valve, and stabilizing force for children and their families. Grandparents are often the backup care provider for an ill child when formal child care is not available for the child. Nurses who understand the influence of grandparenting on childrearing families' health include them in their interventions and family conferences. During situational transitions, such as divorce and remarried blended families, grandparents provide emotional and physical support to divorced parents and children (Smith & Drew, 2002).

Grandparents may be the primary parent or co-parent when they provide full-time care for a grandchild, either temporarily while a teenaged parent finishes high school, or permanently, as may be the case of babies whose parents have addictions (Hayslip & Kaminski, 2005). In 2005, 8% of children in the United States were living in their grandparents' homes (Annie E. Casey Foundation, 2007). In these situations, nurses teach grandparents health-promotion strategies for their grandchildren, referring them to community resources, and discussing strategies for parenting later in life and how to reduce caregiver stress (Smith & Drew, 2002).

Identifying Health Risks and Teaching Prevention Strategies

Because of the relationship between health behaviors and illness or death, increased attention to unhealthy social-emotional behaviors is an important part of nursing practice in families with children. Specifically, nurses assess for, identify, and provide interventions to reduce risk factors associated with morbidity (e.g., sickness) and mortality (i.e., death).

UNINTENTIONAL INJURIES

The leading cause of death among children and youths is unintentional injuries. In 2003, more than 4,000 children, ages 1 to 14 years, died of unintentional injuries (National Center for Injury Prevention and Control, 2006). Motor vehicle crashes are the leading cause of death for children aged 1 to 19 years. The risk for motor vehicle crashes is greater among youths aged 16 to 19 years than for any other group. It is crucial that children of all ages be properly restrained for their age and body size in motor vehicles. Drowning is the second leading cause of injury death in children aged 1 to 11 years, whereas homicide and suicide are the second and third leading causes of death for children aged 12 to 19 (National Center for Injury Prevention and Control, 2006). Family child health care nurses can teach and support families in accident prevention. For example, teaching appropriate car seat restraints and water safety, as well as child-proofing the home prevents poisoning and electrical burns from uncovered electrical outlets in toddlers. Head trauma from bicycle accidents are minimized by teaching the importance of bicycle helmet use and helping families locate resources when they have limited financial means for purchasing helmets. Nurses, either in an informal role as a next-door neighbor or a formal role as working at community or clinic programs, can help parents to understand the importance of and to access approved safety devices such as car seats, helmets, and door/cabinet locks.

OBESITY AND OVERWEIGHT IN FAMILIES WITH CHILDREN

Nurses help families recognize harm and ways to intervene for one of the leading public health problems: obesity and overweight. Childhood obesity is associated with significant health problems. Furthermore, children who are overweight are likely to become overweight adults. In 2006, almost 14% of all children aged 2 to 5 years were overweight (Polhamus, Dalenius, Borland, Smith, & Grummer-Strawn, 2007). Between 1980 and 2004, the percentage of children aged 6 to 11 years who were obese increased from 7% to 19%; for adolescents, it increased from 5% to 17% (Nihiser et al., 2007). Overweight and obese family members, including children, are at increased risk for diabetes type 2, hypertension, hyperlipidemia, cancer, asthma, joint problems, social rejection, and depression (Jeffreys, Smith, Martin, Frankel, & Gunnell, 2004; Miller, Rosenbloom, & Silverstein, 2004; Urrutia-Rojas et al., 2006). Prevention and treatment are crucial to the child's and family's well-being.

The cause of childhood obesity and overweight is complex, involving the environment (e.g., home and society), genetics, family attitudes and beliefs, cultural practices, nutritional practices, and family activities (Baughcum, Burklow, Deeks, Powers, & Whitaker, 1998; Bruss, Morris, & Dannison, 2003; Ritchie, Welk, Styne, Gerstein, & Crawford, 2005). Family beliefs, mediated by cultural and family traditions, are thought to affect family eating behaviors (Baughcum et al., 1998; Bruss et al., 2003). Societal and environmental changes that include decreased physical activity, perceived threats to safety resulting in children playing indoors rather than outdoors, increased interaction with screens of video games and computers, and more consumption of high-calorie fast foods in the community and schools has contributed to the increase in obesity across the world.

Although the incidence of overweight and obesity is increasing at an alarming rate, research about the problem is also increasing. Still, effective strategies to address the problem are not well understood. Because it is difficult to lose weight, prevention of overweight, particularly in the preschool years, a time when children are prone to become overweight or obese, is seen as one important approach (Wofford, 2008). A combined approach of education for families and children, support for changes in policies, such as building safe bike trails, offering better meals at schools, and reducing fast food access while replacing access to healthier foods, will likely have the greatest influence on reducing overweight in families. Parental involvement as role models for physical activity and healthy eating has been found to be essential in prevention of obesity in children (Floriani & Kennedy, 2007; Wofford, 2008). Supporting families in use of an authoritative approach to parenting and helping them to develop sensitive but clear parental expectations regarding self-care, food, and activity choices are important nursing interventions (Luther, 2007). Childhood overweight management in families includes providing children with nutrient-dense foods; reducing children's access to high-calorie, nutrient-poor beverages and food; avoiding excessive restriction of food and use of food as a reward; encouraging children to eat breakfast; finding ways to make physical activity fun; reducing children's television, computer, and video time; and modeling healthful eating practices for children (Hodges, 2003; Ritchie et al., 2005). The American Medical Association (2007) recommends encouraging family meals at home, limiting meals outside the home, and giving children no sugar-sweetened beverages, and specifies that children should get 1 hour or more of physical activity per day. Nurses can influence overweight by helping families consider their eating and exercise activities, as well as by contributing to community actions that will work in concert with family health behavioral changes.

CHILD MALTREATMENT

Nurses recognize situations in which children are in danger because of child maltreatment. In 2006, an estimated 905,000 cases of child abuse and neglect occurred (12.1 cases per 1,000 children), and approximately 1,530 children died of the abuse or neglect (U.S. Department of Health and Human Services Administration on Children Youth and Families, 2008). Children aged birth to 1 year had

the highest rate of victimization at 24.4 per 1,000 cases. Physical abuse is generally defined as a nonaccidental physical injury to the child and can include striking, kicking, burning, or biting the child by a parent, sibling, child care provider, or other caregiver. It represents 16% of child maltreatment. Child neglect is defined as not providing for a child's basic physical, educational, or emotional needs and represents 64% of child maltreatment (National Institutes of Health, 2008). In 2006, almost 9% of all cases of child maltreatment involved sexual abuse, whereas psychological maltreatment was about 7%. Psychological maltreatment is defined as child exploitation (i.e., child prostitution), threats (i.e., threat to kill child), and isolation. Approximately 2% of the cases involved medical neglect. Some children were victims of more than one type of abuse. Children with disabilities are especially vulnerable. Nearly 8% of victims had a reported disability, a figure that is thought to be under-reported. Also at risk are children of unwanted pregnancies, those living in homes with substance abusers, those with a parent with a mental health disorder, and those who have difficult temperaments. Nearly 80% of perpetrators of maltreatment were parents. More than half of all reports of abuse came from professionals involved with the children and families (U.S. Department of Health and Human Services Administration on Children Youth and Families, 2008).

INTERVENING IN CHILD MALTREATMENT. Child maltreatment represents a problem in family behaviors that demands immediate assessment and action/intervention. In most states, nurses are mandatory reporters and are required by law to report to authorities when they suspect that a child is being maltreated. It is important for nurses who work with children and families to understand their legal and ethical responsibilities. (See the Chapter Web Sites section at end of this chapter for more information.)

In addition to identifying children who may be maltreated, nurses screen families for domestic violence by asking questions such as those listed in Box 13-3 (Gedaly-Duff et al., 2000). Unlike family commendations that re-enforce family strength and success, inquiring about family violence can be uncomfortable for nurses and other health professions. Family violence occurs across social economic class and ethnic groups. The standard of practice is to ask *all* families these questions. The stigma of what is

---

BOX 13-3
Family Violence Screening Questions

- Right now, who is living at home with you and your child?
- Is everyone getting along well at home, or is there a lot of stress, arguing, or fighting?
- Has anybody ever been hit or hurt, pushed, or shoved in a fight or argument at your house?
- Has anybody in the family been in trouble with the police or in jail?
- Is anybody worried that your children have been disciplined too harshly?
- Is anybody worried that your children have been touched inappropriately or sexually abused?
- Is there anybody living with you or close to you who drinks a lot or uses drugs?
- Are there guns or knives or weapons at your house?
- Has anything major (e.g., people dying, losing jobs, disasters or accidents) happened recently in your family?
- What is the best part and the worst part of life for you right now?

---

considered intimate questions is now standardized. Families frequently will seek help if given the opportunity to talk about their situations (Hibbard, Desch, Committee on Child Abuse Neglect, & Council on Children with Disabilities, 2007). By screening for family violence, nurses can assess families and children for dangerous situations, teach safety, and make a referral as necessary.

Prevention is the preferred approach for intervening with families for child maltreatment. Nurses identify situations that might foster child maltreatment and intervene accordingly. Risk factors thought to contribute to abuse are categorized into four domains: parent or caregiver, family, child, and environmental factors. *Parent or caregiver factors* include personality characteristics (e.g., low self-esteem, depression, poor impulse control), a history of abuse in the parent's own childhood, substance abuse, attitudes about child behavior, inaccurate knowledge about child development, inappropriate expectations of the child, and younger maternal age. *Family factors* include marital conflict, domestic violence, single parenthood, unemployment, financial stress, and social isolation. *Child factors* include age (with younger children and infants being

the most vulnerable), presence of disabilities or chronic illness, and difficult temperaments. *Environmental factors* include poverty, unemployment, and social isolation. In all cases, it is important to remember that the presence of risk factors is not an indication that the parents or family are, in fact, abusive (U.S. Department of Health and Human Services Administration on Children Youth and Families, 2005). Rather, when the nurse identifies the presence of various stressors and risks, interventions that may decrease the potential for abuse can be evaluated and, if appropriate, initiated.

Protective factors against child abuse and neglect include parental resilience, social connections, knowledge of child development, concrete support in times of need, increased social and emotional competence of children, and nonacceptance of abuse by the community and larger society. Strategies thought to help families are those that facilitate friendships and mutual support, strengthen parenting by teaching and modeling appropriate behavior with children, respond to family crises, link families to services, facilitate children's social and emotional development, and value supporting parents (Horton, 2003). For example, social support has been shown to be positively related to health promotion efforts in adolescent mothers (Black & Ford-Gilboe, 2004). The difference between discipline and abuse may be unclear because of different cultural traditions, but nurses must be alert to helping families learn appropriate discipline measures (Stein & Perrin, 1998). Children's early nurturing experiences and attachment relationships with their caring adults are assumed to affect their future relationships and well-being.

SPECIFIC ADOLESCENT RISKS

Adolescents as a group are especially vulnerable to high-risk behaviors that can lead to illness and death. Data on the prevalence of risk behaviors among adolescents are collected by the Youth Risk Behavior Surveillance (YRBS) System, using a national probability sample of 9th to 12th graders, state and local school-based surveys, and a national household-based survey (Grunbaum et al., 2002). In 2003, in the United States, 71% of all deaths among persons aged 10 to 24 years resulted from only four causes: motor-vehicle crashes, other unintentional injuries, homicide, and suicide (Grunbaum et al., 2004). Health behaviors that contributed to unintentional injury or to violence were use of alcohol and other substances, nonuse of seat belts, and availability of weapons. Other health behaviors that contribute to illness and death were tobacco use, poor nutrition, sedentary lifestyle, and sexual behaviors that led to pregnancies and sexually transmitted infections (Grunbaum et al., 2002).

The 2007 YRBS report shows that youths engage in behaviors associated with significant morbidity and mortality. During the 30 days preceding the survey, 45% had drunk alcohol, 29% had ridden with a driver who had been drinking alcohol, 11% had rarely or never worn a seat belt, and 20% had used marijuana. Twenty-six percent of all adolescents in school currently used tobacco. Forty-eight percent of high-school students had experienced sexual intercourse. Among students who were sexually active, 62% reported using a condom at their last intercourse (Eaton et al., 2008).

Violence is a significant risk for morbidity and mortality for children. In 2003, the second and third leading causes of death for young people aged 15 to 34 years were homicide and suicide. Homicide was the fourth leading cause of death among 4- to 11-year-olds in 2002 (National Center for Injury Prevention and Control, 2006). In 2007, 18% of youths surveyed had carried a weapon on school property. The survey further revealed that close to 8% of students had been threatened or injured on school property at least once in the last year (Eaton et al., 2008). Black male children are four times more likely than white male children aged 1 to 19 years to die (Cook & Ludwig, 2002). Child and youth access to firearms is part of the problem. It is estimated that 50% of parents who own guns keep them unlocked and loaded in the home (Hardy, 2002). The American Academy of Pediatrics (2004) takes a public health position to prevent firearm injuries by removal of guns from families' homes and communities, rather than education in gun use. Although interventions to prevent gun violence have included legislative and community strategies, nurses can assess for presence of guns in the home and provide parental gun safety counseling, reinforcing for parents that children are at risk for injury if a loaded gun is kept in the house (Hardy, 2002). The Centers for Disease Control and Prevention has been testing a school-based violence prevention program in middle schools. The program teaches students conflict resolution and problem-solving skills, trains teachers about violence prevention, and engages family members in program activities (National Center for Injury Prevention and Control, 2006).

The mental health of children and adolescents is a growing concern in terms of increasing incidence, as well as risk for morbidity and mortality. The 2007 YRBS report revealed that during the previous 12 months, 11% had made a suicide plan, and 7% actually attempted suicide (Eaton et al., 2008). Youths susceptible to drug use, unhealthy sexual behaviors, violence/aggression, and suicide often experience mood disorders such as bipolar disorder and depression (Elliott & Smiga, 2003; Houck, Darnell, & Lussman, 2002; Parsons, 2003). In light of these statistics, it is especially important for nurses to use interventions that promote mental health in all family members, to screen for depression and other mental illnesses, and to make referrals as needed. Family child care nurses in school-based health clinics are especially well-placed to participate in health-prevention programs directed at high-risk behaviors leading to sexually transmitted disease and early pregnancy, depression, injuries, substance use, suicide, and violence (Hootman, Houck, & King, 2002).

An alternate approach to risk assessment is to assess what young people need to facilitate their development. The America's Promise Alliance program "Promises" listed the assets believed to protect children and be predictive of positive outcomes and behaviors such as violence avoidance, thriving (i.e., having a special talent or interest that gives them joy), school grades, and frequency of volunteering. The program's five Promises were: (1) presence of caring adults, (2) safe places and constructive use of time, (3) a healthy start, (4) effective education, and (5) opportunities to make a difference. One large study demonstrated that the presence of four to five Promises resulted in positive adolescent development outcomes. The same study found, however, that only a minority of youths experienced enough of the developmental Promises that were related to positive outcomes. Furthermore, non-Hispanic white youths were much more likely to experience the "Promises" than were Hispanic and African American youths (Scales, Benson, Moore, Lippman, Brown, & Zaff, 2008).

INFLUENCE OF POVERTY

Socioeconomic factors, such as poverty, lack of education, little or no health insurance, and immigrant status are strongly related to poor health (Hardy,

2002). Evidence has shown that behavioral symptoms of child psychiatric disorders are associated with poverty, and that those symptoms can be reduced as the family moves out of poverty (Costello, Compton, Keeler, & Angold, 2003). Programs that provide families with employment, adequate income, day care, and health insurance have been shown to have positive effects on academic achievement, classroom behavior, and aspirations (Huston et al., 2001). Children from families from ethnic minority backgrounds are more likely to live below the poverty line (Annie E. Casey Foundation, 2007); thus, they are at risk for health problems.

Families with limited financial resources and those who do not have health insurance have more difficulty with health promotion than families with insurance or other methods of payment. In the United States in 2005, 19% of children (13.4 million) were poor, meaning that they lived in households where the income was less than $19,806 for a family of two adults and two children (Annie E. Casey Foundation, 2007). In the United States in 2006, 9% of all children (6.8 million) were uninsured. Thirteen percent of children who lived in families with incomes at or less than 100% of the federal poverty level were uninsured. About 17% of children who lived in families with incomes at or less than 200% of the federal poverty level were uninsured (Bloom, Cohen, Vickerie, & Wondimu, 2003). Hispanic and African American families are less likely to have health insurance than are white non-Hispanic families. Among children with special health care needs (CSHCNs) and disabilities, offspring from minority groups were more likely to be uninsured and to report being unable to get needed medical care (Newacheck, Hung, & Wright, 2002). Children who have experienced inconsistent parenting (e.g., children whose mothers suffer from chronic depression or have substance abuse problems, foster children, or children whose parents are incarcerated) are at particular risk for poor health outcomes (Kools & Kennedy, 2003). Identification of these high-risk situations, careful assessment of needs, and knowledge of referral resources are integral to high-quality nursing care. Nurses, by exploring parents' perceptions and definitions of health, can develop meaningful health care plans. Health promotion for children occurs during everyday parenting activities. Many North American families are assisted in parenting by other child caretakers, including grandparents, friends and neighbors, and child care and after-school facilities.

Strategies to Support Health Promotion in Families with Children

Families are the major determinant of children's well-being. Nurses and other health professionals collaborate with parents, and do not view parents as secondary and apart from nurses (Bruns & McCollum, 2002). Health promotion and prevention nursing actions are as follows:

1. Write or provide health information for school or community newsletters, e-mail, or online messaging.
2. Demonstrate and teach health-promotion activities, such as family fun night, games, or physical activities that promote health.
3. Provide health messages focusing on strengthening protective factors and cultivating attributes of healthy families that include accountability, self-reliance, informed decision making, access to supportive social networks, and nurturing relationships. Encourage family councils or family nights that provide venues for communications among all the family members.
4. Provide anticipatory guidance about high-risk periods in child and youth development. For example, childproofing the home before the infant begins to crawl or walk, or providing assistance with appropriate limit setting as adolescents get their driver's licenses. The use of a contract for teen driving has reduced teen reports of risky behaviors such as driving under the influence of alcohol or riding with someone who had been drinking (Haggerty, Fleming, Catalano, Harachi, & Abbott, 2006; Novilla, Barnes, De La Cruz, Williams, & Rogers, 2006).
5. Provide connections with school and community services. For example, children learn meanings, responses to, and values about health through their interactions in their school communities. Nurses can refer families to community resources such as the federally funded Head Start programs that serve families of children who are economically disadvantaged and children who have disabilities (American Academy of Pediatrics, 1973). Head Start has been shown to increase high-school graduation rates and reduce rates of juvenile arrests and school dropout rates (Gray & McCormick, 2005).

CARE OF CHILDREN WITH CHRONIC ILLNESS AND FAMILIES

Although most families raising children experience acute illnesses and become familiar with managing these crises, families do not anticipate that their children may have a chronic illness. They are often unprepared for the unknowns and uncertainties of the course of the disease, the effect on their children's development and adulthood, or the effects on each family member and family life.

Defining Chronic Illness in Families with Sick Children

Families of children with chronic illness are diverse, and represent all racial and ethnic groups and income levels. Chronic health problems, long-term condition, disability, and CSHCN are phrases used to describe children with a health problem that cannot be cured. These heterogeneous conditions include, but are not limited to, medical problems (e.g., allergies, asthma, diabetes, congenital heart disease, joint problems, blood disease, spina bifida), disabilities related to developmental delay and rare genetic syndromes (e.g., prematurity, Down syndrome, cerebral palsy, mental retardation), health-related behavioral and educational problems (e.g., attention-deficit and hyperactivity disorder [ADHD], autism, learning disability), social-emotional conditions (e.g., depression and anxiety), and consequences of unintended injuries or acute illness (e.g., head trauma and paralysis). Many children have more than one problem.

To gather data about these diverse families, researchers used the term *children with special health care needs (CSHCNs)* for families whose children "have or are at increased risk for a chronic physical, developmental, behavioral, or emotional condition and who also require health and related services of a type or amount beyond that required by children generally" (McPherson et al., 1998). Approximately 10.2 million children in the United States aged 0 to 17 years have special health care needs (U.S. Department of Health and Human Services, Health Resources and Services Administration, & Maternal and Child Health Bureau, 2008). One in five households with children in the United States have at least one child with special health care needs; this is more than 8.8 million households nationally (Bethell,

Read, Blumberg, & Newacheck, 2008; National Data Resource Center for Child and Adolescent Health, 2007). Between 15% and 22% of the U.S. family population has children and adolescents with a special health care need (Houtrow, Kim, Chen, & Newacheck, 2007; National Data Resource Center for Child and Adolescent Health, 2007; Perrin, Bloom, & Gortmaker, 2007). Forty percent or more of medical expenditures for children overall is spent for families of CSHCNs (Newacheck & Kim, 2005), showing a greater need for mental health care (Spears, 2008), particularly for families of children with chronic emotional, behavioral, or developmental problems (Centers for Disease Control and Prevention, 2005). The 2001 survey of families with CSHCN documented that 86% of the children needed prescription medications, 52% special medical care, 33% vision care, 25% mental health care, 23% specialized therapies, and 11% medical equipment (U.S. Department of Health and Human Services, Health Resources and Services Administration, & Maternal and Child Health Bureau, 2008). Children of African American and Hispanic families have less access to health care and experience more severe illness (Newacheck et al., 2002; Newacheck, Stein, Bauman, & Hung, 2003).

Knowledge of the disease, trajectory, and management is important. The trajectory of the disease or condition, such as a sudden or gradual onset, prognosis of chronicity, relapse or death, a stable or degenerative course over time, the degree of incapacitation, and the amount of uncertainty are as meaningful to families as the specifics of disease management (Rolland, 2005). Families come to know the pattern for their child. Nurses and other health professionals tend to reteach the disease and medicine management when it is the social-emotional and behavioral responses that are troubling families. It may be the degree of unpredictability that interferes with children and their families' abilities to perform age-appropriate and family activities, rather than the degree of severity that explains families' abilities to cope (Rodrigues & Patterson, 2007).

The chronic illness needs vary greatly, ranging from families who are rarely affected by their children's condition, such as mild asthma, to those who are significantly affected, such as children who are ventilator dependent and still attend school. What the families have in common are the consequences of their children's medical conditions (e.g., the reliance on medications and therapies, special education services, medical equipment and devices), as well as the consequences of their children's condition on their family and each member. In families whose children live with a chronic condition into adulthood, the narrow view of disease management needs to shift and broaden to include family and community health.

A noncategorical approach directs attention to the consequences that chronic conditions have on the children, their families, their communities, and health care systems (Perrin et al., 1993; Stein, Bauman, Westbrook, Coupey, & Ireys, 1993). The problem does not go away. The intent is to manage the symptoms so that the children and families can maintain their well-being and move toward each member's and the family's goals. To gain a family perspective, nurses can ask similar questions as the 2001 CSHCN survey (U.S. Department of Health and Human Services, Health Resources and Services Administration, & Maternal and Child Health Bureau, 2008):

- Does the condition limit the child's ability to dress and learn self-care?
- Does the condition interfere with the child's daily activities such as playing and going to school?
- Does the condition require special assistance or technology, medication management, or both?
- Does the condition cause family members to cut back or stop working?
- Can the family access and get a referral for special services for their child, as well as family support services?
- Is the health care insurance adequate for their child and themselves?
- In the case of adolescents, has the young person's health care begun a transfer to adult providers?

Parenting a Child with Chronic Illness

Parenting is the nurturance of children to become healthy, responsible, and creative adults. The interdependencies among child, parents, and the whole family within their community are like a set of Russian nesting dolls. Children with chronic illness are embraced by their parents who share a household and family history, nested in communities and local/national health care systems. The complex, changing interactions among child, family, and community provide the context of parenting a child with chronic illness into adulthood. Tasks specific to health care are integrated with nurturance during their caregiving. Caregiving burden involves both the amount of time spent and the degree of difficulty in caregiving activities; parents have objected to the word *burden* to describe the care they willingly give to their children (Wells et al., 2002). Sullivan-Bolyai, Sadler, Knafl, and Gilliss (2003) describe the parenting responsibilities as taking care of the illness, maintaining family life, and taking care of oneself.

TAKING CARE OF THE ILLNESS

Direct care of their children's illness involves parental time, knowledge, and skills to do technical and nontechnical management (Moskowitz et al., 2007). Technical care and time involves doing procedures and monitoring for changes in their children's illness. This includes specialized care such as administering medications and cleaning indwelling tubes. It accounts for crisis care (e.g., unanticipated seizure, elevated temperature) leading to an ambulance or trip to the emergency department. Nontechnical care is the time and skills needed for feeding, bathing, dressing, grooming, bowel and bladder care, transferring from the bed to a chair, and toileting, together with the necessary extra laundry and house cleaning. The complex illness care (e.g., suctioning tracheotomy tubes, diet and insulin regulation) frightens grandparents and aunts/uncles who are not familiar with the technical care (Nelson, 2002). Finding qualified caregivers whom parents trust has involved educating professionals for the specifics of their child and accepting having strangers in their home (Macdonald & Callery, 2008).

Transportation and waiting time are financial and social costs to families. Parents cut back or quit work to provide care (U.S. Department of Health and Human Services, Health Resources and Services Administration, & Maternal and Child Health Bureau, 2008), or decide against taking a new job if the health insurance benefits will not cover their children's health care needs.

Parents coordinate resources for their CSHCNs. Illness needs involve clinic visits, occupational therapy, community pharmacy stocking medications, and medical equipment delivered to the home.

CSHCNs also need wellness care. The American Academy of Pediatrics recommends a "medical home" in pediatric offices to provide disease prevention through immunizations, promote wellness through anticipatory guidance, address illness questions, and ideally serve as a coordination center for families of CSHCNs (Sadof & Nazarian, 2007; Van Cleave, Heisler, Devries, Joiner, & Davis, 2007). But not all pediatrician offices have the resources or training to provide coordination.

Besides health care, parents advocate for special educational services. The Individuals with Disabilities Education Act (IDEA) passed in 1975 and renewed by The Disabilities Educational Improvement Act of 2004 (U.S. Department of Education, 2004) requires free public education to all eligible children. For children with disabilities, this involves an individual family service plan for children from birth to 5 years, and an individual education program for children 5 to 21 years old. Local school systems' budgets are challenged to meet all the educational and special needs of their students. Some families may not move to another school district if the school has reduced special needs services. Families living in rural areas seem to struggle the most with finding appropriate and available special educational services for their children.

MAINTAINING FAMILY LIFE

Nurturing the family as a whole and keeping each member moving toward family and individual goals are as important as illness management (Sullivan-Bolyai et al., 2003). Parents, as the leaders, help the family find meaning in the situation and ways to include the caregiving into daily life (e.g., a child with Down syndrome who delights in welcoming each visitor to the home enhances the family's joy of the moment, rather than rushing on to the next task). The meaning of the child's illness and the family's identity can change over time. Families may define themselves by the illness such as a "diabetic family." Illness patterns that are chaotic challenge efforts to create family life. For example, children with ADHD, a serious and stigmatizing disorder with symptoms that arise in childhood and continue as adults, can exhibit poor impulse control, learning difficulties, and hyperactivity. Families are constantly adjusting to their child's socially unacceptable behavior. As children with ADHD slowly mature and learn ways to be successful with the help of teachers and health

professionals (National Institute of Mental Health, 2006), the family identity may become "a family" with a CSHCN. Many families try to help their communities by sharing their learning with other families.

Parents maintain the household (e.g., food shopping, meal preparation, laundry, house cleaning, repair of the home, car maintenance) and financial security (Sullivan-Bolyai et al., 2003). Mothers tend to do the immediate household activities and care of the children. Fathers grieve and worry about their children's future, balancing work and time with their family (Chesler & Parry, 2001; Feudtner, 2002). For some households, women are the financial earners whose jobs provide health insurance. In these instances, fathers have done the daily caregiving of the child with the chronic condition and the siblings (Gedaly-Duff et al., 2008). Single-parent households are faced with the demands of caregiving, household management, and earning a living (Ganong, Doty, & Gayer, 2003).

Parents do not want the siblings to be overshadowed by the child with the chronic illness (Hallstrom & Elander, 2007). A "family silence" may be enacted with neither parents nor siblings openly talking about their worries for fear of causing further turmoil. Siblings may assume the responsibilities of the parent, such as the 5-year-old who shares a bedroom alerting his parents that his baby sister needs suctioning (Coffey, 2006). Siblings often try to do well in school to gain parent approval and alleviate parent concern for them because they see their parents working so hard to care for their ill sibling (Hutson & Alter, 2007). They take pride in being able to help their sibling, while simultaneously complaining of doing more than their share of chores and noticing differential treatment from their parents and other relatives. Sibling research has mixed findings that show increased risks for behavior and academic problems on one hand, with improved empathy and independent skills on the other (Sharpe & Rossiter, 2002). Sibling adjustment improved when parents provided problem solving, open communication, and resilience (Giallo & Gavidia-Payne, 2006).

A strong husband-wife relationship is important, but creating opportunities for being a couple is challenging. A ritual such as "date night" fosters closeness (Imber-Black, 2005). Parents sharing time together helps each appreciate the other's contributions. Some parents agree to divide activities, whereas some trade, so that each can learn the other's skills.

Agreement and support of each other's parenting is the anchor for the family.

Parents manage social stigma, most visible in families of children who have visual disabilities such as limb deformities, are technology dependent, have developmental or behavioral disabilities, or have a fear-inducing disease such as HIV infection. Managing stigma means finding safe environments where families can relax and participate, such as Special Olympics or organizations designed to bring similar families together (e.g., National Autism Association). They may find themselves teaching groups (e.g., religious, hobby, school classrooms) about the condition to mediate the stigma and fears when others do not know how to interact with their child and family. Families are also likely to limit social activities or split the family so that the child with the disability is cared for while other family members participate in social events (Rehm & Bradley, 2005a; Sandelowski & Barroso, 2003).

TAKING CARE OF ONESELF

It is difficult for parents to take care of themselves when they are balancing illness care and the ongoing demands of family life (Hallstrom & Elander, 2007; Sullivan-Bolyai et al., 2003). Mothers and fathers, each in their own way, grieve the lost dream of a healthy child. The busyness of daily care can camouflage that the child is not normal. The differences, however, become more evident when the condition worsens or at family events. For example, the "first day of school" is celebrated when boarding the school bus, but using the wheelchair lift makes the child's difference visible. Validating their sadness is a nursing action that gives parents and the children the opportunity to grieve what might have been, and celebrate what is and has been accomplished. Their sadness, called *chronic sorrow,* can recycle at transitions points in the disease (e.g., time of diagnosis, relapse, unexpected hospitalization), developmental benchmarks, and family celebrations (Northington, 2000).

Parents are at risk for social isolation (Wang & Barnard, 2004). Family and friends do not know what to say as the situation continues. Superficial conversations occur as they try to sustain optimism and mask their fear. Neighbors and others may avoid the family. Having the family talk about the illness and its effect on them is an intervention. Questions to ask are, "Who is having the most

difficult time; how is he or she showing it?" "How does [family member] help you the most to deal with stressful situations like this?" "How has the family managed in the past?" "What are the strengths that will help you cope?" Family confidence may be enhanced when the nurse observes and commends them on their strengths. Nurses investing in conversations with families validate that family is important, that each member is affected by the illness, and that they have acquired an expertise through their experiences (Duhamel & Dupuis, 2004).

Conditions that were often fatal in childhood (e.g., premature birth, leukemia, cystic fibrosis) are now considered chronic, managed in outpatient clinics and in the home (Eiser, 1994). Parents feeling guilty about not wanting to take care of their child may see themselves as being a "bad parent" (Nelson, 2002; Wang & Barnard, 2004). Finding appropriate community resources for specialized care is difficult. Respite services and home care are fragmented. Parents dissatisfied by the inconsistent care of various nurses assigned to their home may decide to do their own care (Wang & Barnard, 2004). Parents move between hope and despair, and are at risk for caregiver burnout and depression (Wong & Heriot, 2008). Nurses need to screen and make referrals for families in trouble.

"Living worried" was found to be part of the day-to-day parenting of children with chronic illness (Coffey, 2006). Parents worried about their judgment. When should they call the doctor or go to the emergency department? They worried about their family. Did their in-laws blame their side of the family for the illness (Seligman & Darling, 1997)? They worried that the neighbors would report them for child abuse, as their toddler screamed, "Don't do it, Mommy...please don't hurt me anymore," during an insulin injection. They worried their child was parenting them, after saying, "It's all right, Mommy; don't be sad; it doesn't hurt too bad." Their continued worry has been evident even when the child transitioned from home to an adult independent living situation (Coffey, 2006).

Parents are treated as "heroes" by the families and health professionals who realize the challenges they are expected to overcome. Wanting to be "good parents," they accept the praise and hide their guilt and worry. Connecting a family with another family like it that has experienced the heartache/guilt/failure/fear is an important nursing intervention. They help each other stay in the struggle and share the "tricks of the trade" they learned while caring for their chronically ill child and maintaining family life (Gallo & Knafl, 1998).

Normalization and Family Management Styles in Childhood Chronic Illness

Families are expected to take their children home, master complex treatments, and do it in such a way as not to dominate the child's life, but to integrate the care into daily family life (Knafl, Deatrick, & Kirby, 2001). Interestingly, nurses use the language of sickness or disability, such as "families of children with chronic illness" and "families of children with special health care needs." In contrast, families use the phrase "my child is normal except for [fill in the condition]." Some families, after the crisis of a chronic illness diagnosis, act to normalize their situation. The characteristics of normalization are the following: (1) acknowledging the condition and its potential to threaten family life, (2) adapting a normalcy lens for defining child and family, (3) engaging in parenting behaviors and family routines that are consistent with normalcy, (4) developing management of condition that is consistent with normalcy (e.g., schedule preschool for afternoon session so that physical therapy and medications can be done in the morning), and (5) interacting with others based on view of the child and family as normal (Knafl et al., 2001).

A family's belief about normalcy influences different management styles used to maintain family daily life. The Family Management Style (FMS) describes ways families accommodate day to day (Sullivan-Bolyai et al., 2003; Knafl, Breitmayer, Gallo, & Zoeller, 1996). These include a style called *thriving* (i.e., a philosophy that life is normal and the family feels confident in managing the illness), *accommodating* (i.e., philosophy of normal but having greater difficulty in the day-to-day management), *enduring* (i.e., managing well but with great difficulty and feeling burdened), *struggling* (i.e., experiencing parental conflict over the illness management), and *floundering* (i.e., experiencing confusion, overall negative and uncertain view about how to manage the illness) (p. 459). A more detailed discussion on FMS is provided in Chapter 10.

Not all families have poor outcomes. Families are stressed, but not all are adversely affected, and

some report being stronger from the experience (Hayes, 1997; McClellan & Cohen, 2007; Miles, 2003; Mussatto, 2006; Rodrigues & Patterson, 2007). Nurses knowledgeable about disease, illness, and family interactions can assess the complexity of a family's situation and how it changes over time. A friendly conversation is a nursing intervention where the nurse explores with the family each member's experience and meaning of the situation, validating that it may be different for each person. Sharing each viewpoint facilitates a shared conversation, as even young children can draw and tell a story. Families benefit from identifying their strengths and thinking about their goals as individuals and as a family (Tapp, 2000).

The nurse may observe that family routines have been disrupted. Sharing this observation gives families an opportunity to remake their rituals and holidays. For example, one family used a motorized tricycle at a 4th of July picnic so that the three-year-old could move easily among the family. Nurses can listen for the transitions families are experiencing, validate, and commend the families' efforts to adapt to the changes that may be intersecting among child needs, the illness, and family life. Families raising children who were medically fragile and severely delayed with adequate support and skills and resources found they lived a "good life" but not a normal life (Rehm & Bradley, 2005b). Challenges of families whose children have disabilities and chronic illness are listed in Table 13-2.

CONSENT AND ASSENT IN FAMILY CHILD HEALTH NURSING

Families with children experiencing illness or injury may be asked to make difficult decisions regarding health care. In most instances, when young children are involved, health care providers collaborate with parents to obtain informed consent, except in emergency situations when parents are absent. As children grow and develop, it is important for them to take on more responsibility as primary guardians of personal health and decision making (American Academy of Pediatrics, 2007; American Academy of Pediatrics Committee on Bioethics, 1995). Some family members and health care providers may feel uncomfortable with the inclusion of children in

TABLE 13-2

Stages, Tasks, and Situational Needs of Families of Children with Disabilities and Chronic Illness

STAGES	TASKS	SITUATIONAL NEEDS THAT ALTER TRANSITIONS
1. Beginning family: *Married couple without children*	a. Establish mutually satisfying relationship b. Relate to kin network c. Begin family planning	a. Unprepared for birth of children with disabilities; prenatal testing or visible anomalies at birth begins process b. In the United States, parents usually want to know their infants' diagnosis as early as possible
2. Early childbearing: *First birth up to child's developmental age of 36 months*	a. Integrate new baby into family b. Reconcile conflicting needs of various family members c. Develop parental role d. Accommodate to marital couple changes e. Expand relationships with extended family to adding grandparent and aunt/uncle roles	a. Learn the meaning of infants' behavior, symptoms, and treatments b. Hampered nurturing and parenting, if children are not able to respond to parents' efforts to interact with them (e.g., not smiling or returning sounds in response to parental cooing) c. Search for adequate health care d. Establish Early Intervention Programs (speech and physical therapist, specially trained teachers)
3. Family with preschool children: *First child developmental age 3–5 years*	a. Foster development of children b. Parental privacy c. Increased competence of child d. Socializing children e. Maintenance of couple relationship	a. Formal education of disabled children starts at birth with Early Intervention programs; families may not find adequate programs even into preschool years b. Failure to achieve developmental milestones (toilet training, self-feeding, language) signal chronic sorrow c. Families try to establish routines for themselves and their children
4. Family with school-aged children: *Oldest child developmental age 6–13 years*	a. Letting children go b. Parental needs balanced with children's needs c. Promoting school achievement d. Prepare for high-risk behavior related to drugs and sexual experimentation	a. Move children from family care to community care requires creating new routines and relationships b. Explain to school officials and others the needs of the children c. Negotiate appropriate school services and curriculum d. Behavioral problems may isolate families
5. Family with adolescents: *Oldest child developmental age 13 years until leaves home*	a. Loosening family ties b. Couple relationship c. Parent-teen communication d. Maintenance of family moral and ethical standards e. Promote safe sexual development	a. Continued dependency may mean children never achieve leaving home b. Family examines how to continue family life with increasing physical growth but ongoing dependence of children c. High-risk behavior related to sexual activity and drugs
6. Launching center family: *First through last child to leave home*	a. Promote independence of children while maintaining relationship b. Couple relationship, build new life together c. Midlife developmental crisis for adults	a. Financial costs do not decrease because children still require dependent type care

TABLE 13-2

Stages, Tasks, and Situational Needs of Families of Children with Disabilities and Chronic Illness—cont'd

STAGES	TASKS	SITUATIONAL NEEDS THAT ALTER TRANSITIONS
7. Families in middle years: *Empty nest to retirement*	a. Redefine activity and goals b. Provide healthy environment c. Maintain meaningful relationships with aging parents d. Strengthen couple relationship	a. Redefine relationships with grown children and child with special health care needs
8. Retirement to old age: *Retirement to death of both parents*	a. Deal with losses b. Living place c. Role changes d. Adjust to less income e. Chronic illness f. Mate loss g. Aware of death h. Life review	a. Arrangements for children with special health care needs

Source: Adapted from Gedaly-Duff, V., Stoeger, S., & Shelton, K. (2000). Working with families. In R. E. Nickel & L. W. Desch (Eds.), *The physician's guide to caring for children with disabilities and chronic conditions* (pp. 31–76). Baltimore: Paul H. Brookes.

health care decision making. It is believed by some that children may not make rational decisions, yet adults are not held to the same standard of being rational when they make personal health care decisions (Zawistowski & Frader, 2003). Each child's decision-making capacities should be assessed and given serious consideration (American Academy of Pediatrics, 2007; American Academy of Pediatrics Committee on Bioethics, 1995).

The wishes and concerns of children should be taken into account during decision making, and the assent of children undergoing treatment and procedures is to be solicited. Even when the child's desires cannot be met, the discussion of the situation with the child may help to build child-health provider trust. In the event that an intervention is not essential to the child's welfare, or deferral is possible, a child's objection should be given significant consideration. Regardless of the outcome of any decision, it should be a dialogue rather than a "top-down" conversation, with honest answers provided to the child and family so that the child is never deceived (American Academy of Pediatrics, 2007; American Academy of Pediatrics Committee on Bioethics, 1995).

Laws regarding informed consent and the assent of minors vary from state to state. It is important

that health care providers be knowledgeable of individual state statutes and common law. In Virginia, for example, Abraham's Law was passed in 2007. The catalyst for this statute was the refusal of an adolescent to comply with physician-recommended treatment (*Starchild Abraham Cherrix v. Commonwealth of Virginia, for the County of Accomack*, 2006). This law allows minors age 14 years or older to refuse medical treatment for a life-threatening condition. Children this age may jointly decide with parents, or the parents may make this decision. This law, however, considered a child of this age able to choose the treatment that was in his or her best interest. Some states may consider some minors "emancipated" and give these individuals the authority to make personal health care decisions. They are self-supporting, may not live at home, and may be married, be pregnant, be a parent, be in the military, or be declared emancipated by the courts. Some states also have statutes related to "mature minors." These persons are not emancipated but still have the authority to make health care decisions in certain situations such as addiction, pregnancy, and sexually transmitted disease care (American Academy of Pediatrics, 2007; American Academy of Pediatrics Committee on Bioethics, 1995).

On occasion, the wishes of children, families, and health care providers may differ. It is assumed that all parties will act in the best interest of the child, but best interests are in the eye of the beholder when it comes down to personally held values, such as "what makes a life worth living" (Kon, 2006). Although it is uncommon for parents to be overruled, the courts will invoke the Child Abuse Prevention and Treatment Act in some circumstances, which gives the interests of the state to protect minors greater weight than the rights of parents in decision making (Holder, 1983; Kon, 2006; U.S. Code of Federal Regulations, 2006). In a 2006 case, a mother was charged with second-degree kidnapping when she smuggled her child out of a children's hospital to explore alternative treatments. In situations such as these, health care providers should respect the fact that some patients may need time to understand the situation or come to terms with concerns regarding proposed care (American Academy of Pediatrics, 2007; American Academy of Pediatrics Committee on Bioethics, 1995). Legal intervention should be the last resort, and should occur only when there is a substantial risk to the child, because state intervention can cause serious harm itself (Ostrom, 2006).

CARE OF CHILDREN AND FAMILIES IN THE HOSPITAL

The admission of a child to the hospital is a stressful event for families. Nurses and health care providers have the opportunity to take this crisis situation and make it the best it can be for the child and family by decreasing stressors whenever possible. Viewing the family as essential, full partners in care can help build a trusting relationship between the health care team and the family. This approach decreases the adversarial "us versus them" situation that has the potential to occur when family members are not seen as full team members. Applying the principles of partnering through mutual goal setting with the family, enhancing family connectedness to the child, and assisting the family to understand health care processes and procedures also demonstrates a commitment to mutual interdependence by health care providers (Curley & Meyer, 2001).

Family and child attendance at interdisciplinary team rounds is an ideal place for mutual goal setting to occur, and such rounds have been shown to increase patient and family satisfaction, and decrease intensive care unit (ICU) length of stay (Dutton, Cooper, Jones, Leone, Kramer, & Scalea, 2003; Vazirani, Hays, Shapiro, & Cowan, 2005). Daily interdisciplinary rounds provide a time for education in teaching hospitals and for goal setting for patient care. No one knows the patient better than the family. As participants in the health team rounds, the family can provide insight to their child's responses, assess changes, assist with goal setting, and provide advocacy for their loved one. When families are present for rounds, they have the chance to ask questions of multidisciplinary team members that they may have a hard time connecting with otherwise. Latta, Dick, Parry, and Tamura (2008) identify communication as the most important aspect of rounds for families. Loved ones expressed a need to be included in rounds and found comfort in the fact that they were respected members of the team with an important perspective to share. The American Academy of Pediatrics Committee on Hospital Care (2003) has recommended that parental presence during rounds be standard practice. Groups such as the Joint Commission and the Institute for Healthcare Improvement emphasize the importance of family involvement as a method to improve communication with the health care team. This communication is vital in ensuring patient safety.

Maintaining open communication with the child and family is essential. Nurses can ask how the child and family would like to be addressed instead of defaulting to common terms such as "mom," "dad," "grandma," and so on. Permission needs to be requested before addressing persons by first names. Open communication can be strengthened, trust built, and anxiety lessened if a consistent, limited number of health care providers are assigned to care for the child and family (Mullen & Pate, 2006).

It is important that health care providers refrain from referring to family members as visitors, because this terminology diminishes the significance of the family relationship (Slota, Shearn, Potersnak, & Haas, 2003) and may even be perceived as insulting, because it is the health care providers who are the "visitors" to the family unit. Ensuring that "family" is broadly defined can help to guarantee that support from a wide base of loved ones is available. Close friends and family are seen as sources of security for children, and extended family members can also provide parents or guardians time for self-care and opportunities to address work and home responsibilities.

Health care providers, especially those working with critically ill children, need to be aware that parents may have increased stress because of the severity of illness their child is experiencing, and about their ability to parent and serve as the child's caretaker and protector during hospitalization. This may be especially true if health care providers take on some of the traditional activities the parents are used to doing. Family members may feel uncomfortable with this family boundary ambiguity, as they face uncertainties about who performs which roles and tasks (Boss & Greenberg, 1984). Health care providers can allay much of this stress by assisting the family to maintain parenting and care taking as much as possible during the child's stay. Nurses can assist families to know "how to be" at the bedside as hospital equipment, unit routines, limitations to activity, and the like may be unfamiliar territory. Families need to be oriented to the child's room on admission, and all potentially unfamiliar sights and sounds described. Family members who are unfamiliar with alarms may mistake one that signifies the completion of a medication for something more life-threatening (Board & Ryan-Wenger, 2003). Issues such as the one just described need to be anticipated by the nurse caring for the patient and family. Orientation can provide a time for education, encouragement, and "permission" to participate (Mullen & Pate, 2006).

Partnering with families who have children who are chronically ill or are technology dependent, or both, is of utmost importance. These families are experts in the child's daily care and are acutely aware of subtle changes in the child's condition. If this expertise is not recognized and valued by health care providers, this can become a source of stress for the family and a source of tension as both attempt to control the situation. Candid discussions about how much care the family would like to assume should be negotiated on admission. Responses will vary because some families may welcome the opportunity to take a break from 24-hour caregiving, to obtain much needed uninterrupted sleep and rest. Regardless of the dispersal of caregiving activities, an assessment of the child's usual routine should be obtained on admission and followed as closely as possible (Mullen, 2008).

The needs of siblings should also be addressed during hospitalization. Younger siblings have vivid imaginations and may believe that they caused a brother or sister to become ill or injured, or that the hospitalized child is more acutely ill than is reality. Nurses are equipped to provide parents with information, guidance, and reassurance about the appropriateness of sibling visitation for individual situations. Child life therapists may be available to prepare siblings for visits to the hospital and to assess readiness to visit (Mullen & Pate, 2006). In a study of critically ill children, it was found that best friends had some of the same concerns and needs as siblings, and these should not be dismissed (Lewandowski & Frosch, 2003). Screening siblings and young friends for contagious illnesses before visits can theoretically prevent the spread to hospitalized patients and families. No evidence supports claims that sibling visits increase infection rates, even in the neonatal population (Moore, Coker, DuBuisson, Swett, & Edwards, 2003). Hospital-acquired and endogenous infections pose a greater risk to the hospitalized child (Rozdilsky, 2005). Nevertheless, it is the standard in many pediatric hospitals to complete a screening assessment before a visit. Screening questions address immunization status and any existing symptoms such as rashes, fever, coughs, or other symptoms indicative of a contagion. No reports of siblings acquiring infections from a hospitalized child have been published, but ensuring that siblings' hands are washed after a visit and questioning the appropriateness of sibling visitation for those with immature immune responses (usually younger than 2 years) makes good sense (Rozdilsky, 2005).

Avoiding family separation from the hospitalized child is a priority. Separation increases stress for children and families, and does not encourage a partnership philosophy. The Society of Pediatric Nurses and American Nurses Association (Lewandowski & Tesler, 2003) supports 24-hour parental access to hospitalized children. This access includes giving families the option to remain with their children during procedures, treatments, and resuscitation attempts including in the emergency department. Several professional nursing and medical organizations support this evidence-based data, and patient care units need to have a written procedure to follow practice (American Academy of Pediatrics Committee on Pediatric Emergency & American College of Emergency Physicians Pediatric Emergency Medicine, 2006; American Association of Critical Care Nurses, 2004; Emergency Nurses Association, 2005).

Increasingly, family presence during life-threatening events such as cardiac arrest and resuscitation is supported. Families benefit from presence because doubt is removed about the child's condition, loved ones can see that "everything" was done for the child, and togetherness is supported. In the event of death, families may be comforted by the fact that the child did not die alone with strangers, and loved ones may experience a sense of closure (Bauchner, Waring, & Vinci, 1991; Halm, 2005; Mangurten, et al, 2006). Nurses can assist families by supporting the decision to be present or not, assessing family reactions as needed, answering questions, helping family members to find "a place" in the room, contacting spiritual support as requested, and providing comfort items such as tissues, beverages, and seating. Chapter 11 has an in-depth discussion on nursing intervention.

Transitions during hospital stays can become added stressors for families. For example, those who have been accustomed to one-to-one nursing care for a child in an ICU may find it stressful when transferred to an acute care pediatric unit where the nurses have more patients to attend. Preparation of the families for the differences between units by use of a transfer protocol may help to prevent undue stress and increase family satisfaction (Van Waning, Kleiber, & Freyenberger, 2005).

Although families are glad to have their children discharged from the hospital, stressors can accompany this transition. This is especially true for parents of children who have been in the ICU. Evidence shows that these individuals can experience feelings of uncertainty and unpreparedness as caregivers after discharge home (Bent, Keeling, & Routson, 1996). Adequate time for planning and preparation with families from all hospital stays, well before the time of discharge, can make the transition easier (see Box 13-4). Some patient discharge situations may require collaboration with multidisciplinary team members such as social workers, discharge planners, pharmacist, and home health providers to ensure that the resources needed after discharge are available.

NURSING IMPLICATIONS

Family nurses interact with families and other health professionals, and use a family perspective to guide: (1) health care delivery and practice; (2) education, both for families and for other health care providers;

(3) research, to explore family child health nursing systematically; and (4) health policy proposals and evaluation.

Practice

Family child health nursing must be practiced in collaboration and cooperation with families, as well as other health professionals. In family-centered care, nurses work with families to promote health, prevent disease, and cope with acute, chronic, and life-threatening illnesses. Cooperation means talking "with" rather than "to" families about solving problems and attaining health goals, such as acquiring immunizations for family members. Collaboration with families requires an even more involved relationship wherein ideas, expertise, resources, values, and ways of doing are considered by both nurse and family. The nurse and family initiate actions and solutions, and they work together with this information to address the health needs of the family and its members.

Families in America are diverse in background and lifestyle. Therefore, health care systems and nurses need to understand these differences to be effective in problem solving and health promotion. Rather than have children and families come to hospital clinics, creating school-based and school-linked health clinics in the local schools and communities would decrease transportation barriers and help families access health care. For example, families could receive care for their school-enrolled child and other members of the family at school-based health clinics.

With their close and often frequent contact with families and their children, nurses are in a position to form a partnership with families to promote wellness. Nurses can work collaboratively with families to assist them in taking on self-care responsibilities appropriate to their abilities and developmental levels. For example, a school-aged child is expected to dress, prepare breakfast, and get ready for school. A nurse may find a parent is giving a child with diabetes her morning insulin injection. In this situation, the nurse would recommend that the parent begin preparing the child to do this herself to help her achieve her independence in self-care.

Morbidity and mortality rates in children and adolescents related to behavior and lifestyle may be preventable. Nurses who are aware of these risk factors can intervene with children and families to help prevent or at least minimize situational and developmental-related problems. For example, nurses

BOX 13-4
Preparing Children and Their Families for Surgery Using Hospital Play

Children learn by doing and playing. Using dolls and real equipment helps children know what to expect and act out their fears. Having parents observe helps them learn how to help their child using play.

Before starting, consult with the physician and parent to learn what information the child has been given. Decide the appropriate explanation for age and emotional maturity. For young children, use neutral words such as *opening, drainage,* and *oozing* instead of *cut* and *bleed.* Gather the visual aids (e.g., pictures, doll) and equipment to be used. Do not give too much information because the child may be overwhelmed. Plan for three sessions: why the child needs surgery, what the operating room is like, and what the child will feel and do after surgery.

If a child has never been in the hospital, have toys familiar to the child such as blocks, dollhouses, and stuffed animals together with "real" equipment such as doll with bandages similar to what child will have, operating room masks, scrubs that nurses and doctors wear, and intravenous poles. The child may play with the familiar toys. As the child observes the nurse, tell the story of what will happen to the doll using the "real" equipment on the doll, and the child will learn the equipment is safe.

Session 1: How will the surgery make you better?
a. Ask the child what he or she thinks is going to happen. A child may be silent or say, "I do not know," when talking to a stranger. You can repeat a simple explanation reinforcing what he or she knows.
b. Reassure the child that no one is to blame for his or her condition; make it clear that nothing the child did is responsible.
c. Using the doll, show where the surgery will take place and what the surgery will do to make the child better.

Session 2: What will the surgery be like?
a. Review why surgery will make the child better.
b. Talk about the steps of getting ready for surgery such as not eating or drinking the night before, and what the operating room will smell like (alcohol), feel like (cold), and look like (big lights, a clock, people in special clothes).
c. Child will wear special clothes (hospital gown). Note: Toddlers' body image includes keeping on their underwear, because they have just finished learning toilet training.
d. Put a mask on the face and talk about a "funny smell." Use a real anesthesia mask on the doll and have the child do this too. This gives the child some control.
e. Play with the thermometer, blood pressure cuff, and stethoscope for taking temperatures and listening to heartbeats and breathing on the doll, nurse, and parent.
f. Show pictures of an operating room. Point out the "big lights," the clock, and the nurses and doctors dressed in blue (or whatever color your hospital personnel wear in the operating room suites) clothes and wearing "masks." Talk about the ride on a bed with wheels and doors that open like grocery store doors. These are things the child is familiar with and will notice.
g. Reaffirm that parents will walk with them to the operating room and be with them when they wake up from the surgery. Play with a mommy doll walking with the toy doll going to the operating room. Children need to know that their parents know where they are and will be there for them.

Session 3: Postoperative expectations. Using dolls, act out what will happen after surgery:
a. Soreness at the site of surgery
b. Pain and medication
c. Positioning (how to turn after surgery, deep breathe, and cough)
d. Bandages (the word *dressing* may be understood as *turkey dressing* at Thanksgiving, or playing "dress-up")
e. No eating and drinking right away

can discuss immunizations for vaccine-preventable diseases and safety restraints in automobiles, regardless of the primary reason for the health care encounter. Nurses who explore the situation of the family comprehensively will detect those individual members who are at risk. As another example, in a family whose child has been newly diagnosed with a severe disease such as leukemia, a sibling may begin to fail at school because of the family situation. The nurse who assesses the whole family can identify the new behavior and facilitate a family conference, so that each child understands what is happening and has an opportunity to discuss the meanings of the events, thereby keeping the focus on the family. The family can then see that other family members need attention. The family child health nurse assists the family to construct its career toward more healthy outcomes for all members.

Research

Family nurses need to explore ways that nursing interventions improve family health. For example, when nurses visit homes of families with high-risk infants and children, it improves child and maternal health (Olds et al., 2007). Anticipatory guidance, a commonly used yet underexplored interventional strategy, could be tested. Research could also identify risk factors for families to assist nurses and other health care providers to focus their interactions with clients. One question might be, What is the effect of a child's developmental delay on a family with impaired parents? Family nurses could identify patterns that are cues for future problems and explore the efficacy of interventions. A comprehensive family-centered approach could facilitate early screening and interventions, which could produce efficient and cost-saving strategies. For instance, a 9-year longitudinal study of children in a rural village found that family environment was a more important predictor than socioeconomic conditions in association with glucocorticoid stress and illness, suggesting that family processes may mediate links between poverty and health (Wertlieb, 2003).

The research brief demonstrates how research informs practice and policy. Box 13-5 provides an example of a research brief.

BOX 13-5

Research Brief: Family Experiences During Resuscitation at a Children's Hospital Emergency Department

Introduction: Family presence during cardiopulmonary resuscitation has been recommended by national professional organizations, including the American Association of Critical Care Nurses, the Emergency Nurses Association, and the American Academy of Pediatrics.

Purpose of Study: In an effort to improve the care of families during resuscitation events, the authors of this study examined the experiences of family members whose children underwent resuscitation, and their health and mental health after the episode.

Methodology: Ten family members participated in a 1-hour audio-taped interview in this descriptive, retrospective study. Data collection included both quantitative and qualitative instruments, which contained previously validated and investigator-developed items. Seven family members were present during resuscitation and three were not.

Results: Analysis of interview data revealed that families felt: (1) they had the right to be present during resuscitation; (2) their child wanted them present during resuscitation, and that they were sources of strength for the child; (3) they were reassured by seeing that all possible options to help their child were exhausted; and (4) a facilitator for information-giving would be helpful during the event, because no one was prepared to face resuscitation.

Nursing Implications: Whether present or not, all family members in this study expressed the importance of the option to be present during resuscitation. No indication of post-traumatic stress to family members after the event was reported.

Source: Adapted from McGahey-Oakland, P. R., Lieder, H. S., Young, A., & Jefferson, L. S. (2007). Family experiences during resuscitation at a children's hospital emergency department. *Journal of Pediatric Health Care, 21*(4), 217–225.

Education

Use of the family child health concepts must be based on thorough knowledge of individual and family development, and health and illness patterns. Family-focused care that balances health promotion, disease prevention, and illness management needs to be emphasized in formal and informal settings, as well as in academic and community programs. Educational curricula need case analyses as nurses learn or reformulate their perspectives toward family-centered child health. Family child health nursing involves many areas of knowledge and expertise. Therefore, many educational interactions may be needed for changes in practice to develop. Practicing nurses, as well as those receiving their initial nursing education, need interactions in which to explore a comprehensive framework for constructing effective approaches to family child health.

Policy

Policies made at agency, institutional, regional, state, and national levels influence family health in multiple and diverse ways. For example, public policies often place single-parent families in conflicting circumstances. A parent may find a job but make too much money to qualify for state-assisted health insurance and not have enough to pay for other types of health insurance. Family nurses can influence the development of public policies through their professional organizations, as well as their individual efforts. A professional organization such as the American Nurses' Association develops standards of practice and provides position papers to public servants developing health policies and laws. Policy analysis is, therefore, the job of every nurse.

Family child health nurses practice in many settings; therefore, they need to be aware of policies that apply in and between these settings. At a public policy level, family nurses must advocate for not only "adequate" but "growth-promoting" childcare facilities for the American working family. Another area in need of attention at the policy level is nutrition. Although Americans are slowly changing eating practices toward healthier diets, many gaps exist between the recommendations and actual practices. For example, iron deficiency among infants and young children is decreasing but still needs attention, and the two subgroups who are at greatest risk for nutrition-related problems are people of color and those with low incomes. Family child health nurses are challenged to implement policies to protect and promote nutritional health for these and other populations of children and families.

Family child health nurses can use the goals of current health care leaders and national recommendations on child health issues to guide their own policy evaluations and efforts for change. *Healthy People 2010* and *Healthy People 2020* (U.S. Department of Health and Human Services, 2000, 2008) are examples of national guidelines for family child health nurses to establish priorities of action.

Family Case Study

The purpose of this case study is to apply the family nursing process to a family of Eskimo ethnicity. This case study of the Comantan family demonstrates the use of family systems theory, child health, and a nursing approach to health care. The primary patient is Carl, although other family members have health care issues as well. Figure 13-1 presents the genogram and Figure 13-2 shows the environment ecomap of the Comantan family.

SETTING

Carl Comantan is a 9-year-old boy who lives with his family in their wood-framed house in a coastal, rural area of the northwest region of the United States. He has chronic respiratory illnesses and has been diagnosed by his physician as having asthma. The focus of this case study is his health and the health of his family.

FAMILY MEMBERS

Carl's ethnicity is Alaskan Native, or Inuit. Many people refer to this ethnicity as Eskimo. Their nationality is American, as they were all born in the United States. His father, mother, paternal grandfather, and paternal grandmother are Alaskan Native. His maternal grandfather and grandmother were Alaskan Native; they both passed away several years ago of pneumonia. The remaining family members have light brown skin and dark brown or black hair. The family speaks English, and the elders also speak their native language Inuktitut.

Carl's paternal grandfather, Harry, and grandmother, Relah, are darker brown in skin color than the others. Their skin is also wrinkled. They say it is because they spent many summers fishing on the water and working

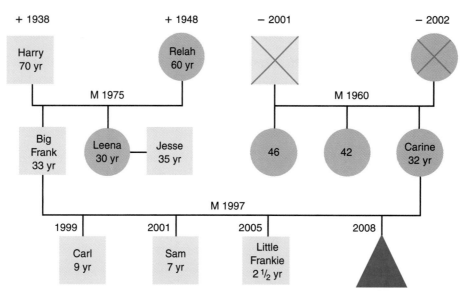

FIGURE 13-1 Comantan family genogram.

on the shore with the fish catches. His paternal grandfather says it is because he looks to the black raven for inspiration and strength. His grandmother says she is dark brown because she is like the brown bear, strong and courageous. They tell many stories of the work and adventures of their lives.

Carl's family consists of his mother, Carine, age 32, his father, Big Frank, age 33, his two brothers, Sam, age 7, and Little Frankie, age 2 and a half. Carine is approximately 4 months pregnant. Big Frank's sister, Leona, age 30, helps with child care. Grandfather Harry and Grandmother Relah are Big Frank's parents. They are very involved with their children and grandchildren. Other extended family members are introduced in their context of functioning. The roles of each person in their work and their community are given later in the case study.

COMANTAN FAMILY STORY

Big Frank and Carine have been married for more than 11 years. The children are their biological children from this marriage. Neither had been married before. They went to high school together and met when Big Frank did business at the gas station where Carine works. They both attend the same church.

Big Frank works part-time as a professional truck driver for a trucking corporation in the region. He is often gone from home for 2 to 3 days at a time for his work. The company offers limited major medical insurance for Big Frank and his family. Office visits and care

less than $800 are not covered. Carine's pregnancy care and births are covered at 60% of the cost. She receives no paid maternity leave benefit from Big Frank's insurance company or from her employer. Carine works at a local gas station that has a small grocery store attached. She manages the grocery store. The store is 5 miles from their home in the nearby village of Anokiviac. Big Frank and Carine are worried that they cannot make enough money to save, let alone pay the ongoing bills for electricity, gasoline for their vehicles, heating oil for their home, and clothing. They feel fortunate to be members of a cohesive community of family and friends, and to have jobs. Many people in their area do not have full-time employment. No family aid programs are in the area. Monthly, they travel to the town an hour's drive away to go to the local food bank. They get a box of staples that includes flour, rice, canned vegetables, and dried milk. The food bank requires that they show bills and pay statements to prove that they qualify for the food. Sometimes the food bank has a limited number of items, and they receive only a few things. They take their large cooler to hold the frozen vegetables and canned fruits from the local grocery store. Because they do not have any credit cards, they only do this when they have enough cash. They often buy groceries for other family members when they go the store. When Carine and Big Frank go to town, they take all the children. They help the children learn how to shop and also to talk with

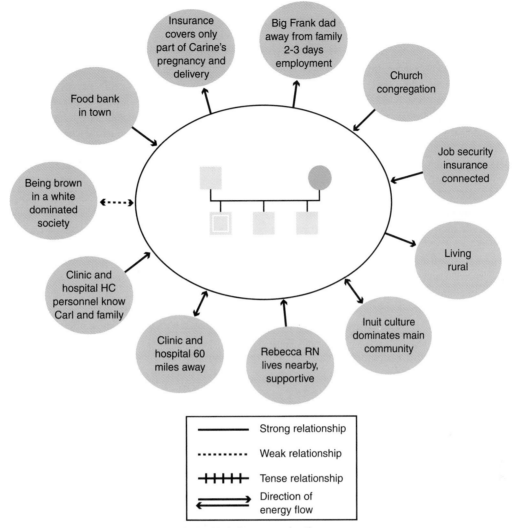

FIGURE 13-2 Comantan family ecomap.

any friends or family seen at the store or clinic. The children were very excited once when they encountered one of their school teachers at the grocery store. They can talk up to 20 minutes or more, sharing stories about events and people.

Big Frank and Carine strongly believe in making and keeping strong relationships with the people in their family and community circles. They talk about how people have helped each other in the past and how they are always on the lookout for someone who needs help. From one conversation with a teacher, Carine learned about a summer program for first graders. She was able to enroll Sam in that 2-week-long program in the town, where he stayed with a cousin's family. In

exchange for the cost of the program, she helped several evenings in their local school program during the school year. These evening programs during the school year were also helpful for Carl, because he missed several days during the school year because of his coughing and respiratory illnesses. As a result of the extra time and attention, he has been able to keep up with his classmates at his school. Carine and Big Frank help the children's Aunt Leona know how to help Carl with his studies, because she cares for the children while the parents are working. Carine and Big Frank believe that if they and a few other people such as Aunt Leona and the school teachers know Carl well, they will notice when he starts to become ill. They believe that they have been able to avert many serious illnesses for Carl because they and the adults he is around know him well. They do not get overly worried if he wheezes a little, which is normal. However, if he gets more short of breath, or if his appetite wanes, he is getting sick. Even his brother Sam knows about Carl being "fever hot" as he calls it, and worries openly about his brother when he is ill. Sam and little Frankie will bring Carl water and crackers when he is sick. The younger children also know about Carl's inhaler and will bring it to him when he is wheezing.

The physicians and nurses at the clinic in the town know that when Carine, Big Frank, Aunt Leona, or other family members call saying Carl is ill, they have assessed his situation to be serious. They listen with high regard.

Big Frank is a partially disabled veteran of the U.S. Army. He served in an international war overseas and was injured in a tank attack. His disability involves his left leg and left arm, both of which are severely scarred from metal and burns. He has decreased range of motion and sensation in both of these limbs. His left chest and face are also scarred; however, he did not lose vision or function of his shoulder or face. He is not overweight and is physically strong and fit. Big Frank receives a monthly disability benefit from Veterans Affairs that covers his health care for military service injuries.

Carine has good health. However, she knows there is a family history of coughing spells. She is not overweight and is physically strong and fit. Both Carine and Big Frank work hard to eat well and feed their children healthy food too. They use frozen vegetables and fruits, and use bread made by various family members. Their protein sources include fish that they catch and either elk or caribou from the annual fall family hunt. Occasionally, they have seal, obtained as a result of traditional hunts by Big Frank and the extended family. Big Frank occasionally talks about the pain in his left arm and leg, but he openly talks about not using medication to ease the pain. Carine will massage and use other comfort measures to help Big Frank with his pain.

Carine and Big Frank will drink an occasional beer but do not drink any other alcoholic beverages. Many of their extended family members and folks in their community drink beer, sometimes to excess, resulting in drunken behavior. Carine and Big Frank worry that their children may drink excessively as adolescents and adults. They do not allow their children to drink any beer or other alcoholic beverage. They are adamant against anyone drinking and then exhibiting irresponsible behavior

such as driving a vehicle, handling a firearm, or looking after children. The extended family members and the folks in the community practice the same behavior. Group disapproval occurs when drunken behavior occurs and those persons are taken home.

Carl is generally healthy except that he suffers frequent episodes of colds, as upper respiratory infections. These often progress into lengthy bouts of wheezing and coughing. He frequently wheezes in the morning on awakening and when he plays outside. He misses all or parts of days from school because of his illnesses. He has an inhaler, but he occasionally forgets to bring it with him to school and church or out to play. He takes his antibiotics and other medications well, reading the labels and talking about the taste. He says out loud, "This is for my breathing!" He also says to little Frankie, "This is not for you; this is my medicine! It is icky; you should never eat it!" He will then give little Frankie a drink of water or play with him to distract him. Carl knows that his mother, Aunt Leona, school teacher, and Sunday school teacher know about each of his medicines. Aunt Leona and his grandmother keep some of his medicines in their refrigerators so he can have them handy when he is with them. Carine and Big Frank are considering sending Carl to asthma camp for 2 weeks in the city during the summer. The physician at the hospital has recommended Carl receive a foundation-funded scholarship at the camp because they note that he learns quickly and likes to help other children. Also, the physician told Carine and Frank that they think Carl could benefit from the time to focus on learning more about managing his own condition.

Sam and Little Frankie are both healthy. They have had occasional respiratory illnesses and a few fractures from playing in the trees. Sam and Carl both had the chickenpox, as the varicella vaccine was not available in their area at the time. Carine and the children are up to date on their vaccines. Big Frank has not had an influenza vaccine and does not recall when he had others since he left the military.

While Carine is at work, all three children go to their Aunt Leona's home either all day or after school, depending on their age. Aunt Leona's home is a 5-minute walk from the school and a 10-minute walk from Big Frank's. Aunt Leona has a car and has driven Carl to the emergency department several times during the last year when he has had severe bouts of wheezing and a fever. Aunt Leona lives with her husband, Uncle Jesse, who works as a truck driver and bush plane pilot in the area. Aunt Leona does not work outside her home. She is involved in the care of her brother's children and is looking forward to the next child. She hopes for a baby girl. She occasionally takes a little gas money when her brother, Big Frank, offers. She is committed to help her brother and his family in any way she can. She and her husband want children but have been unable to conceive.

Grandparents Harry and Relah, who are a 5-minute walk from Big Frank and his family, are also involved in watching, guiding, and helping their three grandchildren. They like Aunt Leona and her husband a lot. Grandmother Relah has learned many treatments for illnesses over her lifetime. She studied for a while with one of the tribal shamans many years ago and maintains contact with the shaman. She makes mint and berry teas for Carl, makes steam for him in the kitchen, and feeds him dried fish for strength and healing. She talks to Carl and his brothers about the herbs she makes from various berries, bark, and leaves in their environment. She also encourages them to think about being strong and quick, wise and caring in their world. She talks to Big Frank about taking Carl to visit the shaman. They have not yet decided whether they will go.

Big Frank and Carine consult extended family members, particularly the elderly parents and other elders in the area, regarding health and family matters of all kinds. They particularly consult regarding Carl's respiratory infections and wheezing. Because the nearest clinic, hospital, or health care facility is more than 60 miles away, they are careful about taking the time and gasoline to drive there. Big Frank and Carine consider themselves equal decision makers in regards to family health matters and will consult providers and family members. Both are held in high esteem in their family and surrounding community. They are supported through congregational prayer in their church, particularly when Carl is ill. Church members, especially direct relatives, often bring cooked or prepared food to the Comantan family home when Carl is ill or when Big Frank is gone for several days on his job. Traditional ingredients of herbs or types of meat are used for these dishes for increased healing power.

One of the Comantan family's neighbors is a registered nurse, Rebecca, who lives about 5 miles away. She works at one of the clinics associated with the hospital that is in the town, which is 60 miles away. One time she took Carl with her to the clinic so that he could see his physician and get a renewal on an anti-inflammatory medication. She often laughs and says she is another "Auntie" for Carl and his siblings.

She says she is at least their cousin, even though she is Salish and not Inuit.

HEALTH CARE GOALS FOR THE COMANTAN FAMILY

1. Reduce the frequency and severity of Carl's respiratory illnesses.
2. Promote Carine's health during her pregnancy.
3. Promote Big Frank's healthy coping with the pain and discomfort of his injuries.
4. Enhance health resources for the family in their community.
5. Reduce the family's barriers to health and increase their strengths for health.

GOALS FOR NURSES

1. Build a therapeutic and collaborative, health-focused relationship with Carl and the Comantan family.
2. Explore ways to reduce the frequency and severity of Carl's respiratory illnesses.
3. Explore with Carl and his family ways to mediate and adapt to the overall effect of his illness on him and his family.
4. Explore the health care resources for the Comantan family.
5. Explore the main strengths and main stressors for Carl and his family.
6. Commend the Comantan family for their current health efforts and outcomes.
7. Focus on maintaining stability in the Comantan family.

FAMILY-SYSTEMS THEORY IN RELATION TO THE COMANTAN FAMILY
CONCEPT 1: ALL PARTS OF THE SYSTEM ARE CONNECTED

Carl and his family are deeply and actively embedded in their family life and their community. Each family and community member contributes to the health of Carl and his family. When Carl is ill, connections are activated to become supportive in a focused manner, according to the needs identified.

One assumption of family systems is that the features of the system are designed to maintain stability of the system, using both adaptive and maladaptive means. The Comantan family is adaptive to Carl's illnesses in their frequent, focused interactions with family and friends. They realize that their situation may change quickly, for example, with finances, and they need lots of resources. For example, their connections with Aunt Leona are part of that adaptation. They realize that with a selected increase in the number of people who know Carl well, a greater likelihood exists that no matter where he is, at relatives' homes, school, or church, he can be quickly and accurately assessed for severity and risk. They believe that by having Carl in several family and school environments, he will learn more and be healthier.

Each family member has many roles, each affecting one another. Big Frank is a provider of financial resources, a responsible adult in his social community, a caring son to his parents, a perpetrator of the culture, and a caring father. These roles influence many aspects of his family. Carine is a provider of financial resources, a responsible adult in her social community, including the school, and a caring mother. These roles influence many aspects of her family. The grandfather passes along to his son and grandsons the stories of the family and society, and helps his grandson progress to choosing an animal to look to for spiritual guidance, strength, and inspiration.

CONCEPT 2: THE WHOLE IS MORE THAN THE SUM OF ITS PARTS

The family members consistently support each other, recognizing the strength of the whole. The Comantan family believes that individuals, doing their part, contribute to the overall health of all and the ability of each to help at various times. The Comantan family adults focus on increasing health of all members in the long term while adapting to Carl's illness. For example, because Carl misses school because of his illness, they plan for Aunt Leona to help him. They also arrange for Sam and Carl to be in summer programs. The Comantan family is a cohesive unit with lots of interdependence. This is consistent with their societal beliefs of helping each other survive and thrive. They believe that each person has value, yet each has responsibilities to all the others in the group. They take great pride in teaching each other necessary and helpful things. This is especially true of the elders to the younger members. However, the elders do listen to the new ideas of the younger members, realizing that all ideas are worth consideration.

The entire family is happily anticipating the arrival of the new baby. They hope it is a girl, but they will be happy whether the baby is a boy or a girl. This normative, expected event may require the three boys, Carl, Sam, and Little Frankie, to stay with Aunt Leona and Uncle Jesse during the birth and early postpartum stage. This will depend on the circumstances, and the aunt and uncle are prepared.

CONCEPT 3: ALL SYSTEMS HAVE SOME FORM OF BOUNDARY OR BORDER BETWEEN THE SYSTEM AND ITS ENVIRONMENT

The Comantan family stays close to family and friends, yet is mindful of the amount and types of contributions made between families. For example, if Carl needs to go to the hospital, Aunt Leona will strive to be the one who takes him, rather than asking Rebecca to do so.

The family has fairly open boundaries within their local community and does reach out to a few resources in the town, which is 60 miles away. The family likes the idea of Sam going to the summer program and staying with his cousins. This was because they knew the teacher and the supervisors. The family would be less trusting with new health care practitioners caring for Carl.

The grandparents help Carl and his brothers find the boundaries of their heritage within the larger White American culture. They are teaching Carl about these boundaries and expect Carl to model these for his two younger brothers, as well as other children in the community.

Rebecca, the nurse, who is Salish and not Inuit, is trusted, and the family is open with her. The family is also open with the members of the congregation of their church.

CONCEPT 4: SYSTEMS CAN BE FURTHER ORGANIZED INTO SUBSYSTEMS

The Comantan family and the family of Aunt Leona and Uncle Jesse are an important subsystem in the Comantan family's overall functioning. Aunt Leona and Uncle Jesse contribute a lot while gaining contact with their beloved nephews. The grandparents, Harry and Relah, are also an important subsystem of the Comantan family.

NURSING PLAN USING FAMILY SYSTEMS APPROACH
NURSE ASSESSMENT (NOTICING/DATA GATHERING AND INTERPRETATION)

1. Explore in detail the expectations the family, including parents, grandparents, aunt, and uncle have for Carl in relation to managing his health, including his illness and illness episodes using affirmations, clarifications, respect, salutations, and honesty.

2. Ask the family to share details of their health practices, including any herbal or practice treatments used by grandparents Harry and Relah.

3. Learn the history and what the family expects about the future of Carl's chronic illness.

4. Explore triggers and factors that worsen his condition.

5. Assess Carl's overall growth and development, his medications, what substances he has used or been given for his health, his health-related behaviors, and his interpretations of all of these.
   a. For example, determine the level of growth and development impairment the family has noticed as a result of his respiratory illnesses and treatment.

6. Discuss the concept of illness trajectory for the Comantan family.

7. Explore what the family thinks is helpful, what might be helpful, and definitely what is not helpful.
   a. For example, they have family and community support, use the clinic in the town, build relationships, have a cohesive family, and Big Frank and Carine are parental partners.
   b. They anticipate that moving, losing employment, or having large unexpected expenses would be a problem.

8. Explore the main adaptive features the family identifies.
   a. For example, they have ongoing relationship-building activities in their daily lives.
   b. They believe that the whole family is actively and explicitly involved in health care of the family.
   c. They actively teach their children about health and healthy behaviors, and they are active in their children's spiritual development.

9. Explore additional health and health cost resources for the family, particularly for the occasions of Carl's potential hospitalizations in the future, for Carine's pregnancy and delivery, and for Big Frank's pain management.

10. Explore any health care disparities the family has experienced or perceived.

11. Assess the family's immunization status, including children's and adult's vaccines.

12. Explore the effect of Big Frank's absence for 3 days at a time when he is driving his truck for work.

13. Notice that various family members have Carl's medications handy at their homes.

14. Assess the boundaries of care and involvement for Aunt Leona and grandparents Harry and Relah.

INTERPRETATIONS

The nurse concludes the following:

1. The Comantan family strengths include their health behaviors, health actions, and beliefs. They reportedly practice health behaviors that help all members without the expense of hurting another family member.

2. The Comantan family has coordinated care for Carl within their family and their community. They are strong advocates for his health and well-being.

3. Members of the extended family are integral to Carl's health and the health of the entire Comantan family.

4. Data so far do not support any major stressors resulting from Big Frank being gone 3 days at a time. This may change with Carine's advancing pregnancy and the birth.

5. The Comantan family has concurrent developmental needs, tasks, and transitions—for example, the dynamics of the transition of the new baby coming via Carine's pregnancy, Carl's chronic illness, and developmental needs of all the family's children.

NURSING ACTIONS AND INTERVENTIONS

1. Use determinants to child's health from earlier in this chapter (see the Strategies to Support Health Promotion in Families with Children section) to guide actions. For example:
   a. Bring appropriate written materials to Carl and his family.
   b. Review with Carl how to use an inhaler, and talk with Carl and his family about recognizing and reducing respiratory triggers.
   c. Commend the family on their management of each illness episode and their overall management of family members' health.
   d. Explore with the family what they believe will be risky times for Carl's health, such as spring when plants are blooming and his asthma symptoms increase.
   e. Support the various roles of family members and subsystems within the family, such as supporting Carl interacting with his uncle and grandfather as adult male role models when his father is away on the road.

2. Use principles of family-centered care in interactions with Carl and his family. For example:

   a. Honor cultural diversity in recognizing and incorporating the extended family as observed in the roles of Aunt Leona and Uncle Jesse.

   b. Understand that the grandparents are important in Carl's cultural upbringing, especially learning about his Inuit culture and history.

   c. Examine the family for its strengths, for example, their efforts to keep Carl successful at his grade level in school.

   d. Collaborate with the family in identifying and evaluating sources of help and support that they already use. Saying, "You need to get Carl admitted at the asthma management center right away; that is the best thing for all of you." is an example of dictating and not collaborating with the family.

   e. Recognize that Carl's family is the constant in his life, as well as his primary caregiver. The nurse should talk with the family, listen to the family, and work collaboratively with the family in regard to his treatments and overall health management. For example, the nurse could first ask Carine or Big Frank where they received their immunizations and other medications before making arrangements for them to secure them in a particular place.

3. Discuss with the Comantan family the advantages and disadvantages of sending Carl to a 2-week residential camp for children with asthma. The camp is near the town that is a 60-minute drive from their home.

EVALUATION

1. Notice how the family has coordinated many people for Carl's care: the nurse, Rebecca, Aunt Leona, and the grandparents.

2. Assess how the family is doing with reducing triggers for Carl's asthma, as well as helping him when he wheezes.

3. Consider the effect on the family if Carl were hospitalized for a severe attack, infection, or both.

4. Consider the question of the projected effect of Carl's illnesses on the new baby: for example, the risks of Carl's infections on a newborn infant.

5. Consider types and potential effects of health-illness transitions for the Comantan family.

6. Consider additional developmental challenges the family may face in the future, such as the increased mobility of Little Frankie and the increased activity needs of Sam.

7. Consider whether any additional foci for the family have not been addressed.

8. Consider asking the family about their plans for financial resources during Carine's maternity leave.

9. Analyze what additional family strengths could be engaged to assist them in the future.

REFLECTION

Consider how the family story about the child's health, as well as their community's health, may or may not fit other families in your practice (Celano, 2006; Dodd et al., 2001; Liu, Stout, Sullivan, Solet, Shay, & Grossman, 2000; Rose & Garwick, 2003; Yoos et al., 2007).

SUMMARY

Families provide constant care for children during health and illness. Nurses and other professionals who are knowledgeable about family tasks, individual development of children and adults, and health policies will provide optimal care of children and their families.

- A major task of families is to nurture children to become healthy, responsible, and creative adults.
- Most parents learn the parenting role "on the job," relying on memories of their childhood experiences in their families of origin to help them.
- Parents are charged with keeping children healthy, as well as caring for them during illness.
- Common health-promotion problems of children and their families occur during transitions as individual members and the family grow and change.
- Because the leading causes of morbidity and mortality among youth are substance use, sexual activity, and violence (both suicidal and homicidal), increased attention to health promotion and prevention in these areas is needed.
- Families are the major determinant of children's health well-being.
- The difference between discipline and abuse may be uncertain because of different cultural traditions, but nurses must be alert to helping families learn appropriate discipline measures.

- Families with children will experience problems specific to a disease or condition, but some have problems with illness transitions through acute, chronic, and palliative/end-of-life phases.
- The health and illness concept can be used by family child health nurses to facilitate and teach healthful activities for growth in families, prevent injury and disease, and manage illness conditions.
- The aim of the nurse is to help families develop appropriate ways to carry out family tasks necessary to promote health and to prevent or handle illness and disease. During the family career, the basic family tasks are: (1) to secure shelter, food, and clothing; (2) to develop emotionally healthy individuals who can manage crisis and experience nonmonetary achievement; (3) to assure each individual's socialization in school, work, spiritual, and community life; (4) to contribute to the next generation by giving birth, adopting a child, or foster-caring for a child; and (5) to promote the health of family members and care for them during illness.
- Although most childrearing families experience acute illnesses and become familiar with managing these crises, families do not anticipate that their children may have chronic illness.
- With their knowledge of family and child development, nurses can collaborate with families with chronically ill children to help them achieve developmental landmarks.
- Family child health nursing practice is affected by health policy decisions relating to legal relationships of stepfamilies and single parents, financing of health care, and services to children.
- Family child health nursing must be practiced in collaboration and cooperation with families, as well as other health professionals. In family-centered care, nurses work with families to promote health, prevent disease, and cope with acute, chronic, and life-threatening illnesses.

REFERENCES

Aldous, J. (1996). *Family careers: Rethinking the developmental perspective.* Thousand Oaks, CA: Sage.

American Academy of Pediatrics. (1973). Day care for handicapped children. *Pediatrics, 51,* 948.

American Academy of Pediatrics. (2004). *Writer bytes...childhood injury: It's no accident.* Retrieved February 1, 2004, from http://www.aap.org/mrt/ciaccidents.htm

American Academy of Pediatrics. (2007). AAP publications retired or reaffirmed, October 2006. *Pediatrics, 119*(2), 405.

American Academy of Pediatrics Committee on Bioethics. (1995). Informed consent, parental permission, and assent in pediatric practice. *Pediatrics, 95*(2), 314–317.

American Academy of Pediatrics Committee on Hospital Care. (2003). Family-centered care and the pediatrician's role. *Pediatrics, 112*(3 Pt 1), 691–697.

American Academy of Pediatrics Committee on Pediatric Emergency, & American College of Emergency Physicians Pediatric Emergency Medicine. (2006). Patient- and family-centered care and the role of the emergency physician providing care to a child in the emergency department. *Pediatrics, 118*(5), 2242–2244.

American Association of Critical Care Nurses. (2004). *Practice alert: Family presence during CPR and invasive procedures.* Retrieved June 2008, from http://www.aacn.org/WD/Practice/Docs/Family_Presence_During_CPR_11-2004.pdf

American Medical Association. (2007, January 25). *Expert committee recommendations on the assessment, prevention, and treatment of child and adolescent overweight and obesity.* Retrieved January 2008, from http://www.ama-assn.org/ama1/pub/upload/mm/433/ped_obesity_recs.pdf

Annie E. Casey Foundation. (2007). *Kids count data book online.* Retrieved July 18, 2008, from http://www.kidscount.org/datacenter/summary07

Barnes, J., Kroll, L., Lee, J., Burke, O., Jones, A., & Stein, A. (2002). Factors predicting communication about the diagnosis of maternal breast cancer to children. *Journal of Psychosomatic Research, 52*(4), 209–214.

Bauchner, H., Waring, C., & Vinci, R. (1991). Parental presence during procedures in an emergency room: Results from 50 observations. *Pediatrics, 87*(4), 544–548.

Baughcum, A. E., Burklow, K. A., Deeks, C., Powers, S. W., & Whitaker, R. C. (1998). Maternal feeding practices and childhood obesity: A focus group study of low-income mothers. *Archives of Pediatrics & Adolescent Medicine, 152*(10), 1010–1014.

Baumrind, D. (1991). The influence of parenting style on adolescent competence and substance use. *Journal of Adolescence, 11,* 56–95.

Baumrind, D. (2005). Patterns of parental authority and adolescent autonomy. In J. Smetana (Ed.), *New directions for child development: Changes in parental authority during adolescence* (pp. 61–69). San Francisco: Jossey-Bass.

Bent, K. N., Keeling, A., & Routson, J. (1996). Home from the PICU: Are parents ready? *Maternal Child Nursing, 21,* 80–84.

Bethell, C. D., Read, D., Blumberg, S. J., & Newacheck, P. W. (2008). What is the prevalence of children with special health care needs? Toward an understanding of variations in findings and methods across three national surveys. *Maternal & Child Health Journal, 12*(1), 1–14.

Bianchi, S. M. (1995). The changing demographic and socioeconomic character of single-parent families. *Marriage and Family Review, 20,* 71–98.

Black, C., & Ford-Gilboe, M. (2004). Adolescent mothers: Resilience, family health work and health-promoting practices. *Journal of Advanced Nursing, 48*(4), 351–360.

Bloom, B., Cohen, R. A., Vickerie, J. L., & Wondimu, E. A. (2003). *Summary health statistics for U. S. children: National Health Interview Survey, 2001.* Washington, DC: National Center for Health Statistics.

Board, R., & Ryan-Wenger, N. (2003). Stressors and stress symptoms of mothers with children in the PICU. *Journal of Pediatric Nursing, 18*(3), 195–202.

Bond, L. A., & Burns, C. E. (2006). Mothers' beliefs about knowledge, child development, and parenting strategies: Expanding the goals of parenting programs. *Journal of Primary Prevention, 27*(6), 555–571.

Boss, P., & Greenberg, J. (1984). Family boundary ambiguity: A new variable in family stress theory. *Family Process, 23*(4), 535–546.

Bright Futures. (2002). *Bright futures: Guidelines for health supervision of infants, children, and adolescents* (2nd ed. rev.). National Center for Education in Maternal and Child Health/Georgetown University. Retrieved July 28, 2008, from http://www.brightfutures.org/bf2/pdf/index.html

Bruns, D. A., & McCollum, J. A. (2002). Partnerships between mothers and professionals in the NICU: Caregiving, information exchange, and relationships. *Neonatal Network Journal of Neonatal Nursing, 21*(7), 15–23.

Bruss, M. B., Morris, J., & Dannison, L. (2003). Prevention of childhood obesity: Sociocultural and familial factors. *Journal of the American Dietetic Association, 103*(8), 1042–1045.

Bukatko, D., & Daehler, M. W. (2004). *Child development: A thematic approach* (5th ed.). Boston: Houghton Mifflin.

Burr, W. R., Herrin, D. A., Beutler, I. F., & Leigh, G. K. (1988). Epistemologies that lead to primary explanations in family science. *Family Science Review, 1*(3), 185–210.

Celano, M. P. (2006). Family processes in pediatric asthma. *Current Opinion in Pediatrics, 18*(5), 539–544.

Centers for Disease Control and Prevention (CDC). (2005). Mental health and well being of children with chronic emotional, behavioral, or developmental problems—United States, 2001. *MMWR Morbidity and Mortality Weekly Report, 54,* 985–988.

Chesler, M. A., & Parry, C. (2001). Gender roles and/or styles in crisis: An integrative analysis of the experiences of fathers of children with cancer. *Qualitative Health Research, 11*(3), 363–384.

Christensen, P. (2004). The health-promoting family: A conceptual framework for future research. *Social Science & Medicine, 59*(2), 377–387.

Coffey, J. S. (2006). Parenting a child with chronic illness: A metasynthesis. *Pediatric Nursing, 32*(1), 51–59.

Cook, P. J., & Ludwig, J. (2002). The costs of gun violence against children. *Future Child, 12*(2), 86–99.

Cooklin, A. (2001). Eliciting children's thinking in families and family therapy. *Family Process, 40*(3), 293–312.

Corlett, J., & Twycross, A. (2006). Negotiation of parental roles within family-centered care: A review of the research. *Journal of Clinical Nursing, 15*(10), 1308–1316.

Costello, E. J., Compton, S. N., Keeler, G., & Angold, A. (2003). Relationships between poverty and psychopathology: A natural experiment. *JAMA, 290*(15), 2023–2029.

Coyne, I. (2006). Consultation with children in hospital: Children, parents' and nurses' perspectives. *Journal of Clinical Nursing, 15*(1), 61–71.

Curley, M. A. Q., & Meyer, E. C. (2001). Caring practices: The impact of the critical care experience on the family. In M. A. Q. Curley & P. A. Moloney-Harmon (Eds.), *Critical care nursing of infants and children* (2nd ed., pp. 47–67). Philadelphia: WB Saunders.

Denham, S. A. (2002). Family routines: A structural perspective for viewing family health. *Advances in Nursing Science, 24*(4), 60–74.

Denham, S. A. (2003). Relationships between family rituals, family routines, and health. *Journal of Family Nursing, 9*(3), 305–330.

Dodd, M., Janson, S., Facione, N., Faucett, J., Froelicher, E. S., Humphreys, J., et al. (2001). Advancing the science of symptom management. *Journal of Advanced Nursing, 33*(5), 668–676.

Driessnack, M. (2005). Children's drawings as facilitators of communication: A meta-analysis. *Journal of Pediatric Nursing: Nursing Care of Children and Families, 20*(6), 415–423.

Duhamel, F., & Dupuis, F. (2004). Guaranteed returns: Investing in conversations with families of patients with cancer. *Clinical Journal of Oncology Nursing, 8*(1), 68–71.

Dutton, R. P., Cooper, C., Jones, A., Leone, S., Kramer, M. E., & Scalea, T. M. (2003). Daily multidisciplinary rounds shorten length of stay for trauma patients. *Journal of Trauma-Injury Infection & Critical Care, 55*(5), 913–919.

Duvall, E. M., & Miller, B. C. (1985). Developmental tasks: Individual and family. In E. M. Duvall & B. C. Miller (Eds.), *Marriage and family development.* New York: Harper & Row.

Eaton, D. K., Kann, L., Kinchen, S., Shanklin, S., Ross, J., Hawkins, J., et al; Center for Disease Control and Prevention. (2008). Youth risk behavior surveillance—United States, 2007. *MMWR Surveillance Summaries: Morbidity and Mortality Weekly Report, 57*(4), 1–131.

Eiser, C. (1994). Making sense of chronic disease. The eleventh Jack Tizard Memorial Lecture. *Journal of Child Psychology and Psychiatry, 35*(8), 1373–1389.

Elliott, G. R., & Smiga, S. (2003). Depression in the child and adolescent. *Pediatric Clinic of North America, 50*(5), 1093–1106.

Emergency Nurses Association. (2005). *Position statement: Family presence at the bedside during invasive procedures and cardiopulmonary resuscitation.* Retrieved June 2008 from http://www.ena.org/about/position/position/Family Presence_-_ENA_White_Paper.pdf

Erikson, E. H. (1973). *Childhood and society.* New York: Norton.

Eshel, N., Daelmans, B., de Mello, M. C., & Martines, J. (2006). Responsive parenting: Interventions and outcomes. *Bulletin of the World Health Organization, 84*(12), 991–998.

Espezel, H. J., & Canam, C. J. (2003). Parent-nurse interactions: Care of hospitalized children. *Journal of Advanced Nursing, 44*(1), 34–41.

Feudtner, C. (2002). Grief-love: Contradictions in the lives of fathers of children with disabilities. *Archives of Pediatrics & Adolescent Medicine, 156*(7), 643.

Floriani, V., & Kennedy, C. (2007). Promotion of physical activity in primary care for obesity treatment/prevention in children. *Current Opinion in Pediatrics, 19*(1), 99–103.

Gallo, A. M., & Knafl, K. A. (1998). Parents' reports of "tricks of the trade" for managing childhood chronic illness. *Journal of the Society of Pediatric Nurses, 3*(3), 93–102.

Ganong, L., Doty, M. E., & Gayer, D. (2003). Mothers in post-divorce families caring for a child with cystic fibrosis. *Journal of Pediatric Nursing, 18*(5), 332–343.

Gedaly-Duff, V., Lee, K. A., Nail, L., Stork, L., Perko, K. P., Anderson, K. D., & Johnson, K. (2008). *Chemotherapy, pain, sleep, fatigue in children & parents* (R01 NR008570, unpublished raw data). Portland: Oregon Health & Science University.

Gedaly-Duff, V., Stoeger, S., & Shelton, K. (2000). Working with families. In R. E. Nickel & L. W. Desch (Eds.), *The physician's guide to caring for children with disabilities and chronic conditions* (pp. 31–76). Baltimore: Paul H. Brookes.

Giallo, R., & Gavidia-Payne, S. (2006). Child, parent and family factors as predictors of adjustment for siblings of children with a disability. *Journal of Intellectual Disability Research, 50*(Pt 12), 937–948.

Gray, R., & McCormick, M. C. (2005). Early childhood intervention programs in the US: Recent advances and future recommendations. *Journal of Primary Prevention, 26*(3), 259–275.

Greening, L., Stoppelbein, L., Konishi, C., Jordan, S. S., & Moll, G. (2007). Child routines and youths' adherence to treatment for type 1 diabetes. *Journal of Pediatric Psychology, 32*(4), 437–447.

Griffin, T. (2003). Facing challenges to family-centered care. II: Anger in the clinical setting. *Pediatric Nursing, 29*(3), 212–214.

Grunbaum, J. A., Kann, L., Kinchen, S., Ross, J., Hawkins, J., Lowry, R., et al. (2004). Youth risk behavior surveillance—United States, 2003 (Abridged). *Journal of School Health, 74*(8), 307–324.

Grunbaum, J. A., Kann, L., Kinchen, S. A., Williams, B., Ross, J. G., Lowry, R., & Kolbe, L. (2002). Youth risk behavior surveillance—United States, 2001. *Journal of School Health, 72*(8), 313–328.

Haggerty, K. P., Fleming, C. B., Catalano, R. F., Harachi, T. W., & Abbott, R. D. (2006). Raising healthy children: Examining the impact of promoting healthy driving behavior within a social development intervention. *Prevention Science, 7*(3), 257–267.

Hallstrom, I., & Elander, G. (2007). Families' needs when a child is long-term ill: A literature review with reference to nursing research. *International Journal of Nursing Practice, 13*(3), 193–200.

Halm, M. A. (2005). Family presence during resuscitation: A critical review of the literature. *American Journal of Critical Care, 14*(6), 494–511.

Hardy, M. S. (2002). Behavior-oriented approaches to reducing youth gun violence. In K. Reich (Ed.), *Children, youth, and gun violence* (Vol. 12, pp. 100–117). Los Altos, CA: From *The Future of Child*, journal publication of The David and Lucile Packard Foundation.

Hayes, V. E. (1997). Families and children's chronic conditions: Knowledge development and methodological considerations. *Scholarly Inquiry for Nursing Practice, 11*(4), 259–290; discussion 291–298.

Hayslip, B., Jr., & Kaminski, P. L. (2005). Grandparents raising their grandchildren: A review of the literature and suggestions for practice. *Gerontologist, 45*(2), 262–269.

Hibbard, R. A., Desch, L. W., Committee on Child Abuse Neglect, & Council on Children with Disabilities. (2007). Maltreatment of children with disabilities. *Pediatrics, 119*(5), 1018–1025.

Hodges, E. A. (2003). A primer on early childhood obesity and parental influence. *Pediatric Nursing, 29*(1), 13.

Holder, A. R. (1983). Parents, courts, and refusal of treatment. *Journal of Pediatrics, 103*(4), 515–521.

Hootman, J., Houck, G. M., & King, M. C. (2002). A program to educate school nurses about mental health interventions. *Journal of School Nursing, 18*(4), 191–195.

Horton, L. (2003). *Protective factors literature review: Early care and education programs and the prevention of child abuse and neglect.* Center for the Study of Social Policy. Retrieved June 2008, from http://www.cssp.org/uploadFiles/horton.pdf

Houck, G. M., Darnell, S., & Lussman, S. (2002). A support group intervention for at-risk female high school students. *Journal of School Nursing, 18*(4), 212–218.

Houtrow, A. J., Kim, S. E., Chen, A. Y., & Newacheck, P. W. (2007). Preventive health care for children with and without special health care needs. *Pediatrics, 119*(4), e821–e828.

Huston, A. C., Duncan, G. J., Granger, R., Bos, J., McLoyd, V., Mistry, R., et al. (2001). Work-based antipoverty programs for parents can enhance the school performance and social behavior of children. *Child Development, 72*(1), 318–336.

Hutson, S. P., & Alter, B. P. (2007). Experiences of siblings of patients with Fanconi anemia. *Pediatric Blood & Cancer, 48*(1), 72–79.

Imber-Black, E. (2005). Creating meaningful rituals for new life cycle transitions. In B. Carter & M. McGoldrick (Eds.), *The expanded family life cycle: Individuals, family, and social perspectives* (3rd ed., pp. 202–214). Boston: Allyn and Bacon.

Jeffreys, M., Smith, G. D., Martin, R. M., Frankel, S., & Gunnell, D. (2004). Childhood body mass index and later cancer risk: A 50-year follow-up of the Boyd Orr study. *International Journal of Cancer, 112*(2), 348–351.

Kirk, S. (2001). Negotiating lay and professional roles in the care of children with complex health care needs. *Journal of Advanced Nursing, 34*(5), 593–602.

Knafl, K., Breitmayer, B., Gallo, A., & Zoeller, L. (1996). Family response to childhood chronic illness: Description of management styles. *Journal of Pediatric Nursing: Nursing Care of Children and Families, 11*(5), 315–326.

Knafl, K. A., Deatrick, J., & Kirby, A. (2001). Normalization promotion. In M. Craft-Rosenberg & J. Denehy (Eds.), *Nursing interventions for infants, children, and families* (pp. 373–388). Thousand Oaks, CA: Sage.

Kohlberg, L. (1984). *The psychology of moral development.* San Francisco: Harper & Row.

Kon, A. A. (2006). When parents refuse treatment for their child. *JONA's Healthcare Law, Ethics, & Regulation, 8*(1), 5–9.

Kools, S., & Kennedy, C. (2003). Foster child health and development: Implications for primary care. *Pediatric Nursing, 29*(1), 39–49.

Latta, L. C., Dick, R., Parry, C., & Tamura, G. S. (2008). Parental responses to involvement in rounds on a pediatric inpatient unit at a teaching hospital: A qualitative study. *Academic Medicine, 83*(3), 292–297.

Lewandowski, L., & Frosch, E. (2003). Psychosocial aspects of pediatric trauma. In P. Moloney-Harmon & S. Czerwinski (Eds.), *Nursing care of the pediatric trauma patient* (pp. 340–354). Philadelphia: WB Saunders.

Lewandowski, L., & Tesler, M. (Eds.). (2003). *Family-centered care: Putting it into action. The SPN/ANA guide to family-centered care.* Washington, DC: Society of Pediatric Nurses/American Nurses Association.

Li, H. C., Lopez, V. (2008). Effectiveness and appropriateness of therapeutic play intervention in preparing children for surgery: A randomized controlled trial study. *Journal for Specialists in Pediatric Nursing, 13*(2), 63–73.

Limacher, L. H., & Wright, L. M. (2006). Exploring the therapeutic family intervention of commendations: Insights from research. *Journal of Family Nursing, 12*(3), 307–331.

Limbo, R., Petersen, W., & Pridham, K. (2003). Promoting safety of young children with guided participation processes. *Journal of Pediatric Health Care, 17*(5), 245–251.

Liu, L. L., Stout, J. W., Sullivan, M., Solet, D., Shay, D. K., & Grossman, D. C. (2000). Asthma and bronchiolitis hospitalizations among American Indian children. *Archives of Pediatrics & Adolescent Medicine, 154*(10), 991–996.

Luther, B. (2007). Looking at childhood obesity through the lens of Baumrind's parenting typologies. *Orthopaedic Nursing, 26*(5), 270–278; quiz 279–280.

Macdonald, H., & Callery, P. (2008). Parenting children requiring complex care: A journey through time. *Child: Care, Health & Development, 34*(2), 207–213.

Mangurten, J., Scott, S. H., Guzzetta, C. E., Clark, A. P., Vinson, L., Sperry, J., et al. (2006). Effects of family presence during resuscitation and invasive procedures in a pediatric emergency department. *Journal of Emergency Nursing, 32*, 225–233.

McClellan, C. B., & Cohen, L. L. (2007). Family functioning in children with chronic illness compared with healthy controls: a critical review. *Journal of Pediatrics, 150*(3), 221–223.

McGahey-Oakland, P. R., Lieder, H. S., Young, A. & Jefferson, L. S. (2007). Family experiences during resuscitation at a children's hospital emergency department. *Journal of Pediatric Health Care, 21*(4), 217–225.

McKinney, E., James, S., Murray, S., & Ashwill, J. (2005). *Maternal-Child Nursing* (2nd ed., pp. 795–801). St. Louis: Elsevier Saunders.

McPherson, M., Arango, P., Fox, H., Lauver, C., McManus, M., Newacheck, P. W., et al. (1998). A new definition of children with special health care needs. *Pediatrics, 102*(1 Pt 1), 137–140.

Meleis, A. I., Sawyer, L. M., Im, E. O., Hilfinger Messias, D. K., & Schumacher, K. (2000). Experiencing transitions: An emerging middle-range theory. *Advances in Nursing Science, 23*(1), 12–38.

Miles, M. S. (2003). Parents of children with chronic health problems: Programs of nursing research and their relationship to developmental science. *Annual Review of Nursing Research, 21*, 247–277.

Miller, J., Rosenbloom, A., & Silverstein, J. (2004). Childhood obesity. *Journal of Clinical Endocrinology & Metabolism, 89*(9), 4211–4218.

Moore, K. A., Coker, K., DuBuisson, A. B., Swett, B., & Edwards, W. H. (2003). Implementing potentially better practices for improving family-centered care in neonatal intensive care units: Successes and challenges. *Pediatrics, 111*(4 Pt 2), e450–e460.

Mosisa, A., & Hipple, S. (2006). *Trends in the labor force participation in the US.* Retrieved July 2008, from http://www.bls.gov/opub/mlr/2006/10/art3full.pdf

Moskowitz, J. T., Butensky, E., Harmatz, P., Vichinsky, E., Heyman, M. B., Acree, M., et al. (2007). Caregiving time in sickle cell disease: Psychological effects in maternal caregivers. *Pediatric Blood & Cancer, 48*(1), 64–71.

Mullen, J. E. (2008). Supporting families of technology-dependent patients hospitalized in pediatric intensive care unit. *AACN Advanced Critical Care, 19*(2), 125–129.

Mullen, J. E., & Pate, M. (2006). Caring for critically ill children and their families. In M. Slota (Ed.), *AAC Core Curriculum*

for Pediatric Critical Care Nursing (2nd ed., pp. 1-39). Philadelphia: WB Saunders.

Mussatto, K. (2006). Adaptation of the child and family to life with a chronic illness. *Cardiology in the Young, 16*(suppl 3), 110–116.

National Center for Injury Prevention and Control. (2006). *CDC injury fact book* (Table 10: Leading Causes of Death by Age Group—2003, p. 2). Retrieved July 28, 2008, from Centers for Disease Control and Prevention Web site: http://www.cdc.gov/ncipc/fact_book/InjuryBook2006.pdf

National Data Resource Center for Child and Adolescent Health. (2007). *Who are children with special health care needs?* Retrieved May 26, 2008, from http://nschdata.org/viewdocument.aspx?item=256

National Institute of Mental Health. (2006, last revised). *The family and the ADHD child. Attention deficit hyperactivity disorder.* U.S. Department of Health and Human Services. Retrieved July 31, 2008, from http://www.nimh.nih.gov/health/publications/adhd/summary.shtml

National Institutes of Health (Medline Plus). (2008). *Child abuse.* Retrieved July 28, 2008, from http://www.nlm.nih.gov/medlineplus/childabuse.html#cat1m.nih.gov

Nelson, A. M. (2002). A metasynthesis: Mothering other-than-normal children. *Qualitative Health Research, 12*(4), 515–530.

Newacheck, P. W., Hung, Y. Y., & Wright, K. K. (2002). Racial and ethnic disparities in access to care for children with special health care needs. *Ambulatory Pediatrics, 2*(4), 247–254.

Newacheck, P. W., & Kim, S. E. (2005). A national profile of health care utilization and expenditures for children with special health care needs [erratum appears in *Archives of Pediatrics & Adolescent Medicine,* 2005 Apr;159(4):318]. *Archives of Pediatrics & Adolescent Medicine, 159*(1), 10–17.

Newacheck, P. W., Stein, R. E., Bauman, L., & Hung, Y. Y. (2003). Disparities in the prevalence of disability between black and white children. *Archives of Pediatrics & Adolescent Medicine, 157*(3), 244–248.

Nihiser, A. J., Lee, S. M., Wechsler, H., McKenna, M., Odom, E., Reinold, C., et al. (2007). Body mass index measurement in schools. *Journal of School Health, 77*(10), 651–671; quiz 722–754.

Northington, L. (2000). Chronic sorrow in caregivers of school age children with sickle cell disease: A grounded theory approach. *Issues in Comprehensive Pediatric Nursing, 23*(3), 141–154.

Novilla, M. L., Barnes, M. D., De La Cruz, N. G., Williams, P. N., & Rogers, J. (2006). Public health perspectives on the family: An ecological approach to promoting health in the family and community. *Family & Community Health, 29*(1), 28–42.

Olds, D. L., Kitzman, H., Hanks, C., Cole, R., Anson, E., Sidora-Arcoleo, K., et al. (2007). Effects of nurse home visiting on maternal and child functioning: Age-9 follow-up of a randomized trial. *Pediatrics, 120*(4), e832–e845.

Ostrom, C. M. (2006, June 27). *Is mom a criminal for not allowing surgery on her son?* Retrieved June 2008, from http://community.seattletimes.nwsource.com/archive/?date=20060627&slug=rileyrogers27m

Parsons, C. (2003). Caring for adolescents and families in crisis. *Nursing Clinics of North America, 38*(1), 111–122.

Perrin, E. C., Newacheck, P., Pless, I. B., Drotar, D., Gortmaker, S. L., Leventhal, J., et al. (1993). Issues involved in the definition and classification of chronic health conditions. *Pediatrics, 91*(4), 787–793.

Perrin, J. M., Bloom, S. R., & Gortmaker, S. L. (2007). The increase of childhood chronic conditions in the United States. *JAMA, 297*(24), 2755–2759.

Piaget, J., & Inhelder, B. (1969). *Psychology of the child.* New York: Basic Books.

Polhamus, B., Dalenius, K., Borland, E., Smith, B., & Grummer-Strawn, L. (2007). *Pediatric nutrition surveillance 2006 report.* Retrieved July 2008, from the Centers for Disease Control and Prevention Web site: http://www.cdc.gov/pednss/pdfs/PedNSS_2006.pdf

Power, N., & Franck, L. (2008). Parent participation in the care of hospitalized children: A systematic review. *Journal of Advanced Nursing, 62*(6), 622–641.

Rankin, S. H. (1989). Family transitions. In C. L. Gilliss, B. L. Highley, B. M. Roberts, & I. M. Martinson (Eds.), *Toward a science of family nursing* (pp. 173–186). Menlo Park, CA: Addison-Wesley.

Rankin, S. H., & Weekes, D. P. (2000). Life-span development: A review of theory and practice for families with chronically ill members. *Scholarly Inquiry for Nursing Practice, 14*(4), 355–373; discussion 375–378.

Rehm, R. S., & Bradley, J. F. (2005a). The search for social safety and comfort in families raising children with complex chronic conditions. *Journal of Family Nursing, 11*(1), 59–78.

Rehm, R. S., & Bradley, J. F. (2005b). Normalization in families raising a child who is medically fragile/technology dependent and developmentally delayed. *Qualitative Health Research, 15*(6), 807–820.

Richaud de Minzi, M. C. (2006). Loneliness and depression in middle and late childhood: The relationship to attachment and parental styles. *Journal of Genetic Psychology, 167*(2), 189–210.

Ritchie, L. D., Welk, G., Styne, D., Gerstein, D. E., & Crawford, P. B. (2005). Family environment and pediatric overweight: What is a parent to do? *Journal of the American Dietetic Association, 105*(5 suppl 1), S70–S79.

Rodrigues, N., & Patterson, J. M. (2007). Impact of severity of a child's chronic condition on the functioning of two-parent families. *Journal of Pediatric Psychology, 32*(4), 417–426.

Rolland, J. S. (2005). Chronic illness and the family life cycle. In B. Carter & M. McGoldrick (Eds.), *The expanded family life cycle: Individual, family and social perspectives* (3rd ed., pp. 492–511). Boston: Allyn and Bacon.

Rose, D., & Garwick, A. (2003). Urban American Indian family caregivers' perceptions of barriers to management of childhood asthma. *Journal of Pediatric Nursing, 18*(1), 2–11.

Rozdilsky, J. R. (2005). Enhancing sibling presence in pediatric ICU. *Critical Care Nursing Clinics of North America, 17*(4), 451–461.

Sadof, M. D., & Nazarian, B. L. (2007). Caring for children who have special health-care needs: A practical guide for the primary care practitioner. *Pediatrics in Review, 28*(7), e36–e42.

Sandelowski, M., & Barroso, J. (2003). Motherhood in the context of maternal HIV infection. *Research in Nursing & Health, 26*(6), 470–482.

Scales, P. C., Benson, P. L., Moore, K. A., Lippman, L., Brown, B., & Zaff, J. F. (2008). Promoting equal developmental opportunity and outcomes among America's children and youth: Results from the National Promises Study. *Journal of Primary Prevention, 29*(2), 121–144.

Schor, E. L. (2007). The future pediatrician: Promoting children's health and development. *Journal of Pediatrics, 151*(5 suppl), S11–S16.

Schultz-Krohn, W. (2004). The meaning of family routines in a homeless shelter. *American Journal of Occupational Therapy, 58*(5), 531–542.

Schumacher, K. L., & Meleis, A. I. (1994). Transitions: A central concept in nursing. *Image Journal of Nursing Scholarship, 26*(2), 119–127.

Segal, R. (2004). Family routines and rituals: A context for occupational therapy interventions. *American Journal of Occupational Therapy, 58*(5), 499–508.

Seligman, M., & Darling, R. B. (1997). *Ordinary families, special children. A systems approach to childhood disability* (2nd ed.). New York: Guildford Press

Sharpe, D., & Rossiter, L. (2002). Siblings of children with a chronic illness: A meta-analysis. *Journal of Pediatric Psychology, 27*(8), 699–710.

Shields, L., Pratt, J., & Hunter, J. (2006). Family centered care: A review of qualitative studies. *Journal of Clinical Nursing, 15*(10), 1317–1323.

Slota, M., Shearn, D., Potersnak, K., & Haas, L. (2003). Perspectives on family-centered, flexible visitation in the intensive care unit setting. *Critical Care Medicine, 31*(5 suppl), S362–S366.

Smith, P., & Drew, L. (2002). *Grandparenthood* (2nd ed., Vol. 3). Mahwah, NJ: Lawrence Erlbaum.

Sorkhabi, N. (2005). Applicability of Baumrind's parent typology to collective cultures: Analysis of cultural explanations of parent socialization effects. *International Journal of Behavioral Development, 29*, 552–563.

Spears, A. P. (2008, February 7). *The healthy people 2010 outcomes for the care of children with special health care needs: An effective national policy for meeting mental health care needs?* Retrieved July 31, 2008, from http://www.ncbi.nlm.nih.gov/entrez/query.fcgi?cmd=Retrieve&db=PubMed&dopt=Citation&list_uids=18256914

Starchild Abraham Cherrix v. Commonwealth of Virginia, for the County of Accomack. (2006). Juvenile and Domestic Relations District Court. Retrieved July 28, 2008, from http://www.oag.state.va.us/LEGAL_LEGIS/CourtFilings/AbrahamCherrixAmicusJuly252006.pdf

Stein, M. T., & Perrin, E. L. (1998). Guidance for effective discipline. American Academy of Pediatrics. Committee on psychosocial aspects of child and family health. *Pediatrics, 101* (4 Pt 1), 723–728.

Stein, R. E., Bauman, L. J., Westbrook, L. E., Coupey, S. M., & Ireys, H. T. (1993). Framework for identifying children who have chronic conditions: The case for a new definition. *Journal of Pediatrics, 122*(3), 342–347.

Sullivan-Bolyai, S., Sadler, L., Knafl, K. A., & Gilliss, C. L. (2003). Great expectations: A position description for parents as caregivers: Part I. *Pediatric Nursing, 29*(6), 457–461.

Tapp, D. M. (2000). The ethics of relational stance in family nursing: Resisting the view of "nurse as expert." *Journal of Family Nursing, 6*(1), 69–91.

Urrutia-Rojas, X., Egbuchunam, C. U., Bae, S., Menchaca, J., Bayona, M., Rivers, P. A., & Singh, K. P. (2006). High blood pressure in school children: Prevalence and risk factors. *BMC Pediatrics, 6*, 32.

U.S. Census Bureau. (2008, February 28). *Nearly half of children receive care from relatives.* Retrieved July 2008, from http://www.census.gov/population/www/socdemo/childcare.html

U.S. Code of Federal Regulations. (2006). Title 42: The public health and welfare. Chapter 67: Child abuse prevention and treatment and adoption reform. Last amended 2006. Retrieved July 24, 2008, from http://www4.law.cornell.edu/uscode/html/uscode42/usc_sup_01_42_10_67.html

U.S. Department of Education. (2004). *Individuals with disabilities education improvement Act of 2004.* Retrieved June 2008, from http://www.nichcy.org/reauth/PL108-446.pdf

U.S. Department of Health and Human Services. (2000). *Healthy people 2010: Understanding and improving health* (Stock No. 017-001-001-00-550-9). Washington, DC: U.S. Government Printing Office.

U.S. Department of Health and Human Services. (2008). *Healthy people 2020: The road ahead.* Retrieved August 2008, from http://www.healthypeople.gov/hp2020

U.S. Department of Health and Human Services Administration on Children Youth and Families. (2005). *Child maltreatment 2003.* Washington, DC: U.S. Government Printing Office. Retrieved July 31, 2008, from http://nccanch.acf.hhs.gov/index.cfm.

U.S. Department of Health and Human Services Administration on Children Youth and Families. (2008). *Child maltreatment 2006.* Washington, DC: U.S. Government Printing Office. Retrieved July 2008, from http://www.acf.hhs.gov/programs/cb/pubs/cm06/summary.htm

U.S. Department of Health and Human Services, Health Resources and Services Administration, & Maternal and Child Health Bureau. (2008). *The national survey of children with special health care needs chart book 2005-2006.* Rockville, MD: Author. Retrieved June 2008, from http://mchb.hrsa.gov/cshcn05

Van Cleave, J., Heisler, M., Devries, J. M., Joiner, T. A., & Davis, M. M. (2007). Discussion of illness during well-child care visits with parents of children with and without special health care needs. *Archives of Pediatrics & Adolescent Medicine, 161*(12), 1170–1175.

Van Waning, N. R., Kleiber, C., & Freyenberger, B. (2005). Pediatric care. Development and implementation of a protocol for transfers out of the pediatric intensive care unit. *Critical Care Nurse, 25*(3), 50–55.

Vazirani, S., Hays, R. D., Shapiro, M. F., & Cowan, M. (2005). Effect of a multidisciplinary intervention on communication and collaboration among physicians and nurses. *American Journal of Critical Care, 14*(1), 71–77.

Wang, K. K., & Barnard, A. (2004). Technology-dependent children and their families: A review. *Journal of Advanced Nursing, 45*(1), 36–46.

Wells, D. K., James, K., Stewart, J. L., Moore, I. M., Kelly, K. P., Moore, B., et al. (2002). The care of my child with cancer: A new instrument to measure caregiving demand in parents of children with cancer. *Journal of Pediatric Nursing, 17*(3), 201–210.

Wertlieb, D. (2003). Converging trends in family research and pediatrics: Recent findings for the American Academy of Pediatrics Task Force on the Family. *Pediatrics, 111*(6 Pt 2), 1572–1587.

Wofford, L. G. (2008). Systematic review of childhood obesity prevention. *Journal of Pediatric Nursing, 23*(1), 5–19.

Wong, M. G., & Heriot, S. A. (2008). Parents of children with cystic fibrosis: How they hope, cope and despair. *Child: Care, Health and Development, 34*(3), 344–354.

Wright, L. M., & Leahey, M. (1999). Maximizing time, minimizing suffering: The 15-minute (or less) family interview. *Journal of Family Nursing, 5*(3), 259–274.

Yoos, H. L., Kitzman, H., Henderson, C., McMullen, A., Sidora-Arcoleo, K., Halterman, J. S., & Anson, E. (2007). The impact of the parental illness representation on disease management in childhood asthma. *Nursing Research, 56*(3), 167–174.

Youngblade, L. M., Theokas, C., Schulenberg, J., Curry, L., Huang, I. C., & Novak, M. (2007). Risk and promotive factors in families, schools, and communities: A contextual model of positive youth development in adolescence. *Pediatrics, 119*(suppl 1), S47–S53.

Zawistowski, C. A., & Frader, J. E. (2003). Ethical problems in pediatric critical care: Consent. *Critical Care Medicine, 31* (5 suppl), S407–S410.

Zigler, E., Pfannenstiel, J., & Seitz, V. (2008). The parents as teachers program and school success. A replication and extension. *Journal of Primary Prevention, 29,* 103–120.

Zuckerman, B., Parker, S., Kaplan-Sanoff, M., Augustyn, M., & Barth, M. C. (2004). Healthy steps: A case study of innovation in pediatric practice. *Pediatrics, 114*(3), 820–826.

CHAPTER WEB SITES

- *Adolescent Health Resources:* http://www.ama-assn.org/ama/pub/physician-resources/public-health/promoting-healthy-lifestyles/adolescent-health.shtml
- *American Academy of Allergy Asthma & Immunology:* http://www.aaaai.org/patients/publicedmat/tips/childhoodasthma.stm
- *American Academy of Pediatrics:* http://www.aap.org
- *American Cancer Society:* http://www.cancer.org
- *American Obesity Association:* http://obesity1.tempdomainname.com/subs/childhood
- *Assets Approach to Promoting Healthy Child Development:* http://www.search-institute.org/assets
- *Association for Children's Palliative Care:* http://www.act.org.uk
- *Bright Futures at Georgetown University:* http://www.brightfutures.org
- *Census Bureau Minority Links for Media, American Indians and Alaskan Natives Minorities:* http://www.census.gov/pubinfo/www/NEWamindML1.html
- *Child Welfare Information Gateway:* http://www.childwelfare.gov/index.cfm
- *Children's Defense Fund:* http://childrensdefense.org
- *Cultural Competence Resources for Health Care Providers:* http://www11.georgetown.edu/research/gucchd/nccc
- *Grandparent Raising Grandchildren:* http://www.usa.gov/Topics/Grandparents.shtml
- *Healthy People 2010:* http://www.health.gov/healthypeople
- *Kids-N-Crisis:* http://www.geocities.com/Heartland/Bluffs/5400/sickkid.html
- *National Center for Cultural Competence:* http://www11.georgetown.edu/research/gucchd/nccc
- *Parents without Partners:* http://www.parentswithoutpartners.org

CHAPTER 14

Nurses and Families in Adult Medical-Surgical Settings

Anne M. Hirsch, DNS, ARNP

Renee Hoeksel, PhD, RN

Alice E. Dupler, JD, APRN-BC

Joanna Rowe Kaakinen, PhD, RN

CRITICAL CONCEPTS

✦ Families who are viewed as part of the health care team are empowered to deal with the stressors of a family member's hospitalization, and are prepared to provide support and aid in their recovery or facilitate a comfortable death.

✦ Supportive actions by family members, as well as conflict and criticism, have an effect on the patients' health behaviors, emotional well-being, immune function, and illness exacerbations.

✦ During the acute illness phase, nursing interventions should focus on patients and their families by providing physical care and emotional support, facilitating family communication, providing timely information, and establishing a collaborative, trusting partnership.

✦ Family nursing is the provision of care to the entire family unit and is an integral aspect of care provided by nurses in adult medical-surgical settings.

✦ Unit or hospital policies may need to be updated so that patient-identified family members are not excluded, which can add stress and trauma for both the patient and their loved ones.

✦ Families are foundational to the comprehensive care of all patients, and it is the responsibility of every nurse and every health care agency to implement and regularly evaluate visitation policies and procedures that reflect this philosophy.

✦ Transferring loved ones from critical care units to the medical-surgical units is stressful for families because it creates a sense of conflict. On one hand, families are glad their loved ones are better, but they also worry that their family members may not be ready to be moved out of such intensive nurse watchfulness.

(continued)

CRITICAL CONCEPTS (continued)

✦ The family member who advocates for his or her loved one in the hospital assumes a difficult, time-consuming, and fatiguing role as he or she often travels long distances to get to the hospital, takes time off work to be there, often stays all night in the hospital, manages the informational needs of the patient and the family, and works through a complex health care system.

✦ Effective communication with patients, families and interdisciplinary health care providers improves client satisfaction, promotes positive response to care, reduces length of stay in care settings, and results in decreased overall cost and resource utilization.

✦ Compassionate communication provides crucial care to families as they are asked to make multiple decisions as their loved one dies in the hospital.

The family is the core of the social environment for most individuals and serves as the foundation for social support during health and illness (Gallant, Spitz, & Prohaska, 2007). Family nursing is the provision of care to the entire family unit and is an integral aspect of care provided by nurses in adult medical-surgical settings. Hospitalization for an acute illness, injury, or exacerbation of a chronic illness is stressful for patients and their families. The ill adult enters the hospital usually in a physiologic crisis, and the family most often accompanies its ill or injured family members into the hospital; both the patient and the family are usually in an emotional crisis (Hudak & Gallo, 1994). Hospitalized family members worry about the effects of their illness and their potentially changed capabilities on the rest of their family members (Perry, Lynam, & Anderson, 2006). The family members also worry about their loved ones, sometimes to the extent of being neglectful of their own needs (Perry et al., 2006). When nurses provide care for the whole family, this allows families to be more supportive of their ill members, to experience less anxiety, and to have less disruption in the family system (Holden, Harrison, & Johnson, 2002; Jansen & Schmitt, 2003). Involving family members in intervention strategies strengthens family relationships and enhances the effects of the interventions (Martire, Lustig, Schulz, Helgeson, & Miller, 2007; Martire & Schulz, 2007). Close social relationships, especially family relationships, affect physical and psychological well-being, and promote adherence to disease management plans that involve changes in health behavior. When family is involved in the care of the loved one in the hospital, the patient has an increased likelihood of positive health outcomes (Martire et al., 2007).

The purpose of this chapter is to describe family nursing in medical-surgical settings where nurses care for adult patients and families, including families in the critical care units and medical-surgical units. A review of literature captures the major stressors families often face during hospitalization of an adult family member: the transfer from one unit to another, being discharged home, participation in cardiopulmonary resuscitation (CPR), withdrawing life support therapy, and organ donation. This chapter includes a family case study that highlights the issues families experience and adapt to when an adult member is ill. The Family Assessment and Intervention Model is applied to a family case study to demonstrate one theoretical approach for working with families. The chapter closes with a discussion of the implications of family nursing on medical-surgical practice, education, and health policy.

FAMILY ADULT MEDICAL-SURGICAL NURSING

Since the late 1970s, progress to move to a more family-centered care model in adult critical care and medical-surgical nursing has been slow but steady (Latour & Haines, 2007). Participating in the care of family members requires accurate and timely information (Fox-Wasylyshyn, El-Masri, & Williamson, 2005). Family members want to be able to ask the following questions about their patient family member: Are they doing as well as can be expected? Are they getting any better? Are they in any pain? Has there been any change? What can I expect in the future? These questions may be expressed in thousands of different ways but stem from the common concern in any language and for any diagnosis that they fear for their loved one's well-being, as well as for their own. The acute phase of illness or injury refers to the period immediately after the onset of the illness or the injury. Family members and significant others of critically ill patients are integral to the recovery of their loved ones (Molter, 1979, 1994; Pearce, 2005). Families with members who are acutely or critically ill are seen in adult medical-surgical units, intensive care or cardiac care units, or emergency departments. Having loved ones in today's acute care hospital can be an upsetting experience at any time, but when a stay in an adult critical care unit occurs (anticipated or not), it can be especially traumatic (Alvarez & Kirby, 2006).

Families in Critical Care Units

Most intensive care units (ICUs) limit visitation to families, but as we have learned, the definition of *family* is complex. This health care situation forces the question, "How close does somebody need to be to the patient to be defined as a 'family member'?" Complicated family structures, such as divorce, blended families, and same-sex partners challenge the biological legal definition of family. "Family" from the patients' perspective is whomever the patient defines as family, but the patient's definition of family can be challenged when the patient's physical condition is such that communication is not possible. Chapter 1 provides a detailed discussion of the definition of *family*.

Unit or hospital policies may need to be updated so that patient-identified family members are not excluded, which adds stress and trauma for both the patient and their loved ones (Harvey, 2004; Rushton, Reina, & Reina, 2007). Such administrative revisions need to take into consideration evidence-based data so that both nursing staff and families can be confident that patient care systems reflect these visionary professional standards even when patients cannot speak for themselves (Latour & Haines, 2007; Verhaeghe, Defloor, Van Zuuren, Duijnstee, & Grypdonck, 2005).

Family visitors in ICUs reported and demonstrated symptoms of anxiety or depression after having their family members in the ICU for a few days (Pouchard et al., 2005). In addition, Azoulay and colleagues (2005) found that family members were at significant risk for development of post-traumatic stress disorder (PTSD) when they had family members in the ICU. The needs of family members with loved ones in the ICU have long been studied (Paul & Rattray, 2008). The classic work of Molter in 1974 first identified the following 10 needs, listed in descending order:

1. Hope
2. Health care provider caring about the patient
3. Having a waiting room near the patient
4. Being called at home for a change in patient condition
5. Knowing about the prognosis
6. Having questions answered honestly
7. Knowing specific facts about prognosis
8. Receiving information about patient once a day
9. Having explanations in understandable terms
10. Seeing patient frequently

Warren developed the Critical Care Family Needs Inventory (CCFNI) based on this work by Molter. The CCFNI has been demonstrated to be a valid and reliable instrument to assess family needs (Paul & Rattray, 2008). These family needs were further collapsed into three categories: assurance, proximity, and information. What is crucial for nurses to know about this research is that health care settings have been only partially responsive to the need of families for information. Nurses in ICU settings are still not practicing family-centered care or family nursing. Table 14-1 shows that, although nurses are providing more information to family members and that families can see their loved ones more frequently, nurses are not providing reassurance to family members or meeting the needs that families identify as important to their own health and well-being (Browning & Warren, 2006). It is worth noting that the language in their work uses the word *patient* and not *family member,* which supports the view that ICU nurses are still focused on the patient and not the family needs.

Families are the primary support for loved ones in the ICU (Verhaeghe et al., 2005; Williams, 2005). Families have been found to experience

TABLE 14-1

Family Needs in the Intensive Care Unit

FAMILY NEEDS ALWAYS/USUALLY MET	FAMILY NEEDS NEVER/SOMETIMES MET
1. Informed about medical treatments	Needs explanations in lay terminology
2. Aware of why and what care is being provided	Need to have access to quality food in the hospital
3. Knows somewhat about the prognosis	Assured it is okay to leave the hospital for a while
4. Allowed to visit in the intensive care unit (ICU) frequently	To be prepared for the ICU environment before entering the unit the first time
5. Understands different types of staff caring for family member	Talk to the same nurse every day
6. Knows who to call in the ICU for information	Have feeling of hope supported
7. Given directions for things to do at bedside while visiting	Share feelings, especially those of guilt, anger, or fear
8. Called at home for condition changes	Feel accepted by the hospital staff
9. Has support of friends and family	Discuss the possibility my family member may die
10. Knows what is being done for their family member	Visit anytime

Source: From Browning, G., & Warren, N. (2006). Unmet needs of family members in the medical intensive care waiting room. *Critical Care Nursing Quarterly, 29*(1), 86–95, by permission.

cognitive, emotional, and social stress when family members are in the ICU. These worries include:

- Information ambiguity
- Uncertain prognosis
- Fear of death
- Role changes
- Financial concerns
- Disruption of normal routines

ICU nurses are in the best position to support these families because they see them often, know the patient intimately, and are called to practice holistically instead of based on a biomedical model. Yet, many ICU nurses continue to view families as obstacles to care and consistently underestimate their professional role in meeting the needs of these families (Verhaeghe et al., 2005; Chesla, 1997). What ICU nurses believe families need does not match what families identify as their needs (Maxwell, Stuenkel, & Saylor, 2007). Therefore, it is important to explore why this dichotomy continues to exist given the evidence that has been known since Molter's work was published in 1974.

Stayt (2007) investigated nurses' perceptions of their ability to practice family nursing in the ICU. Two important findings in this research offer an insight into understanding these nurses' experiences, namely, role ambiguity and role conflict. Role ambiguity was expressed as an unrealistic role

expectation. The nurses were found to believe that it was their responsibility to "make it right" or to "take away the family members' worries" rather than to provide emotional support for families dealing with the uncertainty of outcome for a family member in the ICU. The nurses expressed that they felt guilty for not helping the families. The nurses undervalued their contribution to meeting the family needs during this stressful time. Nurses identified that they felt they lacked training in how to work with families.

Two types of role conflict were identified by ICU nurses (Stayt, 2007). The first role conflict was difficulty in balancing the biomedical technical model of care with the holistic nursing model of care. Chesla (1997) reports a similar role conflict for ICU nurses between technical care and social-emotional care. Nurses are torn between caring for the medically unstable patient, who is their priority, yet recognizing they are responsible for caring for the entire family. The second type of role conflict was the balance of their professional relationship and the family seeking a more personal relationship with the nurse (Stayt, 2007). The nurse-family relationship is established during an intense emotional time for the family. After a period of time, the family was described as seeking too much self-disclosure from the nurses. Nurses found keeping professional boundaries fatiguing and time-consuming. Therefore, the nurses described that they used detachment strategies to keep their relationship professional. They asked for different patients. Nurses physically distanced themselves by focusing only on tasks when they entered the patient's room. They limited conversation with the family. They found themselves emotionally distancing themselves from the family so they would not engage on a personal level.

Nurses recognize the importance of families and wanted to work with them in the ICU, but they found it difficult to provide for the emotional needs of family members. Hospital educational programs are needed to support nurses in providing family-centered care versus patient-centered care. Communication with families can be learned and practiced in the ICU environment (White & Curtis, 2006).

VISITING POLICY

Debate over the "correct" quantity and frequency of visits in adult critical care units continued into the twenty-first century, despite mounting research evidence that a "one size fits all formula" was no more suitable for critically ill adults than it was for ill children (Day, 2006; Miracle, 2005). Policies that have been tried and often revisited have included 10 minutes every hour, 30 minutes several times a day, two visitors at a time, immediate family only, open visiting, closed visiting with rare exceptions, and many more versions of all of the above. Professional nursing organizations, such as the American Association of Critical Care Nurses and the American Nurses Association, have supported the position that, despite being in critical condition, patients cannot be adequately cared for when they are isolated from their families (Bice-Stephens, 2006; Latour & Haines, 2007). Families are foundational to the comprehensive care of all patients, and it is the responsibility of every nurse and every health care agency to implement and regularly evaluate visitation policies and procedures that reflect this philosophy (Pearce, 2005).

WAITING ROOMS

When families of critically ill patients are not in the unit with their loved ones, they are more than likely spending a significant amount of time in the unit's waiting room. Attention to the details that may help relieve family stress is critical. Little research has focused on family comfort and amenities provided in the waiting rooms adjacent to critical care units (Alvarez & Kirby, 2006). Families have consistently voiced desires to have better access to food and drinks, a variety of comfortable seating options to account for all people, available computer access, and nearby rooms for private meetings with physicians, nurses, or other care providers. Providing a beeper system for the family to carry when they leave the unit or waiting room was found to be helpful to families (Deitrick et al., 2005). Receptionists in family room waiting areas are gaining in popularity (Alvarez & Kirby, 2006).

FAMILY INTERVENTIONS

Family intervention strategies that support both nurses and families include shared decision making, ICU family rounds, family conferences, family progress journals, and having a Family Nurse Specialist in the ICU. Shared decision making is crucial in the ICU because patients often cannot speak for themselves; therefore, most treatment decisions should be made from a family perspective (Kaakinen & Hanson, 2005). Family members of patients in the ICU have been found to be at increased risk for experiencing anxiety, depression, and PTSD (Azoulay et al., 2005; Pouchard et al., 2005). Refer to Chapter 4 for detailed information on family shared decision making.

Timed daily family rounds with nurses and physicians decreased family anxiety and increased communication (Mangram et al., 2005). Careful and consistent information can help alleviate these fears. When away from the bedside and the stimulation of the ICU environment, family members are able to hear more clearly and accurately the explanations and answers to their questions and concerns. Therefore, nurses should plan to spend time (e.g., a short 10-minute conference) with families away from the patient's bedside on every shift. Plans for language interpreters should be made ahead of time so that all health care team members meeting with the family can provide culturally competent care.

Encouraging families to keep a family progress journal (Kloos & Daly, 2008) or a computer family blog for extended family and friends was found to decrease family anxiety. Kloos and Daly (2008) have analyzed family progress journals. These authors found the top three family issues addressed in these journals were that the family experienced negative emotions about the physical appearance of their loved one in the ICU, they expressed the need for more regular communication about what was going on, and they worried about the pain their loved ones were experiencing. Families were found to cope with their stress through their faith in God, support of family and friends, and seeing their loved one get physically better. Families wrote that the characteristics of the health care providers that were the most helpful to them were kindness, compassion, watchfulness over their loved one, and availability to answer all their questions.

Families are often overwhelmed and intimidated with the fast-paced, noisy, and highly technologic environments that surround their loved ones (Pikka & Beaulieu, 2004). Patients appear "lost" among all the equipment, tubes, lines, beeping, bonging sounds that can enhance family members' fear that their loved one's identity will be lost in these surroundings, especially when interventions such as dressings or indwelling tubes around the face and head distort facial features (Maxwell et al., 2007). Bringing in individual and family group photographs, which include the hospitalized family member, should become standard practice because this was found to offer comfort to both patients and family members (Bice-Stephens, 2006; Rushton, Reina, & Reina, 2007). Allowing families to participate in the actual care of their family members has been found to offer reassurance as a way to contribute to their family member's recovery (Alvarez & Kirby, 2006). Nurses' careful guidance at the bedside during visits and the family provision of physical care, such as face washing or application of lotion, offers family members and patients a sense of calm reassurance and comfort. Adding a Clinical Nurse Speciality in Family Nursing to the ICU resulted in increased family satisfaction (Nelson & Poist, 2008). As patients improve to the point that they are stable enough to transfer out of the ICU, families experience different stressors as they undergo relocation stress or transfer anxiety (Chaboyer, Kendall, Kendall, & Foster, 2005).

FAMILY RELOCATION STRESS AND TRANSFER ANXIETY

Moving ill family members from the critical care unit to the medical-surgical unit is stressful for families. Even though families report relief that their loved ones are able to transfer out of the ICU, they also fear that the loss of one-to-one nurse-patient vigilance will lead to failure to detect important changes in condition (Chaboyer et al., 2005; Latour & Haines, 2007). Families found that the nursing care on the medical-surgical unit is not as predictable as the ICU and families did not understand the different ratio of nurse-to-patient staffing patterns (Carr, 2002). Families also found the relocation stressful because they missed their relationship with the ICU nurses, the changes in the environment, and the changes in the amount of information they received (Streator et al., 2001).

Chaboyer et al. (2005) classified the families' emotions with relocation stress into four emotions or feelings. Families feel *abandonment* when the transfer is abrupt and not planned. Families describe experiencing *vulnerability*. They are stressed as they felt they had to accept their new responsibility as a different kind of family caregiver within the hospital setting. For example, rather than be a supportive family member from the background, they now had to provide more actual physical care for their loved one as their physical status improved. Their sense of vulnerability was found to be the most intense of these family emotions. The families reported having a feeling of *unimportance*, because of the different staffing ratio on the medical-surgical unit. The last feeling identified was *ambivalence*. The families expressed being caught between the extremes of feeling relieved and happy their loved ones were better, and their fears and doubts that they were well enough to leave the ICU.

Nurses can help families be prepared for the transfer out of the ICU environment. A specific nurse "handover" of the patient and the family was found to decrease family stress (Latour & Haines, 2007). Involving families in the transfer process effectively contributed to less relocation stress (Eldredge, 2004; McKinley, Nagy, Stein-Parbury, Bramwell, & Hudson, 2002). Family conferences scheduled with the health care team are a perfect opportunity for family members to express these concerns, and for team members to respond to all concerns with factual, straightforward information. Ideally, both the nurse manager and supervisor of the sending and receiving hospital units should participate in this transition. A detailed and comprehensive, written patient care plan helps to smooth out this important phase of the patient and family journey (Day, 2006). Family input into this care plan empowers and reassures families during this important transition to the medical-surgical unit.

Families on the Medical-Surgical Units

Families in medical-surgical settings reported numerous stressors and changes in their family environment, and are often desperately in need of support. Nurses are in a position to provide support in the following ways:

- Use effective communication: listen to family's concerns, feelings, and questions; answer all questions or assist the family in finding the answers.
- Respect and support family coping mechanisms and caregiving behaviors.
- Recognize the uniqueness of each family.
- Assist family in decision making by providing information about options.
- Permit the family to make decisions about patient care when appropriate.
- Provide adequate time to visit privately, when possible.
- Facilitate family conferences to allow open sharing of family feelings.
- Clarify information and share resources regarding support groups.
- Foster positive nurse-family relationships through all phases of care.

It is clear that families who have adult members in acute medical surgical areas are stressed by hospitalization, yet this is one of the least studied areas of family nursing. In this section, family visitation, family communication needs, and family needs are explored. Family interventions relative to discharge are discussed.

FAMILY VISITATION

Visitation helps to promote family cohesion and unity (Van Horn & Kautz, 2007). Hospitals have stricter visitation rules in European countries than in the United States (Alvarez & Kirby, 2006). Promotion of family integrity is an actual nursing intervention listed in the book *Nursing Intervention Classification* (McCloskey & Bulechek, 2004). An open family visitation policy supports families by readying them for the role of caregiver, increases family involvement in the care in the hospital, provides for increased communication with nurses and other health care providers, and decreases family anxiety (Van Horn & Kautz, 2007). When families help

provide care to loved ones in the hospital, patients have reported fewer depressive symptoms, less confusion, and less incontinence (Eldredge, 2004).

Many families enact a bedside vigilance that provides a close protective function (Carr & Fogarty, 1999). Families displayed both directive behaviors and supportive behaviors as family caregivers in the hospital, especially when the hospitalized family member was older (Jacelon, 2006). Family directive behaviors were described as follows:

- Acting in place of the ill family member by making decisions about their care without consulting the ill family members, talking to their health care providers, and being the organizer of their care
- Acting as an advisor to the ill family member by working collaboratively with them on decisions
- Not acting in some cases; these family members were found to be available but did not become involved in any decision making

Family supportive behaviors identified by Jacelon (2006) were as follows:

- Keeping the older family members going and active: Families brought items from home, visited daily, and sometimes brought the family pet in for a visit.
- Keeping the older family member's life going: They did many things "behind the scenes" such as running errands, paying bills, keeping up their homes, and keeping friends informed.
- Staying in the background: Some families had family members who were available but not actively involved in daily caregiving.

More specifically, families help their loved ones in the hospital in many ways that enhanced their care in hospitals (MacLeod, Chesson, Blackledge, Hutchison, & Ruta, 2005). Nevertheless, families on medical-surgical units were not seen as partners in patient care in either the United States or the United Kingdom (MacLeod et al., 2005).

Nurses on medical-surgical units are similarly challenged as the nurses in the ICU to provide family-centered care. The floor nurses often carry a heavy nurse-patient caseload. Many of these patients are of high acuity, which challenges these nurses with the same role conflict mentioned earlier: balancing technical needs of their patients and practicing holistic family-centered care. Communication with the family is crucial for the nurses, the patients, and the families so that all parties can work in a partnership to improve the patients' health outcomes.

FAMILY COMMUNICATION NEEDS

Effective communication between and with patients, families, and interdisciplinary health care providers improves client satisfaction, promotes positive response to care, reduces length of stay in care settings, and results in decreased overall cost and resource utilization (Ahrens, Yancey, & Kollef, 2003). Nurses believe that conveying information to families is essential when caring for both acute and chronically ill patients; at the same time, however, they reported refraining from doing so because they do not want to be "in the middle" or cause conflict between the family and the attending physician (Zaforteza, Gastaldo, de Pedro, Sánchez-Cuenca, & Lastra, 2005). They were found to provide basic information and rarely attend to families awaiting news in waiting rooms (Zaforteza et al., 2005).

Nurses identified additional barriers to family communication that included the lack of perceived permission to share information and lack of knowledge regarding what information has already been shared with family members by the physician (Zaforteza et al., 2005). Nurses did not want to contradict physician information and expressed being worried about creating false hopes in the family. Nurses were concerned about families misinterpreting what was said because the nurses lacked training in managing family's emotional responses, especially when the family shared negative emotions. Thus, nurses as part of the interdisciplinary team were found to avoid communication needs of the patients and the families. Rather, nurses focused their communication efforts on the needs of the institution, other health professionals, and themselves (Zaforteza et al., 2005). Nurses must advocate more readily for sharing information with families. Nurses must learn to facilitate patient-family interaction and communication that will increase family support of patients at the bedside (Zaforteza et al., 2005). Clear, concise, timely information has been found to reduce family anxiety and have a calming effect (Zaforteza et al., 2005).

Assessment of patient care needs is integral to nursing and the provision of care at the bedside. It is essential to complete a thorough psychosocial and emotional evaluation to communicate effectively with patients and their families. In particular, nurses should explore family's feelings about the uncertainty of the situation, anxiety, frustration, and fear of losing a family member (Chien, Chiu, Lam, & Ip, 2006; Zaforteza et al., 2005). Clear, concise, timely information has been found to reduce family anxiety and have a calming effect (Zaforteza et al., 2005).

Communicating with families in an empathetic, timely, and sensitive manner is particularly effective to decrease tension, uncertainty, and distress (Zaforteza et al., 2005). Offering systematic, integrated, relevant information provides guidance to family members. Relevant information includes the nature of the illness, prognosis, treatment options, potential complications, care needs after discharge, and alternatives to continued treatment (Nelson, Kinjo, Meier, Ahmad, & Morrison, 2005). In addition, Chien and colleagues (2006) note the importance of communicating specific facts regarding a client's progress and expected outcomes, exploring family feelings including guilt and anger, informing family of what was to be done for the client and why, and providing suggestions to families about actual care they could provide at the bedside to support the patient to help reduce family anxiety (Chien et al., 2006).

Family members find communication from a variety of providers to be worthwhile when health care providers are perceived as sensitive, unhurried, and honest, and as using understandable language (Nelson et al., 2005). Furthermore, follow-up, written verification of information that was shared verbally at patient care conferences was found to be effective in promoting family coping (Kleiber, Davenport, & Freyenberger, 2006; Lautrette et al., 2007). Chien et al. (2006) have determined that conducting a family needs assessment and subsequent systematic education in response to identified issues was an effective means by which to facilitate both patient and family health.

Family-nurse communication is crucial during the hospital stay. Because families are crucial members of the health care team and will be the primary provider of care once the patient leaves the acute setting, addressing the family educational and information needs are critical parts of the discharge process.

FAMILY NEEDS DURING DISCHARGE

Families and patients are excited about leaving the hospital. For some, however, it is a time when anxieties and uncertainties are high; families worry about adding the home caregiver role to their already overburdened load of family responsibilities. For example, families coping with members with traumatic brain injuries reported forgetting what they were taught about what to expect, what resources were available to them, and experienced confusion in the home setting (Paterson, Kieloch, & Gmiterek, 2001). These families actually participated in extensive discharge planning and teaching, yet their severe anxiety inhibited their learning. The families told of not being able to hear the conversations during the care conferences, because they were so worried about how they were going to manage at home. Other families shared that they were so overwhelmed with the complexity of the situation and the health care system, that they could not pay attention in the conferences (Paterson et al., 2001).

Other important factors about these family conferences that hindered family learning were too many people were included, the agenda was too full, and there were time constraints (Paterson et al., 2001). The most important point made was that the health care providers dominated the discussion and allowed little time for the family to voice concerns and pose their questions.

Nurses should be the facilitator at discharge care conferences and help families in the transition to providing caregiving in the home environment. In today's health care scene, families are often caring for very ill family members at home before they are fully recovered and ready to assume their normal family roles (Bjornsdottir, 2002; DesRoches, Blendon, Young, Scoles, & Kim, 2002). Families are providing nursing care at home that is traditionally done by nurses in the hospital, such as assisting with ambulation, transfer, wound care, medication administration, and in some cases, operating high-tech equipment. Hooyman and Gonyea (1999) call this the "Informalization of Health Care."

FAMILY INTERVENTIONS AT DISCHARGE

Family care transition conferences are a valid intervention as long as nurses are aware of the barriers to effective communication during these conferences. Topics to be discussed in these conferences should not focus only on the physical care of the patient, but on ways to assist the family to adjust to having an ill or recuperating family member at home. Ideas to include in this discharge family conference are listed in Box 14-1. Follow-up conversations with

---

BOX 14-1

Addressing Family Needs During Discharge Conference

It is important to talk about the physical care of the family member who is being discharged home and to work with the family about their specific needs. The following points are examples of items to cover with family at discharge:

- Discuss when the family member can be left alone and for how long.
- Help family set up an emergency call system.
- Discuss concerns about modifying the home environment.
- Facilitate setting up a family routine of care.
- Be sure the family knows when to call for help.
- Help family learn to handle visitors, especially children.
- Talk about the balance of sleep and rest for the family caregivers.
- Provide names and numbers for personnel in the billing department for the family to call when they start to receive insurance forms and hospital bills.

---

families indicate that discharge by a nurse who has been trained in transition care helps support families (Coleman, Smith, Frank, Min, Parry, & Kramer, 2004). A 24-hour help line, postdischarge group sessions, and written information were all found to help families adjust to their new situation and roles as family caregivers (Paterson et al., 2001).

End-of-Life Family Care in the Hospital

A different type of transition that occurs in the hospital is from life to the death of a loved one. Regardless of whether the death occurs in the ICU, the emergency department, or on the medical-surgical unit, families are changed by the death of a family member.

Compassionate communication provides crucial care to families as they are asked to make multiple decisions during the dying of their loved ones in the hospital. The more the nurse knows about the family, the better, because the way a family deals with death is affected by cultural background, stage in the family life cycle, values and beliefs, the nature of the illness, whether the loss is sudden or expected, the role played by the dying person in the family, and the emotional functioning of the family before the illness (Artinian, 2005).

Meeting the family needs during the active dying process helps families prepare for their immediate experience. Providing for privacy allows families emotional and physical intimacy. Of utmost concern to family members is to be reassured that the nurse is keeping their loved one comfortable, as pain free as possible, and is continuing to provide comfort nursing care (Artinian, 2005). Keeping the family informed through anticipatory guidance of the physical signs and symptoms they are likely to see is important. Giving family members the option to be present or excused during the actual death is compassionate caring. Ask the family members whether they have any special spiritual or religious rituals and ceremonies that need to be conducted at this time. Most hospitals have various religious services available that can be called in to help the dying patient and their family.

After the death, it is important to allow enough time for questions, allow the family the opportunity to view the body, and describe the events at the time of death (Artinian, 2005). Offering families the choice to participate in after-life preparations, such as bathing the body, is providing culturally sensitive care.

Caring for families when a member is dying is not easy. It is challenging for nurses to help families cope. Rarely do nurses in most medical-surgical units feel comfortable and confident discussing death with patients or families. Several issues are especially difficult for nurses and families: discussions of advance directives, withdrawing or withholding life-sustaining therapies (LSTs), family presence during CPR efforts, and talking with families about organ donation.

ADVANCE DIRECTIVES

The Patient Self-Determination Act was passed in 1991 in the United States requiring hospitals to ensure that patients have been informed of their right to decide on life-preserving measures (Artinian, 2005). This legislation stimulated a host of other documents about end-of-life choices, such as living wills, durable power of attorney for health care, do not resuscitate (DNR) orders, and health care proxies. Despite these efforts, the actual completion rate of such directives among the American population

remains low, with an average completion rate of 20% (Duke, Thompson, & Hastie, 2007).

The barriers to completion that have been identified by individuals and families include lack of knowledge, confusing language, complexity of process, and procrastination until it was too late (Butterworth, 2003). Of those individuals who completed advance directives, they reported doing so because they did not want to be a burden on their family at the time of death and because they had significant health problems over which they wanted to exercise some control (Duke et al., 2007). A signed advance directive implies that families have engaged in discussions about end-of-life choices. These families reported experiencing less of a burden when faced with making end-of-life decisions (Kaufman, 2002).

It is the role of the nurse to talk with families about advance directives. Nurses in the emergency department have expressed that they need more education about the state laws that govern advance directives and both legal and ethical issues of advance directives (Jezewski, Meeker, & Robillard, 2005).

FAMILY PRESENCE DURING CARDIOPULMONARY RESUSCITATION

For many years it was standard practice of both ICUs and emergency departments that family members be removed from the bedside during periods of cardiac arrest, and emergent and invasive procedures. That trend is gradually changing. An increasing number of critical care units and emergency departments allow family members to stay at the patient's bedside no matter what, without putting pressure on the family. This changing trend is due in large part to the work of clinical researchers who have found that family presence does not disrupt patient care and results in positive outcomes for both family members and patients (Tweibell et al., 2008). The Emergency Nurses Association (2005) and the American Association of Critical Care Nurses (2004) have issued position papers calling for the establishment of written hospital policies and standards allowing for the option of family presence during invasive and resuscitation procedures in critical care units.

If family members wish to remain at or return to the bedside while resuscitation efforts are still ongoing, nurses can counsel and coach families members, so that each person can anticipate exactly what they will see and hear (MacLean et al., 2003). Normally, every effort is made to allow family members to be physically close to their loved one, so they can speak into an ear, as well as touch them. Careful and often repeated explanations are necessary by the health care providers, because these are stressful and busy times for all present. Nurses need to be continually assessing how family members are coping and be prepared to intervene as necessary. Recent research demonstrated that nurses are learning to provide more information and comfort to families and patients during times of invasive procedures, including resuscitation efforts (MacLean et al., 2003; Rushton et al., 2007).

FAMILY INVOLVEMENT IN DO NOT RESUSCITATE ORDERS

Handy, Sulmasy, Merkel, and Ury (2008) investigated the experience of surrogate decision makers who are involved in authorizing DNR orders. They described this experience as a process and a cascade of decisions and negotiations, not just making a single decision not to resuscitate. One of the essential elements of this process was honest, sensitive, ongoing communication with the health care team. The surrogates reported a dichotomy of emotions about feeling guilty if they authorized the order and guilty if they did not authorize the order. In the end, the surrogates reported that knowing they were alleviating their loved ones pain was crucial in their decision making. Patients who have family members involved in their care in the hospital were found to be more likely to have a DNR order written (Tschann, Kaufman, & Micco, 2003). The decision process of determining to authorize a DNR order has some similarity to the family decision whether to withdraw or withhold LSTs.

FAMILY EXPERIENCES OF WITHDRAWING OR WITHHOLDING LIFE-SUSTAINING THERAPIES

Families are intricately involved in the decisions to withdraw or withhold LSTs. These types of decisions are complex and occur in phases (Tilden, Tolle, Nelson, & Fields, 2001). The four phases that Tilden and colleagues identified were: (1) recognition of futility, (2) coming to terms, (3) shouldering the surrogate role, and (4) facing the question to withdraw or not withdraw LSTs. Factors that influenced families

to withdraw LSTs were LSTs that were explained and discussed with the families, poor quality of life, poor overall prognosis, and current level of the family members' suffering (Wiegand, 2006). It was noted that, in families where there was a signed advanced directive of some type or where previous conversations occurred about end-of-life choices, this difficult family decision was less of a burden.

Wiegand, Deatrick, and Knafl (2008) have conducted research to describe the different family management styles when faced with making decisions about withdrawing or withholding LSTs. The five family management styles described are progressing, accommodating, maintaining, struggling, and floundering. Families were found to be different in the following areas:

- Their level of understanding of the severity of their loved one's illness
- Their level of hope for recovery
- The tense (past, present, or future) with which they talked about their family member
- Their willingness to engage in a discussion about possibly withdrawing LSTs
- The overall family communication
- The prevalence of facts or emotions in making the decision
- Their actual decision to withdraw LSTs

Table 14-2 shows how families differ in their approach and way of making this crucial family decision. Culture has also been shown to influence family consideration of withdrawing LSTs. For example, African Americans are more likely to continue futile therapies (Hopp & Duffy, 2000).

Family presence during CPR influences decisions to withdraw LST. Tschann, Kaufman, and Micco (2003) compared the prevalence of decisions to withdraw LSTs when families were present and when families were not involved in care. Over a set period of time where withdrawal was considered by the health care team to be appropriate, they found that patients were more likely to be removed from mechanical ventilation if the family was present than if the family was not present. Patients were more inclined to receive narcotics when their families were involved and present during the dying process. In these situations, families work collaboratively with the health care team to determine when and how to withdraw LSTs.

Hsieh, Shannon, and Curtis (2006) analyzed 51 family conferences with the health care team in the

TABLE 14-2

Family Management Styles for Family Decision to Withholding Life-Sustaining Therapies

FAMILY MANAGEMENT STYLE	SEVERITY OF CONDITION UNDERSTOOD	HOPE OF RECOVERY	VERB TENSE USED TO TALK ABOUT FAMILY MEMBER	WILLINGNESS TO ENGAGE IN DISCUSSION OF WITHDRAWAL	FAMILY COMMUNICATION	PRIMARY FACTORS USED IN DECISION MAKING	FAMILY MADE THE DECISION TO SUSTAIN TREATMENTS
Progressing family type	Yes	No/minimal	More past tense used	Willing	Good communication with each other and extended family	Mostly used facts and supported wishes of family member	Planned date and time of withdrawal
Accommodating family type	Yes	No/minimal	More past tense used	Somewhat willing	Fairly good communication	Mostly facts used, mixed with some emotions	Yes, with little-to-moderate conflict
Maintaining family type	Yes	Very hopeful of recovery	Present and past tense used	Undecided	Varied communication, good at times and not good at times	Mixed some facts with emotions	Yes, with moderate-to-extreme difficulty
Struggling family type	Uncertain if understood	Very hopeful of recovery	Present tense used	Not willing	Most family conflict of all styles	Mostly emotions	Some unable to decide, family not in agreement
Floundering family type	No	Believe full recovery was going to happen	Present and future tense used	Not willing	Little family discussion with each other	Emotions only and not follow family members wishes	Decided when dying was active and made with extreme family conflict

Source: From Wiegand, D. L., Deatrick, J.A., & Knafl, K. (2008). Family management styles related to withdrawal of life-sustaining therapy from adults who are acutely ill or injured. *Journal of Family Nursing, 14*(1), 16–32, by permission.

decision-making process to withdraw LSTs. Their insight into this emotional process for these families offers nurses ideas about how to help support families during this difficult time. They identify five contradictory arguments that families often talked about during these family conferences:

- If the family believed that their decision to remove LSTs was actually killing their loved one versus allowing them to die a natural death
- If their decision was viewed as a benefit by alleviating suffering or a burden on the family
- If they were honoring their loved ones end-of-life choices or following their own personal wishes
- If the ill family member expressed several differing end-of-life choices, the family had to work through which one to follow
- Determining whether one family member would be responsible for making the final decision or the family as a whole would make the decision

Regardless of which of these contradictions families discussed during the conference, information-seeking strategies used by the health care team members were found to facilitate these difficult emotional discussions positively. Some of these information-seeking strategies were to acknowledge the contradiction, clarify views, recenter the discussion on the similarity of their desires to help their loved one, and reaffirm their choices.

Once a family decision has been reached to withdraw LSTs, nurses work closely with families to guide them through this difficult procedure. A trusting nurse-family relationship is crucial to the family (Wiegand, 2006). The following nursing actions help prepare the family (Kirchhoff, Palzkill, Kowalkowski, Mork, & Gretarsdottir, 2008):

- Tell the family that the exact time of death cannot be anticipated, but that the nurse will be constantly monitoring the situation and inform them when death appears more imminent.
- Assure the family that the nurse will continue to provide compassionate comfort care.
- Give each family member a choice to watch the actual withdrawal of the therapies.
- Provide for physical and emotional intimacy needs of the family.
- Inform the family of expected signs and symptoms they may see during the active dying process.

- Encourage or give permission for the family to hold, touch, caress, lie with, talk to, and show emotion to the dying family member.

Nurses have been found to be confident in their abilities to talk with families during the process of deciding to withdraw LSTs, authorizing DNR orders, and supporting families during these difficult times (Sulmasy, He, McAuley, & Ury, 2008).

Nurses need to make every effort to keep families involved and informed as death approaches. Providing the ideal level of privacy is not always possible in ICU environments, but every effort needs to be made to allow for families to be with their loved ones, and to remain with their hospitalized family members in a private, unhurried, and quiet environment. Many families and cultures have rituals or spiritual beliefs and procedures that need to be honored. Resources such as Chaplaincy Services and Social Work can offer assistance, especially when death is anticipated. Nurse managers need to relieve bedside nurses from responsibilities of caring for other patients, so that they can remain with families and patients who are dying.

Clarifying information and explanations after physicians have talked with families is an important nursing responsibility. Some family members may wish to participate in postmortem care because this may offer comfort to them. Refer to Chapter 11 for an extensive discussion of family needs at the time of death. Once families and deceased patients have left the hospital unit, it becomes the role of nurse managers to assess the timing and need for debriefing the nursing staff, especially when the patient had a long-term ICU stay, or a particularly complex family situation existed (Maxwell et al., 2007). Simple things such as accompanying families to their car when they leave the hospital helps provide closure for the family and physically supports the family while they transition to their life without their loved one. The Howe family case study (see later) demonstrates family nursing-centered care in the hospital.

OFFERING THE OPTION OF ORGAN DONATION

The number of people who need organs far exceeds the number of donors. In May 2009, in the United States, 110,462 people were waiting for a donor organ (Organ Donor, 2009). It has been shown that when the family knows of a loved ones intent to donate their organs, they have higher rates of donation than when the family is not aware of the loved ones intent to donate organs (Smith, Lindsey, Kopfman, Yoo, & Morrison, 2008).

Discussing organ donation with a family whose loved one has suddenly died or with whom the decision has been made to withdraw LSTs is difficult. The discussion about organ donation should take place separately from the notification of the family member's death, and it should be done by someone who has been specifically trained in asking for organ and tissue donation (Artinian, 2005). Federal regulations now stipulate that hospitals are required to contact their local Organ Procurement Organization (OPC) concerning any death or impending death (Truog et al., 2001). Once contacted, the OPC sends a representative, or a local hospital representative will approach the family at the appropriate time about the option of organ donation and answer all their questions.

If organ donation is viewed as a consoling act, then the option to elect organ donation is easier for the family (Artinian, 2005). Organ donation benefits the donor family, as well as the recipients and their families. Perceiving that organ donation can help someone else live, that functioning organs are not wasted, that something positive can come out of death, or that a family member can live on in someone else through donation helps families cope with their loss (Artinian, 2005).

Many families worry that donation is disfiguring or will delay the funeral, but neither of these worries is valid. The body is not disfigured in the process of removing the organs. If the body parts that are removed have the potential to disfigure the person, then replacement plastic or wooden parts are inserted in the place of those removed so that the person is not disfigured. The organ donation team has a rapid response; therefore, the funeral arrangements are not delayed.

The donor family does not pay for the medical expenses once death has been declared; the costs are paid by the OPC and the recipients. The donor family receives a letter from the OPC informing them of the number of people who received organs from their family members. After time, the donor family can contact the OPC to find out whether the recipient of the organs is interested in corresponding and meeting.

Family Case Study

This case study presents a family dealing with an acute exacerbation of a longstanding chronic illness and hospitalization of one of its members. The Family Assessment and Intervention Model is used as the theoretical approach to the Howe family (refer to Chapter 3 for specific details of this family nursing theory and model). The Howe family genogram and ecomap are presented in Figures 14-1 and 14-2, respectively.

Glenn Howe, a 64-year-old married white male, had his first major myocardial infarction at the age of 41. Since that time, he dutifully embraced numerous lifestyle changes including smoking cessation, diet modifications, and the establishment of a regular exercise regimen. In addition, he took numerous cardiovascular medications to control his blood pressure and enhance his cardiac function. Despite his adherence to his chronic disease management program, Glenn's cardiovascular disease worsened, and he underwent coronary artery bypass surgery 10 years ago. Initial results of the surgery were positive, and Glenn continued to manage his chronic illness well. Recently, however, he experienced another small myocardial infarction, after which his cardiac function declined drastically. His medications were increased, his lifestyle modifications were severe, and his hopes for recovery were dashed.

Glenn's immediate family consists of his wife, Jane, three children—Anne, age 37, Janet, age 35, and Bill, age 32—and six young grandchildren. Glenn is currently retired while Jane continues to work as a special education teacher. All family members are upper middle class and attend the Episcopal Church regularly. All family members are geographically and emotionally close to Glenn, and are quite concerned that he may not survive much longer. Since his first myocardial infarction, the family members have lived their lives in a state of anticipation, feeling as if their time with Glenn is likely to be limited, as if they are on "borrowed time." The benefits of this feeling of anticipation included numerous family vacations, all holidays together, and every chance to be together viewed as special. After Glenn's most recent decline in cardiac function, the family experienced a heightened sense of preciousness, wanting to spend as much time as possible together and wanting every moment with Glenn to be perfect.

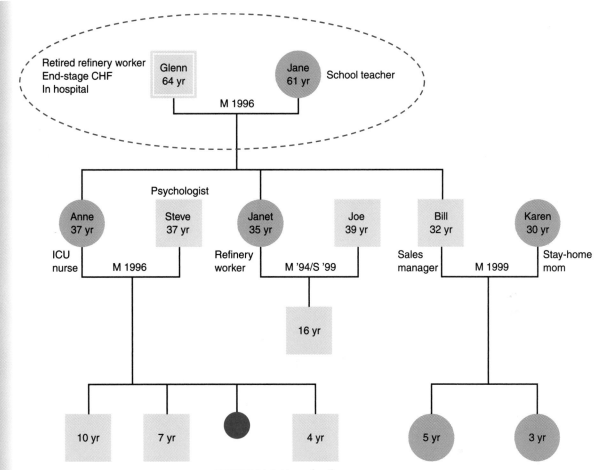

FIGURE 14-1 Howe family genogram.

Before his first myocardial infarction, Glenn was a healthy, robust, active man with many interests and hobbies. After his cardiac surgery, many of his hobbies, including golf, fell by the wayside. He became increasingly short of breath with exertion and resorted to armchair hobbies, such as coin collecting, crossword puzzles, and world history. Family activities changed as well. Family vacations necessarily became sedate and wheelchair oriented, rather than activity-oriented hiking, fishing, and camping trips. The family endeavored, however, to have at least one very special trip every year, the last being a trip to Disney World with Glenn in a wheelchair and a cruise that required very little exertion.

Glenn became more and more debilitated. His cardiac function was so poor he could not eat without becoming short of breath and tachycardic. His appetite decreased dramatically, and he lost more than 60 pounds. He began to suffer from orthopnea and often tried to sleep upright in his recliner all night. As he and Jane tried to cope with his acute and chronic health care needs, their relationship changed. She became a full-time caretaker, trying anything she could to get him to eat and to make him comfortable. A normally unflappable individual, she found herself expressing her frustration at his refusal to eat more than a few bites at a time. Her outburst was distressing to her and her children as it was so out of character. Glenn, usually a more demanding individual, became compliant and resigned as his health deteriorated. The children became hypervigilant and attentive to their parents, making frequent visits on weekends and calling every day. Family roles changed as the stressors affecting the family intensified.

Glenn had been hospitalized on numerous occasions, and he approached the impending admission to a medical-surgical unit with his usual calm and trust in

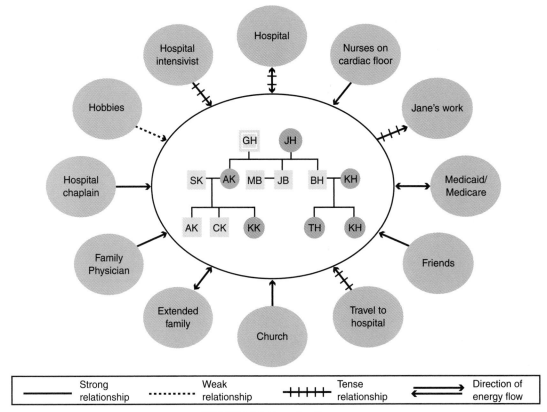

Strong relationship	Weak relationship	Tense relationship	Direction of energy flow

FIGURE 14-2 Howe family ecomap.

his caregivers. He was being admitted for tests because his ventricular function was decreased, his weight decreased from 200 to 140 pounds, and his urine output was declining. He called his oldest daughter, Anne, a cardiovascular intensive care nurse, the morning of his scheduled admission and asked her to meet him at the hospital. She replied that she must travel out of town for an important meeting but would drive up later that night and be with him for the tests the next day. The other children counted on the oldest child to take care of health care needs, and given her education and experience, it was a role she gladly assumed.

Given the chronic nature of Glenn's cardiovascular disease and the life-threatening potential for acute exacerbations requiring frequent hospitalizations, Jane and Glenn had discussed advance directives openly and honestly. Jane was well aware that Glenn did not wish any heroic measures, especially CPR. He felt his two cardiac surgeries were trauma enough and that his heart condition was irreparable. Jane was terrified of losing her husband, best friend, and companion, and was very concerned about having to make the decision that would honor Glenn's wishes.

During this hospital stay, Glenn and Jane renewed their close and trusting relationship with the nurses at their small community hospital. While awaiting his tests and the arrival of their daughters, Glenn experienced a lapse in consciousness with Jane at his bedside. Jane called for help, and two nurses entered the room and quickly assessed the situation. Glenn was in full cardiac arrest. One of the nurses turned to Jane and said, "Do you want us to bring him back? We can bring him back." Jane hesitated, then shook her head no. The nurse asked again, "Are you sure? Do you want us to bring him back?" Once again, Jane answered, "No." She immediately realized the consequences of her decision to deny CPR. Glenn, her husband of 45 years was gone, her children did not expect this hospitalization to result in his death, and she was alone at his bedside.

Jane experienced regret for her decision not to "bring him back." Her decision was so very final. She also regretted the times that she had felt frustrated at his disinterest in eating and his hobbies. Though never an angry person, she had experienced anger at her husband on more than one occasion. The children all felt a measure of guilt as well: Anne for going to a meeting instead of being with her dad, Janet for being at work instead of at her dad's bedside, and Bill for living so far away. Everyone wished they had more time together as a family.

Jane became a grieving widow, very dependent, sad, and indecisive—a person her children barely recognized. At a time when they needed a strong,

supportive mother, that person was absent. The individuals best able to provide support to Jane and her children were the grandchildren and spouses. Having never experienced the death of someone so dear to them, all family members struggled with daily life for several weeks after Glenn's death.

FAMILY ASSESSMENT AND INTERVENTION MODEL AND THE FAMILY SYSTEMS STRESSOR-STRENGTH INVENTORY APPLIED TO THE HOWE FAMILY

The Family Systems Stressor-Strength Inventory (FS³I) was used to assess stressors (problems) and the strengths (resources) that the Howe family had in coping with their situation soon after Glenn's admission to the medical-surgical unit. The patient and his wife, Glenn and Jane, were interviewed together by the nurse, but they each completed their own FS³I. Both Glenn's and Jane's individual scores were tallied using the scoring guide for the FS³I. Anne, the eldest daughter (37 years old), Jan, the middle child (35 years old), and Bill (32 years old) were all present, and all completed the assessment instrument (FS³I).

The general stressors were viewed similarly by both Glenn and Jane, and these stressors were assessed as slightly less serious by the nurse than by the couple. Glenn, Jane, and the nurse concurred that the general stress level was high, which was consistent with their experience. The specific stressors were perceived slightly different by Glenn and Jane. Figures 14-3 through 14-7 summarize the information gained from the Howe family: (1) Figure 14-3 presents their FS³Is; (2) Figure 14-4 provides the Howe family Quantitative Summary of Family Systems Stressors Form: General and Specific; (3) Figure 14-5 lists the Howe family and clinician summary on family strength; (4) Figure 14-6 shows the Howe family Qualitative Summary and Clinician Remarks; (5) and Figure 14-7 presents the Howe Family Care Plan.

The Qualitative Summary Family and Clinician Remarks form in Figure 14-6 serves as the groundwork for the Family Care Plan in Figure 14-7. This form synthesizes information pertaining to general stressors, specific stressors, family strengths, and the overall functioning and physical and mental health of the family members. The nurse completed

this form using her assessment skills with information obtained from the conversation with the family and the data obtained from the written FS³I.

The family members and the nurse perceived that the worsening of Glenn's physical condition because of his chronic heart disease was the major general stressor. Glenn's specific stressors included his growing inability to function as a husband, father, and grandfather, as well as a fear of the unknown. Specific stressors for Jane included concerns regarding the financial impact of Glenn's illness and her inability to provide care for Glenn. The strengths of the family were seen as communication between all family members, religious faith, and the availability of a supportive health care team. The overall family functioning was considered to be as good as could be expected under the circumstances. Whereas Glenn's physical health was compromised, Jane's physical health was good. Both Glenn and Jane expressed mental health concerns, including anxiety, guilt, depression, and fear of the unknown.

Overall, the family members had similar perceptions of their stressors and strengths, and the nurse concurred with their perceptions, although the nurse rated both stressors and strengths lower than the family members. The nurse perceived that the family had the strengths they needed to deal with both the general and specific stressors present when Glenn was hospitalized.

The Howe Family Care Plan (see Fig. 14-7) was developed by the nurse in collaboration with the family members who completed the FS³I. The Family Care Plan includes the Diagnosis of General/ Specific Family Systems Stressors & Family Systems Strengths supporting the Family Care Plan and the Goals of the Family, Primary, Secondary, and Tertiary Interventions and Outcomes/Evaluation. The goals of this Family Care Plan included restoring stable cardiac status sufficient to return home from the hospital, and that all family members will continue to support Glenn and each other.

INSTRUCTIONS FOR ADMINISTRATION

The Family Systems Stressor-Strength Inventory (FS³I) is an assessment and measurement instrument intended for use with families. It focuses on identifying stressful situations occurring in families and the strengths families use to maintain healthy family functioning. Each family member is asked to complete the instrument on an individual form before an interview with the clinician. Questions can be read to members unable to read.

After completion of the instrument, the clinician evaluates the family on each of the stressful situations (general and specific) and the strengths they possess. This evaluation is recorded on the family member form.

The clinician records the individual family member's score and the clinician perception score on the Quantitative Summary. A different color code is used for each family member. The clinician also completes the Qualitative Summary, synthesizing the information gleaned from all participants. Clinicians can use the Family Care Plan to prioritize diagnoses, set goals, develop prevention and intervention activities, and evaluate outcomes.

Family Name _Howe_   **Date** _6/10/08_

Family Member(s) Completing Assessment _Glenn, Jane, Anne_

Ethnic Background(s) _Caucasian-German-English_

Religious Background(s) _Protestant_

Referral Source _Family Physician_

Interviewer _CCU RN_

Family Members	Relationship in Family	Age	Marital Status	Education (highest degree)	Occupation
1. _Glenn_	_Father_	_64_	_Married_	_BS_	_Refinery Worker_
2. _Jane_	_Mother_	_61_	_Married_	_MA_	_Teacher_
3. _Anne_	_Daughter_	_37_	_Married_	_BSN_	_RN_
4. _Janet_	_Daughter_	_35_	_Divorced_	_AA_	_Refinery Worker_
5. _Bill_	_Son_	_32_	_Married_	_PhD_	_Psychologise_
6. _____	_____	___	_____	___	_____

Family's current reasons for seeking assistance:

Glenn's heart disease is worsening, requiring sudden hospitalization for stabilization

Source: Hanson, S. M. H. (2001). *Family health care nursing: Theory, practice, and research* (2nd ed.), pp. 425–437. Philadelphia: F.A. Davis.

FIGURE 14-3 Summary for Howe case study on Introduction Form for the Family Systems Stressor-Strength Inventory.

Part I: Family Systems Stressors (General)

DIRECTIONS: Each of 25 situations/stressors listed here deals with some aspect of normal family life. They have the potential for creating stress within families or between families and the world in which they live. We are interested in your overall impression of how these situations affect your family life. Please circle a number (0 through 5) that best describes the amount of stress or tension they create for you.

STRESSORS	DOES NOT APPLY	LITTLE STRESS		MEDIUM STRESS		HIGH STRESS	CLINICIAN PERCEPTION SCORE
1. Family member(s) feel unappreciated	0	①	2	3	4	5	1
2. Guilt for not accomplishing more	0	1	2	3	4	⑤	4
3. Insufficient "me" time	0	1	2	3	4	⑤	4
4. Self-Image/self-esteem/ feelings of unattractiveness	0	1	2	3	④	5	3
5. Perfectionism	0	1	2	3	④	5	3
6. Dieting	0	①	2	3	4	5	1
7. Health/Illness	0	1	2	3	4	⑤	4
8. Communication with children	0	1	2	3	④	5	4
9. Housekeeping standards	0	1	2	③	4	5	4
10. Insufficient couple time	0	1	2	3	④	5	3
11. Insufficient family playtime	0	1	2	3	4	⑤	4
12. Children's behavior/discipline/ sibling fighting	⓪	1	2	3	4	5	1
13. Television	0	①	2	3	4	5	1
14. Overscheduled family calendar	0	1	2	③	4	5	3
15. Lack of shared responsibility in the family	0	1	2	3	4	⑤	5
16. Moving	⓪	1	2	3	4	5	0
17. Spousal relationship (communication, friendship, sex)	0	1	2	3	4	⑤	4
18. Holidays	⓪	1	2	3	4	5	0
19. In-laws	⓪	1	2	3	4	5	0
20. Teen behaviors (communication, music, friends, school)	⓪	1	2	3	4	5	0
21. New baby	⓪	1	2	3	4	5	0
22. Economics/finances/budgets	0	1	2	3	4	⑤	5
23. Unhappiness with work situation	0	1	2	3	④	5	4
24. Overvolunteerism	⓪	1	2	3	4	5	0
25. Neighbors	0	1	②	3	4	5	2
		$66 \div 18 = 3.6$					$60 \div 18 = 3.3$

FAMILY PERCEPTION SCORE

FIGURE 14-3—cont'd

Additional Stressors: _Uncertainty about the future, spiritual issues_

Family Remarks: _Feeling a sense of urgency related to Glenn's physical condition_

Clinician: Clarification of stressful situations/concerns with family members.

Prioritize in order of importance to family members: _Impact of physical illness on all family activities and interactions_

Part II: Family Systems Stressors (Specific)

DIRECTIONS: The following 12 questions are designed to provide information about your specific stress-producing situation/problem or area of concern influencing your family's health. Please circle a number (1 through 5) that best describes the influence this situation has on your family's life and how well you perceive your family's overall functioning.

The specific stress-producing situation/problem or area of concern at this time is: _Glenn's worsening physical condition, uncertain future and inability to maintain usual family activities_

STRESSORS	FAMILY PERCEPTION SCORE			CLINICIAN PERCEPTION SCORE
	LITTLE	MEDIUM	HIGH	SCORE
1. To what extent is your family bothered by this problem or stressful situation? (e.g., effects on family interactions, communication among members, emotional and social relationships)	1 2 3 4		⑤	_5_

Family Remarks: _"This is huge for our family." "We love Grandpa — we want him to get better."_

Clinician Remarks: _All family members affected by Glenn's physical condition._

2. How much of an effect does this stresssful situation have on your family's usual pattern of living? (e.g., effects on lifestyle patterns and family developmental task)	1 2 3 4		⑤	_5_

Family Remarks: _"We haven't been able to vacation together this year."_

Clinician Remarks: _Normal family activities severely limited by Glenn's illness_

FIGURE 14-3—cont'd

STRESSORS	LITTLE	FAMILY PERCEPTION SCORE			CLINICIAN PERCEPTION SCORE
		MEDIUM	HIGH		

3. How much has this situation affected your family's ability to work together as a family unit? (e.g., alteration in family roles, completion of family tasks, following through with responsibilities)   1   2   3   ④   5   <u>   4   </u>

Family Remarks: <u>"Dad cannot do anything anymore – Mom has to do everything"</u>

Clinician Remarks: <u>All family members helpful to Glenn and Jane</u>

Has your family ever experienced a similar concern in the past?
   YES   If YES, complete question 4
   (NO)   If NO, complete question 5

4. How successful was your family in dealing with this situation/problem/concern in the past? (e.g., workable coping strategies developed, adaptive measures useful, situation improved)   1   2   3   4   5   <u>   </u>

Family Remarks: <u>No experience, with critical illness "Nothing like this has ever happened to us"</u>

Clinician Remarks: <u>New territory for this family.</u>

5. How strongly do you feel this current situation/ problem/concern will affect your family's future? (e.g., anticipated consequences)   1   2   3   4   ⑤   <u>   4   </u>

Family Remarks: <u>Impending loss of head of family will be devastating to entire family</u>

Clinician Remarks: <u>Openly discussing future and ways to be together now</u>

6. To what extent are family members able to help themselves in this present situation/ problem/ concern? (e.g., self-assistive efforts, family expectations, spiritual influence, family resources)   1   2   3   ④   5   <u>   4   </u>

Family Remarks: <u>Rely heavily on one another, friends, clergy and health care-workers</u>

Clinician Remarks: <u>Well informed, knowledgeable, eager to provide care</u>

FIGURE 14-3—cont'd

STRESSORS	FAMILY PERCEPTION SCORE			CLINICIAN PERCEPTION
	LITTLE	MEDIUM	HIGH	SCORE
7. To what extent do you expect others to help your family with this situation/problem/concern? (e.g., what roles would helpers play; how available are extra-family resources)	1 2	3 ④	5	3

Family Remarks: _Neighbors, co-workers, and health care personnel_

Clinician Remarks: _Very trusting, open and cooperative with visitors and nurses_

STRESSORS	POOR	SATISFACTORY	EXCELLENT	SCORE
8. How would you rate the way your family functions overall? (e.g., how your family members relate to each other and to larger family and community)	1 2	3 ④	5	4

Family Remarks: _Recent worsening of physical problems has frightened family members_

Clinician Remarks: _Anxious, asking frequent questions regarding prognosis_

9. How would you rate the overall physical health status of each family member by name?
(Include yourself as a family member; record additional names on back.)

	POOR				EXCELLENT	SCORE
a. _Glenn_	①	2	3	4	5	1
b. _Jane_	1	2	3	④	5	4
c. _Anne_	1	2	3	4	⑤	5
d. _Janet_	1	2	3	④	5	5
e. _Bill_	1	2	3	4	⑤	5

10. How would you rate the overall physical health status of your family as a whole?	1 2 3 ④ 5	4

Family Remarks: _Glenn's deteriorating health is affecting the activities of the entire family_

Clinician Remarks: _Healthy family members are curtailing their usual activities due to Glenn's illness_

11. How would you rate the overall mental health status of each family member by name? (Include yourself as a family member; record additional names on back.)

						SCORE
a. _Glenn_	1	②	3	4	5	2
b. _Jane_	1	2	③	4	5	4
c. _Anne_	1	2	3	④	5	4
d. _Janet_	1	2	③	4	5	3
e. _Bill_	1	2	3	④	5	3

FIGURE 14-3—cont'd

STRESSORS	FAMILY PERCEPTION SCORE					CLINICIAN PERCEPTION SCORE
	LITTLE		MEDIUM	HIGH		
12. How would you rate the overall mental health status of your family as a whole?	1	2	③	4	5	3

Family Remarks: _Glenn is feeling guilty, both Glenn and Jane are anxious, Janet is depressed_

Clinician Remarks: _Glenn's anxiety & fear of the unknown is affecting the entire family_

Glenn 3.6   Clinician 3.3

Part III: Family Systems Strengths

DIRECTIONS: Each of the 16 traits/attributes listed below deals with some aspect of family life and its overall functioning. Each one contributes to the health and well-being of family members as individuals and to the family as a whole. Please circle a number (0 through 5) that best describes the extent to which the trait applies to your family.

MY FAMILY	FAMILY PERCEPTION SCORE						CLINICIAN PERCEPTION SCORE
	DOES NOT APPLY	SELDOM		USUALLY	ALWAYS		SCORE
1. Communicates and listens to one another	0	1	2	3	④	5	5

Family Remarks: _All family members feel they are communicating openly about everything except Glenn's health_

Clinician Remarks: _Need to talk more about Glenn's prognosis and future financial concerns_

2. Affirms and supports one another	0	1	2	3	4	⑤	4

Family Remarks: _All members feel supported especially by Jane_

Clinician Remarks: _Very supportive family_

3. Teaches respect for others	0	1	2	3	4	⑤	4

Family Remarks: _Very respectful of one another_

Clinician Remarks: _Respectful of health care team_

FIGURE 14-3—cont'd

MY FAMILY	DOES NOT APPLY	SELDOM		USUALLY	ALWAYS	CLINICIAN PERCEPTION SCORE
				FAMILY PERCEPTION SCORE		
4. Develops a sense of trust in members	0	1	2	3	4	⑤	4

4. Develops a sense
   of trust in members   0   1   2   3   4   ⑤   4

Family Remarks: _Trust each other and the health care team_

Clinician Remarks: _Work very well with nurses and health care workers_

5. Displays a sense
   of play and humor   0   1   2   3   ④   5   3

Family Remarks: _Less often now as very anxious about Glenn's health_

Clinician Remarks: _Rarely demonstrated_

6. Exhibits a sense of
   shared responsibility   0   1   2   3   ④   5   4

Family Remarks: _Depend on one another_

Clinician Remarks: _Take turns at the bedside_

7. Teaches a sense of
   right and wrong   0   1   2   3   4   ⑤   4

Family Remarks: _"Of course!"_

Clinician Remarks:

8. Has a strong sense of
   family in which rituals and
   traditions abound   0   1   2   ③   4   5   3

Family Remarks: _Holidays very important missing the opportunity for family dinners_

Clinician Remarks:

FIGURE 14-3—cont'd

			FAMILY PERCEPTION SCORE			CLINICIAN PERCEPTION
MY FAMILY	DOES NOT APPLY	SELDOM		USUALLY	ALWAYS	SCORE

9. Has a balance of interaction among members

| | 0 | 1 | 2 | 3 | ④ | 5 | 3 |

Family Remarks: _Balanced responsibilities overall though all very interactive with Jane_

Clinician Remarks: _Anne appears to take the lead interacting with nurses and physicians_

10. Has a shared religious core

| | 0 | 1 | 2 | 3 | ④ | 5 | 3 |

Family Remarks: _Regular church attenders_

Clinician Remarks:

11. Respects the privacy of one another

| | 0 | 1 | 2 | 3 | ④ | 5 | 4 |

Family Remarks: _Not a problem_

Clinician Remarks: _Not observed to be an issued_

12. Values service to others

| | 0 | 1 | 2 | 3 | 4 | ⑤ | 4 |

Family Remarks: _Most in helping professions_

Clinician Remarks: _Very helpful and appreciative of nursing care provided._

13. Fosters family table time and conversation

| | 0 | 1 | 2 | 3 | ④ | 5 | 4 |

Family Remarks: _Missing those opportunities_

Clinician Remarks: _Hospital cafeteria offers some together time_

14. Shares leisure time

| | 0 | 1 | 2 | 3 | 4 | ⑤ | 4 |

Family Remarks: _Usually spend all vacations together_

Clinician Remarks: _Seem to enjoy one another_

FIGURE 14-3—cont'd

MY FAMILY	DOES NOT APPLY	SELDOM	FAMILY PERCEPTION SCORE	USUALLY		ALWAYS	CLINICIAN PERCEPTION SCORE
15. Admits to and seeks help with problems	0	1	2	3	(4)	5	5

Family Remarks: *Rely on family physician and nurses*

Clinician Remarks: *Back help appropriately*

16a. How would you rate the overall strengths that exist in your family?	0	1	2	3	(4)	5	4

Family Remarks: *Excellent, though tested at the moment*

Clinician Remarks: *Very strong*

16b. Additional Family Strengths: *Love and enjoyment of grandchildren*

16c. Clinician: Clarification of family strengths with individual members:

Anne - RN

Bill - Psychologist

FIGURE 14-3—cont'd

Family Systems Stressor-Strength inventory (FS³I) Scoring Summary
Section 1: Family Perception Scores

INSTRUCTIONS FOR ADMINISTRATION

The Family Systems Stressor-Strength Inventory (FS³I) Scoring Summary is divided into two sections: Section 1, Family Perception Scores, and Section 2, Clinician Perception Scores. These two sections are further divided into three parts: Part I, Family Systems Stressors (General); Part II, Family Systems Stressors (Specific); and Part III, Family Systems Strengths. Each part contains a Quantitative Summary and a Qualitative Summary.

Quantifiable family and clinician perception scores are both graphed on the Quantitative Summary. Each family member has a designated color code. Family and clinician remarks are both recorded on the Quantitative Summary. Quantitative Summary scores, when graphed, suggest a level for initiation of prevention/intervention modes: Primary, Secondary, and Tertiary. Qualitative Summary information, when synthesized, contributes to the development and channeling of the Family Care Plan.

Part 1 Family Systems Stressors (General)

Add acores from questions 1 to 25 and calculate an overall numerical score for Family Systems Stressors (General). Ratings are from 1 (most positive) to 5 (most negative). The Does Not Apply (0) responses are omitted from the calculations. Total scores range from 25 to 125.
Family Systems Stressor Score (General)

$(_{25}) \times 1 =$

Graph score on Quantitative Summary, Family Systems Stressors (General), Family Member Perception Score. Color-code to differentiate family members. Record additional stressors and family remarks in Part I, Qualitative Summary: Family and Clinician Remarks.

Part II Family Systems Stressors (Specific)

Add scores from questions 1 through 8, 10, and 12 and calculate a numerical score for Family Systems Stressors (Specific). Ratings are from 1 (most positive) to 5 (most negative). Questions 4, 6, 7, 8, 10 and 12

are reverse scored.* Total scores range from 10 through 50. Family Systems Stressor Score (Specific)

$(_{10}) \times 1 =$

Graph score on Quantitative Summary, Family Systems Stressors (Specific) Family Member Perception Score. Color-code to differentiate family members. Summarize data from questions 9 and 11 (reverse scored) and record family remarks in Part II, Qualitative Summary: Family and Clinician Remarks.

Part III Family Systems Strengths

Add scores from questions 1 through 16 and calculate a numerical score for Family Systems Strengths. Ratings are from 1 (seldom) to 5 (always). The Does Not Apply (0) responses are omitted from the calculations. Total Scores range from 16 to 80.

$(_{16}) \times 1 =$

Graph score on Quantitative Summary: Family Systems Strengths, Family Member Perception Score. Record additional family strengths and family remarks in Part III, Qualitative Summary: Family and Clinician Remarks.

Source: Mischke-Berkey, K., & Hanson, S. M. H. (1991). *Pocket guide to family assessment and intervention.* St. Louis, MO: Mosby.
*Reverse scoring:
Question answered as (1) is scored 5 points.
Question answered as (2) is scored 4 points.
Question answered as (3) is scored 3 points.
Question answered as (4) is scored 2 points.
Question answered as (5) is scored 1 point.

FIGURE 14-3—cont'd

SECTION 2: CLINICIAN PERCEPTION SCORES

Part I Family Systems Stressors (General)*

Add scores from questions 1 through 25 and calculate an overall numerical score for Family Systems Stressors (General). Ratings are from 1 (most positive) to 5 (most negative). The Does Not Apply (0) responses are omitted from the calculations. Total scores range from 25 to 125.

Family systems Stressor Score (General)

$(_{25}) \times 1 =$

Graph score on Quantitative Summary, Family Systems Stressors (General) Clinician Perception Score. Record clinicians' clarification of general stressors in Part I, Qualitative Summary: Family and Clinician Remarks.

Part II Family Systems Stressors (Specific)

Add scores from questions 1 through 8, 10, 12 and calculate a numerical score for Family Systems Stressors (Specific). Ratings are from 1 (most positive) to 5 (most negative). Questions 4, 6, 7, 8, 10, 12 are reverse scored.* Total scores range from 10 to 50.

Family Systems Stressor Score (Specific)

$(_{10}) \times 1 =$

Graph score on Quantitative Summary, Family Systems Stressors (Specific), Clinician Perception Score. Summarize data from questions 9 and 11 (reverse scored) and record clinician remarks in Part II, Qualitative Summary: Family and Clinician Remarks.

Part III Family Systems Strengths

Add scores from questions 1 through 16 and calculate a numerical score for Family Systems Strengths. Ratings are from 1 (seldom) to 5 (always). The Does Not Apply (0) responses are omitted from the calculations. Total scores range from 16 to 80.

$(_{16}) \times 1 =$

Graph score on Quantitative Summary, Family Systems Strengths, Clinician Perception Score. Record clinicians' clarification of family strengths in Part III, Qualitative Summary: Family and Clinician Remarks.

---

*Reverse scoring:
Question answered as (1) is scored 5 points.
Question answered as (2) is scored 4 points.
Question answered as (3) is scored 3 points.
Question answered as (4) is scored 2 points.
Question answered as (5) is scored 1 point.

QUANTITATIVE SUMMARY OF FAMILY SYSTEMS STRESSORS: GENERAL AND SPECIFIC FAMILY AND CLINICIAN PERCEPTION SCORES

DIRECTIONS: Graph the scores from each family member inventory by placing an "X" at the appropriate location. (Use first name initial for each different entry and different color code for each family member.)

	FAMILY SYSTEMS STRESSORS (GENERAL)			FAMILY SYSTEMS STRESSORS (SPECIFIC)	
SCORES FOR WELLNESS AND STABILITY	FAMILY MEMBER PERCEPTION SCORE	CLINICIAN PERCEPTION SCORE	SCORES FOR WELLNESS AND STABILITY	FAMILY MEMBER PERCEPTION SCORE	CLINICIAN PERCEPTION SCORE
5.0			5.0		
4.8	X√4		4.8		
4.6			4.6		
4.4	X√2		4.4	X√4	
4.2	X√3		4.2		
4.0			4.0	X√3	
3.8			3.8	X√5	
3.6	X√1		3.6		
3.4	X√5	X	3.4		X
3.2			3.2	X√2	
3.0			3.0	X√1	
2.8			2.8		
2.6			2.6		
2.4			2.4		
2.2			2.2		
2.0			2.0		
1.8			1.8		
1.6			1.6		
1.4			1.4		
1.2			1.2		
1.0			1.0		

*PRIMARY Prevention/Intervention Mode: Flexible Line   1.0–2.3
*SECONDARY Prevention/Intervention Mode: Normal Line   2.4–3.6
*TERTIARY Prevention/Intervention Mode: Resistance Lines   3.7–5.0
*Breakdowns of numerical scores for stressor penetration are suggested values.
√1 = Glenn √3 = Anne √5 = Bill
√2 = Jane √4 = Janet

FIGURE 14-4 Howe family Quantitative Summary of Family Systems Stressors Form: General and Specific.

FAMILY SYSTEMS STRENGTHS FAMILY AND CLINICIAN PERCEPTION SCORES

DIRECTIONS: Graph the scores from the inventory by placing an "X" at the appropriate location and connect with a line. (Use first name initial for each different entry and different color code for each family member.)

SUM OF STRENGTHS AVAILABLE FOR PREVENTION/ INTERVENTION MODE	FAMILY SYSTEMS STRENGTHS	
	FAMILY MEMBER PERCEPTION SCORE	CLINICIAN PERCEPTION SCORE
5.0		
4.8		
4.6		
	√3	
4.4	√2	
	√1	
4.2		
4.0		
	√5	X
3.8		
	√4	
3.6		
3.4		
3.2		
3.0		
2.8		
2.6		
2.4		
2.2		
2.0		
1.8		
1.6		
1.4		
1.2		
1.0		

*PRIMARY Prevention/Intervention Mode: Flexible Line   1.0–2.3
*SECONDARY Prevention/Intervention Mode: Normal Line 2.4–3.6
*TERTIARY Prevention/Intervention Mode: Resistance Lines 3.7–5.0
*Breakdowns of numerical scores for stressor penetration are suggested values.

√1 = Glenn   √3 = Anne   √5 = Bill
√2 = Jane   √4 = Janet

FIGURE 14-5 Howe family and clinician summary on family strengths.

QUALITATIVE SUMMARY FAMILY AND CLINICIAN REMARKS
PART I: FAMILY SYSTEMS STRESSORS (GENERAL)

Summarize general stressors and remarks of family and clinician. Prioritize stressors according to importance to family members.

The major general stressors of the family is the worsening heart disease and the impact of the disabling stress on the entire family

PART II: FAMILY SYSTEMS STRESSORS (SPECIFIC)

A. Summarize specific stressors and remarks of family and clinician.

Glenn's specific stressors: growing inability to function as a husband, father & grandfather, fear of the unknown

B. Summarize differences (if discrepancies exist) between how family members and clinicians view effects of stressful situation on family.

Concerns regarding financial impact of illness not shared with all family members

C. Summarize overall family functioning.

Functioning fairly well but uncertainty regarding physical health taking a toll on mental health of three family members

D. Summarize overall significant physical health status for family members.

The differences between Glenn's physical health and the physical health of all other family members are significant and problematic for planning family activities

E. Summarize overall significant mental health status for family members.

Glenn's anxieties and Jane's anxiety and Janet's depression are affecting all other family members

PART III: FAMILY SYSTEMS STRENGTHS

Summarize family systems strengths and family and clinician remarks that facilitate family health and stability.

Open communications, supportive family members, religious faith, trust in health care providers, having relationships

FIGURE 14-6 Howe family Qualitative Summary Family and Clinician Remarks.

Family Care Plan*

DIAGNOSIS AND GENERAL AND SPECIFIC FAMILY SYSTEM STRESSORS	FAMILY SYSTEMS STRENGTHS SUPPORTING FAMILY CARE PLAN	GOALS FOR FAMILY AND CLINICIAN	PREVENTION/INTERVENTION MODE		
			PRIMARY, SECONDARY, OR TERTIARY	PREVENTION/ INTERVENTION ACTIVITIES	OUTCOMES EVALUATION AND REPLANNING
Diagnosis of cardiac disease with sudden worsening of symptoms necessitating curtailment of family activities and uncertainty about the future	Family communication, social support, religious faith, good medical care, knowledgeable family members.	Restoration of stable cardiac status sufficient to return home Family members will continue to support Glenn and each other	Education regarding new medications and activity restrictions Home health care & discharge O_2 therapy	Family counseling to deal with anxiety and uncertain future Financial counseling	Evaluation to be done once plan is implemented

*Prioritize the three most significant diagnoses.

FIGURE 14-7 Howe family care plan.

SUMMARY

When medical-surgical nurses view families as partners in the care provided to patients, they are providing unfragmented, holistic, humane, and sensitively delivered health care. When nurses practice family-centered care in the medical-surgical settings, families are empowered to manage the stressors of being in the hospital environment, which is foreign territory to most people. Families then are better prepared to support their loved ones, aid in their recovery, or facilitate a comfortable death. Families are called on to support their ill family member in the hospital, make important life decisions on behalf of or in partnership with the patient, to serve as caregivers, and to advocate for the patient in the complex health care system. The stress families experience when family members are in the hospital is significant. Family members are at risk for depression, anxiety, and PTSD. The role of families in the hospital setting is crucial because patients have been shown to have more positive outcomes when families are involved in their loved one's care while in the hospital. The benefits of practicing family nursing or family-centered care in the hospital setting have been well documented. Yet, health care providers in the hospital environment continue to practice individual patient-centered rather than family-centered care (family nursing).

Some research presented in this chapter indicates that the acute medical-surgical health care system is responding slowly to families' needs for involvement as shared decision makers, for open visitation, and for recognition as team members. It appears that improvements have been made, such as providing information to families, allowing them proximity to their loved ones in hospitals, and communicating changes in conditions. But overall, the evidenced-based literature demonstrates that families, as the focus of practice, remain in the background. According to family studies in the research literature, families believe that they are seldom asked about how they are coping or what they need, and are rarely provided opportunities to talk about their fears and feelings. Nurses in medical-surgical environments recognize and feel responsible to practice family-centered or family nursing. Yet they struggle with role ambiguity and role conflict, as they continue to practice in settings that reward the biomedical model of health care and not a holistic nursing model of care.

Nurses in medical-surgical settings require help and recognition for practicing nursing in their inpatient hospital settings from a family perspective. Medical-surgical nursing cannot be taught in isolation from the perspective of individual patients. Family nursing should be incorporated into every clinical setting, and family assessment frameworks need to be included in the medical-surgical nursing curricula. Often, most family nursing content is relegated to community health, pediatric, or childbearing nursing courses, giving students the impression that families are not as important in medical-surgical settings. Indeed, medical-surgical courses are taught from an individualistic and pathophysiologic perspective. Nurses in medical-surgical settings end up dealing with families every day, despite the fact that they were never educated to do that properly. The strategies and interventions they utilize to help families cope with a very stressful situation need to be taught systematically and then studied, and best practices should be identified. This important information needs to be included in curricula for undergraduate students, graduate students, and graduate nurses already practicing in a myriad of settings.

The environment for providing family-centered nursing care (family nursing) in medical-surgical settings is dependent on hospital policies and procedures that consider the needs of families. Health care policies related to health care access, disparities in health care, lack of insurance to cover the expensive costs of medications and treatment, safe workplace environments, and nurse staffing clearly influence medical-surgical nursing practice. Nurses should strive to assume leadership roles as community role models, legislative advocates, and concerned, informed citizens. Medical-surgical nurses can be involved in many ways, such as joining the American Nurses Association, staying informed about and involved with legislative activities, communicating with political groups and legislators, and joining an active specialty organization, such as the American Association of Critical Care Nurses.

REFERENCES

Ahrens, T., Yancey, V., & Kollef, M. (2003). Improving family communications at the end-of-life: Implications for length of stay in the ICU and resource use. *American Journal of Critical Care, 12*(4), 317–323.

Alvarez, G. & Kirby, A. (2006). The perspective of families of the critically ill patient: Their needs. *Current Opinions in Critical Care, 12*(6), 614–618.

American Association of Critical Care Nurses. (2004, November 11). *Practice alert: Family presence during CPR and invasive procedures.* Retrieved April 1, 2008, from www.aacn.org

Artinian, N. T. (2005). Family-focused medical-surgical nursing. In S. M. H. Hanson, V. Gedaly-Duff, & J. R. Kaakinen (Eds.), *Family health care nursing: Theory, practice and research* (3rd ed., pp. 323–346). Philadelphia: F.A. Davis.

Azoulay, E., Pouchard, F., Kentish-Barnes, N., Chevret, S., Aboab, J., & Adrie, C., et al. (2005). Risk of post traumatic stress symptoms in family members in the intensive care unit patients. *American Journal of Respiratory and Critical Care Medicine, 171*(9), 987–994.

Bice-Stephens, W. (2006). Ownership in the intensive care unit. *Critical Care Nurse, 26*(4), 10–11.

Bjornsdottir, K. (2002). From the state to the family: Reconfiguring the responsibility for long term nursing care at home. *Nursing Inquiry, 9,* 3–11.

Browning, G., & Warren, N. (2006). Unmet needs of family members in the medical intensive care waiting room. *Critical Care Nursing Quarterly, 29*(1), 86–95.

Butterworth, A. M. (2003). Reality check: 10 barriers to advanced planning. *The Nurse Practitioner, 28*(5), 42–43.

Carr, J. M., & Fogarty, J. P. (1999). Families at the bedside: An ethnographic study of vigilance. *Journal of Family Practice, 48*(6), 433–438.

Carr, K. (2002). Ward visits after intensive care discharge: Why. In R. Griffiths & C. Jones (Eds.), *Intensive care aftercare.* Oxford: Butterworth Heinemann.

Chaboyer, W., Kendall, E., Kendall, M., & Foster, M. (2005). Transfer out of intensive care: A qualitative exploration of patient and family perceptions. *Australian Critical Care, 18*(4), 138–145.

Chesla, C. A. (1997). Reconciling technologic and family care in critical care nursing. *Image: Journal of Nursing Scholarship, 28*(3), 199–203.

Chien, W. T., Chiu, Y. L., Lam, L. W. & Ip, W. Y. (2006). Effects of a needs-based education programme for family carers with a relative in an intensive care unit: A quasi-experimental study. *International Journal of Nursing Studies, 43,* 39–50.

Coleman, E. A., Smith, J. D., Frank, J. C., Min, S., Parry, C., & Kramer, A. M. (2004). Preparing patients and caregivers to participate in care delivered across settings: The care transition intervention. *Journal of American Geriatric Society, 52,* 1817–1825.

Day, L. (2006). Family involvement in critical care: Shortcomings of a utilitarian justification. *American Journal of Critical Care, 15*(2), 223–225.

Deitrick, L., Ray, D., Stern, G., Fuhrman, C., Masiado, T., Yaich, S. L., & Wasser, T. (2005). Evaluation and recommendations from a study of critical-care waiting rooms. *Journal for Healthcare Quality, 27*(4), 17–25.

DesRoches, C., Blendon, R., Young, J., Scoles, K., & Kim, M. (2002). Caregiving in the post-hospitalization period: Findings from a national survey. *Nurse economist, 20,* 221–224.

Duke, G., Thompson, S., & Hastie, M. (2007). Factors influencing completion of advanced directive in hospitalized patients. *International Journal of Palliative Nursing, 13*(1), 39–43.

Eldredge, D. (2004). Helping at the bedside: Spouses' preferences for helping critically ill patients. *Research in Nursing and Health, 27,* 307–321.

Emergency Nurses Association. (2005). *Presenting the option for family presence* (3rd ed.). Des Plaines, IL: Emergency Nurses Association.

Fox-Wasylyshyn, S., El-Masri, M., & Williamson, K. (2005). Family perceptions of nurses' roles toward family members of critically ill patients: A descriptive study. *Heart & Lung, 34*(5), 335–344.

Gallant, M., Spitz, G., & Prohaska, T. (2007). Help or hindrance? How family and friends influence chronic illness self-management among older adults. *Research on Aging, 29,* 375–409.

Handy, C. M., Sulmasy, D. P., Merkel, C. K., & Ury, W. A. (2008). The surrogate's experience in authorizing a do not resuscitate order. *Palliative & Supportive Care, 6*(1), 13–19.

Harvey, M. (2004). Evidence-based approach to family care in the intensive care unit: Why can't we just be decent? *Critical Care Medicine, 32*(9), 1975–1976.

Holden, J., Harrison, L., & Johnson, M. (2002). Families, nurses and intensive care patients: A review of the literature. *Journal of Clinical Nursing, 11,* 140–148.

Hooyman, N. R., & Gonyea, J. G. (1999). A feminist model of family care: Practice and policy directions. *Journal of Women and Aging, 11,* 149–169.

Hopp, F. P., & Duffy, S. A. (2000). Racial variations in end-of-life care. *Journal of American Geriatric Society, 48,* 658–663.

Hsieh, H., Shannon, S. E., & Curtis, J. R. (2006). Contradictions and communication strategies during end-of-life decision making in the intensive care unit. *Journal of Critical Care, 21*(4), 294–304.

Hudak, C. M., & Gallo, B. M. (1994). *Critical care nursing: A holistic approach.* Philadelphia: J.B. Lippincott.

Jacelon, C. S. (2006). Directive and supportive behaviors used by families of hospitalized older adults to affect the process of hospitalization. *Journal of Family Nursing, 12,* 234–250.

Jansen, M. P. M., & Schmitt, N. A. (2003). Family-focused interventions. *Critical Care Nursing Clinics of North America, 15*(3), 347–354.

Jezewski, M. A., Meeker, M. A., & Robillard, I. (2005). What is needed to assist patients with advance directives from the perspective of emergency nurses. *Journal of Emergency Nursing, 31*(2), 150–155.

Kaakinen, J. R., & Hanson, S. M. H. (2205). Family assessment and intervention. In S. M. H. Hanson, V. Gedaly-Duff, & J. R. Kaakinen (Eds.), *Family health care nursing: Theory, practice and research* (3rd ed., pp. 215–242). Philadelphia: F.A. Davis.

Kaufman, S. R. (2002). A commentary: Hospital experience and meaning at the end-of-life. *Gerontologist, 42*(3), 449–457.

Kirchhoff, K. R., Palzkill, J., Kowalkowski, J., Mork, A., & Gretarsdottir, E. (2008). Preparing families for intensive care patients for withdrawal of life support: A pilot study. *American Journal of Critical Care 17*(2), 113–121, quiz 122.

Kleiber, C., Davenport, T., & Freyenberger, B. (2006). Open bedside rounds for families with children in pediatric intensive care units. *American Journal of Critical Care, 15*(5), 492–496.

Kloos, J. A., & Daly, B. J. (2008). Effect of family-maintained progress journal on anxiety of families of critically ill patients. *Critical Care Nursing Quarterly, 31*(2), 96–107.

Latour, J., & Haines, C. (2007). Families in the ICU: Do we truly consider their needs, experiences, and satisfaction? *Nursing in Critical Care, 12*(4), 173–174.

Lautrette, A., Darmon, M., Megarbane, B., Joly, L. M., Chevret, S., Adrie, C., et al. (2007). *New England Journal of Medicine, 356*(5), 469–478, 537–540.

MacLean, S., Guzzeta, C., White, C., Fontaine, D., Eichorn, D., Meyers, T., & Desy, P. (2003). Family presence during cardiopulmonary resuscitation and invasive procedures: Practices of critical care and emergency nurses. *American Journal of Critical Care, 12*(3), 246–257.

MacLeod, M., Chesson, R. A., Blackledge, P., Hutchison, J. D., & Ruta, N. (2005). To what extent are carers involved in the care and rehabilitation of patients with hip fracture? *Disability and Rehabilitation, 27*(18–19), 1117–1122.

Mangram, A. J., McCauley, T., Villarreal, D., Howard, D., Dolly A., & Norwood, S. (2005). Families' perception of the value of timed daily "family rounds" in a trauma ICU. *The American Surgeon, 71*(10), 886–891.

Martire, L. M., Lustig, A. P., Schulz, R., Helgeson, V. S., & Miller, G. E. (2007). Is it beneficial to involve a family member? A meta-analysis of psychosocial interventions for chronic illness. *Health Psychology, 23*(6), 599–611.

Martire, L. M., & Schulz, R. (2007). Involving family in psychosocial interventions for chronic illness. *Current Directions in Psychological Science, 16*(2), 90–94.

Maxwell, K., Stuenkel, D., & Saylor, C. (2007). Needs of family members of critically ill patients: A comparison of nurse and family perceptions. *Heart & Lung, 36*, 367–376.

McCloskey, J. C., & Bulechek, G. M. (Eds.). (2004). *Nursing interventions classification (NIC)* (4th ed.). St. Louis, MO: Mosby.

McKinley, S., Nagy, S., Stein-Parbury, J., Bramwell, M., & Hudson, J. (2002). Vulnerability and security in seriously ill patients in intensive care. *Intensive Critical Care Nursing, 18*, 27–36.

Miracle, V. (2005). Critical care visitation. *Dimensions of Critical Care Nursing, 24*(1), 48–49.

Mischke-Berkey, K. & Hanson, S. M. H. (1991). *Pocket guide to family assessment and intervention*. St. Louis, MO: Mosby.

Molter, N. (1979). Needs of relatives of critically ill patients: A descriptive study. *Heart & Lung, 8*(2), 332–339.

Molter, N. (1994). Families are not visitors in the critical care unit. *Dimensions of Critical Care Nursing, 13*(1), 2–3.

Nelson, D. P., & Poist, G. (2008). An interdisciplinary team approach to evidence-based improvement in family-centered care. *Critical Care Nursing Quarterly, 31*(2), 110–118.

Nelson, J. E., Kinjo, K., Meier, D. E., Ahmad, K., & Morrison, R. S. (2005). When critical illness becomes chronic: Information needs of patients and families. *Journal of Critical Care, 20*(1), 79–89.

Organ Donor. (2008). *Donation statistics*. Retrieved July 5, 2008, from www.organdonor.gov

Paterson, B., Kieloch, B., & Gmiterek, J. (2001). "They never told us anything": Postdischarge instruction for families of persons with brain injuries. *Rehabilitation Nursing, 26*(2), 48–53.

Paul, F., & Rattray, J. (2008). Short and long-term impact of critical illness on relatives: Literature review. *Journal of Advanced Nursing, 62*(3), 276–292.

Pearce, L. (2005). Family matters—Liaison nurse offering support to families. *Nursing Standard, 20*(12), 22–24.

Perry, J., Lynam, J., & Anderson, J. M. (2006). Resisting vulnerability: The experiences of families who have kin in the hospital—a feminist ethnography. *International Journal of Nursing Studies, 43*(2), 173–184.

Pikka, L., & Beaulieu, M. (2004). Experiences of families in the neurological ICU: A "bedside phenomenon." *Journal of Neuroscience Nursing, 36*(3), 142–155.

Pouchard, F., Darmon, M., Fassier, T., Bollaert, P., Cheval, C., Coloigner, M., et al. (2005). Symptoms of anxiety and depression in family members of intensive care unit patients before discharge or death: A prospective multicenter study. *Journal of Critical Care, 20*(1), 90–96.

Rushton, C., Reina, M., & Reina, D. (2007). Building trustworthy relationships with critically ill patients and families. *AACN Advances in Critical Care, 18*(1), 19.

Smith, S. W., Lindsey, L. L., Kopfman, J. E., Yoo, J., & Morrison, K. (2008). Predictors of engaging in family discussion about organ donation and getting organ donor cards witnessed. *Health Communication, 23*(2), 142–152.

Stayt, L. (2007). Nurses' experiences of caring for families with relatives in intensive care units. *Journal of Advanced Nursing, 57*(6), 623–630.

Streator, C., Golledge, J., Sutherland, H., Easton, J., MacDonald, R., McNamara, R., et al. (2001). The relocation experiences of relatives leaving a neurosciences critical care unit: A phenomenological study. *Nursing in Critical Care, 6*, 163–170.

Sulmasy, D. P., He, M. K., McAuley, R., & Ury, W. A. (2008). Beliefs and attitudes of nurses and physicians about do not resuscitate orders and who should speak to patients and families about them. *Critical Care Medicine, 36*(6), 1817–1822.

Tilden, V. P., Tolle, S. W., Nelson, C. A., & Fields, J. (2001). Family decision-making to withdraw life-sustaining therapies from hospitalized patients. *Nursing Research, 50*(2), 105–115.

Truog, R. D., Cist, A. F. M., Bracket, S. E., Burns, J. P., Curley, M. A. Q., Danis, M., et al. (2001). Recommendations for end-of-life care in the intensive care unit: The Ethics Committee of the Society of Critical Care Medicine. *Critical Care Medicine, 29*(12), 2332–2348.

Tschann, J. M., Kaufman, S. R., & Micco, G. P. (2003). Family involvement in end-of-life hospital care. *The American Geriatric Society, 51*(6), 835–840.

Tweibell, R. S., Siela, D., Riwitis, C., Wheatley, J., Riegle, T., Rouseman, D., et al. (2008). Nurses' perceptions of their self-confidence and the benefits and risks of family presence during resuscitation. *American Journal of Critical Care, 17*(2), 101–111.

Van Horn, E., & Kautz, D. (2007). Promotion of family integrity in the acute care setting. *Dimensions of Critical Care Nursing, 26*(3), 101–107.

Verhaeghe, S., Defloor, T., Van Zuuren, F., Duijnstee, M., & Grypdonck, M. (2005). The needs and experiences of family members of adult patients in an intensive care unit: A review of the literature. *Journal of Clinical Nursing, (14)*, 501–509.

White, D., & Curtis, J. R. (2006). Establishing an evidence base for physician-family communication and shared-decision making in the intensive care unit. *Critical Care Medicine, 34*(9), 2500–2501.

Wiegand, D. L. (2006). Families and withdrawal of life-sustaining therapy: State of the science. *Journal of Family Nursing, 12*(2), 165–184.

Wiegand, D. L., Deatrick, J. A., & Knafl, K. (2008). Family management styles related to withdrawal of life-sustaining therapy from adults who are acutely ill or injured. *Journal of Family Nursing, 14*(1), 16–32.

Williams, C. M. A. (2005). The identification of family members' contribution to patients' care in the intensive care unit: A naturalistic inquiry. *Nursing in Critical Care, 10*(1), 6–14.

Zaforteza, C., Gastaldo, D., de Pedro, J. E., Sánchez-Cuenca, P., & Lastra, P. (2005). The process of giving information to families of critically ill patients: A field of tension. *International Journal of Nursing Studies, 42*(2), 135–145.

CHAPTER 15

Gerontological Family Nursing

Diana L. White, PhD

Jeannette O'Brien, PhD, RN

CRITICAL CONCEPTS

✦ In most care settings, a majority of those receiving care are older than 65 years. Although most older adults are healthy and independent, many become more limited in activities of daily living with advanced age as a result of chronic illnesses.

✦ Most older adults have family ties that are positive, meaningful, and supportive. It is rare for older adults to be neglected or uncared for by their families.

✦ Like all families, families of older adults are diverse. This diversity is influenced by history, race, class, and sex, as well as by individual family history and traditions. These factors influence family composition, health status, health beliefs, and capacity to support each other during times of illness or stress.

✦ Older adults in families are givers of care as well as receivers. Until very old age, older family members provide more economic, social, and emotional support to adult children than they receive; they step in to assist families members in crisis (e.g., because of divorce, illness, or addiction), and most caregivers of older adults are spouses.

✦ Families provide most of the care to older adults, regardless of the care setting. The ways families organize and structure care varies (e.g., primary caregiver vs. collective caregiving). Nursing care is most effective when done in partnership with families.

✦ All families experience transitions over the life course (e.g., births, deaths, school, work, retirement, forming partnerships). Some are expected and some are not. Each transition is influenced by health status, culture, financial security, and social supports.

✦ Gerontological nursing takes place in all care settings, although the specific needs of older adults and their families vary. Most older adults live and receive care in community settings.

This chapter explores families in later life and the implications for nursing care. When we think about aging families, we often think of individuals or couples who are older than 65 years. These individuals, however, are embedded within a larger family system that includes different and intersecting generations. For example, a 75-year-old couple today may be newlyweds and have living parents. They may be completely healthy with no chronic conditions and spend some of their family time supporting themselves and others. In contrast, a 75-year-old person may be widowed and isolated from other social support, may have multiple chronic conditions, experience several limitations in activities of daily living (ADL), and require significant help from others. In either case, if the 75-year-olds have children, they are likely to be grandparents and even great-grandparents, and they may be the primary caregivers to one or more of those grandchildren. If help is needed, it will come most often from family members. When older adults need care, whether at home, in the hospital, or in a range of long-term care (LTC) settings, families will be participating in that care in most circumstances. Some family members will be active leaders in that care, whereas others will require substantial support from nurses and other professionals. A minority of older adults will have weak social ties and may be isolated from family and friends in old age.

The aging population is diverse, and family systems are complex. Family gerontologists (those who study aging) often use a life course perspective as a way to understand this complexity (Settersten, 2006). The life course perspective recognizes that individuals are embedded in a family system, and that individuals and the family as a whole develop and change over time. This outlook is compatible with many family and social science theories, and is often used in conjunction with other theories, including the theories that guide this book. This chapter discusses the life course perspective in relation to family systems, Family Life Cycle Theory, and the ecology model of family development. Family systems theories emphasize connections among family members. When something happens to or is experienced by one family member, others are affected in some way. It is useful to consider older family systems broadly. Connidis (2001) describes family relationships in terms of "family ties," which helps us think about families that extend beyond households

and the nuclear family. Family ties include extended family members and those who are "like family" but are not connected through blood or marriage.

As described throughout this chapter, the character of family ties varies within and between families. Responses to life events among family members are influenced by a history of family rules and traditions that have developed over time (Hanson, 1995), and the quality and characteristics of family ties. Family breakdown may occur when rules and traditions are not adequate to a particular situation. For example, in some families, this may occur when siblings disagree strongly on how to provide support to frail, cognitively impaired parents. One may stress the importance of a parent remaining in her own home, whereas another may feel that the unique health and safety needs of her mother demands nursing home care. At the same time, neither can agree on how to spend scarce resources to make either option workable.

THEORETICAL FRAMEWORK

Like the family development models, the life course perspective follows families over time, considering both continuity and change. This perspective is useful for assessing families across time and evaluating health care changes related to development, transitions, experiences, and events within a family. Families change as individual members grow and change, although the affective nature of relationships is likely to remain relatively constant over time. The family development model helps to predict when normative, or expected, changes will occur. For example, many middle-aged and older adults experience their children leaving home and establishing their own households. Adult children form partnerships through marriage or cohabitation. They also begin to achieve financial independence through work. Middle-aged adults who are parents can expect to become grandparents. Retirement is an expected and often desired transition for those with an adequate income and retirement savings. More now than ever before, however, many family transitions are occurring at less predictable times. The life course concepts of "off-time" or "non-normative" life experiences are significant to understanding these changes. For example, young adults leave home and then return. Women and men go to college in midlife to begin new careers. Many couples in middle age are beginning their families, not "launching them." Some in their 50s adopt young children, sometimes their own grandchildren. Those in their 70s may seek paid employment because of a desire to work or because of financial necessity. According to Quadagno (2008), after several years of declining labor force participation by those older than 60, trends now for both women and men are to remain in the labor force longer. More than 30% and 10% of men (and about 22% and 8% of women) 65 to 69 years old and older than 70 years, respectively, continue to work full-time or part-time. Finally, some transitions, although common, are not expected and may cause difficulties for families. These include divorce, involuntary job loss, declining health or disability, and providing care for ill or dependent family members. Nurses should be aware that entry into the health care system by an older adult may represent an unwelcome and unanticipated life transition for the entire family. All families experience losses through death, but when death occurs suddenly and unexpectedly, especially the loss of a child within a family, the loss can be particularly traumatic for all family members, including the older adults. The loss of a child or grandchild is one of the hardest off-time events for older adults to bear (de Vries, Lana, & Falch, 1994; White, 1999).

The life course perspective, like ecology models, emphasizes the social context in which families are located (Bengtson & Allen, 1993). Individuals and families are influenced by the historical times in which they live. For example, those who are currently in their 80s experienced the Great Depression if they lived in the United States when they were children or young adults. Many served in World War II, and later were parents of the baby boom generation. The baby boom represented a reversal in the trend toward smaller families, resulting in a population bulge that has dominated family life and public policy in the United States ever since. Baby boomers had a different set of challenges and opportunities than their parents. Young adults now in their 20s have grown up in a technologic and global age quite different from either their parents or grandparents. They have experienced households in which both parents are more likely to work outside the home, divorce is more common, and so is postponing or forgoing childbearing. This generation has also seen a growth in health and economic disparities among various segments of the population, and to varying degrees, have experienced the Iraqi and Afghanistan wars.

In all phases of history, societal issues related to race, class, sex, abilities, and immigration have influenced the kinds of opportunities and barriers individuals experience throughout their lives. The life course perspective is useful in understanding how changing environments, cultural norms, economic conditions, and political circumstances affect families. Such influences can be seen in work and family decisions, access to health care, and educational opportunities. At the same time, individuals are not passive but are active in shaping their lives through their own actions, even as those actions may be constrained or enhanced by broader societal circumstances (Settersten, 2006). Decisions made at one point in time often have significant lasting consequences for close relationships, work, and living situations throughout the life course. This can be seen in lifestyle choices that affect health in older age, consequences of divorce that influence care received in later life, and decisions about work and family that determine adequacy of retirement income. The life course perspective will be used to guide understanding of families with older adults and the family ties that influence their health. This perspective will be used to guide nursing care for these families, using the nursing process. This perspective will also be used to explain current social policies impacting older adults and their families, and recommendations for the future.

PROFILE OF AGING FAMILIES

Families are changing in structure and function at a rapid pace. One of these changes is the increased numbers of adults older than 65 years within all Western societies. These adults are part of families, offering historical context, developmental perspective, and support for younger adults and children. At the same time, older adults are living longer, and as they grow older, often require the assistance of younger adults to maintain independent living or care for progressive chronic illnesses. Several trends have emerged as our population ages, and many of these trends impact families and nursing care of families. These trends include increasing diversity in later life, increasing numbers of older adults living with chronic illnesses, changing family structure including increased numbers of divorced older adults and increased numbers of grandparents living with and/or raising grandchildren, and changing family relationships, including increased reliance on support across generations and the challenge of intergenerational conflicts. Caregiving has also grown and includes the unpaid assistance provided by family members for an individual with one or more chronic conditions.

Demographic Profile

The aging of the population worldwide is an unprecedented historical tide that has implications for all aspects of society. The 37.3 million adults older than 65 in the United States represent 12% of the population (Federal Interagency Forum on Aging Related Statistics, 2008). By 2050, numbers will more than double, resulting in an aging population comprising 21% of the population. The fastest growing segment of the population is those older than 85 years (Administration on Aging, 2004). As a group, older adults are healthier, better educated, and more financially secure than in previous generations. People throughout the world are living longer than ever before. At 65 years, an individual in the United States can expect to live nearly 19 more years; women reaching age 85 can expect to live more than 7 more years, whereas men are likely to exceed 6 more years of life (Federal Interagency Forum on Aging Related Statistics, 2008). Most, even those who are very old, live independently and in good health. Nearly three quarters of those older than 65 years report having good, very good, or excellent health (Federal Interagency Forum on Aging Related Statistics, 2008). In fact, the prevalence of older adults with chronic disabilities has declined steadily, particularly since the 1980s, with the greatest rate of decline between 1999 and 2004 (Manton, 2008). About 75% of older adults, including those with chronic conditions, report no difficulty or disability related to ADL or in instrumental activities of daily living (IADL) (Spillman, 2004). Declines in the need for assistance with IADL may be explained in part by use of technology, including new mobility devices. Declines in disabilities related to ADL are due to improved management of chronic disease, particularly cardiovascular disease (Manton, 2008). Given the growing issues related to obesity,

however, it is uncertain whether these trends will continue.

Older adults are more diverse than in previous generations. This includes growing proportions of minority older adults in the population. The older African American population will quadruple between 2000 and 2050, whereas the Hispanic and Asian/Pacific Islander populations will be seven and six-and-a-half times larger, respectively (Dilworth-Anderson, Williams, & Gibson, 2002). Minority older adults have shorter life expectancies and report poorer health throughout the life course. A majority of Hispanics who are 85 years or older describe themselves to be in poor health, more than any other racial or ethnic group (Federal Interagency Forum on Aging Related Statistics, 2008). In addition, racial and ethnic minority groups tend to receive poorer quality care than whites, even controlling for socioeconomic status and severity of illness or condition (Kronenfeld, 2006).

Although the outlook for a healthy old age is generally positive, older adults have the greatest need for health care and are the major users of health care services, especially those older than 85 years. Approximately 25% of older adults have chronic conditions that interfere with daily activities (Kronenfeld, 2006). This means that close to 7 million older adults in the United States have significant chronic disabilities (Manton, 2008; Spillman, 2004). In 2002, about half of hospital patients were older than 65 and accounted for 41% of all hospitalizations (Kleinpell, Fletcher, & Jennings, 2008). Unlike younger adults and children, older adults are more likely to have chronic illnesses, and most with chronic illnesses have more than one. In 2004, six of the top seven causes of death were due to chronic illnesses: heart disease, malignant neoplasms, cerebrovascular diseases, chronic lower respiratory diseases, Alzheimer disease, and diabetes mellitus (Federal Interagency Forum on Aging Related Statistics, 2008). Other chronic diseases common in old age include arthritis and hypertension. Older adults also experience sensory impairments with age. Kronenfeld reports that, in 2002, nearly half of older men and about one third of older women indicated they had trouble hearing. Vision problems, even after correction from glasses or contact lenses, occurred in 16% of men and 19% of women (Kronenfeld, 2006). Between 9% and 21% of those older than 70 years have both hearing and vision loss (Saunders & Echt, 2007). Sensory changes may interfere with abilities to function or to interact socially. Hearing loss can be particularly difficult, leading to social isolation or mistaken perceptions by others that the elder is cognitively impaired. Vision loss can affect or prohibit the ability to drive, which can increase dependency on others. Senses related to smell and taste generally remain stable into old age when one is healthy, but can be negatively affected by disease or medications. This in turn may lead to poor nutritional status, which will adversely affect health status (Maas, Buckwalter, Hardy, Tripp-Reimer, Titler, & Specht, 2001; Mattes, 2002).

All nurses will work with increasing numbers of older adults simply because the population is aging so rapidly. Even nurses who focus on maternal and child or pediatric nursing are likely to encounter grandparents in the course of their work more often now than in the past, because of increased longevity of grandparents and the increasing numbers of grandparents raising their grandchildren. As discussed later in this chapter, more grandparents are assuming parenting roles because their adult children are unable to function as parents (Dolbin-MacNab, 2006; Uhlenberg & Kirby, 1998).

Family Structure

With increasing life expectancy, family relationships now last for decades. It is increasingly common to see newspaper photos of couples celebrating their 60th anniversaries, and to know "children" in their 60s or 70s who have living parents. We now encounter siblings with relationships of 80 or 90 years, and even grandparent-grandchild relationships that extend five or more decades. These long-lasting relationships with their histories of shared experiences, traditions, and exchanges of help will most often be an asset to the older adult as illnesses or functional declines occur. With declining birth rates, however, older adults in the future will have a smaller pool of family members to draw on for help.

Differences in life expectancy by sex influence family structures and functions in old age. Women outlive men across all ethnic groups and in all age groups. Women are more likely than men to be widowed throughout the life course, but especially in the oldest age groups: 76% of very old women (those 85 years and older) and 34% of very old men are widowed (Federal Interagency Forum on Aging

Related Statistics, 2008). Living arrangements show a similar pattern, with men more likely to live with their spouses and women more likely to live alone or with other relatives in older age. When caring for older adults, therefore, men are much more likely to have a spouse caregiver than women (Connidis, 2001). Though they are similar with respect to being divorced or never married, men are much more likely than women to be married in old age due in part to greater rates of remarriage after widowhood or divorce for men. For example, more than 75% of men 65 to 74 years old are married compared with 57% of women. By the time they reach old age, the disparity is even greater; 60% of men 85 years and older are married, whereas only 15% of women in that age group are married. Marital status varies by ethnicity, with a greater proportion of African American and Hispanic adults widowed or divorced than whites. In addition, African Americans have greater rates of cohabitation than the general population throughout adulthood. Asian, African American, Hispanic, and Native American elders are more likely to live with nonspouse kin and less likely to live alone than whites. Function changes as structure changes. For example, sexuality changes are dependent on age, health, attitudes toward sexuality, developmental behaviors, and availability of a partner. DeLamater (2002) encourages an integrated model of assessing sexuality in later life, including:

- Biological influences: physical health (i.e., presence of chronic conditions that impact sexual function or desire, or both), age, hormonal levels, medical treatments that may impact sexual function
- Psychological: attitudes toward sexuality, role of sexual relationships, knowledge, past experiences, mental health
- Social: availability of partner, including duration and quality of relationship, societal views and influences on sexuality in later life, socioeconomic status

In a study of 1,384 older adults, DeLamater and Moorman (2007) have found that sexuality continues into later life, and is most dependent on an interplay between physical health, quality and availability of relationships, change in role from procreation to pleasure and validation, societal influences, and previous sexual experiences. These researchers emphasize the danger of viewing sexuality from only a biological or medical perspective, noting that attitude is more salient in predicting continued sexual desire and behavior than presence or absence of chronic illness or age. Women and men continue to desire sexual relationships well into later life, with many reporting increased freedom to explore sexuality because of decreased concern over procreation and decreased family responsibilities.

Women's marital status is closely linked to financial status in old age. Widows, especially minority women, experience significant losses in income and net worth (Angel, Jimenez, & Angel, 2007). Compared with men, today's oldest women have not had careers or worked in jobs with pension benefits. Those with a history of low-wage jobs, more frequent marital disruption, and fewer opportunities to accumulate assets during their working years are especially vulnerable. More than 12% of older women are poor compared with 7% of men. On average, Social Security provides 60% of income for most older women, and it is the sole source of income for 20% of older women (Herd, 2005). Disparities by race and ethnicity are even greater. For example, older African American women are more than twice as likely to live below the poverty level than are older white women (Herd, 2005).

Divorce rates increased dramatically during the 20th century, more than doubling between the 1960s and 1980s before stabilizing in the 1990s; most divorces occurred in young or middle adulthood (Faust & McKibben, 1999). Only about 20% of marriages are expected to survive for 50 years because of divorce or widowhood (Wu & Schimmele, 2007). Although many will enter old age as divorced persons, divorce occurring in late life is a growing phenomenon, with many older adults no longer willing to live another 20 or 25 years in a poor and unsatisfying relationship. Reasons for late-life divorce are similar to those found in other age groups, including falling out of love, emotional or physical abuse, substance abuse, or infidelity. Women tend to leave their spouses more frequently than men (Wu & Schimmele, 2007).

Family Relationships

A prevailing myth in the United States is that older adults, particularly those who are part of the dominant culture, are isolated from and neglected by their younger family members, and ultimately are abandoned in nursing homes. Study after study has demonstrated that most family ties are strong and characterized by affection, caring, and many shared values (Rossi & Rossi, 1990). Furthermore, families have demonstrated remarkable adaptability to social change. Although the family structure has changed in recent decades, much about family life has remained the same, including valuing families. Individuals continue to travel through life in the company of others, which Antonucci and Akiyama (1995) describe as "social convoys." Some people come and go in our convoys, but many, especially family members, remain constant social companions for decades. Families value providing family members with emotional and practical support, with women typically taking the lead in this aspect of family life throughout the life course (Walker, Manoogian-O'Dell, McGraw, & White, 2001).

Intergenerational relationships may be of growing importance in family life, particularly as divorce becomes more common. Bengtson and Harootyan (1994) describe linkages between generations as "solidarity" with six distinct but interdependent dimensions: proximity, contact, emotional closeness, similarity of opinions, giving help, and feelings of responsibility. Based on a national representative sample, Bengtson and his colleagues found evidence of solidarity in most families, a finding that supports previous research and continues to be reported in the family literature. Most older adults have one grown child who lives within an hour's drive. This has remained relatively constant despite the often cited geographic mobility of younger generations. At the same time, adult children with college degrees are more likely to live farther away (Uhlenberg, 2005). Contact between generations is common, with the majority of adult children reporting contact with their parents at least once a week. Contact with mothers is more frequent than contact with fathers, and contact between mothers and daughters is the most common intergenerational interaction, reflecting that the strongest intergenerational tie is between mothers and daughters. Contact between grandparents and grandchildren is similar to that between parents and adult children, with 66% of grandparents living within an hour's drive from at least one set of grandchildren. The strongest predictor of grandparent-grandchild relationships is the quality of relationships between parents and grandparents (Monserud, 2008; Thiele & Whelan, 2006). The amount of contact by adult children is influenced by parental marital status, with the lowest contact being with fathers who are widowed, divorced, or remarried, and with remarried mothers.

Relationship quality is as important as contact. Feelings of closeness between generations are the norm, with most adult children reporting feeling very close to parents, especially to mothers. The older generation, even more frequently than their children, report feeling very close to their adult children. When adult children report that they are not close to their parents, they are more likely to be describing their relationships with their fathers than their relationships with their mothers. This likely reflects the way that relationships developed over time, as well as issues related to marital transitions described earlier. In addition, men tend to focus more on same-generation relationships, and women are more involved with intergenerational relationships (Uhlenberg, 2005). Exchanges of help and support between generations occur throughout the life course and are motivated by affection, as well as by a sense of obligation. Until late old age, older adults provide more help than they receive in all areas of support, including caring for family members, financial support, and instrumental support (Bengtson & Harootyan, 1994). We further explore exchanges among generations later in our discussion of caregiving.

Although family relationships are generally strong and characterized by affection and caring, family gerontology researchers have increasingly focused on more complex aspects of family life. The concept of ambivalence has received increasing attention, recognizing that family members can simultaneously hold positive and negative feelings about one another (Connidis & McMullin, 2002; Pillemer & Suiter, 2005). Fingerman (2001) studied relationships between mothers and their adult daughters. Relationships were complex, involving both positive and negative feelings toward one another, although they were generally more positive than negative. Adult daughters tended to express more ambivalence about their mothers than mothers expressed about their daughters. Pillemer and Suiter (2005) report that the majority of parents felt "torn in two directions" about their adult children. They found that ambivalence was frequently related to their adult children's achievements, particularly

achievements of their oldest child. More ambivalence was expressed toward those who did not attain normative adult statuses, such as completing college, getting married, or becoming financially independent. Peters, Hooker, and Zvonkovic (2006) conclude that ambivalence is a normal part of family life. In their study, older adults experienced ambivalence surrounding their adult children's busy lives and boundaries related to communication (e.g., holding back on opinions and feelings about being left out). Unexpressed to adult children were uncertainties older adults had about the availability of help from children should they need it, though Peters and her colleagues found that those who needed help received it.

Though less common than solidarity or ambivalence, family conflict, or negative social interactions, can have serious consequences for family relationships. Furthermore, negative aspects of relationships may lead to poorer health, and may decrease the amount and quality of support available when needed (Lachman, 2003; Rook, 2003). Newsom, Rook, Nishishiba, Sorkin, and Mahan (2005) report on a growing body of research that describes the disproportionate effect of negative social exchanges on psychological health when compared with positive social exchanges. They found that failure of those in one's social network to provide help when it was needed was evaluated most negatively. Umberson, Williams, Powers, Liu, and Needham (2006) have examined marriage quality and health over the life course, finding that poor marriage quality was associated with accelerated health declines in old age. They suggest that stress related to marital conflicts undermines immune functioning and has a cumulative effect on health over time. Conflicted families are less likely to provide assistance to each other throughout the life course and may have little contact, share few values, and generally are more detached. As such, they are less likely to be resources to older family members in need (Scharlach, Li, & Dalvi, 2006). Divorce is often a factor in these situations and has implications for intergenerational relationships throughout the life course. Although not focusing on conflict specifically, Bucx, van Wel, Knijin, and Hagendoorn (2008) report less contact by adult children with divorced mothers and fathers overall. Moreover, mothers may be mediating relationships between fathers and adult children, as indicated by increased contact between adult children with widowed mothers, but not with widowed fathers. Less contact was also reported with divorced and remarried fathers, although no differences were found in contact with widowed and remarried mothers (Bucx et al., 2008).

An extreme consequence of family conflict is elder abuse or mistreatment, estimated to affect 1.3% to 5.4% of older adults (Fulmer, Guadagno, Bitondo, & Connolly, 2004). Elder mistreatment includes physical pain or injury, psychological anguish, neglect or abandonment, and financial exploitation. Its causes remain poorly understood, but risk factors include unhealthy dependency of the perpetrator or victim; disturbed psychological state of the perpetrator; frailty, disability, or impairment of the victim; and isolation of the family (Wolf, 1996). In addition to mistreatment by family members, frail older adults are also at risk for mistreatment by care providers. Nurses and other professionals have a responsibility to screen and assess elders for abuse. Fulmer and her colleagues (2004) have reviewed and evaluated several assessment tools. One of the recommended tools is the Elder Assessment Instrument, which can be found on the *Try This* section of the Hartford Institute for Geriatric Nursing (HIGN) Web site (Fulmer, 2008).

This section began by stating that most family relationships are strong, characterized by affection and exchange. As illustrated by the discussions on ambivalence and conflict, however, it is evident that many family relationships are more complex and the strengths of association may vary considerably over time. Those who are most vulnerable with respect to family relationships are divorced men. As discussed later in this chapter, divorced men, especially those who do not remarry, may have fewer ties that connect them to informal care and may rely more on formal services such as nursing homes than their married counterparts.

To add to the complexity, we have found that levels of ambivalence and conflict vary within families. An individual may have conflicted feelings about one family member and close, affectionate feelings about another. Both ambivalence and conflict may be apparent for nurses and other health providers when an older adult needs care. Nurses must be sensitive to underlying tensions and be able to provide support in nonjudgmental ways, remembering that the current family dynamics are embedded in a lifetime of relationships and actions.

Family Case Study

Throughout this chapter, Maria and her family illustrate experiences common to older adults who need nursing and family care. Using the life course perspective illustrated by Maria and her family, we explore transitions families experience as a result of declining health and increasing dependency common in old age, and the intersection of older families with the health care system.

OLDER ADULT: INDEPENDENT LIVING

Maria, age 60, is the oldest of four siblings. She has two brothers, James and Paul, and a sister, Ruth. Maria always counts Jane as her sister, too. Jane is a year younger than Maria and is the daughter of one of her mother's closest friends. When Jane needed a home as a young teenager, Maria's parents, Sarah and Louis, took her in, and Jane lived with them for 5 years. She and Maria became especially close, and now Jane and her family participate in all of Maria's and her extended family's gatherings.

Sarah, age 82, and Louis, age 84, have lived in their community since their marriage 60 years earlier. They enjoy good health, except for Sarah's arthritis and mild hearing loss, and Louis's diabetes and hypertension, which are well controlled. They experience no limitations in ADL, although both complain that it takes them longer to get things done. Still, they both volunteer for several different organizations and spend time with their friends. Maria lives 40 miles away, closer than the rest of her siblings. Maria and her parents talk on the phone about twice a week and they get together for dinner every couple of weeks.

Maria was divorced when her children, Jason and Kyra, were in elementary school. She still maintains connections with her ex-mother-in-law, Carol, who is now 87 years old. Carol has been widowed for 40 years. When Maria and her husband were divorced, Carol was determined that she would not lose contact with her grandchildren, as she had seen that happen with some of her friends. Maria had always been on good terms with Carol and felt it important that her children know their paternal grandmother, so both Maria and Carol made the effort to maintain contact. Carol lived about an hour away, but Maria and her children would spend at least one Saturday a month with her until the children entered into high school and were involved with multiple high-school activities. Their visits became more sporadic, but Carol would come and watch her grandchildren's games and music concerts whenever she could.

When Carol was diagnosed with Parkinson disease about 10 years ago, Maria became part of a community support system. Her role was to visit monthly, purchase groceries, and do some housekeeping. In addition to Parkinson disease, Carol began to have problems with her memory and could no longer live alone. With some reluctance, she moved into an assisted living facility (ALF) in her community. Maria has continued to visit her nearly every month. Carol usually knows Maria, but sometimes forgets she is divorced from her son. They mostly reminisce about the grandchildren.

Maria's life is quite busy. She is the office manager of a small business, and in addition to her parents and mother-in-law, Maria is involved in her children's lives. Jason and his partner live several hundred miles away, but Maria talks with him every couple of weeks. Maria often spends her vacations with them. Kyra is married and has two children of her own. Because Kyra lives close, Maria frequently baby-sits and delights in having each child spend the night about once a month. Maria enjoys being a grandparent, yet feels bad for her sister, Ruth, who has had sole responsibility for raising her own grandchildren for the past two years.

DISCUSSION

Maria's family is reflective of many older families (Fig. 15-1). At 60 years old, Maria is on the leading edge of the baby boomers, and like many in her generation, she has several siblings who represent potential support systems for both Maria and her parents. Typical for most older families, Maria lives relatively close to her parents and is in regular contact with them. Generally, they have a good relationship, characterized by affection, a history of mutual exchanges of help, and many shared values. Maria and her children are especially close to her parents because they provided considerable support as Maria was going through her divorce. Support included temporary housing, child care, and some financial assistance. Now, Sarah and Louis (Maria's parents) are close to becoming the "old-old" generation, that is, those older than 85 years. Although they are independent, engaged in their community, and consider themselves in good health, both have several chronic illnesses that could cause them problems in the future. Maria's former mother-in-law, Carol, has not been as fortunate. She was widowed "off-time" in her 40s and has lived alone since her son grew up and left home. Her activities have been limited for many years because of Parkinson disease and, more recently, cognitive impairment. She has resided for several years in an ALF that accepts Medicaid clients.

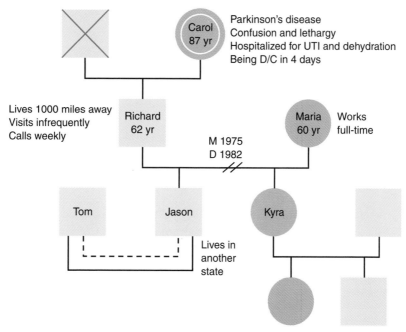

FIGURE 15-1 Hooper family genogram.

TYPES OF CARE

Much of the care that older adults receive is related to needs associated to chronic illness or disability. This LTC encompasses a wide range of services, both paid and unpaid. Although the term *long-term care* (LTC) is sometimes used interchangeably with nursing home care, nursing homes represent only one type of LTC service. A variety of community-based care services are available, including home care, adult day care, and a range of residential care. Residential care includes assisted living, board and care, and adult foster homes (Stone, 2006). Descriptions of home- and community-based LTC services are presented in Table 15-1. We begin our discussion with family caregiving in the context of

---

TABLE 15-1

Home- and Community-Based Services

Home- and community-based services (HCBS) describe a range of personal, support, and health services provided to individuals in their homes or communities to help them stay at home and live as independently as possible. Most people who receive long-term care at home generally require additional help either from family or friends to supplement services from paid providers. This is because so much of the care needed is personal care: help with activities such as bathing and dressing, help managing medications, or supervision for someone with a condition such as Alzheimer's disease.

Some of the most common home and community services are as follows:

Adult day service (ADS) programs are designed to meet the needs of adults with cognitive or functional impairments, as well as adults needing social interaction and a place to go when their family caregivers are at work. They provide a variety of health, social, and other support services in a protective setting during part of the day. Adult day centers typically operate programs during normal business hours 5 days a week; some have evening and weekend hours. These programs do not provide 24-hour care.

Case managers/geriatric care managers are health care professionals (typically nurses or social workers) who specialize in assisting you and your family with your long-term care needs. This includes, but is not limited to assisting, coordinating, and managing long-term care services; developing a plan of care; and monitoring your long-term care needs over extended periods.

Emergency response systems provide an automatic response to a medical or other emergency via electronic monitors. If you live alone, you wear a signaling device that you activate when you need assistance.

Friendly visitor/companion services are typically staffed by volunteers who regularly pay short visits (less than 2 hours) to someone who is frail or living alone.

Home health care and home care are two different services; they may be provided by a single agency or separate agencies. Home health care typically includes skilled, short-term services such as nursing, physical therapy, or other therapies ordered by a physician for a specific condition. Home care services are most often limited to personal care services such as bathing and dressing, and often also include homemaker services such as help with meal preparation or household chores.

Homemaker/chore services can help you with general household activities such as meal preparation, routine household care, and heavy household chores such as washing floors, washing windows, or shoveling snow.

Meals programs include both home-delivered meals (so called Meals-on-Wheels) or congregate meals, which are provided in a variety of community settings.

Respite care gives families temporary relief from the responsibility of caring for family members who are unable to care for themselves. Respite care is provided in a variety of settings including in the home, at an adult day center, or in a nursing home.

Senior centers provide a variety of services including nutrition, recreation, social and educational services, and comprehensive information and referral to help people find the care and services they might need.

Transportation services can help you get to and from medical appointments and shopping centers, and access a variety of community services and resources.

Source: Adapted from National Clearinghouse for Long-Term Care (Administration on Aging). (2008). *Understanding Long-Term Care.* Retrieved July 14, 2008, from http://www.longtermcare.gov/LTC/Main_Site/Understanding_Long_Term_Care/Services/Services.aspx, by permission.

community-based LTC, where most care to older adults is provided. With our discussion of caregiving, we examine the unpaid LTC system, which occurs mostly in the older adult's or a family member's home. We next move on to a discussion of acute care, followed by LTC in assisted living and nursing homes settings. We have chosen this order because it reflects the trajectory of care experienced by many older adults and their families.

Family Caregiving

As described earlier, family life is characterized by exchanges of help and support throughout the life course. Until very old age, older adults are more often givers than receivers in this exchange. They provide financial assistance to younger adults in college or those who are making major purchases such as cars or homes (Bengtson & Harootyan, 1994). Grandparents are a frequent source of childcare for grandchildren, particularly in their first three years (Vandell, McCartney, Owen, Booth, & Clarke-Stewart, 2003). They provide child care for their grandchildren while their adult children work or are unable to care for their children because of illness or planned absences (i.e., vacations). Less typical is providing care for dependent adult children with cognitive or physical disabilities. In some cases, caring for dependent children can be a lifelong role (Bilmes, 2008; Pruchno & Meeks, 2004; Seltzer, Greenberg, Floyd, & Hong, 2004; Yeoman, 2008). Grandparents also are often a source of stability when parents divorce, and growing numbers of grandparents are filling parenting roles for grandchildren because their parents are unable or unwilling to fulfill their parental obligations (Hayslip & Kaminski, 2005).

Regardless of the type of care provided, family caregiving grows out of ongoing family relationships and refers to support given to those who are dependent on that support for everyday functioning (Waldrop, 2003). The transition from the normal and mutual aid to support that is defined as caregiving is often a gradual process. Many wives, for example, do not describe what they do as caregiving, because the work they do in support of their increasingly dependent husbands is part of their ongoing family roles related to meal preparation, housework, and laundry. Walker, Pratt, and Eddy (1995) note that adult daughters do similar things

for dependent mothers as they do for mothers who are more self-sufficient, including running errands, preparing meals, and assisting with housework. Caregiving may simply mean "keeping an eye on" an older adult to monitor well-being (Messecar, 2008). As dependency increases, the time spent on these activities increases, and at some point the now caregiver recognizes that the care recipient is no longer able to perform these tasks without help.

In contrast, transitions to caregiving can happen suddenly if an otherwise healthy older adult has a traumatic injury, or experiences a stroke or cardiac arrest. The older adult may die as a result of the crisis or may recover independence, making the caregiving experience relatively short term. For many older adults, however, the health crisis may signal an end to independence or ability to live alone. In this case, a variety of decisions are made regarding informal and formal care services. Depending on the situation, which includes the nature of the disability, availability of services, and personal resources, the older person may receive support services in several places. The majority (55%) receive care in their own home, and about a third live with someone else, usually in the caregiver's home (National Alliance for Caregiving and AARP, 2004).

Whether the onset of caregiving is sudden or gradual, most caregivers will be family members, accounting for 80% or more of care received by older adults (Messecar, 2008). Few older adults who live in their own or in their caregiver's home rely on formal services, with fewer than 40% using any type of paid care. The most frequent paid care involves a direct care worker, nurse, or housekeeper (National Alliance for Caregiving and AARP, 2004). Estimates of the prevalence of caregiving range widely depending on how caregiving is defined. Care may support IADL, which consist of functions related to laundry, housekeeping, transportation, food preparation, shopping, handling finances, using the phone, and medication management (Graf, 2007). Increasing dependency requires care specific to ADL, which involves intimate, personal care related to bathing, dressing, eating, toileting, transferring, and mobility (Wallace & Shelkey, 2007). Messecar (2008) estimates that between 22.4 and 52 million people provide some care to family members every year. The smaller estimates are related to the more intense ADL care, whereas the larger estimates include those who receive assistance with IADL only. About 10% of care recipients require extensive assistance with multiple ADL (National Alliance for Caregiving and AARP, 2004). Combining all levels of care, Reinhard, Given, Petlick, and Bemis (2008) cite the statistic of 44 million caregivers, which is about 20% of the adult population. Increasingly, providing care to an older adult is becoming part of the normative life experience in families, as up to 75% of adults will experience caring for another adult family member at least once in their lifetime.

Most caregivers are middle aged or older. Most care is provided by wives and daughters, although men are increasingly assuming this role. Research has consistently shown that women provide more personal care, more hours of caregiving, and more housekeeping, whereas men more typically provide financial assistance (such as money management), make arrangements for formal care, and do home and yard maintenance work. These historically gendered roles, however, are becoming less distinct. Reinhard and her colleagues (2008) report a 50% increase between 1984 and 1994 in the number of caregiving men doing more physical care. Similarly, Neal and Hammer (2007) report that men in dual-earner couples are taking on substantially more parent care responsibilities, including ADL care, even as their wives are providing about 2 more hours of caregiving per week than husbands. Women continue to provide more care than men even when the person cared for is the husband's relative. The trend of increasing involvement by men in all facets of caregiving likely will continue as the number of older adults needing support increases.

Duration of caregiving may last for days or decades, with the average length of time being 4.3 years. Twenty percent of caregivers have been providing care for 10 years or longer (Reinhard et al., 2008). About half of caregivers provide 8 hours of care or more each week, with 20% of caregivers providing 40 hours or more. As in families who Neal and Hammer (2007) have described, working couples are often involved in providing parent care for more than one person, such as providing care to both parents or to one's parent and a parent-in-law. Referring to the earlier family case study, we illustrate the multiple caregiving demands as Maria provides care to both her father and her mother-in-law.

Estimates of the value of unpaid family care range from annual costs of $257 billion (National Alliance for Caregiving and AARP, 2004) to more than $300 billion (Messecar, 2008). Out-of-pocket medical expenses are 2.5 times greater for caregivers than noncaregivers (Family Caregiver Alliance, 2006). Furthermore, caregiving often results in lost income if spouses and adult children leave the workforce early to care for older family members. Those who maintain their jobs often lose time and, therefore, wages, promotions, or other job opportunities because of parent care responsibilities. As discussed earlier, the loss of income may be particularly difficult for those with low incomes to begin with. Family members are often faced with the difficult decision of less income because of less time in the workforce versus the expense of paid care either in the home or at a residential care facility.

The experience of caregiving differs by role. Spouses are generally the first line of caregivers. Because women live longer than men, wives are more likely than husbands to become caregivers. Spouse caregivers, in particular, may have their own health concerns that are exacerbated by strains related to caregiving. Messecar (2008) reports that caregiving spouses have a 63% greater mortality rate than others their age who are not caregivers. At times, the spouse who is designated as caregiver is also in need of support services. It is not unusual for husbands and wives to support each other; they are both caregivers and care recipients. These situations are often tenuous but can work for a while. Spouses typically experience greater burden and depression than adult children who provide care (Messecar, 2008). Spouses are more likely to experience chronic illnesses and frailty themselves. Because spouse caregivers typically live with the care recipient, they are at risk for not getting rest, not having time to recuperate from illnesses, and experiencing health declines. This is particularly true if the person they are caring for has Alzheimer disease or some other kind of dementing illness (Reinhard et al., 2008). Those who care for someone with dementia are at increased risk for depression, greater levels of stress, and lower levels of subjective well-being. This is particularly true for wives (Pinquart & Sorensen, 2006). Adult children, particularly daughters, experience the stresses of care in other ways. More than half are working while providing care, and most have to make a range of adjustments at work. This may include going in late or leaving early, cutting down on hours worked, or leaving the labor force entirely (National Alliance for Caregiving and

AARP, 2004). Adult children have to balance caregiving and other family obligations. Some are doing substantial caregiving for parents while caring for young children at home (Neal & Hammer, 2007).

Caregiving is influenced by culture. It is important to be aware of and sensitive to possible ethnic differences in caregiving experiences and resources. At the same time, it is important not to stereotype and make assumptions based on race or ethnicity. More differences are found within ethnic groups than between them. With that caution, Dilworth-Anderson and her colleagues (2002) argue that "culture affects caregiving experiences. Findings on values and norms provide evidence that individuals and groups use explicit rules and guidelines that influence who provides care to elders as well as interactions between caregivers, family members, and social institutions" (p. 264). From their review of the literature, it appears that minority caregivers often have a more diverse group of extended helpers than do white caregivers. But although more people might be involved in providing care to a dependent family member, minority caregivers are no more likely to feel supported by their social network than are caregivers from the dominant culture. Whites are more likely to care for a spouse, which is related to whites having more married couples in later life and a longer life expectancy for men. African Americans are more likely to include church connections to assist with caregiving tasks. They are also more likely to have a network of kinship relationships that assist with caregiving. African Americans and Hispanics are least likely to use formal services and yet are most likely to express the need for assistance with caregiving responsibilities. Cultural values do influence who takes on the leadership role of caregiving within a family (Dilworth-Anderson et al., 2002). These values are affected by a sense of filial obligation and a sense of responsibility, cultural norms regarding who provides care (i.e., daughter or daughter-in-laws), values of giving back, culturally based illness meanings (e.g., a view that disease is normal or that there is a stigma), and larger belief systems such as religion. Because of lower health status found in most minority populations, caregiving is often started at a younger age, but the duration is shorter.

African American caregivers are more likely to have children younger than 18 years living in the household than other ethnic groups. They are more likely to be working and caring for a family member, and also spending more time and money to support the person they care for. This commitment contributes to the financial burden for the family, increasing their risk for living at a low socioeconomic level. African American caregivers are more likely to say caregiving is a financial hardship. Asian American caregivers are found, as a rule, to have more education and higher incomes when compared with other racial ethnic groups. This group is less likely to report emotional stress and be more able to pay for assistance with caregiving. White caregivers tend to be older and also living in a higher income bracket when compared with other racial groups (Dilworth-Anderson et al., 2002).

Our discussion of providing care to frail older adults reflects the research in this area, as well as the population most at need of family caregiving. It is important to emphasize, however, that many older adults are primary caregivers of younger members of their families.

GRANDPARENTS CARING FOR GRANDCHILDREN

Almost all older adults with children are likely to become grandparents, usually around the age of 50, although the transition occurs both earlier and later in the life course. It is a role that is contingent on the actions of others for timing, number, location, and amount of contact (Thiele & Whelan, 2006). Sometimes called a "roleless role," grandparents are often faced with creating their role within the family based on the family's stage in the life course and the family history of grandparenting roles. Grandparents are influenced by experiences with their own grandparents and with their parents as grandparents. Also, relationships with grandchildren are strongly shaped by the quality of relationships with adult children. When the grandparent-parent relationship is strong, grandparents and grandchildren are also likely to enjoy strong connections. If the role is perceived to come too early, as in the case of teenage pregnancy, the transition to grandparenthood may be altered by disappointment, anxiety, and emotional and financial distress. As in other family relationships, the ways that grandparents relate to grandchildren vary widely among families (Silverstein & Marenco, 2001; Thiele

& Whelan, 2006). Most older adults, however, find grandparenting meaningful and experience the role with both satisfaction and pleasure (Roberto, 1990; Szinovacz, 1998). Grandparents are often an important resource for their adult children. For example, they are a major provider of child care when grandchildren are young (Vandell et al., 2003). With aging of both grandparents and grandchildren, the nature of relationships will change. Older grandparents, for example, are more likely to provide money and gifts as grandchildren get older rather than direct care (Thiele & Whelan, 2006).

Unlike caregiving for older adults, which often evolves over time, grandparents may suddenly find themselves in the role of raising their grandchildren. This may occur when teenagers have children or as a result of traumatic circumstances surrounding the parent generation, including divorce, substance abuse, incarceration, child abuse or neglect, or death. The number of grandparents who are raising their grandchildren has risen dramatically, increasing 30% between 1990 and 2000 (Hayslip & Kaminski, 2005). Lumpkin (2008) reports that this accounts for 11% of grandparents in the United States. In 2002, 2.4 million children younger than 18 were under the care of their grandparents (Goodman & Silverstein, 2006). These grandparent-grandchild families are more likely to live below the poverty line and lack health insurance. Some grandparents leave the workforce to care for grandchildren, whereas others feel that they cannot retire for financial reasons. Grandparent caregivers are most often women, are in poorer physical health, and have a greater incidence of depression than other grandparents. Ongoing conflict with adult children is common, with accompanying feelings of disappointment, resentment, feeling taken advantage of, and grief. If parents have been substance abusers, grandchildren may have physical and behavioral problems that cause further anxiety for grandparents (Hayslip & Kaminski, 2005; Leder, Grinstead, & Torres, 2007). Those who co-reside with grandchildren may be less likely than those who live in separate households to hold a self-identify as grandparents. Many custodial grandparents are saddened by the loss of the traditional grandparent role that emphasizes indulgence and fun, instead of being responsible for discipline, financial support, and a myriad of activities related to daily care. Caregiving grandparents may be isolated from their age peers who are pursuing more traditional grandparent-, work-,

or retirement-related activities. They also may have little in common with the parents of their grandchildren's friends (Landry-Meyer & Newman, 2004). Most grandparents who raise grandchildren are non-Hispanic whites, yet the largest proportion of any ethnic or racial group of grandparents raising grandchildren are African Americans. African American and Latino grandparents are more likely to assume the responsibility because of economic conditions and teen pregnancies, whereas white grandparents are more likely to be parenting because of substance abuse by their adult children. They are also more likely to report greater levels of burden and more intergenerational conflict than those in other ethnic groups. This may be because of combined circumstances of normative expectations and issues related to substance abuse (Goodman & Silverstein, 2006).

As with caregiving in general, grandparents and their grandchildren experience many benefits from grandparents parenting. Grandparents are often a stabilizing influence, and their grandchildren generally do well in school, are less likely to be on welfare, and have fewer negative behaviors. Grandparents, in spite of their grief and the burdens associated with care, report benefits such as realizing their inner strength, close relationships with their grandchildren, and a sense of accomplishment and purpose (Hayslip & Kaminski, 2005; Waldrop, 2003).

OLDER ADULTS CARING FOR ADULT CHILDREN

Much of the literature addresses parents caring for adult children with developmental disabilities or mental illness. Seltzer and her colleagues have followed aging mothers of adults with mental retardation or severe mental illness for many years. Their research indicates many similarities and also some important differences between these mothers (Seltzer et al., 2004; Seltzer, Greenberg, Krause, & Hong, 1997). The onset of disability occurred at different times in the life course—at birth for those with mental retardation and in young adulthood for those with mental illness. Mothers of those with mental retardation experienced more gratification and less subjective burden than mothers of those with mental illness. They also received more social support and had developed more effective coping skills. Mothers of children with mental illness experienced greater levels of stress and burden. The course of the child's illness was less predictable, sometimes including repeated crises involving hospitalization or incarceration. As mothers aged, they required additional supports, including placement of their children in residential care. Reasons leading to placement varied. For mothers of children with mental retardation, placement often occurred because of poor health and declining abilities of the mothers. Mothers in both groups maintained a high frequency of contact (Seltzer et al., 1997). Magana, Seltzer, and Krause (2002) focus on Latino populations, finding that they had higher service needs than the general population, in part because of lack of knowledge and the difficulty of navigating the system. When programs were culturally sensitive and provided opportunities for peer support, however, Latinos did increase use of services.

An aftermath of the Iraqi and Afghanistan wars is that many parents are finding themselves caring for disabled war veterans (Yeoman, 2008). In April 2008, Yeoman reported that nearly 32,000 servicemen had been wounded, and that 38% of soldiers and 49% of national guardsmen had psychiatric symptoms consistent with chronic mental illness. Nearly half of the soldiers in the armed forces are not married, so when they are disabled, their parents become caregivers and advocates. Parents of soldiers who are parents may also see increased involvement during deployment and, in the case of disability and death, a greater role in raising grandchildren.

NURSING ROLE IN ASSESSING AND SUPPORTING CAREGIVERS

Many caregivers are unprepared for their role. Lack of experience or knowledge involved with physical care can lead to medication errors, inability to monitor for adverse or toxic effects, injury and/or exhaustion for the caregiver, or uncertainty about when medical or emergency care is needed. In addition to issues of physical health and health care delivery, most are also unprepared for handling health insurance, managing the care recipient's assets such as selling a home, or finding and moving the care recipient to another living situation. As we have seen, caregivers themselves are at risk for negative outcomes. The degree of risk is influenced by the context of caregiving including family history and dynamics, the nature of impairment such as behavioral problems related to dementia, the level of care

recipient dependency, and a wide range of personal and financial resources. Caregivers may not be able to care emotionally or deal with stresses of caregiving (Messecar, 2008).

Nurses and other health and social service providers can assist family caregivers by teaching them caregiving skills, providing information to support the care receiver, providing emotional support, connecting them to services and resources, and through other ways. Coehlo, Hooker, and Bowman (2007) emphasize the importance of forming partnerships between formal care providers, including nurses, to support caregivers in using in-home care services, adult day care facilities, respite care, and residential care as determined by the complexity of care needed and the caregiver's abilities. Yet, needs of caregivers are not assessed routinely, and caregivers remain at risk for burnout and care recipients at risk for not receiving appropriate care, either at home or in another setting. Reinhard and her colleagues (2008) recommend that assessments be done for families as clients and for families as providers of care, and that they go beyond a listing of ADL and IADL needs for the following reason:

> [T]hose concepts do not adequately capture the complexity and stressfulness of caregiving. Assistance with bathing does not capture bathing a person who is resisting a bath. Helping with medications does not adequately capture the hassles of medication administration, especially when the care recipient is receiving multiple medications several times a day, including injections, inhalers, eye drops, and crushed tablets (p. 2).

To address the lack of systematic attention to assessing caregiver needs, the National Center on Caregiving, at the Family Caregiver Alliance, convened a National Consensus Development Conference for Caregiver Assessment. The conference resulted in a report published in 2006 documenting key issues in assessment and recommendations from the panel. The fundamental principles for caregiver assessment are presented in Table 15-2. Domains to be included in assessments are context; caregiver perception of health and functional status of the care recipient; caregiver values and principles; well-being of the caregiver; consequences of caregiving; skills, abilities, and knowledge to provide care; and potential resources that the caregiver could choose to use (Family Caregiver Alliance, 2006).

TABLE 15-2

Fundamental Principles for Caregiver Assessment

1. Because family caregivers are a core part of health care and long-term care, it is important to recognize, respect, assess, and address their needs.

2. Caregiver assessment should embrace a family-centered perspective, inclusive of the needs and preferences of both the care recipient and the family caregiver.

3. Caregiver assessment should result in a plan of care (developed collaboratively with the caregiver) that indicates the provision of services and intended measurable outcomes.

4. Caregiver assessment should be multidimensional in approach and periodically updated.

5. Caregiver assessment should reflect culturally competent practice.

6. Effective caregiver assessment requires assessors to have specialized knowledge and skills. Practitioners' and service providers' education and training should equip them with an understanding of the caregiving process and its impacts, as well as the benefits and elements of an effective caregiver assessment.

7. Government and other third-party payers should recognize and pay for caregiver assessment as a part of care for older people and adults with disabilities.

Source: From Family Caregiver Alliance (2006). *Caregiver assessment: Principles, guidelines and strategies for change. Report from a National Consensus Development Conference* (Vol. I, p. 12). San Francisco: Author.

Multiple interventions have been developed and tested to address the needs of caregivers both as clients and as providers. Pinquart and Sorensen (2006) have conducted a meta-analysis of interventions designed to assist caregivers of persons with dementia. They categorize interventions as psychoeducational, cognitive behavioral therapy (CBT), counseling/case management, support, training the care recipient, respite care, and multicomponent interventions. Outcomes of interest include reducing burden, depression, care recipient symptoms, and institutionalization of the care recipient, as well as increasing subjective well-being and caregiver knowledge and ability. They found the largest effects were with CBT, which helped to reduce depression and, to a lesser extent, helped reduce feelings of burden. CBT concentrates on helping caregivers identify and modify beliefs related to the

situation, and develop new behaviors to cope with caregiving demands. Psychoeducational programs contributed to small-to-moderate effects related to decreasing burden, depression, subjective well-being, and care receiver symptoms. Only care receiver education and multicomponent interventions were successful in reducing institutionalization. Other interventions that show some promise in reducing stress include moderate intensity exercise programs, and yoga and meditation activities (Messecar, 2008).

Teaching caregivers to be providers of care can be powerful interventions that contribute to feelings of mastery. Those with high mastery have more positive experiences with caregiving and more positive health behaviors (Reinhard et al., 2008). They are also more likely to provide safe care and develop critical thinking skills. Pinquart and Sorensen (2006) suggest that more effort needs to be given to designing multicomponent interventions that target individual caregiver needs. Working in partnership with the caregiver to individualize interventions tends to be more successful in meeting needs as defined by the caregiver and care recipient (Archbold et al., 1995). Nursing care strategies to support caregivers that can improve caregiver outcomes are presented in Table 15-3.

TABLE 15-3

Nursing Care Strategies to Support Caregivers

1. Identify content and skills needed to increase preparedness for caregiving.

2. Form a partnership with the caregiver before generating strategies to address issues and concerns.

3. Identify the caregiving issues and concerns on which the caregiver wants to work and generate strategies.

4. Assist the caregiver in identifying strengths in the caregiving situation.

5. Assist the caregiver in finding and using resources.

6. Help caregivers identify and manage their physical and emotional responses to caregiving.

7. Use an interdisciplinary approach when working with family caregivers.

Source: From Messecar, D. C. (2008). Family caregiving. In E. Capezuti, D. Zwicker, M. Mezey, & T. Fulmer (Eds.), *Evidence-based geriatric nursing protocols for best practice* (3rd ed.). New York: Springer, by permission.

Acute Care

Hospitalization puts older adults at great risk for functional decline. This is especially true for frail elders who have mobility or cognitive impairments before hospitalization. Kleinpell, Fletcher, and Jennings (2008) report that, after 2 days of bed rest, 71% of older patients experienced declines in mobility, transferring, toileting, feeding, and grooming. This deconditioning is also responsible for accelerated bone loss, reduced cardiovascular efficiency, and decreased muscle strength. As a result, older adults are at increased risk for falls, delirium, nosocomial infections, adverse drug reactions, and pressure ulcers. Furthermore, after discharge, they continue to experience functional decline and prolonged recovery.

Comprehensive assessment is essential to identify potential problems and design interventions to prevent complications and maintain function. Four areas are critical: (1) ADL, (2) IADL, (3) cognitive status, and (4) presence of sensory impairments. Although nurses are always assessing through observations and interactions with clients, the use of standardized tools facilitates consistent data collection over time to be able to evaluate baseline status, detect changes, and evaluate response to interventions. Several tools are available to assess an older adult admitted to acute care (Graf, 2006). As described previously, ADL assessment includes bathing, dressing, eating, toileting, hygiene, and mobility. This information is important for planning care during hospitalization and for discharge. IADL function often determines a person's ability to continue to live independently, as these include areas such as shopping, managing finances, meal preparation, driving, and managing medications. Persons with visual or hearing impairments will also have difficulty participating in assessment of ADL and IADL. Failure to recognize hearing and visual impairments risks making erroneous diagnoses. Providing the person with her glasses and hearing aides are easy but important interventions.

Cognitive assessment serves two purposes. First, this assessment identifies the presence of any of the "3 D's": dementia, delirium, and depression. Although some symptoms are similar, these disorders are distinct and require very different kinds of interventions. Dementia is a group of several progressive cognitive disorders that results in memory loss, confusion, loss of judgment, and various executive functions such as ability to plan or organize activities. Onset is slow and insidious. Alzheimer disease is the most common form of dementia and risk increases with age; estimates are that 50% or more of those older than 85 years have the disease (Doerflinger, 2007). Early detection is important to begin treatment to slow progression, and allow the individual and families to plan ahead for care. Delirium also involves confusion, though onset occurs rapidly. Symptoms also include inattention, disorganized thinking, and altered level of consciousness (Waszynski, 2007). Because of their more fragile physiologic balance, older adults are more susceptible to delirium, which is usually due to physiologic causes such as infection, adverse effects of medications, dehydration, and fluid and electrolyte imbalance. With estimates of 14% to 56% of older patients experiencing delirium in hospitals, it is extremely important to be alert to symptoms. Postoperative patients appear to be especially vulnerable. Family members can be especially important in providing baseline information about cognitive status. It is important to remember that delirium is usually reversible if detected, underlying causes are identified, and it is then treated early. If it is not detected, morbidity and mortality rates are high.

Depression, common in older adults, is often not recognized and consequently is under-treated, diminishing quality of life. Depression is a mood disorder with affective, cognitive, and physical symptoms (Greenberg, 2007). Depression is responsive to treatment, though left untreated, it may persist or progress.

In addition to timely and appropriate treatment of these disorders, artful cognitive assessment is needed to determine the older adult's ability to participate in assessment of ADL and IADL. For example, a person with dementia may have difficulty remembering complex directions, and will need these provided using single words or short phrases and demonstration. The Hartford Insititue for Geriatric Nursing (HIGN) has developed a resource called *Try This*, which is composed of several assessment tools to guide nurses, including those related to delirium, depression, or dementia (Table 15-4). The *American Journal of Nursing* has partnered with HIGN to develop a series of articles that provide more in-depth information regarding the development of the *Try This* assessment tools. For example, see Doerflinger (2007) for

TABLE 15-4

The *Try This: Best Practices in Nursing Care to Older Adults* Series of Assessment Tools is to Provide Knowledge of Best Practices in the Care of Older Adults

1. SPICES: An Overall Assessment Tool of Older Adults
2. Katz Index of Independence in Activities of Daily Living
3. Mental Status Assessment of Older Adults: The Mini-Cog
4. The Geriatric Depression Scale (GDS)
5. Predicting Pressure Ulcer Risk
6.1. The Pittsburgh Sleep Quality Index
6.2. The Epworth Sleepiness Scale
7. Assessing Pain in Older Adults
8. Fall Risk Assessment
9. Assessing Nutrition in Older Adults
10. Sexuality Assessment for Older Adults
11.1. Urinary Incontinence Assessment in Older Adults: Part I—Transient Urinary Incontinence
11.2. Urinary Incontinence Assessment in Older Adults: Part II—Persistent Urinary Incontinence
12. Hearing Screening in Older Adults
13. Confusion Assessment Method (CAM)
14. The Modified Caregiver Strain Index (CSI)
15. Elder Mistreatment Assessment
16. Beers Criteria for Potentially Inappropriate Medication Use in the Elderly
17. Alcohol Use Screening and Assessment
18. The Kayser–Jones Brief Oral Health Status Examination (BOHSE)
19. Horowitz's Impact of Event Scale: An Assessment of Post Traumatic Stress in Older Adults
20. Preventing Aspiration in Older Adults with Dysphagia
21. Immunizations for the Older Adult
22. Assessing Family Preferences for Participation in Care in Hospitalized Older Adults
23. The Lawton Instrumental Activities of Daily Living (IADL) Scale
24. The Hospital Admission Risk Profile (HARP)
25. Confusion Assessment Method for the Intensive Care Unit (CAM-ICU)
26. Issues on Dementia:

    D1 Avoiding Restraints in Patients with Dementia

    D2 Assessing Pain in Persons with Dementia

    D3 Brief Evaluation of Executive Dysfunction

    D4 Therapeutic Activity Kits

    D5 Recognition of Dementia in Hospitalized Older Adults

    D6 Wandering in the Hospitalized Older Adult

    D7 Communication Difficulties: Assessment and Interventions

    D8 Assessing and Managing Delirium in Persons with Dementia

    D9 Decision Making in Older Adults with Dementia

    D10 Working with Families of Hospitalized Older Adults with Dementia

    D11.1 Eating and Feeding Issues in Older Adults with Dementia

Source: Adapted from Hartford Institute for Geriatric Nursing. (2009, September). *TRY THIS: and How To Try This Series Assessment Tools on the Care of Older Adults.* Retrieved September 27, 2009, from http://hartfordign.org/try this

information about the Mini-Cog assessment tool for dementia, Greenberg (2007) for a description of the Geriatric Depression Scale, and Waszynski, (2007) who presents the Confusion Assessment Method for identifying delirium.

Families need to be included in assessing hospitalized older adults. They are key informants regarding the elder's baseline cognitive status and prior IADL abilities, which are key factors in predicting functional decline. Family members also need information about the risks of bed rest, and can help encourage mobility and self-care during hospitalization. As described previously, hospital staff must assess caregiver needs and abilities. Too often, older adults are discharged to home where a caregiver is not physically, emotionally, or cognitively able to provide care needed. Fortunately, several programs and models for providing nursing care to hospitalized older adults have been developed (see Table 15-5 for a summary of these programs and models).

Family Case Study, cont'd

TRANSITION 1: HOME TO HOSPITAL

Sarah (now age 83) spent most of the day at a friend's house. When she returned home about 4 p.m., she found her husband, Louis (age 85), on the floor in the garage. He told her that he tripped on the stairs while carrying a chair that needed repair to the garage; this occurred about 9:30 a.m. He tried to get up or crawl up the three steps from the attached garage to the kitchen, but he could not move because the pain was too great. Sarah called 911, and Louis was taken to the emergency department. Fortunately, it was a relatively uncomplicated fracture of his hip. He was able to have a surgical repair later the next morning. Because he experienced some confusion after surgery, the nurses were reluctant to give him pain medication, believing the medication would cause more confusion. He started physical therapy the day after surgery but could participate only to a limited extent because of

---

TABLE 15-5

Programs and Models to Improve Quality of Care for Older Adults in Hospitals

Nurses Improving Care to Health System Elders (NICHE): Initiated in 1992, this is a nation-wide program of staff education and system evaluation to deliver "sensitive and exemplary nursing care" to older adults (Mezey et al., 2004, p. 452). As of 2008, more than 200 hospitals were participating in this effort.

Geriatric Resource Nurse (GRN) Model: In this unit-based model, staff nurses with an interest in working with older adults are provided with additional knowledge and skills for working with this specialized population. They serve as resources for other nurses on their units by implementing best practices and providing consultation to their peers. The GRN is usually a key component in hospitals that have implemented the NICHE program (Mezey et al., 2004).

Geriatric Syndrome Management Model: This model uses advanced practice nurses, usually gerontological clinical nurse specialists (GCNSs), as consultants to assess and manage problems common to hospitalized older adults, such as delirium, falls, and incontinence. They also provide staff education and evaluate policies, procedures, and other system issues to identify barriers to design strategies to provide optimal care for older adults (Mezey et al., 2004).

Acute Care for the Elderly (ACE) Model: These are hospital units designed specifically to meet the needs of older adults. An interdisciplinary team approach is used, often with a GCNS as the team coordinator. The goal is to prevent loss of function while being hospitalized for an acute health problem.

Hospital Elder Life Program (HELP): This model also uses an interdisciplinary approach with a focus on ongoing assessment to identify and treat problems promptly. Volunteers are also incorporated in this model (Inouye, Bogardus, Baker, Leo-Summers, & Cooney, 2000).

Family-Centered Geriatric Resource Nurse (FCGRN) Model: This combines the GRN role with concepts from the Family-Centered Care (FCC) Model. The FCC Model, previously used for working with chronically ill children, was adapted for care of hospitalized older adults. The focus is on assessment of the family, as well as the individual older adult (Salinas, O'Connor, Weinstein, Lee, & Fitzpatrick, 2002). This model is used in the case study example.

Older Adults Services Inpatient Strategies (OASIS): This program was developed at a hospital in Atlanta and combined features from other programs based on the local needs and resources. It used an interdisciplinary approach with a GCNS as the team coordinator (Tucker et al., 2006). *Note:* This should not be confused with the OASIS (Outcome Assessment and Information Set), a comprehensive assessment and database used in home health care.

the pain. He was also started on insulin to control his diabetes (he previously took an oral medication). After 4 days in the hospital, Louis was discharged to the skilled care unit of a nursing home for additional rehabilitation, with the goal of returning to his own home.

Louis's needs are common. As an older adult, Louis was at a greater risk for falls and related injuries. Hospital care by those unfamiliar with the needs of older adults can exacerbate rather than prevent negative outcomes. Knowing, for example, that untreated pain can increase confusion and delay successful rehabilitation is important for nurses caring for Louis. Sarah needs support to bring Louis home as quickly and successfully as possible. Sarah will need instruction on insulin, changing the home environment to prevent falls, and managing Louis's pain while his hip heals. Without including Sarah in the transition plan, Louis is likely to spend longer time in the skilled facility or return home without sufficient support. Without support, Sarah is likely to experience greater levels of stress and caregiver burden in her expanded role as caregiver.

Facility-Based Long-Term Care

We now turn to the formal care system of nursing home and other residential settings where LTC services are provided. Although the term *long-term care* (LTC) is sometimes used interchangeably with nursing home care, nursing homes represent only one type of LTC service. Residential care includes assisted living, board and care, and adult foster homes (Stone, 2006). Descriptions of facility-based LTC options for services are presented in Table 15-6. The number of older adults who reside in nursing home settings has declined as more residential care options have become available (Stone, 2006). This section describes two aspects of LTC: (1) the development of assisted living models of care, and (2) the broader cultural change movement regarding care of older adults that is sweeping the country. Throughout this discussion, we examine the changing role of LTC nurses, and the partnership of nurses with LTC consumers, their family members, and other LTC providers. As explained later, families continue to be integrally involved in all of these care settings, and nurses play a vital role in shaping care and supporting older adults and their families.

Assisted Living

ALFs were developed in part as a response to the institutional environment of nursing homes. Nursing homes were considered to function under a medical model that was unresponsive to the quality-of-life needs of its residents. In contrast, the new assisted living approach was described as a social model of care that would serve as an extension of "home." Wilson (2007) was a pioneer in this effort in the early 1980s. She was interested in creating housing that would match the needs of frail elders for support whereas maintaining their autonomy, privacy, and a sense of home. The idea was to provide help to people who required some assistance because of physical or cognitive impairment and could not live safely at home. At the same time, they did not require levels of nursing care found in traditional nursing home settings. The key features of this assisted living model included a private living space with locking doors, a kitchenette, and the right of residents to make a wide range of choices about their lives, including visits from friends and family, and their health care. The state of Oregon supports this and other community-based models of care. Oregon obtained a Medicaid Waiver to support low-income clients in using assisted living and other community-based care settings. Oregon administrative rules identify five values that are necessary for assisted living: independence, choices, dignity, homelike environments, and privacy (Carder, 2002). In contrast, most other states use LTC Medicaid funds predominantly for nursing home care. The Medicaid Waiver allowed Oregon to use Medicaid funds to support individuals in assisted living, adult foster care (homes with five or fewer residents), and a variety of other home care services. Evaluations of these services indicated that these new forms of community-based care were generally viewed positively by consumers, and they were substituting for nursing home care (Wilson, 2007).

Other assisted living models were developing independently and simultaneously around the United States (Stone & Reinhard, 2007; Wilson, 2007; Zimmerman & Sloan, 2007). By the 1990s, the number of assisted living housing units and those served by them had exploded to become the fastest growing type of LTC service. By 2005, the number of residential or assisted living beds was similar to the number of nursing home beds (Sloane, Zimmerman, & Sheps 2005). With this growth came increasing divergence

TABLE 15-6
Facility-Based Long-Term Care Options

Numerous types of facility-based programs provide a range of long-term care services. Some facilities provide only housing and related housekeeping, but many also include help managing medications, assistance with personal care, supervision and special programs for individuals with Alzheimer's disease, or 24-hour nursing care. The services available in each facility are often regulated by the state in which the facility operates (e.g., some states do not allow some types of facilities to include residents who are wheelchair bound or who cannot exit the facility on their own in an emergency). Facility-based care is known by a wide variety of names, including board and care, assisted living, adult foster care, continuing care retirement communities (CCRCs), and nursing homes.

Facility-based service providers include the following:

Adult Foster Care
Adult foster care can be provided for individuals or for small groups of adults who need help functioning or who cannot live safely on their own. The foster family provides room and board, 24-hour availability, help managing medications, and assistance with activities of daily living. Licensure requirements and the terminology used for this type of facility vary greatly from state to state.

Board and Care Homes
Board and care homes, also called *residential care facilities* or *group homes,* are smaller private facilities, usually with 20 or fewer residents. Most board and care homes accept six or fewer residents. Rooms may be private or residents may share rooms. Residents receive meals, personal care, and have staff available 24 hours a day. Nursing and medical attention are usually not provided on the premises. State licensure and the terminology used for this type of facility vary greatly.

Assisted Living
Assisted living is designed for people who want to live in a community setting and who need or expect to need help functioning, but who do not need as much care as they would receive at a nursing home. Some assisted living facilities are quite small, with as few as 25 residents, whereas some can accommodate 120 or more units. Residents often live in their own apartments or rooms but enjoy the support services that a community setting makes possible, such as:

- Up to three meals a day

- Assistance with personal care

- Help with medications, housekeeping, and laundry

- 24-hour security and onsite staff for emergencies

- Social programs

The cost of assisted living varies widely, depending in part on the services needed by the resident and the amenities provided by the facility. Assisted living is regulated in all states; however, the requirements vary.

Continuing Care Retirement Communities (CCRCs)
CCRCs are also called *life care communities.* They offer several levels of care in one location. For example, many offer independent housing for people who need little or no care, but also have assisted living housing and a nursing facility, all on one campus, for those who need greater levels of care or supervision. In a CCRC, if you become unable to live independently, you can move to the assisted living area, or sometimes you can receive home care in your independent living unit. If necessary, you can enter the onsite or affiliated nursing home. The fee arrangements for CCRCs vary by the type of community. In addition to a monthly fee, many CCRCs also charge a one-time "entrance fee" that may be partially or completely refundable (often on the sale of the unit).

Nursing Homes
Nursing homes, also called *skilled nursing facilities* (SNF) or *convalescent care facilities,* provide a wide range of services, including nursing care, 24-hour supervision, assistance with activities of daily living, and rehabilitation services such as physical, occupational, and speech therapy. Some people need nursing home services for a short period for recovery or rehabilitation after a serious illness or operation, whereas others need longer stays because of chronic physical, health, or cognitive conditions that require constant care or supervision. Families typically seek nursing home care when it is no longer possible to care for a person at home safely or when the cost of round-the-clock care at home becomes too great. Nursing homes are highly regulated. They must be licensed by state governments.

Source: Adapted from National Clearinghouse for Long-Term Care (Administration on Aging). (2008). *Understanding Long-Term Care.* Retrieved July 14, 2008, from http://www.longtermcare.gov/LTC/Main_Site/Understanding_Long_Term_Care/Services/Services.aspx, by permission.

in the definitions of assisted living and the services associated with it. In some instances, private units were no longer emphasized, and the types of supportive services ranged from medication reminders only to a full range of ADL and dementia care services. Each state has developed its own definitions and regulations that influence how assisted living is implemented. Financing varies widely, with some states using Medicaid dollars to fund assisted living, whereas in other states, only those with financial means have assisted living as a housing option. State regulations also vary regarding nurse delegation, which affects the type of services that can be provided (Stone & Reinhard, 2007). For example, ALFs in states permitting nurse delegation of medication administration to unlicensed personnel can provide a broader range of services than those in states requiring nurses only to administer medications. This does not preclude involvement of nurses in providing education and overseeing and monitoring care to unlicensed personnel. When considering assisted living services as a housing option, therefore, it is important to understand the context, including state and local definitions and models of care supported. Currently, most assisted living housing has been developed by for-profit companies serving private-pay consumers.

Although research is limited, it appears that assisted living residents tend to be women in their 80s who have two or more chronic illnesses, require assistance in one to three ADL, and have some level of dementia (Maas & Buckwalter, 2006). Beel-Bates, Ziemba, and Algase (2007) surveyed family members of assisted living residents, mostly residing in Michigan. These family members identified resident needs for an average of 18 services related to ADL and IADL. Even more service needs were anticipated by family members as residents grew older. Generally, family members of residents in the ALFs represented in this study felt the ALFs met the needs of residents in their care with respect to ADL. The service needed by most and received by most residents was related to medication management. Family members felt that resident needs, however, exceeded services available or provided by the ALFs for many aspects of nursing assessment services, including assessing the effectiveness of medications and monitoring residents to identify adverse effects of the medications. Other unmet needs included assessments of overall health, new health problems, and urgent situations (Beel-Bates et al., 2007). The availability and provision of advocacy services by nurses also fell short of needs related to care management, teaching, referrals, first aid, and evaluating the plan of care.

As reflected by Beel-Bates and her colleagues (2007), health care for assisted living residents is of growing concern. As residents age, they become increasingly frail and dependent, which may make it difficult for them to age in place if the ALF does not provide comprehensive support services, either through their own programs or through contracts with other agencies. Some ALFs make extensive efforts to help residents "age in place" by providing of a variety of support services, including medication management, personal care, and nursing case management. Also, many of these models have step up programs, with the ability of residents who are no longer able to live in the independent part to move up to a level with more assistance, with the final level including nursing care in a more traditional nursing home setting. If services are limited, residents or their family member frequently contracts with outside agencies or care providers to meet the gap between ALF services and resident needs. This option, however, may be prohibitively expensive.

ALFs were developed, in part, to be different from nursing homes; they are less of a medical model and more of a social model. As a result, many do not have the resources or staffing needed to provide a full range of health care and support services. In their review of research, Stone and Reinhard (2007) found that a sizable number (75% in one study) of ALFs would not keep residents who required nursing home care for more than 2 weeks. In contrast, Stone and Reinhard described another study that suggested that as residents become increasingly frail and dependent, ALFs can and do become substitutes for nursing home care, providing additional services as the need arises. This occurs most freqently in ALFs with full-time RNs. Most people who move into assisted living apartments do not expect to move into nursing homes as they experience physical and cognitive declines. Yet, because of the gap between needs and services that exist in many facilities, individuals may be asked to move, with their only options being a nursing home or perhaps a foster care placement.

The extent to which nursing services are available within an ALF is a function of state regulations, as well as organizational policy. Some ALFs include full-time or part-time RNs as part of their staff, some do not employ nurses, and still others contract with nurses to provide assessment or delegation services (i.e., medication administration) as needed. The role of nurses in addressing health needs of residents is as variable as the models of assisted living, although all nurses in assisted living settings clearly have a different role from nurses in nursing homes, in acute care settings, or even nurses in home care. Nurses in assisted living conduct assessments, offer health-promotion interventions, identify ways to help maintain function, and provide education to the frontline staff who is working most directly with residents (Maas & Buckwalter, 2006). Additional nursing activities, often initiated at the requests of families who do not live with the older adult, include assisting direct care workers with documentation; teaching paid care workers what to expect in caring for residents; and advocacy, monitoring, and support through long-term trusting relationships. Delegation and assignment of various nursing or basic tasks are also key to the role (Caffrey, 2005).

When a nurse is employed as part of the staff of a community-based care facility, outcomes for residents improve. For example, Maas and Buckwalter (2006) report that residents are less likely to leave an ALF because of impairment if a full-time nurse is on staff. Nurses are able to help maintain function and prevent exacerbations of chronic illness episodes requiring hospitalization. Although evidence exists about the efficacy of employing full-time nurses, most ALFs opt to contract for these services on a part-time basis.

Despite concerns about meeting the care needs of frail elders, residents and staff alike are generally positive about working and living in ALFs. According to Sikorska-Simmons (2006b),

> The success of AL [assisted living] as a person-centered model of care will greatly depend on its ability to create a pc [person centered] organizational culture that values both residents and staff and recognizes the key role of staff in the provision of quality care (p. 27).

She reports that staff generally had favorable perceptions of the organizational culture, including higher levels of job satisfaction, satisfaction with coworkers, and greater organizational commitment. Especially important to staff outcomes are teamwork, participation in decision making, and supportive relationships among staff. Sikorska-Simmons

(2006a) also reports positive relationships between resident satisfaction and the quality of work environment for staff in assisted living settings, and found greater resident satisfaction associated with higher aggregate levels of staff job satisfaction and more positive views of organizational culture. These findings, however, had no relationship to job commitment. The only significant resident characteristic was education, with residents with more education being less satisfied than those residents with less education.

Family Case Study, cont'd

TRANSITION 2: APARTMENT TO ASSISTED LIVING

Recall from the earlier case study that Carol, Maria's former mother in-law, had been living in an ALF for several years (see Fig. 15-1). She initially moved there because her worsening Parkinson disease made it impossible to remain at home in her apartment. In the community, Carol's main support system came from friends and neighbors, with Maria and her children helping when they could. Richard, Carol's son and Maria's ex-husband, lived in another state but would visit two or three times a year to fix things around the apartment and to handle Carol's finances. The year before Carol moved into the ALF, she began losing weight because she was not able to prepare meals. In response, Maria and some of Carol's friends often prepared meals and froze these meals in individual portions. Maria also did grocery shopping during her monthly visits. A local volunteer organization provided some house cleaning, and friends from Carol's church would take her to lunch or bring her dinner at least once a week. At Maria's urging, Richard arranged for meals-on-wheels from a local community center. However, Carol often did not eat the food from this service (her reasons included "It's not like my own cooking," and "It all tastes the same."). Several times, when the volunteer delivered the meal, she found Carol on the floor because she had fallen. Concern about Carol's safety prompted Richard, her friends, and Maria to convince her to move to the ALF, which was also closer to Maria's home. Although Carol had limited income from Social Security, the ALF accepted residents receiving housing subsidy as a Medicaid benefit.

Carol was initially reluctant to move to the ALF. She was not familiar with assisted living and thought her family wanted her to move to a nursing home, which she strongly opposed. She changed her mind after visiting a few ALFs and learned that she could still have her own apartment. After moving in, she discovered she enjoyed the opportunities to participate in many of the activities. Her strength also improved; at her apartment, it had been difficult to get regular exercise because of limited space and a short flight of stairs to get outside. At the ALF, the long hallways provided a safe walking space, and with the elevator she did not need to worry about stairs. As a result, she was able to go outside more often. Carol developed close friendships with several other residents during the time she lived at the ALF. She recognized that she had become somewhat isolated in her apartment because of her increasing difficulty with mobility. As she received three meals daily in the dining room, her weight improved. She also received assistance with bathing twice a week. Bathing had been a challenge in her apartment because she had only a tub and shower combination, and the owner would not allow her to have safety bars installed in the bathroom.

TRANSITION 3: ASSISTED LIVING TO HOSPITAL

After living successfully in the ALF for three years, Carol gradually experienced development of memory problems; her physician was not sure whether it was Alzheimer disease or dementia secondary to the Parkinson disease. The ALF staff frequently had to go find her at mealtimes. Like many older adults, Carol took several medications, both prescription and over-the-counter drugs. She had been able to take them safely and accurately once the med-aide had set them up for her in a pill box, but now when Maria visited, she found Carol has not taken about half of the doses. When cleaning her apartment, the staff also noted clothes soiled with urine in her bathroom. One morning, when she did not come to breakfast, the resident assistant found her still in bed. She was very difficult to wake up, she had been incontinent and could not stand even with the assistance of the resident assistant. When the ALF nurse came on duty, she assessed Carol and suspected she had an infection. She contacted Richard, who lives several hundred miles away. He called Maria, who arranged to take time off work and took Carol to see her physician. The physician determined that Carol was dehydrated and had a urinary tract infection (UTI). He had her admitted to the hospital for treatment. Figure 15-2 presents the Hooper family ecomap.

COMMENTARY

Incontinence is not "normal" for older adults; development of incontinence may indicate a change in health status. For example, it may be a sign of a UTI. Other changes in urinary elimination such as burning or frequency may also be signals that further evaluation is warranted. Because of her memory problems, Carol may not have remembered to mention these symptoms to Maria or the ALF nurse. If identified early, the UTI could probably have been successfully treated with oral antibiotics and hospitalization avoided.

Unlike nursing homes, ALFs do not have nurses available 24 hours per day; other staff may have limited training and experience working with older adults (e. g., unlike nursing homes, they are not required to have a structured training for direct care workers). Staff training should focus on normal aging and health-related changes. Staff should also understand the importance of reporting changes in the resident's usual condition, such as a change in continence, or behaviors to the nurse, who will then follow up with additional assessments and evaluations. For example, although Carol had memory problems, she was usually awake and alert, so for the resident assistant to find her difficult to awaken represented a significant change.

TRANSITION 4: HOSPITALIZATION

Carol was admitted to a general medical-surgical unit of a community hospital later that afternoon. The hospital recently implemented a program similar to the Family-Centered Geriatric Resource Nurse model that Salinas, O'Connor, Weinstein, Lee, and Fitzpatrick (2002) describe (see Table 15-5). This model incorporates the acronyms SPICES and FAMILY as frameworks for assessing both the older adult and her family. Susan Jones, the admitting nurse, obtained the information from Maria and also from the ALF nurse as Carol was still quite lethargic when she first arrived at the hospital. An explanation for the acronym SPICES is as follows:

Sleep disorders: No problems.

Poor nutrition: Carol has a history of problems, but over the past year her weight has been stable and within the ideal weight range for her height.

Incontinence: As noted earlier, this is a recent development. The bathroom in Carol's apartment has safety bars and is arranged in a manner that makes it easily accessible for persons with mobility problems.

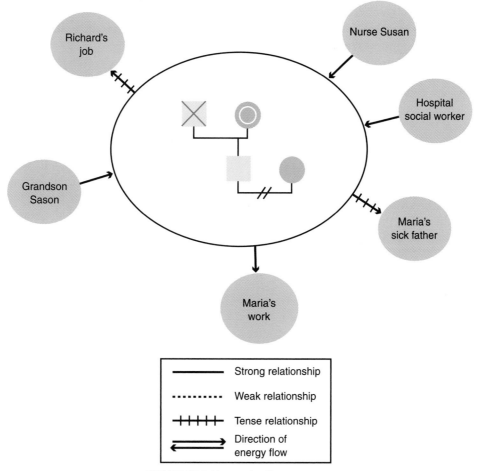

FIGURE 15-2 Hooper family ecomap.

Confusion: The admitting nurse recognizes that Carol is experiencing the "hypoactive" form of delirium as demonstrated by lethargy (it was difficult for the resident assistant to get her to wake up) and is at risk for it worsening.

Evidence of falling: Carol has a history of falls but none in the past year. She has not sustained any serious injuries from falling.

Skin breakdown: No problems.

An explanation for the acronym FAMILY is as follows:

Family involvement: Carol has regular contact with Maria, who provides assistance with a variety of needs. Carol also has come to consider her close friends at the ALF as part of her family. Her son Richard calls about once a week but visits infrequently. Susan learns that Maria is also involved with her own parent care activities as her father Louis is recovering from his hip fracture. Maria has used most of her vacation days providing parent care and cannot afford to take many days without pay.

Assistance needed: Because of her current mental status changes, Carol needs extensive assistance with eating and drinking, changing position, hygiene, and other activities. Because Carol has missed some doses of her anti-Parkinson medication, her mobility is not as good as usual. This is more assistance than her family or the ALF staff can provide at this time.

Members' needs (what family members need from staff to be able to continue to provide care): Maria needs to be updated regularly about Carol's condition so she can keep other family members informed (particularly Carol's son, Richard). She also needs to know whether Carol will be able to return to the ALF, and if not, what options are available. At the same time, Maria expresses some resentment to Susan about Richard's apparent lack of willingness to step up and take more responsibility for the care of his mother. She reports feeling pulled by the needs of her parents, Carol, her grandchildren, and her sister, who is raising her grandchildren.

Integration into care plan (inclusion of family in planning and teaching activities): Susan gives Maria a business card for the unit social worker; she also shares Maria's contact information with the social worker. The team will meet the following day to evaluate Carol's situation. She will probably be in the hospital for only 2 to 4 days; therefore, it is important to start planning for discharge as soon as possible.

Links to community support: Before the team meeting, Susan will follow up with the ALF nurse to learn what care can be provided after discharge. One option could be for Carol to return to the ALF and receive home health care from an outside agency for additional support and follow-up.

Your intervention: On admission, Susan completed the Confusion Assessment Method (Waszynski, 2007). She also knows that Carol has a diagnosis of dementia. Carol is too lethargic to participate in any structured assessments of ADL or IADL function. Susan will reassess her in the morning. By then, Carol should have improved hydration and will have received a few doses of the antibiotic to treat the UTI and may be alert enough for further assessment. This will be important information to have before the team meeting.

TRANSITION 5: HOSPITAL TO NURSING HOME

Carol's condition did improve by the next day, but she was not able to return to the ALF because she needed more assistance than could be provided. She was transferred to the rehabilitation unit of a nearby nursing home with the long-term goal to have her return to the ALF. She received physical therapy twice daily. Another important aspect of her care was to get her re-established on her medication regimen to manage the symptoms of her Parkinson disease to improve her mobility. The nursing staff also used scheduled voiding to help Carol regain continence.

CULTURE CHANGE MOVEMENT IN LONG-TERM CARE

Nursing home care was the focus of initial efforts to change organizational cultures in LTC. Although the movement has expanded to include all types of formal support to older adults, this section emphasizes nursing homes. Efforts to change nursing homes have been made for decades because of widespread recognition that care frequently was inadequate or substandard, and that virtually no one wanted to live in a nursing home. The Nursing Home Reform Act, passed in 1987 as part of the Omnibus Reconciliation Act (OBRA 1987), attempted to address shortcomings by changing practice and systems of care. Practice changes included reducing restraint use, and addressing psychosocial and physical care (Sloane, Zimmerman, & Sheps, 2005). OBRA also resulted in the development of a national data system, known as the Minimum Data Set. Although there have always been nursing homes where excellent, nurturing care was provided, and although extensive federal and state regulations have attempted to address shortcomings, the prevailing public view and experience of LTC for many older adults, their families, and nurses and others remained negative.

In 1995, a group of individuals who had been working independently to change the prevailing culture in their own nursing home settings were invited to present on a panel organized by the National Citizens Coalition for Nursing Home Reform. Although they were all doing different things, they recognized their common purpose. In 1997, 28 individuals representing regulation, law, advocates, and nursing home administration gathered in Rochester, New York. The Pioneer Network was born from this movement (Lustbader, 2001). Pioneers questioned why nursing homes had to be institutional, lacking in respect and dignity, and why efforts such as those of ALFs could not be applied to nursing homes as well with its emphasis on respect, dignity, choice, independence, and home-like or home environments. Today, the Pioneer Network has a large following, with its annual conference attracting hundreds of attendees. The mission and values of the Pioneer Network are presented in Table 15-7.

Person-directed care is central to the culture change movement. It is a way of thinking about care that honors and values the person receiving

TABLE 15-7
Pioneer Network: Toward a New Culture of Aging: Mission, Vision and Values

The new culture of aging involves a transformation based on person-directed values, where the voices of elders and those working closest with them are honored and respected. We seek to promote an inclusive grassroots movement where new ways of deinstitutionalizing services and individualizing care are shared freely. The Pioneer Network is the common ground where we gather to foster new innovations and promote growth.

Our Vision
The Pioneer Network's vision is a culture of aging that is life-affirming, satisfying, humane, and meaningful.

Our Mission
The Pioneer Network advocates and facilitates deep system change and transformation in our culture of aging.

Our Values and Principles
- Know each person.
- Each person can and does make a difference.
- Relationship is the fundamental building block of a transformed culture.
- Respond to spirit, as well as mind and body.
- Risk taking is a normal part of life.
- Put person before task.
- All elders are entitled to self-determination wherever they live.
- Community is the antidote to institutionalization.
- Do unto others as you would have them do unto you—yes, the Golden Rule.
- Promote the growth and development of all.
- Shape and use the potential of the environment in all its aspects: physical, organizational, psycho/social/spiritual.
- Practice self-examination, searching for new creativity and opportunities for doing better.
- Recognize that culture change and transformation are not destinations but a journey, always a work in progress.

When we transform nursing homes into human communities, places for living and growing, we will ultimately change the very nature of aging in America.

Source: Pioneer Network. (1997). *Toward a new culture of aging: Mission, vision and values.* Retrieved September 27, 2009, from http://www.pioneernetwork.net/AboutUs/Values

care, with an emphasis on both quality of care and quality of life so that the individual is not lost in the process of providing care. An example of a person-directed care approach for Maria's mother in-law is illustrated in the case study. Consensus on definitions of person-directed care and culture change are still being developed. Other terms used include person-centered care, resident-centered care, individualized care, and person-centered thinking. Person-directed care is consistent with nursing values, in that nursing strives to individualize care and put the individual ahead of the task (Robinson & Rosher, 2006; Talerico, O'Brien, & Swafford, 2003), but common elements include personhood, knowing the person, autonomy/choice, comfort, and relationships (White, Newton-Curtis, & Lyons, 2008).

Definitions of person-directed care are listed in Table 15-8.

A major part of the culture change movement in LTC is the parallel effort to create person-centered work environments for staff in addition to creating person-centered living environments for residents (Tellis-Nayak, 2007). This is particularly important for direct care workers who provide the vast majority of hands-on care. Turnover in all aspects of LTC is high, because of the hard work, limited pay and benefits, and alternative employment. A major factor in turnover, however, has to do with the climate of the organization. Staff at all levels is more likely to leave the workforce if they do not feel valued, do not feel empowered to advocate for residents, feel inadequately prepared to care for residents, or do

TABLE 15-8

Person-Directed Care

Person-directed care is a way of thinking about care that honors and values the person receiving care. Well-being and quality of life are what the person receiving services say it is. Helping people get care the way they want to get care is more important than completing care tasks.

1. **Personhood.** Each person:
   - Has value and deserves respect
   - Has abilities and can contribute to those around them
   - Has his or her own feelings about living in this place

2. **Knowing the Person.**
   - Each person has a different life story—who was in their family, who was important to them, what did they do during their lives, and their cultural heritage.
   - Everyone has their own ways of doing things (e.g., eating, doing personal care, spending time).
   - Knowing people's life stories and how they like to do things are important for understanding what kind of care they need now.

3. **Choice.**
   - Most people like to make their own choices about how they live.
   - Most people like to control their situation, and they are happier and function better when they can.
   - People have the right to make choices even if it puts them at risk.
   - Although safety is important, it must be balanced with the person's choices.

4. **Comfort.**
   - Both emotional and physical comfort are emphasized.
   - The highest standards of practice are used (e.g., pain control, alternatives to restraints, appropriate medications, exercise, bathing, dressing, eating, toileting, skin care, wheelchair seating, appropriate touch, calming people when they are agitated or worried).

5. **Relating to others.**
   - Each person has relationships with others, including family members, friends, or staff.
   - Relationships between staff and the person receiving care contributes to better care.
   - Relationships with family members and friends help to reduce isolation and provide continuity in the person's life.

6. **Supportive environment.** The ability to provide person-directed care depends on the organization. For the direct care worker, this means:
   - Adequate information and training
   - Ability to be an advocate for residents
   - Ability to make decisions about resident care
   - Having the time and support to work with residents
   - Teamwork
   - Good supervisors
   - Staffing

Source: From White, D. L., Newton-Curtis, L., & Lyons, K. S. (2008). Development and initial testing of a measure of person-directed care. *The Gerontologist, 48(Special Issue 1),* 114-123, by permission.

not feel cared about by supervisors. Nurses of the 21st century will play an increasing role in supervising, teaching, and guiding direct care staff. An organizational environment that supports nurses, direct care workers, and the rest of the staff (e.g., housekeeping, therapists, social services, maintenance, administrative staff) provides adequate education and training, fosters teamwork, and provides skilled supervisors and adequate staffing. Much of this is directed at empowering staff to advocate for residents and having time to develop relationships with residents. Through these relationships, staff, especially direct care workers, are able to know residents, their values, preferences, and interests, and then make decisions with residents about their care (White, Newton-Curtis, & Lyons, 2008).

The key role of nursing in improving quality care and quality of life in nursing homes is illustrated by the Well Spring Model developed in Wisconsin (Stone, Reinhard, Bowers et al., 2002). A group of 11 facilities made a commitment to sharing resources and working together to meet education and practice goals. A geriatric nurse practitioner (GNP) was key to the project. The GNP developed training modules and presented them to Care Resource Teams (CRTs) from each facility. The CRTs were composed of all levels of nursing staff and were responsible, under the guidance of the facility's Wellspring Coordinator, to plan and implement educational modules in their own nursing homes. The GNP also provided consultation to the participating facilities. Over a 6-year period, Wellspring facilities had fewer deficiencies compared with other nursing homes in Wisconsin and compared with their own baseline. Wellspring facilities also had greater staff retention rates (Stone et al., 2002).

The Commonwealth Fund recently sponsored a national study to examine the impact of culture change on nursing home practice (Doty, Koren, & Sturla, 2008). Many aspects of culture change have not been implemented widely, including changes focused on empowering direct care workers with more decision-making authority or in redesign of the management or the physical environment. The authors did find, however, that progress was being made in involving residents in decision making. Based on perceptions of directors of nurses regarding the organization's commitment to culture change, the authors categorized nearly one third of nursing homes as "culture change adopters," 25% as culture change strivers, and 43% as traditional nursing homes. Cultural change adopters were more likely and traditional nursing homes least likely to have changed practices to make resident care more person centered. These practices included increasing the ability of residents to direct their own schedules, and participate in decisions about their care such as sleeping, bathing, and eating choices (Doty et al., 2008). All nursing homes, however, continue to fall short in areas such as organizational redesign to foster practices such as empowering direct care workers, increasing flexibility in staff roles, and creating self-managed work teams.

Family Involvement in Facility-Based Care Settings

Contrary to prevailing myths, families typically do not abandon their older members once they move into facility-based care, nor do they cease providing care, although the nature of that care will be different (Keefe & Fancey, 2000). Decades of research in nursing homes have revealed that family members continue to visit and provide emotional support, as well as some types of informal care, after transition into a nursing facility. A similar pattern is emerging in research examining families and assisted living. Family members generally visit or call frequently. Compared with nursing homes, families of residents in assisted living are somewhat more likely to supplement facility care, for example, assisting with grooming, bathing, or medication management (Gaugler & Kane, 2007).

Although residents are more likely than their community-dwelling counterparts to not have family available, many residents do have close ties to families. In many cases, family members have been providing care for many years. Entry into a LTC facility often occurs after a health crisis, such as a broken hip, acute care illness, or worsening of a chronic disease. Other people enter care because functional declines become too much for caregivers to manage (e.g., incontinence, wandering or aggressive behaviors). Assisted living, nursing home, or other placements are often difficult transitions for residents and family members alike. Nursing home placement can be especially difficult for family members who may feel they have failed their elder family member.

Nurses and other LTC personnel can do a lot to create a welcoming environment for residents and family members, and engage family members as partners in providing care (Logue, 2003; Pillemer et al., 2003; Reuss, Dupuis, & Whitfield, 2005). Providing person-directed care as defined by White and her colleagues (2008) is consistent with the type of care preferred by families of those receiving LTC services. Duncan and Morgan (1994) describe elements of *personhood* in their descriptions of what families want from care. This included the resident being treated with respect and as a person rather than an object of care. Family members wanted paid caregivers to care about their loved one. Friedmann, Montgomery, Maiberger, and Smith (1997) found families who described problems with resident care most often described staff's failure to support personhood, including meeting needs unique to the individual and failure to maintain their family member's dignity. As residents experience declines and various social and physical losses, they often use their past as a way to maintain their identities. Iwasiw, Goldenberg, Bol, and MacMaster (2003) report that facility staff rarely asked residents about their former roles and contributions, undermining residents' sense of personhood.

As indicated earlier, *knowing the person* is valued by residents and families, and contributes to personhood. Duncan and Morgan (1994) found that family members want staff to gain knowledge about the resident, often striving to be role models in demonstrating how to give care to the individual. Partnerships between families and staff are particularly important to enabling staff to know residents in meaningful ways. Families are key informants with respect to the individual's history, likes and dislikes, personality, routines, and what is and has been important to them (Boise & White, 2004; Iwasiw et al., 2003; Logue, 2003; Reuss et al., 2005). This knowledge is critical when residents have dementia and cannot clearly communicate this information themselves. Family members can provide insight into resident actions, which in turn can help the staff respond more quickly to resident needs as conveyed through their behavior.

Comfort care is composed of quality nursing care and emotional support. Families provide considerable psychological support through their visits. Another important role of family members is in monitoring this care and advocating for the resident if needed. Advocacy will become a primary role, if families are concerned about quality care (Friedmann et al.,

1997). In addition, family members continue to provide a lot of hands-on care, including helping a family member eat, attend activities, and handle personal care. White, Newton-Curtis, Lyons, and Boise (manuscript in preparation) found an important family indicator of satisfaction with care was their ability to go on vacation or be absent from the facility and not feel worried or concerned because they knew that the family member would be well cared for, and that staff would make the right decisions in the event of emergency.

AUTONOMY AND CHOICE

Although autonomy and choice are central to the culture change movement, families tend to stress autonomy less than other features of person-directed care. At the same time, by helping staff members learn to know the resident, families facilitate decision making by residents with respect to preferred routines and activities. Examples include getting ice water rather than tap water, having a specific type and brand of tea, and choosing to walk independently rather than using a walker or wheelchair. Occasionally, families might disagree with resident choice out of concerns for safety or a desire to maintain prior levels of activities. Nursing staff can help mediate disagreements by helping families to understand the importance of autonomy and choice, and helping to balance this aspect of care with safety issues.

RELATIONSHIPS

Families are key members of the resident's social network, contributing to identity, dignity, and quality of life (Boise & White, 2004; Iwasiw et al., 2003). Families help the resident to maintain connections with the larger community by taking them to public events such as concerts, parks, shopping, and to family gatherings. Family members desire positive relationships between staff and residents. They facilitate this by expressing appreciation and encouragement to staff, offering gifts, showing empathy, and helping out when workers are busy (Gladstone & Wexler, 2000). Many studies indicate that families are generally positive toward staff, especially direct care staff. Families relate to the hard work of caregiving because they have been doing it before their family member moved into the care facility (Gladstone & Wexler, 2000). At the same time, relationships between staff and families may be strained. Heiselman and Noelker (1991) found that nearly half of the nurse's assistants in their study reported lack of respect by family and residents toward them. Nearly a third described verbal abuse and insults. Most (95%), however, said they expected to be like family to residents. Facilities can inadvertently set up barriers that decrease the ability of family members to participate in the life of the resident, thereby decreasing attachments between staff and family. Several models have been developed to strengthen staff-family relationships to the benefit of residents, staff, and families. Keefe and Fancey (2000) recommend that family members who wish to be involved in care should be considered part of the care team and be fully involved in making care planning decisions. They also note that families need to be educated about the health status of residents, including expected changing health needs. Finally, they suggest that facilities could assist family members to visit with their relatives, especially those with dementia, by including families in facility-sponsored activities. Similarly, Logue (2003) has found that many facilities lacked institutional encouragement for family involvement, insufficient staff and program resources addressing social and emotional needs of the family, and ineffective communication between staff and families. This can be addressed successfully by inviting families to participate at mealtimes, providing private areas for family meals and celebrations, encouraging drop-in visits, and encouraging continuation of pre-established caregiving activities. As a final example, Pillemer and his colleagues (2003) developed the Partners in Caregiving program. The program involves a series of communication workshops held separately for family members and staff followed by a joint meeting at the conclusion of the program to discuss facility policies and procedures. In testing the effectiveness of the program, perceptions of one another had changed: Family members perceived more empathy from staff, and staff were more positive about family behaviors toward them.

SUMMARY

This chapter has described the aging population in the United States and provided an overview of family ties of older adults. Using the life course perspective, we discussed the diversity of family structure in later life and how it has been influenced by societal trends such as increasing life expectancy, increasing divorce rates, changing fertility patterns, greater ethnic diversity, and changes in economic status and work patterns. Most elders are embedded in social networks in which kin are important sources of emotional and instrumental support. Given the diversity of family life, many configurations of "family" exist. In most families, individuals enjoy strong and affectionate relationships, and can count on family members to provide care and support when needed. Nonetheless, it is also common for families to have both positive and negative feelings toward one another because they are providing support. In some families, negative feelings may predominate, which will have consequences for health, well-being, and availability of support.

Throughout this chapter, we have considered where nurses are most likely to encounter older adults and their families. Even the very old are relatively healthy and function independently. Still, older adults, especially those of advanced years, have unique health care needs that must be addressed whether in clinics, at home, in hospitals, or through a variety of LTC services. Nursing and other professionals in gerontology have developed evidence-based assessment tools and interventions that are the basis for optimal care. Nurses must be familiar with these tools and apply them routinely and appropriately. Professionals must also recognize that older adults, including many care recipients, are also providers of care to their spouses, children, grandchildren, or friends. In fact, the majority of care is delivered by family members.

As the population ages, it is increasingly important that nurses develop expertise in geriatric care, regardless of setting. Nurses with strong leadership skills are needed, especially in community-based care and nursing home settings. In all of these settings, nurses must partner with elders and their family members in designing and providing care that addresses unique needs and supports relationships.

REFERENCES

Administration on Aging. (2004). *Statistics: Aging into the 21st century*. Retrieved June 20, 2008, from http://www.aoa.gov/prof/Statistics/future_growth/aging21/demography.asp

Angel, J. L., Jimenez, M. A., & Angel, R. J. (2007). The economic consequences of widowhood for older minority women. *The Gerontologist, 47,* 224–234.

Antonucci, T. C., & Akiyama, H. (1995). Convoys of social relations: Family and friendships within a life span context. In

R. Blieszner & V. H. Bedford (Eds.). *Handbook of aging and the family*. Westport, CT: Greenwood Press.

Archbold, P. G., Stewart, B. J., Miller, L. L., Harvath, T. A., Greenlick, M. R., Van Buren, L., et al. (1995). The PREP system of nursing interventions: A pilot test with families caring for older members—preparedness (PR), enrichment (E), and predictability (P). *Research in Nursing & Health, 18,* 3–16.

Beel-Bates, C. A., Ziemba, R., Algase, D. L. (2007). Families' perceptions of services in assisted living residences [electronic version]. *Journal of Gerontological Nursing, 33*(12), 5–12.

Bengtson, V. L., & Allen, K. R. (1993). The life course perspective applied to families over time. In P. G. Boss, W. J. Doherty, R. LaRossa, W. R. Schumm, & S. K. Steinmetz (Eds.), *Sourcebook of family theories and methods: A contextual approach* (pp. 469–498). New York: Plenum Press.

Bengtson, V. L., & Harootyan, R. A. (1994). (Eds.). *Intergenerational linkages: Hidden connections in American society.* New York: Springer.

Bilmes, L. J. (2008). Iraq's 100-year mortgage. *Foreign Policy, March/April,* 84–85.

Boise, L., & White, D. (2004). The family's role in person-centered care: Practice considerations. [Electronic version]. *Journal of Psychosocial Nursing, 42,* 12–20.

Bucx, F., Van Wel, F., Knijin, T., & Hagendoorn, L. (2008). Intergenerational contact and the life course status of young adult children. *Journal of Marriage and Family, 70,* 144–156.

Caffrey, R. A. (2005). Community care gerontological nursing: The independent nurse's role. [Electronic version]. *Journal of Gerontological Nursing, 31 (7),* 18–25.

Carder. P. C. (2002). The social world of assisted living. *Journal of Aging Studies, 16,* 1–18.

Coehlo, D. P., Hooker, K., & Bowman, S. (2007). Institutional placement of persons with dementia: What predicts occurrence and timing. *Journal of Family Nursing, 13,* 253–277.

Connidis, I. A. (2001). *Family ties & aging.* Thousand Oaks, CA: Sage.

Connidis, I. A., & McMullin, J. A. (2002). Sociological ambivalence and family ties: A critical perspective. *Journal of Marriage and the Family, 64,* 558–567.

DeLamater, J. (2002). *Sexuality across the life course: A biopsychosocial perspective.* Paper presented at the Midcontinent and Eastern regions meeting of the Society for the Scientific Study of Sexuality, Big Rapids, MI.

DeLamater, J., & Moorman, S. M. (2007). Sexual behavior in later life. *Journal of Aging and Health, 19*(6), 921–945.

de Vries, B., Lana, R. D., & Falch, V. T. (1994). Parental bereavement over the life course: A theoretical intersection and empirical review. *Omega, 29,* 47–69.

Dilworth-Anderson, P., Williams, I. C., & Gibson, B. E. (2002). Issues of race, ethnicity, and culture in caregiving research: A 20-year review (1980-2000). *The Gerontologist, 42,* 237–272.

Doerflinger, D. M. C. (2007). How to try this: The Mini-Cog. *American Journal of Nursing, 107*(12), 62–71.

Dolbin-MacNab, M. L. (2006). Just like raising your own? Grandmothers' perceptions of parenting a second time around. *Family Relations, 55,* 564–575.

Doty, M. M., Koren, M. J., & Sturla, E. L. (2008). *Culture change in nursing homes: How far have we come? Findings from the Commonwealth Fund 2007 national survey of nursing homes.* [Electronic version]. New York: The Commonwealth Fund. www.commonwealthfund.org

Duncan, M. T., & Morgan, D. L. (1994). Sharing the caring: Family caregivers' views of their relationships with nursing home staff. *The Gerontologist, 34,* 235–259.

Family Caregiver Alliance. (2006). *Caregiver assessment: Principles, guidelines and strategies for change. Report from a National Consensus Development Conference* (Vol. I). San Francisco: Author.

Faust, K. A., & McKibben, J. N. (1999). Marital dissolution: Divorce, separation, annulment, and widowhood. In M. B. Sussman, S. K. Steinmetz, & G. W. Peterson (Eds.), *Handbook of marriage and the family* (2nd ed.). New York: Plenum.

Federal Interagency Forum on Aging Related Statistics. (2008). *Older Americans 2008: Key indicators of well-being. CB08-FF.06.* Retrieved on June 5, 2008, from http://www.agingstats.gov/ agingstatsdotnet/main_site/default.aspx

Fingerman, K. L. (2001). *Aging mothers and their adult daughters: A study in mixed emotions.* New York: Springer.

Friedemann, M. L., Montgomery, R. J., Maiberger, B., & Smith, A. A. (1997). Family involvement in the nursing home: Family oriented practices and staff-family relationships. *Research in Nursing & Health, 20,* 527–537.

Friedemann, M. L., Montgomery, R. J., Rice, C., & Farrell, L. (1999). Family involvement in the nursing home. *Western Journal of Nursing Research, 21,* 549–567.

Fulmer, T. (2008). Elder mistreatment assessment. In M. Boltz (Series Ed.), *Try this: Best practices in nursing care to older adults* (Issue No. 15). Retrieved May 28, 2009, from http:// consultgerirn.org/uploads/File/trythis/issue15.pdf

Fulmer, T., Guadagno, L., Bitondo, C., & Connolly, M. T. (2004). Progress in elder abuse screening and assessment instruments. [Electronic version]. *Journal of American Geriatrics Society, 52,* 297–304.

Gaugler, J. E., & Kane, R. A. (2007). Families and assisted living. *The Gerontologist, 47*(Special Issue III), 83–99.

Gladstone, J., & Wexler, E. (2000). A family perspective of family/staff interaction in long-term care facilities. *Geriatric Nursing, 21*(1), 16–19.

Goodman, C. C., & Silverstein, M. (2006). Grandmothers raising grandchildren: Ethnic and racial differences in well-being among custodial and coparenting families. *Journal of Family Issues, 27,* 1605–1626.

Graf, C. (2006). Functional decline in hospitalized older adults. *American Journal of Nursing, 106*(1), 58–67.

Graf, C. (2007). The Lawton instrumental activities of daily living scale. In M. Boltz (Series Ed.), *Try this: Best practices in nursing care to older adults* (Issue No. 23). Retrieved May 28, 2009, from http://consultgerirn.org/uploads/File/trythis/issue23.pdf

Greenberg, S. A. (2007). How to try this: The geriatric depression scale: Short form. *American Journal of Nursing, 107*(10), 60–69.

Hanson, B. G. (1995). *General systems theory beginning with wholes.* Washington, DC: Taylor & Francis.

Hayslip, B., & Kaminski, P. L. (2005). Grandparents raising their grandchildren: A review of the literature and suggestions for practice. *The Gerontologist, 45,* 262–269.

Heiselman, T., & Noelker, L. S. (1991). Enhancing mutual respect among nursing assistants, residents, and residents' families. *The Gerontologist, 31,* 552–555.

Herd, P. (2005). Ensuring a minimum: Social Security reform and women. *The Gerontologist, 45,* 12–25.

Inouye, S. K., Bogardus, S. T., Baker, D. I., Leo-Summers, L., & Cooney, L. M. (2000). The Hospital Elder Life program: A model of care to prevent cognitive and functional decline in older hospitalized patients. [Electronic version]. *Journal of the American Geriatrics Society, 48,* 1697–1706.

Iwasiw, C., Goldenberg, D., Bol, N., & MacMaster, E. (2003). Resident and family perspectives: The first year in a long-term care facility. *Journal of Gerontological Nursing, 29,* 45–54.

Keefe, J., & Fancey, P. (2000). The care continues: Responsibility for elderly relatives before and after admission to a long term care facility. *Family Relations, 49,* 235–244.

Kleinpell, R. M., Fletcher K., Jennings, B. M. (2008). Reducing functional decline in hospitalized elderly. In Hughes, R. G. (Ed.), *Patient safety and quality: An evidence-based handbook for nurses.* Rockford, MD: Agency for Healthcare Research and Quality. Retrieved May 25, 2008, from http://www.ahrq.gov/qual/nurseshdbk/docs/KleinpellR_RFDHE.pdf

Kronenfeld, J. J. (2006). Changing conceptions of health and life course concepts. [Electronic version]. *Health, 10,* 501–517.

Lachman, M. E. (2003). Negative interactions in close relationships: Introduction to a special section. *Journal of Gerontology: Psychological Sciences, 52B,* P69.

Landry-Meyer, L., & Newman, B. M. (2004). An exploration of the grandparent caregiver role. *Journal of Family Issues, 25,* 1-5–1-25.

Leder, S., Grinstead, L. N., & Torres, E. (2007). Grandparents raising grandchildren: Stressors, social support, and health outcomes. *Journal of Family Nursing, 13,* 333–352.

Logue, R. M. (2003). Maintaining family connectedness in long-term care. *Journal of Gerontological nursing, 29*(6), 24–31.

Lumpkin, J. R. (2008). Grandparents in a parental or near-parental role: Sources of stress and coping mechanisms. *Journal of Family Issues, 29,* 357–372.

Lustbader, W. (2001). The pioneer challenge: A radical change in the culture of nursing homes. In L. S. Noelker & Z. Harel (Eds.), *Linking quality of long-term care and quality of life* (pp. 185–203). New York: Springer.

Maas, M. L., & Buckwalter, K. C. (2006). Providing quality care in assisted living facilities: Recommendations for enhanced staffing and staff training. [Electronic version]. *Journal of Gerontological Nursing, 32*(11), 14–22.

Maas, M. L., Buckwalter, K. C., Hardy, M. D., Tripp-Reimer, T., Titler, M. G., & Specht, J. P. (2001). *Nursing care of older adults: Diagnoses, outcomes, & interventions.* St. Louis: Mosby.

Magana, S., Seltzer, M. M., & Krauss, M. W. (2002). Service utilization patterns of adults with intellectual disabilities: A comparison of Puerto Rican and non-Latino White families. *Journal of Gerontological Social Work, 37*(3/34), 65–86.

Manton, K. G. (2008). Recent declines in chronic disability in the elderly U.S. population: Risk factors and future dynamics. *Annual Review of Public Health, 29,* 91–113. Retrieved May 28, 2008, from arjournals.annualreviews.org

Mattes, R. D. (2002). The chemical senses and nutrition in aging: Challenging old assumptions. [Electronic version]. *Journal of the American Dietetic Association, 102,* 192–196.

Messecar, D. C. (2008). Family caregiving. In E. Capezuti, D. Zwicker, M. Mezey, & T. Fulmer (Eds.), *Evidence-based geriatric nursing protocols for best practice.* New York: Springer.

Mezey, M., Kobayashi, M., Grossman, S., Firpo, A., Fulmer, T., & Ethel, M. (2004). Nurses improving care to health system elders (NICHE): Implementation of best practice models. *Journal of Nursing Administration, 34*(10), 451–457.

Mezey, M., Kobayashi, M., Grossman, S., Firpo, A., Fulmer, T., Mitty, E. (2004). Nurses Improving Care to Health System

Elders (NICHE): Implementation of Best Practice Models. *The Journal of Nursing Administration, 34,* 451–457.

Monserud, M. A. (2008). Intergenerational relationships and affectual solidarity between grandparents and young adults. *Journal of Marriage and Family, 70,* 182–195.

National Alliance for Caregiving and AARP. (2004). *Caregiving in the U.S.* Bethesda, MD. Retrieved May 28, 2009, from http://www.caregiving.org/data/04finalreport.pdf

National Clearinghouse for Long-Term Care (Administration on Aging). Understanding LTC Services. Retrieved July 14, 2008, from http://www.longtermcare.gov/LTC/Main_Site/index.aspx

Neal, M. B., & Hammer, L. B. (2007). *Working couples caring for children and aging parents: Effects on work and well-being.* Mahwah, NJ: Lawrence Erlbaum Associates.

Newsom, J. T., Rook, K. S., Nishishiba, M., Sorkin, D. H., & Mahan, T. L. (2005). Understanding the relative importance of positive and negative social exchanges: Examining specific domains and appraisals. *Journal of Gerontology: Psychological Sciences, 60B,* P304–P312.

Peters, C. L., Hooker, K., & Zvonkovic, A. M. (2006). Older parents' perceptions of ambivalence in relationships with their children. *Family Relations, 55,* 539–551.

Pillemer, K., & Suiter, J. J. (2005). Ambivalence and the study of intergenerational relations. In M. Silverstein (Ed.), Focus on intergenerational relations across time and place, [Electronic version]. *Annual Review of Gerontology and Geriatrics, 24,* (pp. 3–28). New York: Springer.

Pillemer, K., Suitor, J. J., Henderson, C. R., Meador, R., Schultz, L., Robison, J., et al. (2003). A cooperative communication intervention for nursing home staff and family members of residents. *The Gerontologist, 43,* 96–106.

Pinquart, M., & Sorensen, S. (2006). Helping caregivers of persons with dementia: Which interventions work and how large are their effects? [Electronic version]. *International Psychogeriatrics, 18,* 577–595.

Pioneer Network. (1997). *Toward a new culture of aging: Mission, vision and values.* Retrieved September 27, 2009, from http://www.pioneernetwork.net/AboutUs/Values

Pruchno, R. A., & Meeks, S. (2004). Health-related stress, affect, and depressive symptoms experienced by caregiving mothers of adults with a developmental disability. [Electronic version]. *Psychology and Aging, 19,* 394–401.

Quadagno, J. (2008). *Aging & the life course: An introduction to social gerontology* (4th ed.). New York: McGraw Hill.

Reinhard, S. C., Given, B., Petlick, N. H., & Bemis, A. (2008). Supporting family caregivers in providing care. *Patient safety and quality: An evidence-based handbook for nurses.* Agency for Health Research & Quality. Retrieved May 28, 2009, from http://www.ahrq.gov/qual/nurseshdbk

Reuss, G. F., Dupuis, S. L., & Whitfield, K. (2005). Understanding the experience of moving a loved one to a long-term care facility. [Electronic version] *Journal of Gerontological Social Work, 46,* 17–46.

Roberto, K. A. (1990). Grandparent and grandchild relationships. In T. H. Brubaker (Ed.), *Family relationships in later life* (2nd ed., pp. 100–112). Newbury Park, CA: Sage.

Robinson, S. B., Rosher, R. B. (2006). Tangling with the barriers to culture change. *Journal of Gerontological Nursing, 32*(10), 19–25.

Rook, K. S. (2003). Exposure and reactivity to negative social exchanges: A preliminary investigation using daily diary data.

[Electronic version]. *The Journals of Gerontology. Series A, Biological Sciences and Medical Sciences, 58,* P100–P111.

Rossi, A. S., & Rossi, P. H. (1990). *Of human bonding.* New York: Aldine de Gruyter.

Salinas, T. K., O'Connor, L. J., Weinstein, M., Lee, S. Y. V., & Fitzpatrick, J. J. (2002). A family assessment tool for hospitalized elders. *Geriatric Nursing, 23,* 316–319.

Saunders, G. H., & Echt, K. V. (2007). An overview of dual sensory impairment in older adults: Perspectives for rehabilitation, *Trends in Amplification, 11,* 243–258.

Scharlach, A., Li, W., Dalvi, T. B. (2006). Family conflict as a mediator of caregiver strain. *Family Relations, 55,* 625–635.

Seltzer, M. M., Greenberg, J. S., Floyd, F. J., & Hong, J. (2004). Accommodative coping and well-being of midlife parents of children with mental health problems or developmental disabilities. *American Journal of Orthopsychiatry, 74,* 187–195.

Seltzer, M. M., Greenberg, J. S., Krause, M. W., & Hong, J. (1997). Predictors and outcomes of the end of co-resident caregiving in aging families of adults with mental retardation or mental illness. *Family Relations, 46,* 13–22.

Settersten, R. A. (2006). Aging and the life course. In R. H. Binstock & L. K. George (Eds.), *Handbook of aging and the social sciences* (6th ed., pp. 3–19). New York: Academic Press.

Sikorska-Simmons, E. (2006a). Linking resident satisfaction to staff perceptions of the work environment in assisted living: A multilevel analysis. *The Gerontologist, 46,* 590–598.

Sikorska-Simmons, E. (2006b). Organizational culture and work-related attitudes among staff in assisted living. [Electronic version]. *Journal of Gerontological Nursing, 32*(2), 19–27.

Silverstein, M., & Marenco, A. (2001). How Americans enact the grandparent role across the family life course. [Electronic version]. *Journal of Family Issues, 22,* 493–522.

Sloane, P. D., Zimmerman, S., & Sheps, C. G. (2005). *Improvement and innovation in long-term care: A research agenda report and recommendations from a national consensus conference.* University of North Carolina at Chapel Hill. Retrieved May 28, 2009, from http://www.pragmaticinnovations.unc.edu/FinalReport/Pragmatic%20Innovations%20Final%20Report%201-9-05.pdf

Spillman, B. C. (2004). Changes in elderly disability rates and the implications for health care utilization and cost. [Electronic version]. *The Milbank Quarterly, 82,* 157–194.

Stone, R. I. (2006). Emerging issues in long-term care. In R. H. Binstock & L. K. George (Eds.), *Handbook of aging and the social sciences* (6th ed., pp. 397–418). New York: Academic Press.

Stone, R. I., Reinhard, S. C., Bowers, B., Zimmerman, D., Phillips, C. D., Hawes, C., et al. (2002). *Evaluation of the Wellspring Model for improving nursing home quality.* [Electronic version]. New York: Commonwealth Fund.

Stone, R. I., & Reinhard, S. C. (2007). The place of assisted living in long-term care and related service systems. *The Gerontologists, 47*(Special Issue III), 23–32.

Szinovacz, M. E. (Ed.). (1998). *Handbook of grandparenthood.* Westport, CT: Greenwood Press.

Talerico, K. A., O'Brien, J. A., & Swafford, K. L. (2003). Person-centered care: An important approach for 21st century health care. *Journal of Psychosocial Nursing, 41,* 12–16.

Tellis-Nayak, V. (2007). A person-centered workplace: The foundation for person-centered caregiving in long-term care. [Electronic version]. *Journal of the American Medical Directors Association, 8*(1), 46–54.

Thiele, D. M., & Whelan, T. A. (2006). The nature and dimensions of the grandparent role. *Marriage & Family Review, 40,* 93–108.

Tucker, D., Bechtel, G., Quartana, C., Badger, N., Werner, D., Ford, I. F., et al. (2006). The OASIS Program: Redesigning hospital care for older adults. *Geriatric Nursing, 27,* 112–117.

Uhlenberg, P. (2005). Historical forces shaping grandparent-grandchild relationships: Demography and beyond. In M. Silverstein (Ed.), Focus on intergenerational relations across time and Place. [Electronic version]. *Annual Review of Gerontology and Geriatrics, 24,* (pp. 77–97). New York: Springer.

Uhlenberg, P., & Kirby, J. P. (1998). Grandparenthood over time: Historical and demographic trends. In M. E. Szinvocz (Ed.), *Handbook of grandparenthood* (pp. 23–39). Westport, CT: Greenwood Press.

Umberson, D., Williams, K., Powers, D. A., Liu, H., & Needham, B. (2006, March). You make me sick: Marital quality and health over the life course. [Electronic version]. *Journal of Health and Social Behavior, 47,* 1–16.

Vandell, D. L., McCartney, K., Owen, M. T., Booth, C., & Clarke-Stewart, A. (2003). Variations in child care by grandparents during the first three years. *Journal of Marriage and Family, 65,* 375–381.

Waldrop, D. P. (2003). Caregiving issues for grandmothers raising their grandchildren. *Journal of Human Behavior in the Social Environment, 7,* 201–223.

Walker, A. J., Manoogian-O'Dell, M., McGraw, L. A., & White, D. L. (2001). *Families in later life: Connections and transitions.* Thousand Oaks, CA: Pine Forge Press.

Walker, A. J., Pratt, C. C., Eddy, L. (1995). Informal caregiving to aging family members: A critical review. *Family Relations, 44,* 402–411.

Wallace, M., & Shelkey, M. (2007). Katz Index of independence in activities of daily living (ADL). In M. Boltz (Series Ed.), *Try This: Best Practices in Nursing Care to older adults* (Issue No. 2). Retrieved July 14, 2008, from http://consultgerirn.org/uploads/File/trythis/issue02.pdf

Waszynski, C. M. (2007). Detecting delirium. *American Journal of Nursing, 107*(12), 50–59.

White, D. L. (1999). Grandparent participation in times of family bereavement. In B. de Vries (Ed.), *End of Life Issues: Interdisciplinary and Multidimensional Perspectives* (pp. 145–165). New York: Springer.

White, D. L., Newton-Curtis, L., & Lyons, K. S. (2008). Development and initial testing of a measure of person-directed care. *The Gerontologist, 48*(Special Issue 1), 114–123.

White, D. L., Newton-Curtis, L., Lyons, K. S., & Boise, L. (unpublished manuscript). *A measure of family perspectives of person-directed care in long-term care facilities.* Manuscript in preparation, June 2009.

Wilson, K. B. (2007). Historical evolution of assisted living in the United States, 1979 to the present. *The Gerontologist, 47*(Special Issue III), 8–22.

Wolf, R. S. (1996). Understanding elder abuse and neglect. [Electronic version]. *Aging, 367,* 4–9.

Wu, A., & Schimmele, C. M. (2007). Uncoupling in late life. [Electronic version]. *Generations, 31*(3), 41–46.

Yeoman, B. (2008, July/August). When wounded vets come home. *AARP Magazine,* 60.

Zimmerman, S., & Sloane, P. D. (2007). Definition and classification of assisted living. *The Gerontologist, 47*(Special Issue III), 33–39.

CHAPTER 16

Family Mental Health Nursing

Darcy Copeland, PhD, RN

Diane Vines, PhD, RN

CRITICAL CONCEPTS

+ All parts of the family system are interconnected; therefore, all members are affected when a member has a mental disorder.

+ The family of a person with a mental disorder is more than the sum of its parts, so the family needs to be involved in treatment.

+ The boundaries of self and others within a family system are dysfunctional when a member has a mental disorder.

+ Family systems of families with a member who has a mental disorder can be further organized into subsystems. These subsystems must be understood to treat the family effectively.

+ The involvement of families in the treatment of a family member with a mental disorder enhances the effectiveness of the treatment.

*I*n the United States, the diagnosis of a mental disorder is made based on criteria from the American Psychiatric Association's (APA's) *Diagnostic and Statistical Manual of Mental Disorders* (DSM-IV-TR). The DSM provides a classification system used in many countries around the world that categorizes and describes the array of mental conditions. These conditions are assigned diagnostic codes/numbers based on their classification. The DSM creates a common language and diagnostic coding system that can be understood across disciplines and by mental health providers around the world. In this

respect, it is similar to the International Classification of Disease (ICD). The DSM is currently in its fourth edition, because of the changing way mental health providers understand mental disorders, their symptomology, and diagnosis.

The DSM describes mental disorders as conditions characterized by alterations in thinking, mood, or behavior that cause a person distress, impaired occupational or social functioning, or significant risk for experiencing death, pain, disability, or a loss of freedom (APA, 2000). Individuals are affected by these disorders across the life span. It is estimated that 21% of children aged 9 to 17 (Shaffer et al., 1996) and 26% of Americans 18 years and older are affected by a diagnosable mental disorder (Kessler, Chiu, Demler, & Walters, 2005). That is, approximately one in four American adults and one in five children experience distress or impaired functioning as a result of a mental disorder.

One way the impact of this impairment may be measured is by looking at the effect of a mental disorder on years of life lost to premature death and years lived with a disability. According to the Global Burden of Disease study conducted by the World Health Organization (WHO), the World Bank, and Harvard University, this measure of disease burden is known as the *disability-adjusted life-year* (Murray & Lopez, 1996). Using this measure in established countries such as the United States, researchers found that mental illnesses rank second, only behind cardiovascular conditions, with respect to disease burden (Murray & Lopez, 1996). In fact, worldwide, among people aged 15 to 44 years, mental disorders account for 4 of the top 10 causes of years of life lived with a disability (WHO, 2001).

Given the fact that such a large segment of the population is living with a disabling mental disorder, it is important to address care and treatment not only from the perspective of preventing and treating these disorders at the individual level, but from a broader perspective as well. Equally important is the effect on family members and caretakers of those with these disorders. All members of the family are affected when any of its members experiences a chronic mental illness. Family members of individuals who are mentally ill provide an enormous amount of support and encouragement to their relatives. These valuable familial resources accent the care provided by mental health professionals. The support they provide, however, is often not appreciated or even acknowledged by mental health professionals. It is also frequently associated with significant stress for these familial caretakers themselves.

This chapter intends to provide nursing students with a brief history of mental health policy in the United States and a literature review of issues significant to family members of individuals with a mental illness. Practice strategies nurses can implement in the provision of family mental health nursing both for the patient and the family are provided, together with a case study illustrating some of these strategies.

HISTORY OF MENTAL HEALTH CARE POLICY

A brief discussion of the history of mental health care policy and civil commitment helps to frame the current mental health system and its effect on mentally ill individuals and their families who now assume a primary caretaking role. As far back as the 1820s, specialized residential institutions were created to provide services for socially "abnormal" people, including the mentally ill, orphans, and criminals (Burt, 2001). Insane asylums, orphanages, and penitentiaries were designed to provide treatment and enable people to return to society once their deviant behaviors were cured. Unfortunately, these institutions became custodial warehouses fraught with brutality, violence, and a variety of inhumane and nontherapeutic treatments.

Historically, the provision of mental health services to U.S. citizens was the responsibility of individual states. Throughout the late 1800s and early 1900s, mental health services primarily consisted of institutional care. This institutionalization occurred in large, state-run hospitals. During this time, loose justification was necessary to involuntarily hospitalize individuals with mental illness. In addition, because of beliefs that mental illnesses could not be cured, once individuals were hospitalized, it was not uncommon for them to be confined indefinitely. Consequently, the peak of institutionalized individuals in 1955 found an estimated 560,000 U.S. citizens were housed in these huge institutions (Urff, 2004).

After World War II, the idea spread that it was possible to recover from mental illness, resulting in improvements in psychopharmacologic agents, particularly antipsychotic drugs. In addition, social reform movements began to take shape. Involuntary hospitalization was perceived as a denial of civil rights. Previously, medical, not legal, professionals made the decisions to commit people to institutions. Patient rights advocates began to argue that this decision implicated a loss of liberty. This perspective reframed the issue as a constitutional one. Consequently, the legal system became responsible for overseeing commitment decisions.

The attention placed on civil liberties, coupled with a growing sentiment that large, state-run institutions were ineffective in providing meaningful treatment, contributed to restructuring the United States' mental health delivery system. In 1963,

President Kennedy passed the Community Mental Health Centers Construction (CMHC) Act (Urff, 2004). This law was pivotal in shifting the treatment of people with mental illness from large, state-run institutions to smaller, community-run mental health centers. The intent of the CHMC Act was to create a network of community mental health centers that could provide services to people who had previously been institutionalized in state hospitals. The existence of community-based programs, however, was not a prerequisite for releasing patients from state hospitals. As a result, state hospitals downsized or closed their doors and previously institutionalized individuals flooded communities that were not prepared to provide services to the large number of people in need of services. Whereas state institutions provided housing, food, clothing, education, social interaction, and employment opportunities to patients, community-based mental health centers were not designed to meet these needs of formerly institutionalized individuals (Urff, 2004).

Community mental health systems have continued to be underfunded and overwhelmed by demand. In response, family members of mentally ill individuals have taken on greater caretaking responsibilities (Solomon, 1996).

Various reforms have been made to the CMHC Act throughout the years since its passage. Not one has been successful in repairing the fractured service delivery system that currently exists. Most recently, in 2002, President George W. Bush established the New Freedom Commission on Mental Health to study the mental health delivery system in the United States. This commission identified six goals to transform mental health care in this country. These goals are presented in Table 16-1.

In addition, the recovery movement has begun to transform the structure of mental health care in the United States. This evolving movement holds as central the goal of transforming the lives of those affected by mental illness (Green-Hennessy & Hennessy, 2004). The historically negative and hopeless views of mental illness are shifting. Recovery models are patient-focused, and emphasize skill development, empowerment over mental illness, and a reawakening of hope (American Psychiatric Nurses Association [APNA], 2007). They necessitate a transformation in the way patients, family members, mental health professionals, and society as a whole view mental illness. Rather than being

TABLE 16-1
Goals Identified by the New Freedom Commission on Mental Health

- Americans understand that mental health is essential to overall health.
- Mental health care is consumer and family driven.
- Disparities in mental health services are eliminated.
- Early mental health screening, assessment, and referral to services are common practice.
- Excellent mental health care is delivered and research is accelerated.
- Technology is used to access mental health care and information.

New Freedom Commission on Mental Health. (2003). *Achieving the Promise: Transforming Mental Health Care in America*. Rockville, MD: U.S. Department of Health and Human Services, 2003. Retrieved February 20, 2008, from http://www.mentalhealthcommission.gov/reports/FinalReport/toc.html

characterized as diagnosed with a "life sentence" as they were in the past, individuals with mental disorders are experiencing a sense of optimism and acceptance that personal and professional opportunities still exist.

FAMILY MEMBERS OF INDIVIDUALS WITH A MENTAL ILLNESS

Given the important role familial caregivers now play in the care and treatment of mentally ill individuals, a large body of scientific literature is available that describes their experiences and needs. This chapter presents a brief review of this literature, divided into the following prominent themes: family impact, social support and stigma, coping, and assistance from mental health professionals.

Family Impact

The term *burden* is used widely in the literature as a means of describing the impact of having a family member with a mental illness. It has been suggested that the term *burden* itself implies that the person with the mental illness is responsible in some way for problems within the family (Corrigan & Miller, 2004). For this reason, when possible, the term *impact* will be used instead of burden. An early study with family members of people who had schizophrenia differentiated the impact experienced by relatives as either objective or subjective (Hoenig & Hamilton, 1966). Objective impact can be described as tangible or observable adverse effects on family members that result from mental illness. Examples of objective impact include financial loss, physical strain, effects on the health of other family members, or disruption to the lives of family members caused by the behavior of the person with a mental illness. *Subjective impact,* in contrast, refers to how family members feel about and perceive the burden they experience.

Although the objective and subjective impact of caregiving may be heightened among family members living with their ill relative (Hoenig & Hamilton, 1966; Jones, Roth, & Jones, 1995), the impact is thought to be attributed more to the level of caregiving responsibility assumed by the family members (Reinhard & Horwitz, 1995). Caregiving has been described as a role including providing nursing care, social work, psychiatric services, and cooking (Veltman, Cameron, & Stewart, 2002). It has been suggested that assisting with activities of daily living, including grooming, preparing meals, providing transportation, doing housework, managing time, and managing money are more objectively burdensome to caregivers than attempting to control troublesome behaviors exhibited by family members with mental illnesses (Jones et al., 1995).

Meanwhile, the subjective impact of caregiving has been associated with feeling unable to cope, trapped, and unknowledgeable about how to respond to symptoms that their relatives exhibit (Ferriter & Huband, 2003). Psychological distress has also been associated with the experience of providing care to individuals with a mental illness (Bibou-Nakou, Dikaiou, & Bairactaris, 1997; Olridge & Hughes, 1992). Family members have attributed some of their own mental health problems to their mentally ill relatives. In one study, 40% of family members felt that dealing with their relatives' mental illnesses led to mental health problems of their own, and 10% reported feeling that the burden they experienced was so great that they had suicidal thoughts themselves (Ostman & Kjellin, 2002).

In addition to caregiving responsibilities, social factors such as social isolation and social stigma have been identified as significant sources of family impact (Tsang, Tam, Chan, & Chang, 2003). Familial caregivers with little social support from other family members or mental health agencies report greater impact (Biegel, Milligan, Putnam, & Song, 1994). In fact, familial caregivers reported feeling "taken for granted" as if they "don't exist" (Veltman et al., 2002, p. 110). One stated that "[people] can sympathize or empathize with a caregiver for someone with cancer or dementia or a stroke, but they just don't get mental illness. They don't appreciate how difficult it is to be in this position" (Veltman et al., 2002, p. 110).

Social Support and Stigma

The social stigma experienced by people with mental disorders has been the focus of research for many decades. More recently investigated, however, is the stigma associated with being the family member of a person with a mental illness. In *Mental Health: A Report of the Surgeon General,* stigma associated with mental illness is described as follows:

> [M]anifested by bias, distrust, stereotyping, fear, embarrassment, anger, and/or avoidance. Stigma leads others to avoid living, socializing or working with, renting to, or employing people with mental disorders....It reduces patients' access to resources and opportunities (e.g., housing, jobs) and leads to low self-esteem, isolation, and hopelessness. It deters the public from seeking, and wanting to pay for, care. In its most overt and egregious form, stigma results in outright discrimination and abuse. More tragically, it deprives people of their dignity and interferes with their full participation in society (U.S. Department of Health and Human Services, 1999, p. 6).

In one study, nearly half of all caregivers of individuals with a serious mental disorder believed that most people devalued family members of people with a mental illness (Struening, Perlick, Link, Hellman, Herman, & Sirey, 2001). In addition to feeling devalued by the public, shame is a contributing factor to stigma associated with being a family member of a person with a mental illness. In studies conducted in the United States and across the globe, family members reported that being related to a person with a mental illness is a source of shame that influences their disclosure of that relationship to others (Ohaeri

& Fido, 2001; Phelan, Bromet, & Link, 1998; Phillips, Pearson, Li, Xu, & Yang, 2002; Shibre et al., 2001).

Family members of people with mental illnesses reported that their relationships with other people are affected, including their ability to have company in their own home (Ostman & Kjellin, 2002). Caregiving can be an isolating experience. As one caregiver reported, "The stigma of mental illness is always there. People don't understand, you don't know who you can trust to understand, so you don't tell anyone" (Veltman et al., 2002, p. 111). Family members said they do not have friends as a result of the "secret" they keep, or that they have lost friends because of their relatives' illness (Veltman et al., 2002).

Dually diagnosed clients (those with co-occurring mental illnesses and substance disorders) often experience a double stigma—against mental illness and against substance abuse. For example, Camilli and Martin (2005) found that emergency room personnel had "negative or apathetic attitudes" toward intoxicated or psychiatric patients (p. 313). In addition, family members expressed more negative feelings about mentally ill relatives who abuse substances. One study found that relatives of dually diagnosed individuals perceived their ill family member as having greater control over, and being more responsible for, their psychiatric symptoms than did relatives of those without a co-occurring substance disorder (Niv, Lopez, Glynn, & Mueser, 2007). Despite the stigma, social support is extremely important for dual-disorder families and patients. Warren, Stein, and Grella (2007) report that social support facilitates both improved mental health status and less drug use among those with dual diagnoses, emphasizing the importance of the patient's personal resources, including the family.

Coping

Among familial caregivers of individuals with a mental illness, many claim that their role as caregiver has made them stronger, more patient, or more appreciative of time with their families (Veltman et al., 2002). Caregivers reported feeling less judgmental of others and sensing that their own ability to care about people has increased. The quality of familial relationships may affect the entire family unit's ability to function and cope. The establishment of mutually satisfying relationships helps families to connect more with their ill family member rather than perpetuating relationships based solely on familial obligation (Acton, 2002; Johnson, 2000).

In general, families cope with stressors in many ways. Coping related to mental illness in a family may include actions aimed at reducing the number of and intensity of demands placed on the family, acquiring additional resources, managing ongoing stressors, and making situations manageable and acceptable for all members of the family (Saunders, 2003). Establishing realistic behavioral expectations for each family member may aid families as they cope with the presence of a chronic mental illness. In addition, preserving a sense of hopefulness about the future helps families to maintain balance (Doornbos, 1997). Balance within families can be conceptualized in multiple ways. It may refer to a balance between familial stressors and resources or coping mechanisms to manage those stressors. It may involve trade-offs in family members sacrificing their own needs to meet the needs of other family members. Family members of individuals with a mental illness may neglect their own needs, if only temporarily, to meet the needs of their ill relative. It is important, however, for all family members to have the opportunity to have their individual needs met. In fact, family members who practice health-promoting self-care are found to be better protected from stress (Acton, 2002).

The literature has identified several additional coping mechanisms to help families affected by mental illness manage stress. Caregivers of young adults with a mental illness identified facilitative attitudes, reliance on faith, the use of support groups, and increasing knowledge about mental illness as effective coping strategies (Doornbos, 1997). Consequently, nurses acting as teachers, referral agents, and spiritual caregivers were identified in this study as assisting families in coping.

Cuijpers and Stam (2000) have found that family members' abilities to cope with patient behaviors, worry about patients, and strain on the relationship were three elements of objective family impact that strongly influenced subjective impact. Therefore, they recommend concentrating family psychoeducational programs on these elements by teaching family members how to cope with their relatives' behaviors and their own feelings of worry, and how to improve their familial relationship. In addition, using problem-solving and coping strategies assists families in functioning more effectively (Saunders, 1999). Among caregivers of individuals with schizophrenia, these strategies included mobilization of resources, search for spiritual support, reframing (thinking about the situation from a different perspective), internal and external patterns, passivity, and social support (Saunders, 1999). In fact, social support has been shown to be one of the most influential factors in family coping (Solomon & Draine, 1995). Specifically, staying connected in peer support groups, such as the National Alliance on Mental Illness (NAMI), and with family or friends helps families cope (Harvey, Burns, Fahy, Manley, & Tattan, 2001; Doornbos, 2002; Saunders, 2003; Saunders & Byrne, 2002).

Unfortunately, some family members may use coping strategies that are maladaptive and do not enhance family functioning. For example, a sample of fathers of adult children with a mental illness was found to use isolating coping strategies (Wintersteen & Rasmussen, 1997). Furthermore, mental health professionals did not recognize or acknowledge the depth of emotional stress that these fathers experienced (Wintersteen & Rasmussen, 1997).

Assistance from Mental Health Professionals

Family members frequently report dissatisfaction with their level of involvement in their relatives' care. Familial caregivers report feeling unappreciated, blamed, and misunderstood by the public, and sometimes by mental health professionals themselves (Veltman et al., 2002). Parents of children with schizophrenia, for example, reported that they had to convince health care professionals of their children's need for help (Czuchta & McCay, 2001). With respect to communication between family members and mental health professionals, in one study with community mental health providers, 40% of therapists reported having no contact with their clients' family within the previous year. Among those who had contact with family members, it typically involved telephone contact during periods of crisis. The majority of these providers were satisfied with the level of contact they had with family (Dixon, Lucksted, Stewart, & Delahanty, 2000).

A disconnect exists between what mental health providers feel is satisfactory and what families

desire in terms of communication. Research with familial caregivers revealed that 85% of participants felt that interaction with mental health providers was the least supportive aspect of the mental health system (Doornbos, 2002). These caregivers perceived an overall lack of support from mental health professionals and even reported feeling blamed for the illness. Greater than one-third of these caregivers found nothing supportive in the mental health system to which they belonged. The mental health providers perceived as most supportive to these caregivers were those who affirmed the positive impact of their caregiving efforts and who showed empathy regarding the challenges the caregivers faced themselves (Doornbos, 2002).

Issues of confidentiality are an additional source of frustration for those wishing to be involved in the care and treatment of their family member. Although individuals receiving mental health treatment have a right to confidentiality, family members responsible for providing support to these individuals desire information and input regarding their loved one's care. Although shifts in child mental health policy have led to viewing parents as resources who have the right to be involved in treatment, and whose involvement is perceived as necessary for successful treatment (Friedman et al., 2004), this concept has not sufficiently been embraced by the adult mental health community. Familial caregivers continue to voice frustration regarding their inability to obtain pertinent information and to be involved in care planning (Doornbos, 2002).

Family members also experience a lack of services available to them as caregivers. In a study with relatives of people with a mental illness, only 24% felt that psychiatric service staff members were supportive in carrying the burden of having a relative with a mental illness, and 28% felt inferior during conversations with psychiatric service staff members (Ostman & Kjellin, 2002). Among another sample of familial caregivers, 41% reported never receiving assistance in identifying resources for themselves, and 36% had never been encouraged to recognize the effectiveness of their role as caregiver (Doornbos, 2001). The services they do receive provide family members with little emotional support. In fact, the most common service provided to family members is illness/medication education when what they report needing more of are practical problem-solving solutions and support for themselves.

DUAL DIAGNOSES

The National Mental Health Association (2008) estimates that 75% to 80% of adolescents receiving inpatient substance abuse treatment have a coexisting mental health disorder. The most common diagnoses are conduct disorder and depression. The diagnosis of both types of disorders is complicated by the fact that the symptoms of some mental disorders are similar to the effects of substance misuse (Hawkings, 2005). In fact, researchers and clinicians sometimes disagree about which came first, the mental illness or the substance abuse. Most experts believe that mental illness typically precedes substance abuse, and that the abuse is an attempt to "self-medicate" or control the psychiatric symptoms (Deykin, Levy, & Wells, 1987; Kandel, Kessler, & Margulies, 1978). Some do believe the reverse is true, however; that the substance abuse triggers or accompanies the mental illness (Bukstein, Brent, & Kaminer, 1989).

With respect to the care and treatment of those with a substance disorder, some mental health professionals feel that abstinence may not be appropriate or achievable for some dual-disorder patients, and that harm reduction, stabilization of consumption, and education on risk, mental illness, care, and support systems may be more realistic (Hawkings, 2005). When planning care for individuals with dual diagnoses, it is important to negotiate a plan of care that is achievable and includes a logical appraisal of the risks of substance abuse (Barrett, 2005). In addition, the earlier in their lives or in the life of their substance abuse a person begins treatment, the more likely he or she is to continue treatment, resulting in better outcomes (Hawkings, 2005). Most experts recommend integrated rather than parallel or sequential treatment for the mental illness and the substance abuse (Barrowclough et al., 2001; Tiet & Mausbach, 2007; Walsh & Frankland, 2005). For many people, it is not realistic to attempt to recover from one disorder before working on recovering from the other. The National Mental Health Association of the United Kingdom maintains the position that "treatment programs designed primarily for people with substance abuse problems may not be appropriate for people who also have a diagnosed mental illness because of their reliance on confrontation techniques and their counsel against the use of prescription medications. The most effective programs address the care and treatment of both disorders in an integrated manner" (National Mental Health Association, 2008, p. 2). This care, however, does not necessarily need to be provided in residential settings. Timko, Chen, Sempel, and Barnett (2006) have found that patients with dual diagnoses treated in community residential facilities experienced comparable psychiatric outcomes and less substance use than those who were hospitalized. In addition, duration of treatment may have more of an impact on outcomes than intensity of treatment, and Barrowclough, Haddock, Fitzsimmons, and Johnson (2006) emphasize that brief therapy is not adequate for these patients and their families.

With respect to family members of those with dual diagnoses, their need for information, skill building, and support should be addressed. Nurses can teach affected families problem solving, parenting, coping, and communication skills (O'Connell, 2006) in addition to providing diagnosis- and treatment-specific information. Referrals to organizations such as Al-Anon or other support groups may also be helpful for family members wishing to connect with people with similar experiences. Integrated treatment may be beneficial in promoting the involvement of family members. Because of multiple stressors in their own lives, it is often difficult for family members to attend treatment, particularly when separate systems are providing that treatment (Esposito-Smythers, 2005). Family members wishing to be involved may be more willing and able to participate in their loved one's care if it can all be provided by one system.

FAMILY MENTAL HEALTH NURSING PRACTICE

In its most recent *Psychiatric and Mental Health Nursing Scope and Standards of Practice*, the APNA defines psychiatric-mental health nursing as follows:

A specialized area of nursing practice committed to promoting mental health through the assessment, diagnosis, and treatment of human responses to mental health problems and psychiatric disorders. Psychiatric-mental health nursing, a core mental health profession, employs a purposeful use of self as its art and a wide range of nursing, psychosocial, and neurobiological theories and research evidence as its science (APNA, 2007, p. 1).

Baccalaureate education is preferred within the specialty of psychiatric mental health nursing because of the complexity of care it involves. The practice of psychiatric-mental health nursing may occur in a variety of settings, including emergency departments, acute inpatient care, long-term care, partial hospitalization or intensive outpatient programs, residential facilities, primary care facilities, community-based centers, integrative programs for those dually diagnosed with a substance abuse disorder, telehealth centers, forensic settings such as jails or prisons, or disaster mental health settings. Regardless of the practice setting, embedded within the practice of psychiatric-mental health nursing is the involvement of family members or significant others throughout the nursing process.

In accordance with the identified goal of the New Freedom Commission to make the provision of mental health services consumer and family driven, nurses must listen to and address the needs of both mental health consumers and their family members. One mechanism that has the potential to address family members' needs is providing family psychoeducation. *Family psychoeducation* is a term used to describe various family programs that incorporate the following three elements: family education, training in coping skills, and social support (Schock & Gavazzi, 2005). The time commitment and emphasis on each of these elements is what differs among the diverse psychoeducational models. Currently, these interventions offered may continue for months or years. Because psychoeducational programs are multifaceted and involve such long-term relationships, they are typically delivered by teams of professionals working together (Marsh & Johnson, 1997). Nurses' training and education make them well suited to participate in such interdisciplinary teams emphasizing client and family education, enhancing coping skills, and developing supportive networks.

The educational element of these programs involves providing information to relatives regarding diagnoses, cause of mental illness, prognosis, and treatment. Skills training may include coping skills for family members and social skills training for the family member with the mental illness. In addition, the entire family may work on developing communication skills so they may communicate more effectively with one another. Social support for family members is enhanced by actively including relatives as members of the treatment team. Social support is also established through connections to other families with similar experiences. Through networking with one another, families can find support and share problem-solving strategies. A local chapter of the NAMI is one support and advocacy organization that families may find helpful.

In addition to family psychoeducation, nurses can provide family mental health care through the use of home-based programs. Simply meeting families in their homes acknowledges their important role in treatment decision making. In hospital and office settings, control lies with the professional, whereas home visits provide individuals who are mentally ill and their families some control (Finkelman, 2000). The home is also frequently the location in which familial stressors arise and where coping with these stressors takes place. The nurse may be better equipped to place these stressors and coping strategies in context by visiting patients and families where they live.

Regardless of the location or structure of care delivery, two goals of working with family members of mentally ill individuals exist: first, to achieve the best possible outcome for the patient through collaborative treatment and management; and second, to minimize the suffering of family members by supporting their efforts to aid the recovery of their ill family member (Dixon et al., 2001). As family members have increasingly assumed the role of primary caregivers for mentally ill individuals, it is more important than ever to include them as partners in the delivery of mental health care. Care delivery systems that involve family members acknowledge the effect mental disorders have on entire family systems. They seek to prevent the return or exacerbation of a disorder, and alleviate pain and suffering experienced by family members. To fulfill these goals, researchers have identified 15 evidence-based principles for involving families of individuals with a mental illness (Table 16-2) (Dixon et al., 2001). These principles can be incorporated into the family nursing process at each step: assessment, diagnosis, outcome identification, planning, implementation, and evaluation.

Assessment

Before discussing assessment in detail, it is important to note that patients with mental illnesses have a right to privacy regarding their health information.

TABLE 16-2

Evidenced-Based Principles for Working with Families of Individuals with a Mental Illness

- Organize care so that everyone involved is working toward the same treatment goals within a collaborative, supportive relationship.
- Attend to both the social and clinical needs of the primary patient.
- Provide optimal medication management.
- Listen to family's concerns and involve them in all elements of treatment.
- Examine family's expectations of treatment and expectations of the primary patient.
- Evaluate strengths and limitations of family's ability to provide support.
- Aid in the resolution of family conflict.
- Explore feelings of loss.
- Provide pertinent information to patients and families at appropriate times.
- Develop a clear crisis plan.
- Help enhance family communication.
- Train families in problem-solving techniques.
- Promote expansion of the family's social support network.
- Be adaptable in meeting the family's needs.
- Provide easy access to another professional if current work with the family ceases.

Source: From Dixon, L., McFarlane, W., Lefley, H., Lucksted, A., Cohen, M., Falloon, I., et al. (2001). Evidence-based practices for services to families of people with psychiatric disabilities. *Psychiatric Services, 52*(7), 903–910, by permission.

Laws may differ from state to state, but in general, health care professionals can receive information from family or other individuals without consent from the patient. They cannot, however, provide information or in any way discuss a person's private health information without consent. In addition, in the absence of an emergency, a health care provider cannot actively seek out or request information from family or other sources without consent. With respect to children and adolescents, parents and legal guardians may have access to their children's health information without consent. Regardless of whether the individual with the mental illness is a child, adolescent, or adult, the ideal situation is to create an atmosphere of trust and teamwork among the individual, their family members, and professional mental health providers. The identified "patient" can sign a release of information form authorizing information to be shared by mental health providers with specified family members. The release of information can be presented as a means of enhancing treatment. Patients and their family members can decide what types of information may be shared and under what circumstances.

Regardless of the setting in which assessment occurs, nurses can exhibit respect to family members by allowing time for them to discuss their understanding of the relevant mental illness, how their relative's illness has affected them, past treatment experiences from their perspective, and their treatment goals for their family member (Finkelman, 2000). The APNA Standards of Practice and Standards of Care articulate that assessment data are collected from multiple sources in a systematic and ongoing manner (APNA, 2007). It is during this phase of the nursing process that a therapeutic alliance is established. Ideally, a therapeutic alliance can be established with the individual and any family members involved in his or her care. Assessment data from the perspective of the individual who is mentally ill or family members, or both, may include the following (APNA, 2000; Finkelman, 2000):

- Perception of and understanding of the illness
- The primary complaint, symptoms, or concerns
- Physical, developmental, cognitive, mental, and emotional health status
- Health history
- Treatment history
- Family, social, cultural, racial, ethnic, and community systems
- Activities of daily living and health habits
- Substance use history
- Interpersonal and communication skills
- Sources of stress
- Coping mechanisms used
- Spiritual and religious beliefs or values
- Economic, legal, or other environmental factors that affect health
- Health-promoting strengths
- Complementary therapies utilized
- Family conflicts
- Familial roles and responsibilities
- Treatment goals
- The person's ability to remain safe

Diagnosis

Once the nurse has conducted a thorough assessment, the nurse determines relevant diagnoses. During this process, the nurse "identifies actual or potential risks to the patient's health and safety or barriers to mental and physical health which may include but are not limited to interpersonal, systematic, or environmental circumstances" (APNA, 2007, p. 31). Once these risks and barriers are identified, the nurse discusses and validates them with the individual and his or her family members. Family-specific nursing diagnoses recognized by the North American Nursing Diagnosis Association include the following (Ackley & Ladwig, 2006):

- Risk for caregiver role strain
- Caregiver role strain
- Compromised family coping
- Disabled family coping
- Readiness for enhanced family coping
- Dysfunctional family process
- Interrupted family process
- Readiness for enhanced family process
- Supportive family role performance
- Ineffective family therapeutic regimen management

Outcome Identification

The formulation of desired outcomes is an individualized process. The patient, nurse, family members, and other members of the interdisciplinary team work collaboratively to identify measurable, realistic, attainable, and cost-effective outcomes or goals. Outcomes may be directed to the patient's or the family's needs and are evidence-based. These outcomes may be modified based on changes in the patient's or family's situation. In revisiting these expected outcomes periodically, the direction for continuity of care is established.

Planning

After identifying and agreeing on expected outcomes, an individualized, strategic plan is developed to facilitate the attainment of these goals. Again, this planning involves a collaborative effort among the patient, family, and health care providers. Each of these "stakeholders" is allowed an opportunity to prioritize elements of the plan. This plan articulates direction of patient care activities, and the responsibilities of the patient, family, and health care providers in meeting the identified outcomes.

The strategic plan addresses each identified diagnosis and assigns evidence-based interventions to promote or restore health. The plan also includes approaches geared toward the prevention of illness or injury (APNA, 2007). An educational program may be related to the patient's health problems, or it may specifically address the individual or family's needs with respect to topics such as stress management, treatment regimen, relapse prevention, self-care activities, or quality of life. In addition to this educational component, the nurse assists the patient and family in identifying and securing services available and meaningful to them given their individual situation. The patient's and family's motivation, health beliefs, and functional capabilities are reflected in the plan (APNA, 2000). When appropriate, the plan includes referrals to other resources and case management.

Implementation

Nurses can help individuals with mental illness and their family members develop interventions specific to the problems they identify. A variety of family intervention strategies are outlined in Table 16-3. A place to begin working with families is to discuss and create ways for them to manage the treatment plans that affect the everyday family routines. Nurses can help families negotiate problem behaviors that interrupt the family, such as smoking or pacing. The family can keep a log of disruptive behaviors, especially when a medication has been changed, added, or deleted. Nurses may help families develop plans to provide increased structure in the home during periods of stress, to identify when to see a physician for medication adjustments, or to know when to take the ill individual to the hospital or call the police for assistance (Finkelman, 2000).

It may be useful to aid families in identifying ways that the mentally ill family member can realistically participate and contribute to the family so that he or she can feel and be viewed as a contributing member. This may include helping families understand specific challenges faced by the individual who is mentally ill within the context of the family. For example, anxiety and an inability to cope with overstimulation, such as at large family events, are

TABLE 16-3
Family Intervention Strategies

- Coordinate information and treatment plans across settings and with multiple health care providers.
- Ensure that communication is bidirectional from health care providers to families and from families to health care providers.
- Provide validation for commitment and work being done by all family members.
- Create ways for families to manage treatment plans that affect everyday routines.
- Identify realistic ways that the mentally ill family member can participate and contribute to the family.
- Articulate an action plan to implement during times of crisis.
- Negotiate ways to manage specific problem behaviors.
- Connect with appropriate social resources (individual/group therapy, support groups, extended family, friends, religious organizations).
- Provide diagnostic and treatment-related education.
- Encourage self-care behaviors for all family members.
- Identify effective coping skills for individual family members.
- Advocate for policy changes that benefit individuals with mental illnesses and their family members.
- Challenge detrimental stereotypes of mental illness.

common for people with some mental illnesses. Nurses can work with families to create ways for the mentally ill member to participate in such events, but it is critical to success that there be a planned escape route if the situation becomes intolerable.

Nurses can also facilitate families in identifying their social support resources. Families may need assistance in drawing support from friends or extended family. Nurses help families get connected with various support groups in the community, such as diagnosis-specific support groups or Al-Anon. Families may benefit by connections to religious organizations or the NAMI.

The interventions used by the psychiatric-mental health nurse depend partially on the practice setting of the nurse. In the 2000 edition of the *Scope and Standards of Psychiatric-Mental Health Nursing Practice* (APNA), the following interventions were described as available to nurses who do not possess advanced education and training: counseling, promotion of self-care activities, health teaching, case

management, health promotion and maintenance, crisis intervention, community-based care, and psychiatric home health. Each of these interventions can easily be extended to include family members.

Counseling may assist people in improving their coping skills. This intervention may be helpful to families during times of crisis. It may be used to engage people in problem-solving activities or explore stress management and relaxation techniques. Counseling provided by nurses can also emphasize grief, assertiveness training, conflict resolution, or behavior modification (APNA, 2000). It is also a powerful strategy when used to commend all members of the family for their commitment, compassion, and interest in learning ways to help each other adjust and adapt to living with a chronic illness. Providing recognition and acknowledgment for their hard work validates their feelings and demonstrates empathy and understanding.

The promotion of self-care activities is aimed at improving functional status and quality of life. Again, this intervention can be applied to an entire family unit. The nurse may assist the primary patient in assuming responsibility for activities of daily living and medication management, whereas assisting family members in engaging in other health-promoting behaviors that target the maintenance of their own quality of life.

It is necessary to involve family members in teaching regarding diagnosis, treatment options, and symptom identification and management. Teaching provided by nurses often involves providing information patients and families need to make informed decisions regarding the course of treatment. In addition, family members of individuals with a mental illness often express a need for education in problem-solving techniques. As a primary role of the nurse, teaching often incorporates health promotion and skills training. As such, nurses can assist family members in defining the unique problems they experience and lead families to find solutions that are feasible within the context of the particular family. Families may need assistance in finding ways to cope with day-to-day disruptions in their lives, or they may need to develop more specific ways to manage crisis situations or solve housing dilemmas. In addition, conflict resolution, coping, and communication skills can be taught to entire families.

Case management as an intervention involves the coordination and assurance of continuity of care. Being mindful of family needs and resources, the nurse assists families in establishing linkages with other providers or service agencies. Similarly, in the role of health promoter, the nurse assists families in identifying community resources. The psychiatric mental health nurse takes an active role in the community to identify problems in the mental health system and work toward addressing those problems by reaching out to consumer alliances and advocacy groups.

Nurses have a responsibility to advocate for patients and their families, including lobbying policymakers. Supporting legislation such as the Mental Health Parity Act is one way to advocate for patients and their families. The intent of the Mental Health Parity Act (1996) was to have equitable coverage for mental health issues and physical health issues, but limited coverage and lifetime capped service costs continue (Bomar, 2004). Challenging stereotypes and discriminatory practices involving individuals with mental illness and their family members will help change the stigma associated with these disorders. Landlords, employers, health care providers, criminal justice professionals, policymakers, and the media can all be held accountable by psychiatric-mental health nurses for discriminatory practices and targeted to help change the stigma of mental illness in our society.

Evaluation

Periodically, the patient, family, and mental health professionals evaluate the effectiveness of the treatment plan in relation to attainment of the expected outcomes. Evaluation is a continuous, systematic, and criterion-based process. During evaluation, the patient and family have the opportunity to share their feelings with respect to satisfaction of the care they received. The costs and benefits of treatment are discussed. Taking this information into account, diagnoses, outcomes, and treatment plans are once again revised and mutually agreed on.

BENEFITS OF AND BARRIERS TO INVOLVING FAMILY

Family interventions have beneficial effects on relatives' subjective and objective impact, psychological distress, relationships with the ill relative, and family distress and functioning (Cuijpers, 1999). Providing services to family members of individuals with mental illness has been shown to reduce rehospitalization rates, reduce symptomology, and increase medication compliance and quality of life for the ill family member (Solomon, 1996; Young & Magnabosco, 2004).

Involving the family in the treatment of dual disorders has many benefits. Family involvement may contribute to engaging treatment-resistant individuals, promote treatment adherence, reduce relapse, reduce substance use, and improve the well-being of both clients and their family members (Moore, 2005). Additional benefits of involving family that have been reported in the literature include decreasing family conflicts and violence, decreasing enabling behaviors in family members, and positively influencing the course of both the mental illness and the substance abuse (Mueser & Fox, 2002). If family members are involved in treatment, they are more likely to continue to remain involved, and are specifically more likely to offer financial assistance and assistance with tasks of daily living (Clark, 2001; Warren et al., 2007). Families are helped by developing a consistent interpretation of the causes of the illnesses and new ways of managing situations that arise (Ahlstrom, Skarsater, & Danielson, 2007). The structure of family involvement may play an important role in the treatment of individuals with dual diagnoses. It has been suggested that family participation in multiple family groups, as opposed to single family groups, extended remission, particularly for patients at high risk for relapse (McFarlane et al., 1995).

Unfortunately, despite the benefits noted earlier, few families receive services (Dixon et al., 1999). Family members may find it difficult to participate in family-oriented services because of transportation issues, or lack of time or energy to devote to such activities (Solomon, 1996). As mentioned earlier, the stigma associated with mental illness may prevent some family members from becoming involved because of a sense of shame or embarrassment. A history of failed attempts to be involved or negative experiences, including blame, with mental health professionals may also discourage family members. Loss of hope or emotional burnout and difficulty communicating with their ill family member are additional barriers families may encounter (Kaas, Lee, & Peitzman, 2003).

Among mental health professionals, a lack of time and resources, coupled with high caseloads, can prevent them from actively including family members in decision making and treatment. Lack of funding and reimbursement for services rendered to family members of mentally ill individuals may also prevent implementation of family-based care (Dixon et al., 2001). Concern about issues related to confidentiality of patient information may complicate family involvement. Mental health professionals may wish to uphold their clients' right to confidentiality and treatment autonomy, but in the process, they shut out concerned family members who are requesting involvement. Lack of training and resources to manage family issues are cited as barriers to implementing family-focused mental health care (Mason & Subedi, 2006). Additional barriers include conflicting feelings about treating the client versus treating the family, beliefs that family involvement is not necessary or potentially harmful to clients, and a lack of visible or measurable results of the benefits of including family members (Kaas et al., 2003).

Family Case Study

The following case study of the Johnson family demonstrates the assessment, diagnosis, outcome identification, planning, implementation, and evaluation for care of a family with a member who has a mental illness.

SETTING: Inpatient acute care hospital, cardiac intensive care unit (ICU).

NURSING GOAL: Work with the family to assist them in planning for discharge to a less intensive care facility that is planned to occur in the next 3 days.

FAMILY MEMBERS:
 + Steve: father, 55 years old, small businessman
 + Mary: mother, 49 years old, stay-at-home mother
 + Debbie: stepmother, 54 years old, schoolteacher
 + Harold: stepfather, 60 years old, successful building contractor
 + Tony: identified patient, 23 years old, oldest child, son, unemployed, sleeping on couches of friends
 + Susie: younger daughter, Tony's sister, 14 years old, eighth grader, overachiever and "perfect" child
 + Bobby: Tony's half-brother, mother's son, 12 years old
 + Rachael: stepmother's daughter from previous marriage, 30 years old
 + Thomas: Mary's father, 86 years old, wealthy businessman
 + Emma: Mary's mother, 85 years old, abuses alcohol

JOHNSON FAMILY STORY

Tony Johnson is a 23-year-old man who was admitted to the hospital cardiac ICU through the emergency department in acute cardiac distress from an accidental methamphetamine overdose. He arrived at the emergency department by ambulance from his drug-free friend Doug's single-room occupancy hotel room. Tony is currently homeless. He had been sleeping on his drug dealer's couch for a week until he was arrested for assault. Since his arrest a few days ago, he has been sleeping on Doug's floor.

Tony has been in and out of substance abuse treatment programs since he was 17 years old. He was diagnosed with bipolar disorder at the first treatment program he attended. His father and stepmother convinced him to enter that program just before his 18th birthday and paid for the expensive 3-month program. As with all of the programs he has attended, he left soon after admission to the program.

During a previous emergency room admission, Tony got angry at his family, tore off his electrocardiogram leads and oxygen mask, and left the hospital against medical advice. During the present hospitalization, Tony called his father from the emergency department to ask him to come and help get him admitted to another treatment facility. Tony has agreed to see his sister and stepmother, but not his stepfather or stepsiblings. He also refuses to see his mother because he says she "is the cause of all my problems." His mother and father separated, and later divorced, when Tony was 10 years old and his younger sister was about 1 year old. He and his mother fought constantly when he was a child, and she was overprotective of him. Tony was an obedient child who then began using alcohol and drugs and stealing from family members beginning in his early teens.

Tony's father has maintained Tony on his small business's health insurance policy. Tony is eligible for short-term residential treatment if he can prove to the director of the program that he intends to cooperate this time. His father is again willing to pay for longer term drug and psychiatric treatment if Tony proves that he is intent on cooperating with his treatment plan.

Tony stopped taking his mood-stabilizing medications approximately 2 weeks ago, when his most recent binge use of methamphetamine started. Currently, the doctors are reluctant to prescribe his mood-stabilizing medications while the methamphetamine is still affecting his major systems.

FAMILY MEMBERS

The admitting nurse and the ICU social worker have gleaned the following familial information from Steve, Mary, and Debbie. The Johnson family genogram is illustrated in Figure 16-1. The Johnson family ecomap is illustrated in Figure 16-2.

Steve is very concerned about his son's health and reminds him that the doctors have said he will not survive another year if he continues to use methamphetamine. Steve recognizes his son's depression and anger, and feels guilty that he did not notice sooner that Tony was depressed and "self-medicating" with alcohol and drugs. He blames himself for the divorce, which he believes precipitated Tony's alcohol and drug abuse. He also regrets his workaholism during Tony's early years and for being a co-dependent, allowing Tony to live at home when he was drinking and using drugs to excess, and sleeping round the clock between drug-induced manic episodes. Steve initiated the divorce when he discovered his ex-wife was having affairs and using cocaine. Steve was diagnosed at the time of the divorce as having bipolar disorder, with a manic episode that resulted in his hospitalization. He is maintained on medications and has had no further episodes.

Mary, Tony's mother, became a stay-at-home mom when she gave birth to Tony. She was overprotective with him but secretly resented that he was not a good student. She punished him severely for his learning difficulties, especially when she was drinking. Her closet drinking became cocaine use after Tony's sister Susie was born, when Tony was 9 years old. Tony both resented his sister for taking his mother's attention away from him and was relieved not to be the sole focus of her anger. Mary is currently recovering from drug abuse but drinks wine still, even drinking with Tony when they are speaking to one another.

Debbie, Tony's stepmother, met Tony's father about a year after his divorce. Tony was living with his father at the time and refused to accept his stepmother as a mother figure for him for several years. Debbie is a better limit-setter than Steve, and is often more practical about recognizing and addressing Tony's needs. She is influential with both Steve and Mary in making decisions about Tony. She has a daughter from a previous marriage, *Rachael,* who is 30 years old.

Harold, Tony's stepfather, is 11 years older than Mary and, in many ways, is a father figure for his wife. He dotes on his 12-year-old son and largely ignores his stepson and stepdaughter; he does brag about Susie's successes. He is a successful building contractor and is able to provide a luxurious life for his wife and son.

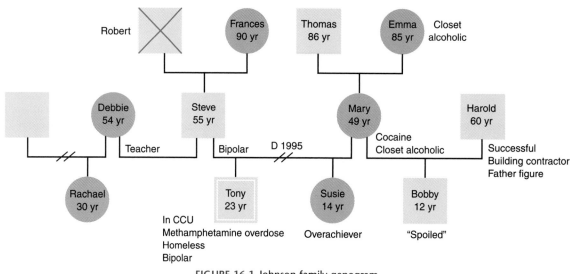

FIGURE 16-1 Johnson family genogram.

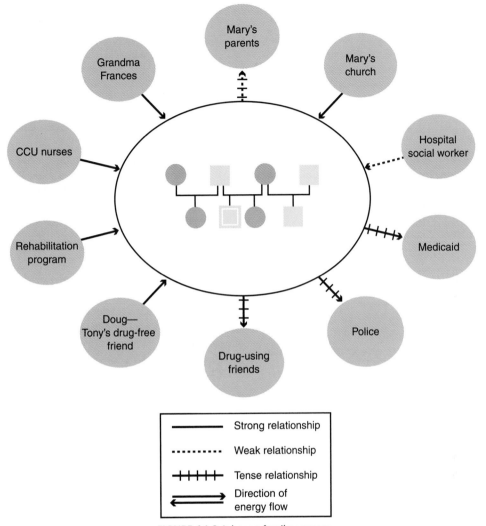

Strong relationship

Weak relationship

Tense relationship

Direction of energy flow

FIGURE 16-2 Johnson family ecomap.

Susie, 14 years old, is bright and well-behaved. Tony calls her the "perfect" child he never was. She is an honor student, talented in music and art, and well-liked by her fellow students and by adults. She worries about Tony and has always tried to please him. She can't understand why he gets so mad at his parents and her; she tries to encourage him to enter treatment and tells him she misses him very much. Her parents divorced when she was about a year old, and she has lived most of the time with her mother who remarried and had another son soon after the divorce. Her step-father is very attached to her half-brother and takes him with him to work and on fishing trips. Susie loves her father very much but sees him only every other weekend and holidays.

Steve's mother, *Frances,* lives about an hour away, is 90 years old, and is very fond and sympathetic of Tony. Steve's father died when Tony was young. His parents owned a grocery store that they ran as a family.

Mary's parents, *Thomas* and *Emma,* live nearby. Thomas is a wealthy but distant businessman who gave money rather than time to his wife and children. Emma was a stay-at-home wife and mother; she is a drinking alcoholic who fairly successfully hides her alcoholism except on family occasions when she often makes a scene.

DISCHARGE PLANS: Tony will be discharged from the ICU in 3 days; his insurance does not cover a longer hospital stay once his acute methamphetamine poisoning is treated.

FAMILY SYSTEMS THEORY IN RELATION TO THE JOHNSON FAMILY

The health event the Johnson family is managing will be viewed through the lens of a nurse that used family systems theory as the foundational approach to working with this family. A more detailed discussion of the family nursing system can be found in Chapter 3.

CONCEPT 1: ALL PARTS OF THE SYSTEM ARE INTERCONNECTED

In the Johnson case, all members of the family are affected by Tony's dual DSM-IV diagnoses of amphetamine dependence and bipolar disorder, and his dramatic overdoses and near-death experiences. His father feels enormous guilt and is afraid to confront and set limits with his son for fear of sending him to his death. His mother reluctantly verbalizes feeling guilty but lacks sincerity. Her son feels she does not want to change her own behavior; thus, admitting guilt is not possible for her. His stepmother is more realistic because she is not as emotionally attached to Tony, but she worries about the effects of Tony's drug use and the worry it causes Steve, and she fears a relapse of Steve's own bipolar symptoms.

CONCEPT 2: THE WHOLE IS MORE THAN THE SUM OF ITS PARTS

In the Johnson family case study, the complexity of the blended family increases the interconnectedness and interdependence of the family members. It is not just parents and children or grandparents and parents, but a complex system that deteriorates over time as the stress of Tony's illness takes its toll on the entire system.

CONCEPT 3: ALL SYSTEMS HAVE SOME FORM OF BOUNDARIES OR BORDER BETWEEN THE SYSTEM AND ITS ENVIRONMENT

In the Johnson family, the normal boundaries of self and others, and of family and outsiders are dysfunctional. Spousal boundaries are violated by infidelity; parent-child boundaries are violated by theft and parents drinking with substance-abusing children. Some of the boundaries are closed by distant, aloof parents and spouses. Tony demonstrates some flexible boundaries by refusing to allow visits by some family members but allowing visits by others.

CONCEPT 4: SYSTEMS CAN BE FURTHER ORGANIZED INTO SUBSYSTEMS

The Johnson family has many subsystems: parent, parent-stepparent, parent-child, grandparent-parent, sibling, grandparent, and in-law. Each of these subsystems can be mobilized to help with the goals defined for the family. Specifically, the mother-father-stepmother-son subsystem will probably prove most influential in discharge planning.

FAMILY IMPACT

In the Johnson family, objective impact includes the financial costs of treatment, physical strain and damage, effects on the health of other family members, and disruption in the daily lives of many of the family members. The subjective impact is the enormous guilt and fear felt by the family members, the damage to Tony's mental and social health, the disruption felt by other children in the family, the strain placed on the marriages, and the disrupted family routines such as regular mealtimes and leisure time.

SOCIAL SUPPORT AND STIGMA

The Johnson family has been moderately successful in previous generations at hiding the substance abuse and dysfunction. Although more acceptable now than in previous generations, some social stigma is attached to divorce, remarriage, alcoholism, drug addiction, and mental illness—all of which affect the Johnson family. Methamphetamine addiction carries a large social stigma today as the enormous physical, mental, social, and physical damage is better understood.

COPING AND RESILIENCY

The Johnson family is in need of intervention to teach them more successful ways of dealing with Tony's and others' behaviors, and their feelings of worry and concern. Most mental health professionals would suggest that they attend 12-step meetings for families of substance abusers, and that they have family counseling with Tony. All subsystems need help learning more effective coping strategies, from those who remain aloof from the problems to those who become overenmeshed in the lives of other family members.

ASSISTANCE FROM MENTAL HEALTH PROFESSIONALS

The Johnson family needs referral to a treatment facility that focuses on the needs of the family and the enabling behaviors of family members. In addition, the extended family needs counseling concerning the impact of these disorders on their family and the maladaptive coping styles being used. Tony needs treatment for both his substance abuse and his bipolar disorder.

Family psychoeducation for the Johnson family would include education about substance abuse and bipolar disorders, coping skills for Tony and the family members, especially in dealing with grief and anger, and effective communication skills to express feelings constructively.

MENTAL HEALTH CARE NURSING FROM A FAMILY SYSTEMS PERSPECTIVE

The needs of each member of the Johnson family will be identified and the family as a whole will be addressed by looking at the family from a Family Systems perspective.

Assessment

The assessment of the Johnson family is conducted by the ICU nurse and social worker with Tony, Steve, Mary, and Debbie and includes the following:

+ Perception of and understanding of the illness: The Johnson family has some experience with substance abuse and bipolar disorder. The nurse assesses whether the knowledge is accurate and current.
+ The primary complaint, symptoms, or concerns: The Johnson family believes that Tony's illness is their "problem," but their dysfunctional family dynamics are at the heart of their needs. Since this crisis has arisen, their biggest concern is Tony's safety. They now fear that Tony will either end up dead or in prison.
+ Physical, developmental, cognitive, mental, and emotional health status: The Johnson family is in a great deal of emotional pain and is in a crisis state at this time. The family's stress level is at an all-time high.
+ Health history: The Johnson family has a history of mental health problems but appears to be physically healthy otherwise.
+ Treatment history: Tony has a history of unsuccessful treatment attempts, with brief periods of abstinence from alcohol and drugs, and minimal treatment for his bipolar disorder. Tony takes mood-stabilizing medication intermittently but has not had a long-term relationship with a psychiatrist since he was 20.
+ Family, social, cultural, racial, ethnic, and community systems: The Johnson family systems have been described and are reflected in the ecomap of the family (see Fig. 16-2). Mary is involved with church activities. Tony is in contact with friends from high school in addition to his friends who use drugs.
+ Activities of daily living and health habits: These activities are seriously disrupted for Steve, Debbie, Mary, and Susie. The stress, worry, and concern

they have for Tony, and the time and energy they are using to help Tony find a place to live and get into treatment are affecting their own abilities to spend time focusing on their own health and well-being.

+ Substance use: The Johnson family has alcohol, cocaine, and methamphetamine abuse in its history.
+ Coping mechanisms used: Although some healthy mechanisms are used by the Johnson family, they also use rationalization, projection, denial, and substance use as ways of coping.
+ Spiritual and religious beliefs or values: The Johnson family members state they are Christians, but the only family members to attend services or admit to spiritual practices are Steve, Mary, and Frances. Steve uses meditation to maintain focus in his life but has been unable to do so for many months as a result of his increased time spent on attempting to keep track of Tony.
+ Economic, legal, or other environmental factors that affect health: Steve's finances have been strained by Tony's illness. Harold and Mary refuse to accept any of the monetary burden of his care, saying that "he needs to take care of himself," but they remain emotionally involved.
+ Health-promoting strengths: There is obvious love between Tony and his father and stepmother, and between Tony and his grandmother, Frances; this can be mobilized to promote healthy family behaviors and communication.
+ Complementary therapies used: Tony's friends have recommended acupuncture for his addictions, but he has not been clean long enough to try it. Debbie is trying meditation to ease the stress and is trying to get Steve to join a yoga group with her.
+ Family conflicts: Numerous unresolved family conflicts continue in the Johnson family.
+ Familial roles and responsibilities: In the Johnson family, Mary alternates between being overprotective and harsh and critical with her children. Steve is an enabler and unable to set appropriate limits. Susie is pseudomature in her relationship with Tony.
+ Treatment goals: The treatment goals for the Johnson family are to get Tony into a short-term residential treatment facility and to find a long-term treatment program for families with a member with dual diagnoses. They desire social support from others with similar experiences, education regarding Tony's ongoing treatment options, and skills training that will help them communicate

better with one another and teach them to manage the impact of these disorders on the family in between these intermittent crises.

+ The person's ability to remain safe: Without long-term treatment and medication management, Tony is at great risk for harm.

Diagnosis

Tony's dual diagnosis of bipolar disorder with methamphetamine dependence helps determine the best treatment approach for Tony as an individual. His dual disorder probably began when he was an adolescent. For Tony, he describes the feelings of depression and hopelessness preceding his misuse of drugs.

But it is often said that the "mentally ill" patient is just the "delegate to the convention" for the family; most experts advocate for the inclusion of the family in treatment. In addition to the plan of care that staff nurses have established to address Tony's individual nursing diagnoses, family diagnoses for the Johnson family include:

1. Compromised family coping related to situational crisis as evidenced by Tony's overdose and hospitalization, the family's disruption in their daily activities, and their increased need for support

2. Dysfunctional family process related to drug abuse as evidenced by familial conflict and ineffective problem solving

3. Ineffective family therapeutic regimen management related to decisional conflict (discharge decision), economic difficulty, and excessive demands on family as evidenced by verbalization of desire to manage Tony's treatment and prevent the negative sequelae of his methamphetamine abuse and untreated bipolar disorder

Outcome Identification

For the Johnson family and Tony, treatment attempts have failed to date, and it appears that Tony will need to aim for abstinence and control of his mental illness to survive. The desired outcomes for the Johnson family include but are not limited to the recovery of Tony from his methamphetamine addiction/abuse and control of his bipolar disorder. Outcomes for the family include identifying familial support systems in the community, exploring financial options for paying for Tony's treatment, making a family decision regarding the best treatment option available for Tony, Tony's acceptance into a residential treatment facility, expressing anger appropriately, discussing openly substance abuse and other "family secrets," setting limits on inappropriate

and enabling behavior, and honoring individual and family boundaries and needs.

Planning

For the Johnson family, an integrated program in the community is most appropriate but not easy to find and often quite expensive. Discharge planning for the Johnson family includes the following: the family will be given information about appropriate referrals for residential care, the family (and Tony) will seek out and accept an appropriate referral, and Tony will be discharged to the referral facility. The family will also be given referrals to the Meth Family and Friends Support Group, as well as the NAMI. The family will also be referred for counseling to a therapist/counselor who is available through Steve's insurance plan so they may work on their communication and coping skills, develop more appropriate boundaries with one another, and address some of their own needs.

Implementation

Tony and his family accepted a referral to a Volunteers of America drug-free facility/treatment program in which family members participate on a regular basis. This program is free to Tony as long as he continues to work at the facility. He was willing to accept this placement, and it did not burden Steve economically.

Evaluation

Follow-up would be needed to determine the effectiveness of the referral in assisting the family to function more appropriately, helping Tony to be drug free, and providing treatment for Tony's bipolar disorder.

Benefits of Involving Family

In the Johnson family, Tony is reaching out for help from his family. He has been unsuccessful in receiving and accepting treatment on his own, and he needs the resources of his family (insurance and finances) to get the treatment he needs. The family needs him healthy to improve their self-image and their own successful functioning and vice versa.

Barriers to Involving Family

Many of the barriers to involving the Johnson family are a result of the family dynamics that the family exhibits. The family has a pattern of rescuing Tony during periods of crisis, and has difficulty setting appropriate limits and insisting that Tony take responsibility for his actions. They tend to become overly involved during periods and remain aloof at others, resulting in inconsistent participation. They are in need of long-term partnership with a treatment team. Tony's lack of commitment to treatment hinders any type of long-term relationship being established with his family. In addition, Steve may experience a sense of guilt that Tony may have inherited the bipolar disorder from him, and he may need counseling to express some of these feelings. Also, the stress of Tony's illness and recent crisis may exacerbate Steve's own disorder.

SUMMARY

Involving clients and their family members in mental health care and treatment maximizes the knowledge and experience of those involved. As has been demonstrated, the presence of disabling mental disorders has a devastating effect on individuals and their families. This chapter reviews the history of mental health policy and provides a discussion of the issues that families of individuals with mental illness face. These issues include the family impact, stigmatization, a need for social support, and coping/resiliency. Using evidenced-based theory and a family case study, we discuss how mental health professionals, especially nurses, can assist these families most effectively. Based on the principles for working with families of individuals with mental illness, we apply these principles to the assessment, diagnosis, outcome identification, planning, implementation, and evaluation of families. We make the case for involving the family, citing ways to overcome barriers to such involvement. Family involvement is essential to the successful treatment of persons with severe and persistent mental illness.

REFERENCES

Ackley, B., & Ladwig, G. (2006). *Nursing diagnosis handbook: A guide to planning care* (7th ed.). St. Louis, MO: Mosby.

Acton, G. (2002). Health-promoting self care in family caregivers. *Western Journal of Nursing Research, 24*(1), 73–86.

Ahlstrom, B., Skarsater, I., & Danielson, E. (2007). Major depression in a family: What happens and how to manage—A case study. *Issues in Mental Health Nursing, 28,* 691–706.

American Psychiatric Association (APA). (2000). *Diagnostic and statistical manual-IV-TR* (4th ed., text revision). Washington, DC: American Psychiatric Association.

American Psychiatric Nurses Association (APNA). (2000). *Scope and standards of psychiatric-mental health nursing practice.* Washington, DC: American Nurses Publishing.

American Psychiatric Nurses Association (APNA). (2007). *Psychiatric-Mental health nursing: Scope and standards of practice.* Silver Spring, MD: American Nurses Association.

Barrett, A. (2005). Rationalizing risk: The use of non- prescribed substances in severe and enduring mental illness. *Journal of Substance Use, 10*(6), 341–346.

Barrowclough, C., Haddock, G., Fitzsimmons, M., Johnson, R. (2006). Treatment development for psychosis and co-occurring substance misuse: A descriptive review. *Journal of Mental Health, 15*(6), 619–632.

Barrowclough, C., Haddock, G., Tarrier, N., Lewis, S., Moring, J., O'Brien, R., et al. (2001). Randomized controlled trial of motivational interviewing, cognitive behavior therapy, and family intervention for patients with co-morbid schizophrenia and substance use disorders. *American Journal of Psychiatry, 158*(10), 1706–1713.

Bibou-Nakou, I., Dikaiou, M., & Bairactaris, C. (1997). Psychosocial dimensions of family burden among two groups of carers looking after psychiatric patients. *Social Psychiatry and Psychiatric Epidemiology, 32,* 104–108.

Biegel, D., Milligan, S., Putnam, P., & Song, L. (1994). Predictors of burden among lower socioeconomic status caregivers of persons with chronic mental illness. *Community Mental Health Journal, 30*(5), 473–494.

Bomar, P. (2004). Influences of social and health policy on family health. In P. Bomar (Ed.), *Promoting health in families: Applying family research and theory to nursing practice* (3rd ed., pp. 607–633). Philadelphia: Saunders.

Bukstein, O., Brent, D., & Kaminer, Y. (1989). Co-morbidity of substance abuse and other psychiatric disorders in adolescents. *American Journal of Psychiatry, 146*(9), 1131–1141.

Burt, R. (2001). Promises to keep, miles to go: Mental health law since 1972. In L. Frost & R. Bonnie (Eds.), *The evolution of mental health law* (pp. 11–30). Washington, DC: American Psychological Association.

Camilli, V., & Martin, J. (2005). Emergency department nurses' attitudes toward suspected intoxicated and psychiatric patients. *Topics in Emergency Medicine, 27*(4), 313–316.

Clark, R. (2001). Family support and substance use outcomes for persons with mental illness and substance use disorders. *Schizophrenia Bulletin, 27*(1), 93–101.

Corrigan, P., & Miller, F. (2004). Shame, blame, and contamination: A review of the impact of mental illness stigma on family members. *Journal of Mental Health, 13*(6), 537–548.

Cuijpers, P. (1999). The effects of family interventions on relatives' burden: A meta-analysis. *Journal of Mental Health, 8*(3), 275–285.

Cuijpers, P., & Stam, H. (2000). Burnout among relatives of psychiatric patients attending psychoeducational support groups. *Psychiatric Services, 51*(3), 375–379.

Czuchta, D., & McCay, E. (2001). Help-seeking for parents of individuals experiencing a first episode of schizophrenia. *Archives of Psychiatric Nursing, 15*(4), 159–170.

Deykin, E., Levy, J., & Wells, V. (1987). Adolescent depression, alcohol and drug abuse. *American Journal of Public Health, 77,* 178–182.

Dixon, L., Lucksted, A., Stewart, B. & Delahanty, J. (2000). Therapists' contacts with family members of persons with severe mental illness in a community treatment program. *Psychiatric Services, 51*(11), 1449–1451.

Dixon, L., Lyles, A., Scott, J., Lehman, A., Postrado, L., Goldman, H., et al. (1999). Services to families of adults with schizophrenia: From treatment recommendations to dissemination. *Psychiatric Services, 50*(2), 233–238.

Dixon, L., McFarlane, W., Lefley, H., Lucksted, A., Cohen, M., Falloon, I., et al. (2001). Evidence-based practices for services to families of people with psychiatric disabilities. *Psychiatric Services, 52*(7), 903–910.

Doornbos, M. (1997). The problems and coping methods of caregivers of young adults with mental illness. *Journal of Psychosocial Nursing and Mental Health Services, 35*(9), 22–26.

Doornbos, M. (2001). Professional support for family caregivers of people with serious and persistent mental illnesses. *Journal of Psychosocial Nursing, 39*(12), 39–47.

Doornbos, M. (2002). Family caregivers and the mental health care system: Reality and dreams. *Archives of Psychiatric Nursing, 16*(1), 39–46.

Esposito-Smythers, C. (2005). From the field. Adolescent substance abuse and co-morbid conditions: An integrated treatment model. *The Brown University Digest of Addiction Theory and Application, 24*(7), 8.

Ferriter, M., & Huband, N. (2003). Experiences of parents with a son or daughter suffering from schizophrenia. *Journal of Psychiatric and Mental Health Nursing, 10*, 552–560.

Finkelman, A. (2000, August). Psychiatric patients and families: Moving from a catastrophic event to long-term coping. *Home Care Provider*, 142–147.

Friedman, R., Best, K., Armstrong, M., Duchnowski, A., Evans, M. & Hernandez, M., et al. (2004). Child mental health policy. In B. Levin, J. Petrila, & K. Hennessy (Eds.), *Mental health services: A public health perspective* (2nd ed., pp. 129–153). Oxford: Oxford University Press.

Green-Hennessy, S., & Hennessy, K. (2004). The recovery movement: Consumers, families, and the mental health system. In B. Levin, J. Petrila, & K. Hennessy (Eds.), *Mental health services: A public health perspective* (2nd ed., pp. 88–105). Oxford: Oxford University Press.

Harvey, K., Burns, T., Fahy, T., Manley, C., & Tattan, T. (2001). Relatives of patients with severe psychotic illness: Factors that influence appraisal of caregiving and psychological distress. *Social Psychiatry and Psychiatric Epidemiology, 36*, 456–461.

Hawkings, C. (2005). Dual diagnosis: developing a practical toolkit. *Mental Health Review, 10*(2), 15–18.

Hoenig, J., & Hamilton, M. (1966). The schizophrenic patient in the community and his effect on the household. *International Journal of Social Psychiatry, 12*, 165–176.

Johnson, E. (2000). Differences among families coping with serious mental illness: A qualitative analysis. *American Journal of Orthopsychiatry, 70*(1), 126–134.

Jones, S., Roth, D., & Jones, P. (1995). Effect of demographic and behavioral variables on burden of caregivers of chronic mentally ill persons. *Psychiatric Services, 46*(2), 141–145.

Kaas, M., Lee, S., & Peitzman, C. (2003). Barriers to collaboration between mental health professionals and families in the care of persons with serious mental illness. *Issues in Mental Health Nursing, 24*, 741–756.

Kandel, D., Kessler, R., & Margulies, R. (1978). Antecedents of adolescent initiation into stages of drug use. In D. Kandel (ed.), *Longitudinal research on drug use: Empirical findings and methodological issues* (pp. 73–100). Washington, DC: Hemisphere Wiley.

Kessler, R., Chiu, W., Demler, O., & Walters, E. (2005, June). Prevalence, severity, and comorbidity of 12-month DSM-IV disorders in the national comorbidity survey replication. *Archives of General Psychiatry, 62*, 617–627.

Marsh, D., & Johnson, D. (1997). The family experience of mental illness: Implications for intervention. *Professional Psychology: Research and Practice, 28*(3), 229–237.

Mason, C., & Subedi, S. (2006). Helping parents with mental illnesses and their children: A call for family-focused mental health care. *Journal of Psychosocial Nursing, 44*(7), 36–41.

McFarlane, W., Lukens, E., Link, B., Dushay, R., Deakins, S., Newmark, M., et al. (1995). Multiple-family groups and psychoeducation in the treatment of schizophrenia. *Archives of General Psychiatry, 52*, 679–687.

Moore, B. (2005). Empirically supported family and peer interventions for dual disorders. *Research on Social Work Practice, 15*(4), 231–245.

Mueser, K., & Fox, L. (2002). A family intervention program for dual disorders. *Community Mental Health Journal, 38*(3), 253–271.

Murray, C., & Lopez, A. (1996). The global burden of disease: A comprehensive assessment of mortality and disability from diseases, injuries, and risk factors in 1990 and projected to 2020. *Global burden of disease and injury series* (Vol. 1). Boston: Harvard University, School of Public Health.

National Mental Health Association. (2008). *Youth with co-occurring mental health and substance abuse disorders in the juvenile justice system.* Retrieved February 15, 2008, from www1.nmha.org/children/justjuv/co_occurring_factsheet.cfm

New Freedom Commission on Mental Health. (2003). *Achieving the Promise: Transforming Mental Health Care in America.* Rockville, MD: U.S. Department of Health and Human Services. Retrieved February 20, 2008, from http://www.mentalhealthcommission.gov/reports/FinalReport/toc.html

Niv, N., Lopez, S., Glynn, S., & Mueser, K. (2007). The role of substance use in families' attributions and effective reactions to their relative with severe mental illness. *Journal of Nervous and Mental Disorders, 195*(4), 307–314.

O'Connell, K. (2006). Needs of families affected by mental illness: Through support, information and skill training, advocacy, and referral, nurses can help families put the pieces together. *Journal of Psychosocial Nursing and Mental Health Services, 44*(3), 40–51.

Ohaeri, J., & Fido, A. (2001). The opinion of caregivers on aspects of schizophrenia and major affective disorders in a Nigerian setting. *Social Psychiatry and Psychiatric Epidemiology, 36*(10), 493–499.

Olridge, M., & Hughes, I. (1992). Psychological well-being in families with a member suffering from schizophrenia. *British Journal of Psychiatry, 161*, 249–251.

Ostman, M., & Kjellin, L. (2002). Stigma by association. *British Journal of Psychiatry, 181*, 494–498.

Phelan, J., Bromet, E., & Link, B. (1998). Psychiatric illness and family stigma. *Schizophrenia Bulletin, 24*(1), 115–126.

Phillips, M., Pearson, V., Li, F., Xu, M., & Yang, L. (2002). Stigma and expressed emotion: A study of people with schizophrenia and their family members in China. *The British Journal of Psychiatry, 181*, 488–493.

Reinhard, S., & Horwitz, A. (1995). Caregiver burden: Differentiating the content and consequences of family caregiving. *Journal of Marriage and the Family, 57*(3), 741–750.

Saunders, J. (1999). Family functioning in families providing care for a family member with schizophrenia. *Issues in Mental Health Nursing, 20*(2), 95–113.

Saunders, J. (2003). Families living with severe mental illness: A literature review. *Issues in Mental Health Nursing, 24,* 175–198.

Saunders, J., & Byrne, M. (2002). A thematic analysis of families living with schizophrenia. *Archives of Psychiatric Nursing, 14*(5), 217–223.

Schock, A., & Gavazzi, S. (2005). Mental illness and families. In P. McKenry & S. Price (Eds.), *Families & change: Coping with stressful events and transitions* (3rd ed., pp. 179–204). Thousand Oaks, CA: Sage.

Shaffer, D., Fisher, P., Dulcan, M., Davies, M., Piacentini, J., Schwab-Stone, M., et al. (1996). The NIMH Diagnostic Interview Schedule for Children Version 2.3 (DISC-2.3): Description, acceptability, prevalence rates, and performance in the MECA study. Methods for the Epidemiology of Child and Adolescent Mental Disorders Study. *Journal of the American Academy of Child and Adolescent Psychiatry, 35,* 865–877.

Shibre, T., Negash, A., Kullgren, G., Kebede, D., Alem, A., Fekadu, A., et al. (2001). Perception of stigma among family members of individuals with schizophrenia and major affective disorders in rural Ethiopia. *Social Psychiatry and Psychiatric Epidemiology, 36*(6), 299–303.

Solomon, P. (1996). Moving from psychoeducation to family education for families of adults with serious mental illness. *Psychiatric Services, 47*(12), 1364–1370.

Solomon, P., & Draine, J. (1995). Adaptive coping among family members of persons with serious mental illness. *Psychiatric Services, 46*(11), 1156–1160.

Struening, E., Perlick, D., Link, B., Hellman, F., Herman, D., & Sirey, J. (2001). The extent to which caregivers believe most people devalue consumers and their families. *Psychiatric Services, 52*(12), 1633–1638.

Tiet, Q., & Mausbach, B. (2007). Treatments for patients with dual diagnosis: A review. *Alcoholism: Clinical and Experimental Research, 31*(4), 513–536.

Timko, C., Chen, S., Sempel, J., & Barnett, P. (2006). Dual diagnosis patients in community or hospital care: One year outcomes and health care utilization and costs. *Journal of Mental Health, 15*(2), 163–177.

Tsang, H., Tam, P., Chan, F., & Chang, W. (2003). Sources of burdens on families of individuals with mental illness. *International Journal of Rehabilitative Research, 26*(2), 123–130.

Urff, J. (2004). Public mental health systems: Structures, goals, and constraints. In B. Levin, J. Petrila, & K. Hennessy (Eds.), *Mental health services: A public health perspective* (2nd ed., pp. 72–87). Oxford: Oxford University Press.

U.S. Department of Health and Human Services. (1999). *Mental health: A report of the Surgeon General.* Rockville, MD: U.S. Department of Health and Human Services, Substance Abuse, and Mental Health Services Administration, Center for Mental Health Services, National Institutes of Health, National Institute of Mental Health.

Veltman, A., Cameron, J., & Stewart, D. (2002). The experience of providing care to relatives with chronic mental illness. *The Journal of Nervous and Mental Disease, 190*(2), 108–114.

Walsh, Y., & Frankland, A. (2005). Dual diagnosis 2005. *Mental Health Review, 10*(2), 7–14.

Warren, J., Stein, J., & Grella, C. (2007). Role of social support and self-efficacy in treatment outcomes among clients with co-occurring disorders. *Drug and Alcohol Dependence, 89*(2–3), 267–274.

Wintersteen, R., & Rasmussen, K. (1997). Fathers of persons with mental illness: A preliminary study of coping capacity and service needs. *Community Mental Health Journal, 3*(5), 401–413.

World Health Organization. (2001). *The world health report 2001. Mental health: New understanding, new hope.* Geneva: World Health Organization.

Young, A., & Magnabosco, J. (2004). Services for adults with mental illness. In B. Levin, J. Petrila, & K. Hennessy (Eds.), *Mental health services: A public health perspective* (2nd ed., pp. 177–208). Oxford: Oxford University Press.

CHAPTER WEB SITES

- *Al Anon:* www.al-anon.alateen.org
- *American Psychiatric Association:* www.psych.org
- *American Psychiatric Nurses Association:* www.apna.org
- *American Psychological Association:* www.apa.org
- *Family Caregiver Alliance:* www.caregiver.org
- *Federation of Families for Children's Mental Health:* www.ffcmh.org
- *International Society of Psychiatric-Mental Health Nurses:* www.ispn-psych.org
- *National Alliance on Mental Illness:* www.nami.org
- *National Institute of Mental Health:* www.nimh.nih.gov
- *National Mental Health Association:* www.nmha.org
- *World Health Organization:* www.who.int

CHAPTER 17

Families and Community/Public Health Nursing

Linda L. Eddy, PhD, RN, CPNP

Dawn Doutrich, PhD, RN, CNS

CRITICAL CONCEPTS

- ✦ Community is a mindset, not a place.
- ✦ Transitioning from individually focused nursing care to care of families and communities is a process.
- ✦ Community/public health nurses care for families in a variety of settings.
- ✦ Community/public health nurses view families as subunits of the community or as client in the context of the community.
- ✦ Community/public health nurses shift between holistic, family-focused, supportive care to more biomedically oriented tasks, depending on need and priority.
- ✦ Healthy families contribute to healthy communities.
- ✦ Community/public health family nursing is grounded in social justice and culturally safe, ethical practice.
- ✦ Rather than blaming families for their situations, nurses strive to empower them and activate upstream system and policy change.
- ✦ Nurses foster interconnectedness among families in the community.
- ✦ Family interventions in the community are targeted toward primary, secondary, and tertiary prevention.
- ✦ The nurse-family relationship is central in interventions at all three levels of prevention.
- ✦ Community/public health nursing is evidence based and policy driven.
- ✦ Viewing the family in an ecological context can help community/public health nurses derive plans and interventions, and evaluate them.

*H*ealthy communities are composed of healthy families. Community/public health nurses understand the effects that families have on individuals, and the relationship between the health of the family and the health of the community (U.S. Department of Health and Human Services [DHHS], 2001). As community/public health nurses move between focusing on the health of individuals toward a focus on population health, we must pay close attention to family health.

The health of communities is measured both formally and informally by the health of its members, especially its most vulnerable members (e.g., homeless families, refugees, victims of intimate partner violence, low-birth-weight infants, families in poverty, and families of individuals with chronic health problems). Many community/public health nurses are called to the community and public health through their commitment to social justice. The degree to which community/public health nurses can contribute positively to the well-being of families in their communities may influence nurses' decisions to choose community/public health nursing as a primary focus. This chapter integrates principles of family nursing with those of community/public health nursing and offers suggestions for working with families in the community.

COMMUNITY/PUBLIC HEALTH NURSING

Nurses desiring to practice community/public health nursing need to shift their perception of 'community' from a geographic place to a mindset, a focus on the interconnectedness of individuals and families wherever they are. Community/public health nurses care for families in a variety of settings, such as in their homes, schools, clinics, adult day care or retirement centers, correctional facilities, under bridges, or in temporary housing during transitional or recovery programs.

The World Health Organization (WHO) defines a community as a group of people who have something in common and who will act together in the common interest (WHO, 2000, p.6). This WHO definition helps to view community as connection with others wherever they may be, and reminds us that individuals and families are often parts of several communities: the place where they live, their workplace or school setting, as well as other social or religious groups. In a study of the transition from acute care to community nursing, Zurmehly (2007) finds that a successful role transition required conceptual and emotional adjustments for the nurse. Nurses described community nursing as a holistic, multidimensional practice that relied on the interaction between nurse and client (family).

Acute care typically expects nurses to focus care with a biomedical orientation, whereas in family nursing, as in other areas of community nursing practice, nurses shift the focus of their care back and forth between holistic and biomedical depending on context (Berg, Hedelin, & Sarvimaki, 2005). For example, Tuffrey, Finlay, and Lewis (2007) describe how the nurses working with families at the end of a child's life engaged in both biomedical tasks, such as direct care, documentation, and medication administration, and provided holistic, family-oriented care coordination and supportive interventions.

Doane and Varcoe (2007) state that, in the current health care context, nurses' attention to relationships and implementing nursing values and goals "are becoming increasingly challenging" because they are managing increased patient acuity, high nurse/patient ratios, and large workloads (p. 192). Nursing practice requires a "deep sensitivity to what is significant" (p. 194). They focus on relationships in context and term it *relational practice*. Relational practice is necessary for holistic, family-oriented care (Tuffrey et al., 2007).

SmithBattle, Diekemper, and Leander (2004a, 2004b) have conducted a study describing the process of becoming a public health nurse. In their qualitative, longitudinal, interpretive research, they note that beginning public health nurses learn a "situated understanding of practice," and develop the perceptual skills and responsiveness to clients that allowed them to grasp the "big picture." Participants in their study described giving up a "predetermined, nurse directed agenda" (2004b, p. 97). Nurses questioned "the prevailing ideology in which health and lifestyle choices are promoted in a vacuum, regardless of a person's or family's history, resources, and understandings of what are worthy ends and commitments" (2004b, p. 96). Notably, it was this change in understanding the context of families that contributed to the nurses being less likely to blame families for their circumstances.

Doutrich and Marvin (2004) paired community students with local public health nurses in their clinical rotation. The students reported that they learned to value relationship building with community clients as critical to practice. They described this relationship as the key to "finding the door," getting through it, and establishing a trust relationship with clients. Other important skills these students identified included becoming aware of their own biases, getting the client's story, and not blaming or judging the clients. This ability to remain nonjudgmental usually occurred when the students were truly engaged with families and understood the family's context.

THEORY AND CONCEPTS

According to the American Public Health Association (APHA, 2008), "Public health nurses integrate community involvement and knowledge about the entire population with personal, clinical understandings of the health and illness experiences of individuals and families within the population" (p. 1). This description contributes to understanding the interconnectedness of individual health with the health of families and communities. Specifically, it helps nurses to understand the critical nature of fostering care for families on the margin—that is,

those without human or financial resources that allow for true integration into communities.

Assessment, Assurance, and Policy Development

Community/public health nurses are engaged in the core public health functions of assessment, assurance, and policy development. *Assessment* is facilitated by the trust that public health nurses have earned from their clients, agencies, and private providers, trust that provides ready access to populations that are otherwise difficult to access and engage in health care. In addition, they have knowledge of current and emerging health issues through their daily contact with high-risk and vulnerable populations. This trust and knowledge provides the foundation for ways nurses work with communities (populations) and families and individuals in the community. Table 17-1 lists the different assessment approaches nurses can use in the community, based on the focus of the health care.

Assurance activities are the direct individual-focused services that public health nurses have provided over the past several years. Provision of these services was due, in large part, to programmatic funding and Medicaid reimbursement that focused on the individual rather than population-focused services. Measuring health department performance

TABLE 17-1		
Comparison of Assessment Approaches		
COMMUNITY	**FAMILY**	**INDIVIDUAL**
1. Analyze data on and needs of specific populations or geographic area.	1. Evaluate a specific family's strengths and areas of concern. This involves a comprehensive assessment of the physical, social, and mental health needs of the family.	1. Identify individuals within the family who are in need of services.
2. Identify and interact with key community leaders, both formally and informally.		2. Evaluate the functional capacity of the total individual through the use of specific assessment measures, including physical, social, and mental health screening tools.
3. Identify target populations that may be at risk. These populations may include families living in high-density low-income areas, preschool children, primary and secondary school children, and elderly adults.	2. Evaluate the family's living environment, looking specifically at support, relationships, and other factors that might have a significant impact on family health outcomes.	3. Develop a nursing diagnosis for the individual that describes a problem or potential problem, causative factors, and contributing factors.
4. Participate in data collection on a target population.	3. Assess the larger environment in which the family lives (their block or specific community) for safety, access, and other related issues.	4. Develop a Nursing Care Plan for the individual.
5. Conduct surveys or observe targeted populations, such as preschools, jails, and detention centers, to gain a better understanding of needs.		

is another example of assurance (Novick, 2003; Zahner & Vandermause, 2003). Although the current shift in emphasis is toward assessment and policy development, critical assurance activities remain for the public health nurse. The Centers for Disease Control and Prevention and Robert Wood Johnson Foundation recently funded the project "Exploring Accreditation" (U.S. DHHS Centers for Disease Control, 2005). This program has helped fuel a movement toward accountability and evaluation as it pushed for voluntary accreditation within state and local boards of health (Bender, Benjamin, Fallon, Jarris, & Libbey, 2007). Assurance activities at the community, family, and individual levels are outlined in Table 17-2.

Policy development at the family level relies on data collected from individuals, families, and communities. The information obtained in the assessment will be used to help families make decisions at the community level. Table 17-3 demonstrates how activities influence policy development.

Theories and Models

FAMILY CAREGIVING MODEL FOR PUBLIC HEALTH NURSING

The Core Public Health Functions Model (Novick, 2003) provides guidance in the provision of nursing care for families (Fig. 17-1). This model addresses both views of the family as the client within the community and the family as a part of the community client. At any level or in any setting, the role of the community/public health nurse is targeted toward

TABLE 17-2

Assurance Activities in Community, Family, and Individual Care

COMMUNITY	FAMILY	INDIVIDUAL
1. Provide service to target populations such as child care centers, preschools, worksites, minority communities, jails, juvenile detention facilities, and homeless shelters. Interventions may include health screening, education, health promotion, and injury prevention programs.	1. Provide services to a cluster of families within a geographic setting. Services may be provided in a variety of settings including homes, child care centers, preschools, and schools. Services may include physical assessment, health education and counseling, and health and developmental screening.	1. Provide nursing services based on standards of nursing practice to individuals across the age continuum. These services may encompass a variety of programs including, specifically, First Steps and Children With Special Health Care Needs, and more generally, child abuse prevention, immunizations, well child care, and HIV/AIDS programs.
2. Improve quality assurance activities with various health care providers in the community. Examples include education on new immunization policies, educational programs for communicable disease control, assistance in developing effective approaches, and support techniques for high-risk populations.	2. Provide care in a nursing clinic to a specific group of families in a geographic location.	2. Assess and support the individual's progress toward meeting outcome goals.
3. Maintain safe levels of communicable disease surveillance and outbreak control.		3. Consult with other health care providers and team members regarding the individual's plan of care.
4. Participate in research or demonstration projects.		4. Prioritize individual's needs on an ongoing basis.
5. Provide expert public health consultation in the community.		5. Participate on quality-assurance teams to measure the quality of care provided.
6. Assure that standards of care are met within the community.		

TABLE 17-3

Activities that Influence Policy Development

COMMUNITY	FAMILY	INDIVIDUAL
1. Provide leadership in convening and facilitating community groups to evaluate health concerns and develop a plan to address the concerns.	1. Recommend new or increased services to families based on identified needs.	1. Recommend or assist in the development of standards for individual client care.
2. Recommend specific training and programs to meet identified health needs.	2. Recommend programs to meet specific families' needs within a geographic area.	2. Recommend or adopt risk classification systems to assist with prioritizing individual client care.
3. Raise awareness of key policymakers about health regulations, budget decisions, and other factors that may negatively affect the health of communities.	3. Facilitate networking with families with similar needs or issues. Guide policymakers on specific issues that affect clusters of families.	3. Participate in establishing criteria for opening, closing, or referring individual cases.
4. Recommend programs to target populations such as child care centers, retirement centers, jails, juvenile detention facilities, homeless shelters, worksites, and minority communities.	4. Request additional data and analyze information to identify trends in a group or cluster of families.	4. Participate in the development of job descriptions to establish roles for various team members who will provide service to individuals.
5. Act as an advocate for the community and individuals who are not willing or able to speak to policymakers about issues and programs of concern.	5. Identify key families in a community who may either oppose or support specific policies or programs, and develop appropriate and effective intervention strategies to use with these families.	
6. Work with business and industry to develop employee health programs.		

promotion and maintenance of health, and prevention of illness, disability, or injury. Community/public health nurses must remain current on social and political policies as they assist members of the community to voice their needs and concerns (APHA, 2008).

A number of family theories inform the practice of community/public health nurses. One of these models is the Family Caregiving Model for Public Health Nursing (Fig. 17-2; Zerwekh, 1991). This model continues to be a useful framework for providing care to families in the community (Ackerman, 1994; Collins & Reinke, 1997). Expert community health nurses described the care they provided to their maternal-child clients. From these descriptions, researchers identified 16 competencies that became the foundation of this model. The focus of this model is the family and developing the ability of members to take charge of their lives and make their own choices. Nurses' actions are aimed at

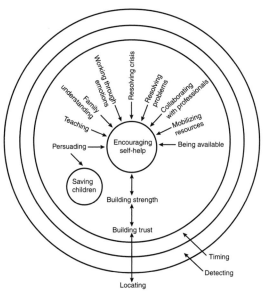

FIGURE 17-1 Core Public Health Function Model.
Source: Novick, L. F. (2003). Core public health functions: 15 year update. *Public Health Management Practice, 9*(1), 5.

encouraging family self-help through believing in the family's ability to make choices and aiding them to believe in themselves. Appropriate nursing actions include listening to the family's needs, expanding the family's vision of choices, and feeding back reality so that the family sees patterns in their lives and the consequences of their decisions.

The first three competencies establish the foundation for family caregiving: (1) locating the family, (2) building trust, and (3) building strength. After laying this foundation, community nurses use eight encouraging self-help competencies when working with families:

- Being available
- Mobilizing resources
- Collaborating with other professionals
- Resolving problems
- Working through emotions
- Fostering family understanding
- Teaching
- Persuading

Three of these competencies help to foster community: being available, mobilizing resources, and collaborating with other professionals. Thus, the model acknowledges that the community is the context for family care.

If family self-help cannot be achieved and the nurse finds that a family member is still at risk, the nurse can use two additional forceful competencies: (1) persuading, which includes the use of reasoning, confronting, and threatening action (e.g., calling child protective services); and (2) saving the children (e.g., arranging for out of home placement). In these at-risk situations, the nurse's responsibility for children (or individuals at risk) becomes primary.

Two other competencies, called *encompassing competencies,* are used simultaneously with the other competencies and are ongoing during the care of the family. The first of these, timing, relates to the speed of introducing an intervention and has three dimensions: (1) identifying the right time to initiate the action; (2) persisting in implementing the intervention; and (3) "futuring," whereby the nurse considers the present action based on a view of the future (e.g., the child's development). The second encompassing competency, detecting, uses comprehensive assessment to identify potential and actual health problems.

BIOECOLOGICAL THEORY

Another theory that fits well with the practice of family nursing in the community is Urie Bronfenbrenner's bioecological theory (e.g., Bronfenbrenner, 2004). See

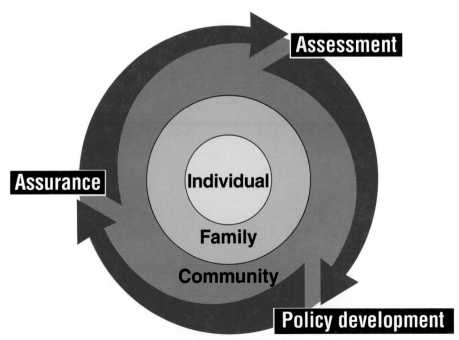

FIGURE 17-2 Zerwekh Family Caregiving Model.
Source: Zerwekh, J. V. (1991). A family caregiving model for public health nursing. *Nursing Outlook,* 39(5), 213–217.

Chapter 3 for foundational concepts of bioecological theory. One level of interaction between the family and outside influences is the microsystem, which includes the settings in which daily life is experienced: interactions with other family members, peers, schools, churches, neighborhoods, and other settings with which families have direct interaction. Nurses help families mediate interaction between these relationships. For example, the family of a child newly diagnosed with type I diabetes must learn to work with the school environment. The community/public health nurse can strengthen this family-school mesosystem by designing interventions that educate the child's peers and teachers. The bioecological theory fits well with the community/public health nurse's obligation to help families in the community. In the bioecological framework, what happens outside of family units, including in the community, is as important as what happens within family units.

CONCEPTS IN COMMUNITY/ PUBLIC HEALTH NURSING

This section discusses the way community and public health nurses work with families.

Definition and Role of "Family"

A broad definition of the *family* guides community/ public health nurses toward inclusiveness in working with and understanding complex family systems. McDaniel, Cambell, Hepworth, and Lorenz (2005) define family as "as any group of people related either biologically, emotionally, or legally that an individual defines as significant for his or her well-being" (p. 2). It is important that nurses ask families whom they consider family.

Nursing models for families reflect two prevalent schools of thought in community/public health nursing. One view sees the family as the unit of care and the community as context. The other view is to focus on the community as client and view the family as context. According to Shuster and Goeppinger (2004), actualizing community as client occurs when the nursing focus is on the collective good of the population. What is common among these views is that a reciprocal relationship exists between healthy families and healthy communities. What nurses do for families will affect all of their communities.

Although the notion of community as client is understood by nurses at a conceptual level, it is less clear what kind of effect this understanding has on everyday practice. St. John (1998), in a qualitative study examining practicing nurses' definitions of community, found that, although instances existed where community was described as client or entity, these examples were not universal, and most nurses described community in terms of geography and provision of resources.

Kaiser, Hays, Cho, and Agrawal (2002) have described the complexity of nursing care based on "family as client" in community/public health nursing. Two key issues that contribute to this complexity are: (1) labeling family health problems, and (2) identifying the level of need of the family as a whole. Developing a plan of care for families based solely on medical problems addresses only one area of family need. When working with families, nurses need to consider environmental, psychological, and behavioral health issues, as well as those of a more physiologic nature. In addition, Kaiser and colleagues suggest that providing family-focused nursing care in the community requires a very different set of skills from those required in acute care nursing.

For some clients, the definition of self is wrapped up in the family (Doutrich, Wros, Valdez, & Ruiz, 2005). For example, *familismo* has been reported as a typical feature of Hispanic families (Vega, 1990). In a classic work, Sabogal, Marín, Otero-Sabogal, Marín, and Pérez-Stable (1987) find that *familismo* included three specific types of value orientations: (1) obligations to provide support; (2) perceived high levels of help and support from family; and importantly, (3) the perception of relatives as behavioral and attitudinal referents, meaning that one's family determines how one is perceived and perceives the world. With some Latino clients, relational practice will include attention to these values and the understanding that family is the unit of care rather than the individual. For the community/ public health family nurse, this definition of self that is inclusive of family will influence the provision of culturally congruent care. In addition, recently immigrated Japanese clients (Wros, Doutrich, & Izumi, 2004) or clients from the former Soviet Union may expect the family nurse to consult the non-ill adult family member(s) rather than the ill member, particularly if the prognosis is poor. With U.S. Health Insurance Portability and Accountability Act laws and legal constraints, this expectation could result in ethical concerns for the relationally astute nurse.

The role of the family with respect to individual family members is situational. What this means is that with one family the nurse may focus on wellness care on one family member, knowing that the family will have some influence on the health of the person (family as context), and for another situation the nurse will focus wellness care on the family as a whole (family as client). See Chapter 1 for different approaches to practicing family nursing. For example, a nurse caring for a child with Down syndrome who has an ear infection might consider family as context for overcoming the ear infection in the child during one visit. In this situation, educating caregivers about proper medication administration would be important to the prevention of secondary complications. During another encounter, however, the nurse may focus on supporting the whole family as the parents are faced with the reality that their daughter will not start kindergarten with her peers.

Cultural Competence

Many families that community/public health nurses care for may not speak English well. For providers without language competencies, this creates challenges to developing good communication, a prerequisite to trust. The Institute of Medicine (IOM) report, "Unequal Treatment: Confronting Racial and Ethnic Disparities in Healthcare" (Smedley, Stith, & Nelson, 2003), found that ethnic and racial minority populations "tend to receive a lower quality of health care" than majority populations even when access and income were controlled (p. 1). The reasons for this finding are complex but include bias, time pressures, and lack of language and cultural understanding (Smedley et al., 2003). Increasing the numbers of bilingual, bicultural, under-represented providers is identified as one of the IOM solutions aimed at improving health disparities.

In 2001, the Office of Minority Health (OMH) published 14 standards for Culturally and Linguistically Appropriate Services (CLAS). Standards four through seven address language access services, which are required if organizations want to receive federal funds (Cassey, 2008). Standard 4 reads: "Health care organizations must offer and provide language assistance services, including bilingual staff and interpreter services, at no cost to each patient/consumer with limited English proficiency at all points of contact, in a timely manner during all hours of operation" (OMH, U.S. DHHS, 2001, p. 10). This means that family nurses in the community must plan ahead for visits with non-English-speaking families. It is the professional responsibility of nurses to ensure that families understand what is going on in the meeting, either through an interpreter or other means. For details about selecting the appropriate interpreter for working with families, reference Chapter 4.

The Joint Commission began to study issues related to the CLAS standards in 2004, and in 2007 developed the document "Office of Minority Health National Culturally and Linguistically Appropriate Services Standards Crosswalked to Joint Commission 2007 Standards" (Cassey, 2008; Joint Commission: Division of Standards and Survey Methods, 2007). This document suggests putting into operation the CLAS standards in a variety of settings (Cassey, 2008) to ensure that patients receive "effective, understandable, and respectful care" (Cassey, 2008, p. 133) congruent with their health beliefs, practices, and preferred language (OMH, U.S. DHHS, 2001).

Internet resources provide the public/community health family nurses with multiple supportive options for increasing their understanding of minority families. The OMH offers language and cultural sites that are updated often and are freely accessible; two examples are "Culturally Competent Nursing Care: A Cornerstone of Caring" (OMH, U.S. DHHS, 2007a) and "Cultural Competency CME Portal" (OMH, U.S. DHHS, 2007b). To strengthen their relational practice, nurses should understand that their cultural competence begins by reflecting on their own prejudices, and having a deep awareness of how their own culture has informed their worldview, including those biases.

Refugee families may comprise a subset of those with limited or no English abilities that community/public health family nurses will serve. Although it is important to understand the background and perspective of all families, refugee families may have added to this context surviving war, disaster, and devastating trauma such as torture, rape, and/or watching family members or others die. Often, these families are enduring post-traumatic stress disorder, depression, or both, which may intensify the life challenges they face. In understanding the family's context, nurses need to be aware of such circumstances.

Nurse-Client Relationship in the Community

Community/public health nurses caring for families in the community rely on the nurse-client relationship as the foundation of their care for at-risk families (McNaughton, 2000, 2005). In fact, the early phase of home visiting programs is based on the development of trust through helping clients identify problems, engaging in mutual problem solving, making decisions about necessary health services, and adopting health-promoting behaviors. Zerwekh (1992) claims that this trust-building phase is crucial to the success of longer term intervention programs because the efficacy of home visiting programs seems to be greater in longer-term, relationship-based home visiting programs than in shorter-term interventions (Koniak-Griffin et al., 2003; McNaughton, 2004; Zotti & Zahner, 1995).

The nurse-client relationship makes the crucial difference in the success of intervention programs. McNaughton (2005) tested Peplau's Theory of Interpersonal Relations in Nursing as the framework for successful home visits. Using this theoretical framework, she underscored the development of successful nurse-client relationships between public health nurses and pregnant women at risk. The results of this study suggested that the greater number of interactions over time contributes to more effective home visiting programs.

Family Empowerment in the Community

Helping families to become empowered toward living in a healthier way requires development of a partnership between nurse and family. Empowerment can be facilitated by nurses but not "given," and it is a process as well as an outcome. Empowering families can be difficult because of the complex and changing nature of the family in its unique environment. Family interventions must be tied to problems as they are voiced by the family (Kaiser et al., 2002). Nurses must have the skills to build trusting, nonjudgmental relationships that empower families to tell their stories so they can jointly uncover the family's needs. Although hierarchical relationships still characterize many provider-client relationships in health care, a significant number of nurses incorporate family empowerment into their community/public health practice. In shared care planning, nurses begin with the client's knowledge of his or her situation first because this approach recognizes and validates that clients have extensive knowledge about their own health (Anderson, Capuzzi, & Hatton, 2001). Falk-Rafael (2001) has investigated the relationship between and among the meaning, practice, and outcomes of empowerment. This study revealed that active participation enabled individuals to increase control over their own health (see Box 17-1 for a Research Brief).

Community/public health nurses must have skills that facilitate empowering families to make decisions about their health (Aston, Meagher-Stewart, Vukic, Sheppard-Lemoine, & Chircop, 2006). For example, nurses can adopt the role of mediator or

---

BOX 17-1

RESEARCH BRIEF: Eddy, L. L., & Engel, J. M. (2008). The Impact of Child Disability Type on the Family. *Rehabilitation Nursing*, **33(3), 98–103.**

Quality of life in children with a variety of physical and developmental challenges, and the families of those children is a growing area of research emphasis for community/public health nurses caring for families. In a study of the impact of type of physical disability on family processes and outcomes, Eddy and Engel (2008) have found that parents of children with conditions that were less stable medically, such as neuromuscular disease, spina bifida, or cerebral palsy, experienced more worry and concern than did parents of children with more stable conditions, such as congenital limb deficiency or amputation. Families whose children had those "stable" conditions such as amputation and congenital limb deficiency, though, were more likely to be limited in the type of activities they participated in or to have family activities interrupted.

Because findings varied by child diagnosis on five of the eight variables measured, it seems clear that plans for family advocacy and care need to be somewhat individualized based on diagnosis. In particular, families

BOX 17-1

RESEARCH BRIEF: Eddy, L. L., & Engel, J. M. (2008). The Impact of Child Disability Type on the Family. *Rehabilitation Nursing,* 33(3), 98–103.—cont'd

of children with conditions such as muscular dystrophy that may become worse over time indicated concern about worsening health of their child. These families need a care team that would be able to recognize when care needed to intensify. For this reason, child health care team members need to work together to assure that a comprehensive pediatric health care "home" is available to all families with youths with special needs.

In keeping with the concept of community as mindset rather than geographic place, the authors propose a team-based, family-driven model that could respond to individualized needs identified by this and other studies because of its flexibility in composition and intensity of services. The family HOMETEAM would include usual aspects of care coordination such as assessment, planning, implementation, evaluation, monitoring, support, education, and advocacy (Lindeke, Leonard, Presler, & Garwick, 2002), but would differ in that the single point of contact would be the HOMETEAM rather than a single health care professional. The team, a small group of professionals headed by the family and in regular communication, could interact flexibly to meet ongoing and changing needs. Local families and health care team members interested in this concept suggested weekly phone or in-person meetings, with additional communication as needed. Team composition would be dependent on family needs and may change over time.

coach rather than director or decision maker, and focus on starting where families are and help them problem-solve by building on their strengths. Rather than thinking of clients and families as "powerless" or the nurse as having "power over" them, Falk-Rafael (2001) conceptualizes power as coming from within the person and depending on the situation.

Community family nurses must learn to speak out and are obligated to be actively involved in issues and policies that affect their family clients. Bekemeier and Butterfield (2005) point out that "social justice is 1 of the 5 core values of baccalaureate nursing education" (p. 154), and that nurses have a responsibility to social action and collaboration, including with the "people and populations most impacted by the negative social conditions" (p. 154). They call to question the lack of population focus in the Code of Ethics for Nurses. Family community health nurses, in concert with their clients, are most intimate with the issues experienced by families in the community. Therefore, they must give voice to the policy and environmental factors that affect U.S. families.

FAMILY NURSING ROLES IN THE COMMUNITY

This section examines common family nursing roles in the community, including health appraisal, education, and ensuring access to care.

Health Appraisal Through Nurse Home Visiting Programs

When possible, community/public health nurses working with families make home visits to assess family health status, needs, and their environment to develop specific interventions and identify available resources. Assessment of the physical environment of the home includes examination of safety hazards, such as the condition of paint, age of housing, availability of smoke detectors and fire extinguishers, any dangerous playground equipment, and the adequacy of running water and indoor plumbing. In addition, they inventory items to meet basic needs, such as food, heating, cooking facilities, and refrigeration, and objects that promote social, emotional, and physical development, such as toys and books. Community health nurses assess clients for health literacy so they can tailor interventions and promote self-advocacy. The neighborhood should be assessed for level of violence, safety hazards, availability of transportation, access to needed goods and services, access to recreational facilities, and the presence of environmental pollutants (Clark, 1998). For example, do the elevators in single-room occupancy hotels work? Are there underpasses that residents need to use? Are they safe? Do they smell of urine or feces? Community health nurses also appraise the family's psychological, social, and economic environment. In the home, nurses directly assess family communication patterns, role relationships, family dynamics, emotional strengths, coping strategies, and childrearing and discipline practices. The effects of the social environment (e.g., religious practices, culture, social class, economic status, and social support system) on health can and should be assessed during a home visit.

It is important for community/public health nurses to evaluate their work with families. Community/public health nurses must base their practice on current evidence-based practices. A review of the literature on the efficacy of nurse home visiting programs suggests that regardless of the specific intervention, the fact that interventions were implemented is crucial to long-term health outcomes for families.

The work of David Olds and his colleagues (Olds, 2002; Olds, Kitzman, Cole, & Robinson, 1997) shows the effectiveness of family-centered care and the effectiveness of community/public health nursing home visitation. Nurses visited low-income, unmarried mothers and their children. The families with home visitation had significantly improved health outcomes. The home visitation was found to contribute to the reduced number of the mothers' subsequent pregnancies, use of welfare, child abuse and neglect, and criminal behaviors for up to 15 years after the first child's birth. The home visit nursing program was found to reduce serious antisocial behavior and substance use as the high-risk children in the study entered adolescence (Olds et al., 1998). As adolescents, they ran away less often, were arrested and convicted less frequently, were less promiscuous, and smoked and drank alcohol less than comparable adolescents who did not receive home visits. The results of this work illustrate how community/public health nurse home visits in the community are beneficial for high-risk families.

More recently, Olds and colleagues (2004) have reported on the outcomes of a longitudinal study of prenatal and infancy home visits by nurses with a primarily African American, urban sample. Their results indicate that, compared with the control group, women involved in the nurse home visiting program had fewer subsequent pregnancies and births, longer relationships with partners, and less use of welfare. In addition, children of families in the intervention (home visit) group were more likely to be involved in formal out-of-home care between ages 2 and 4 ½ years, and demonstrated higher intellectual functioning and fewer behavioral problems than did control children.

Empirical evidence for the efficacy of home visit programs shows that further research is necessary, however. A recent search of the Cochrane Database of Systematic Reviews revealed two reviews specific to nursing. Hodnett & Fredericks (2003) found that, although the evidence did not support the effectiveness of programs of nurse home visits during pregnancy in reducing the number of babies born too early or with low birth weight, the interventions probably resulted in reduced maternal anxiety and lower cesarean birth rates. Doggett, Burrett, and Osborn (2005) developed programs for postpartum women with drug and alcohol issues. They found evidence that home visits after the birth increased the engagement of these women in drug treatment services, but insufficient data were reported to confirm whether this improved the health of the baby or the mother. Further research is needed, with visits starting during pregnancy. It is important to note that both reviews also involved interventions by a variety of health care professionals, as well as trained lay health workers. In both of theses situations, therefore, it is difficult to determine the individual effect of nursing interventions on families.

In contrast, McNaughton (2004) reviewed 13 home visiting interventions by registered nurses with maternal-child clients during 1980 to 2000 and found that about half of the interventions reported were effective in achieving the desired outcomes. This author calls for more research tying theory to interventions and for specifying more accurately the intervention and its dosage.

Nurse home visit programs have demonstrated efficacy in preventing child abuse and neglect (e.g., Olds et al., 1997; Olds, Henderson, Kitzman, & Cole, 2005), a finding that has been successfully replicated in many settings internationally. Unfortunately, attempts to use these models to prevent recidivism in families with a history of abusing their children have not shown to be efficacious (MacMillan, Thomas, Jamieson, & Walsh, 2005). MacMillan and colleagues postulate that interventions for the group of families already in the child protection system are complicated, and although a more intensive program of longer duration might have resulted in better outcomes, no data substantiate this, and the cost might be prohibitive. Their take-home message is that prevention was key to improved health outcomes.

Although most studies of nurse home visiting programs focus on maternal-child health, a few studies in other populations have been reported. Most studies of home visiting programs for community-dwelling older adults reported satisfaction but are less rigorous with respect to clinical outcomes than are maternal-child studies. Masters (2005) reports on an innovative student nurse home visiting program with older adults and finds that the adults reported satisfaction with the educational interventions by the students but were most satisfied by having someone to talk with.

Health Appraisal and Education in Community Settings Outside of the Home

The role of the nurse in working with families in settings other than their homes are explored in this section.

COMMUNITY NURSING CENTERS

One model of family nursing in the community occurs within community nursing centers. These unique centers, found in rural and urban communities, offer the public access to a wide array of nursing services in a single setting. These programs typically provide services that are not available elsewhere and are likely to focus on the needs of underserved populations (Glick, 1999). Family-focused services that might be provided at community nursing centers include health-promotion and disease-prevention interventions, such as health screening, education, and well-child care. In addition, such centers may offer secondary and tertiary prevention services, such as management of acute and chronic health conditions, and mental health counseling.

The model for these centers is usually multidisciplinary and strives to provide affordable, accessible, acceptable care that serves to empower individuals to meet their own health care goals. The focus on social justice in many of these centers is realized by attempts to reach out to marginalized populations and to provide comprehensive, quality, nonjudgmental health care. In keeping with the community-as-mindset concept, community nursing centers may be either physical places or they may be embedded in more traditional health care settings. Some community nursing centers provide

educational experiences for nursing students and students from other disciplines, making these centers a place where nursing practice, theory, and research can blend in a model that serves those who need health care the most.

PUBLIC HEALTH DEPARTMENTS

Probably the most widely known and accepted model for center-based services for families is that used by county and state departments of health services. Public health clinics serve the needs of clients across the life span in both center- and home-based models. These clinics include services to vulnerable groups, such as pregnant and childbearing families (women, infants, and children programs [WIC]), children with special health care needs, individuals at risk for or diagnosed with infectious diseases, and those with chronic conditions. Lahr, Rosenberg, and Lapidus (2005) document an example of effective public health nursing practice with families. These investigators found that, compared with parents receiving newborn care and education from private clinics, those receiving care and education in public health departments were less likely to choose prone sleeping positions for their infant, a major public health initiative to reduce sudden infant death syndrome.

Public health departments care for high-risk clients and are in a unique position to address issues of intimate partner violence. Shattuck (2002) reports positive outcomes from an intervention program targeted toward better preparing family planning nurses who work in a public health department to recognize domestic violence. The intervention, which consisted of a formal curriculum offered to nursing staff, increased intimate partner violence screening from 0% before the program to 16% in a 4-week period, and resulted in approximately 12% of women who screened positive for violence. With respect to reducing intimate partner violence, a goal for *Healthy People 2010* (U.S. DHHS, 2000), a role clearly exists for family-focused community nurses to make a difference.

Although many public health department services are aimed at childbearing and childrearing families, there are programs for older adults with chronic illness. An example is a public health nursing program aimed at educating older adults about their high blood cholesterol levels, implementing better dietary practices, and reducing cholesterol levels. This nursing intervention consisted of three individual diet counseling sessions given by public health nurses. The nurses used a structured dietary intervention (Food for Heart Program), referred elders to a nutritionist if they did not reach lipid goals at 3-month follow-up, made reinforcement phone calls, and sent newsletters. Although blood cholesterol reduction was similar between the groups who received the special interventions and those who received a minimal intervention, the special intervention group had significantly lower dietary risk assessment scores (Ammerman, Keyserling, Atwood, Hosking, Zayed, & Krasny, 2003).

Chronic pain management in older adults living in the community is a pervasive public health problem that can be amenable to public health nursing interventions aimed at individuals and families. Dewar (2006) has reviewed the literature about chronic pain management by nurses in the community. Dewar found that most studies focused on pain assessment tools, and that less focus was on how older adults managed pain and what community resources were available to help these families with pain-management issues. In both of the earlier community health nursing programs, the nurse-client relationship was an integral component to the success of these programs.

The relationship between community nurses and families of older adults was also found to be important in a study of community nurses working with older clients in Sweden (Weman & Fagerberg, 2006). Nurses in this qualitative study claimed that the family was important in the successful care of their older family members. The nurses reported feeling conflicted at times in relationship with the families, however, especially when family members did not take the side of the older adult or paid no attention to them at all. Registered nurses often felt pressure when they needed to take action that family members opposed and spent considerable effort on forging cooperative partnerships with family. Nurses in this study noted the importance of clinical competence by community nurses.

Caring for older families in the community requires nurses to be alert for signs of elder abuse. Potter (2004) notes that community nurses were often the only professionals invited into peoples' homes, so they must be alert to the many forms abuse takes: physical, psychological, financial,

sexual, and verbal. Nurses also must be aware of omission of needed support and attention as a type of abuse. Nurses need to know how to report elder abuse in their communities and be willing to take quick action to prevent further abuse.

Education in the Home and in Community Settings Outside the Home

Education is essential to the promotion of health and the prevention of disease in families. Using information gained through family health appraisals, community health nurses reinforce health-promoting behaviors, and provide health information and teaching in identified at-risk areas. The four determinants of health include: (1) environment (including socioeconomic status), (2) social/lifestyle, (3) biology, and (4) health care (University of Southern Mississippi School of Nursing, 2003). Community health nurses use a variety of strategies to modify risky lifestyles identified in the health appraisal. Teaching and health information can be used to discuss immunizations, nutrition, rest, exercise, use of seat belts, and abuse of harmful substances, such as alcohol and drugs. Community health nurses may refer families to programs and resources that assist in their lifestyle modifications (e.g., smoking cessation classes, exercise programs).

One example of this is the "Biggest Loser" intervention program that was designed to assist clients in a West Virginia county to lose weight. This intervention was developed in response to high obesity rates and included a program based loosely on the television show of the same name. Specific social supports, weigh-ins, exercise, and dietary help were provided for the participants, though in the public health intervention, no one was "voted off the show."

While designing/referring clients to lifestyle modification programs, it is important for nurses to keep in mind policy- and community-level changes that might affect the participants or family lifestyle changes. For instance, in the case of obesity, King County in Washington state and New York City instituted regulation so that fast-food outlets with 10 to 15 franchises are required to provide caloric information to help consumers make informed choices. Moreover, some city and county planners have been involving public health community nurses in the planning of environments (including wetlands, walkable areas, and access to gardens and fresh food) as part of the zoning and development process (Dannenberg et al., 2003).

Health teaching based on appraisal of the physical environment might also include information on child safety and prevention of falls. Other teaching might focus on psychological or social environmental problems, such as family communications or dealing with peer pressure. In some situations, community health nurses promote a healthy environment by providing information to community members outside the family. For example, community health nurses working in schools might need to inform officials about playground hazards or poor food-handling practices.

Although most often community health nurses will understand issues of significance to "their" families, sometimes they may need to research their clients' health priorities. In this instance, community-based participatory research (CBPR) can be used to identify issues of significance (Minkler & Wallenstein, 2003). Partnerships between academia and local public health providers can be transformational for both institutions (Doutrich & Marvin, 2004; Doutrich & Storey, 2006; Gebbie, Rosenstock, & Hernandez, 2003; Minkler, Frantz, & Wechsler, 2006). For example, Minkler, Frantz, and Wechsler (2006) describe a CBPR program that took place in San Francisco's Tenderloin District single-room occupancy hotels, one of America's large "gray ghettos." Through meetings and focus groups, community students and faculty members found that the elderly occupants were most concerned about crime and victimization, and thus the "crime project" was born. With support from community health students (and faculty), residents became politically active, meeting with the police chief and mayor, and were eventually successful in lobbying for added police to walk the Tenderloin beat. At the same time, residents developed connections and a lasting interhotel coalition that became an empowered force for change within the community.

Access to Resources

A major health-promotion strategy is to ensure access to health promotion and prevention services, including immunizations, family planning, prenatal care, well-child care, nutrition, exercise classes, and dental hygiene. These services may be provided directly by community health nurses in the home or in clinics, schools, or work settings. In some cases, community health nurses facilitate access to these services through referrals, case management, discharge planning, advocacy, coordination, and collaboration.

Nevertheless, access to resources must be considered within a context where, according to the 2006 U.S. census report, 47 million Americans do not have health insurance (Anonymous, 2007). *The Nation's Health* recently published a "Families USA" report that suggests that this number most likely grossly underestimates the U.S. uninsured because the census counted only those without health insurance for the full calendar year. When all Americans younger than 65 years who were without health insurance at some point during 2006 to 2007 were counted, the number burgeoned to 90 million, or 1 in 3 people without health insurance (Bailey, 2007).

Not only are many U.S. families at risk for little access to health care, but many lack stable housing or adequate food. The Homeless Research Institute of the National Alliance to End Homelessness released a report revealing that, in 2005, one of the fastest growing segments of the homeless population was homeless families with children, and that these families accounted for 41% of the total counted homeless population (Cunningham & Henry, 2007). Despite years of a strong economy, in 2004, Siefert, Heflin, Corcoran, and Williams (2004) estimated that food insecurity was a problem in 31 million U.S. households, meaning that in some time during the year, they were unable to acquire or were uncertain of having enough food to meet their basic needs because of inadequate household resources. It is critical to understand that these families were disproportionately made up of women and people of color. For example, low-middle-income, single, female heads of households with children were 5.5 times more likely than other families to be without adequate food (Siefert et al., 2004). Significantly, many of the homeless and hungry were working families.

Though reasons for these dismal statistics are many and complex, several national policies have not adequately addressed the issues and concerns. Welfare caseloads declined significantly since the federal Personal Responsibility and Work Opportunity Reconciliation Act of 1996 (PRWORA) was enacted. The title of the law leaves no question about how the Clinton White House and Congress framed ideas about cause and effects of poverty (Shipler, 2004). This act ended the federal guarantee of income support to low-income families with children and established a 5-year lifetime limit on benefits (Siefert et al., 2004). Recipients of Temporary Assistance for Needy Families (TANF) have to meet work requirements to receive aid. The assumption behind this act is that people will choose welfare over work unless forced into the workforce (Anderson, Halter, & Gryzlak, 2004).

The reform has been credited by some former welfare recipients as inducing them to move away from dependence into active participation in the workplace (Shipler, 2004). Certainly since reform, welfare caseloads have declined. But a study of returnees to welfare revealed that reasons for their return included low wages and unstable or seasonal positions. Difficulty obtaining health care and child care while working also appeared to be an obstacle (Anderson et al., 2004). And although fewer families are receiving welfare (typically a single mother with two children), the numbers and rates of homeless and hungry families without access to health care have increased. Indeed, these increases came *before* the housing crisis and economic downturn of 2008.

Widener (2007/2008) suggests that the United States is lagging behind Europe in family-friendly policies. Around the world, 163 countries guarantee paid leave to women, as well as men in some countries, in connection with childbirth. The United States does not offer anything close to this type of family assistance. In addition, at least 37 countries guarantee some paid leave when children are ill. Again this family assistance is not offered in the United States. Yet, it has been shown that mothers with access to paid leave have better health outcomes, as do their children (Widener, 2007/2008). Forty percent of job loss stems from taking care of family members. Still, despite being introduced, the Healthy Families Act (2007) and Family Leave Insurance Act (2007) have yet to be passed by the U.S. Congress. Wage inequity between men and women persists (Widener, 2007/2008), and as the TANF returnees stated, minimum wage is often not a living wage (Anderson et al., 2004).

Paul Farmer, a physician and author best known for his medical work in Haiti and worldwide with tuberculosis and AIDS, wrote about structural violence in his book, *Pathologies of Power: Health, Human Rights and the New War on the Poor* (2003). Structural violence refers to historical, economic, and political roots of generational oppression. It is about unequal treatment, racism, classism, and discrimination. In short, it refers to systematized, unequal access to resources. Working toward social justice requires a partnership between families and professionals. The community/public health nurses' responses to the structural violence perpetuated by policy, the myth of meritocracy (that anyone hardworking and deserving can succeed), and our biases make it an ethical obligation to engage in deep relational practice with the families we serve.

Family Case Study

CARING FOR THE JAMISON-JENSEN FAMILY AT HOME

With Bioecological Theory as a framework for evaluating a family over time, we visit the Jamison-Jensen family in their home. Stacie Jensen is a 21-year-old high-school graduate, sometimes girlfriend of Griff Jamison, and now a first-time mom. Her daughter, Danni Jensen-Jamison, was born prematurely at 27 weeks gestation, and weighed barely 2 ½ pounds at birth. Danni remained in the neonatal intensive care unit (NICU) for 10 weeks and encountered many complications of her preterm birth, including infection, difficulty being weaned from the ventilator, respiratory compromise, and vision difficulties. As she was moved from the NICU to intermediate care for her last 3 weeks of hospitalization, the NICU staff made a referral to the Children with Special Healthcare Needs program at the local public health department. The Children with Special Healthcare Needs nurse assigned to care for the family visited them briefly 1 week before Danni's hospital discharge to establish a relationship, and to describe the program and in-home and clinic-based nursing advocacy services for families.

The Children with Special Healthcare Needs nurse's next visit to Stacie and Danni occurred 1 week after Danni's arrival home, 14 weeks after her birth, and when she would have been 41 weeks gestation. On the initial home visit, Stacie and Danni seemed to be settling into their new routines at home fairly well, but concern about Danni's well-being had relegated Stacie to being a captive in her own home. She was so worried about Danni contracting an illness that she had asked friends not to visit at a time when she needed all the support she could get. When asked about supportive people in her life, she reported that Griff, her 22-year-old sometimes boyfriend and the father of the baby, had been close to her and excited about Danni's birth until the reality of caring for a very premature baby hit him. At this point, Stacie and Griff have had very little contact with each other. Because Stacie was unable to work, she had moved into a small house with her stepfather, mother, and brother, but Stacie's relationships with them were tenuous, and she did not find them supportive; Figure 17-3 presents the Jamison-Jensen family genogram. In fact, she felt trapped by the small house with all those people in it and yearned for a home of her own. The home environment was clean and neat but very crowded with the oxygen and monitoring equipment required for Danni's care. Stacie was overwhelmed by the physical care of Danni, and worried that she would do something wrong. With these issues so all-consuming, the idea of filling out the many forms required for various types of financial support and medical insurance to which Danni was entitled was too much. Stacie had tears in her eyes when she told the Children with Special Healthcare Needs nurse, "I don't think I can do this, but what would it mean to NOT do it?"

A plan of care for the Jamison-Jensens, developed in partnership with the family, required a family-as-client perspective and attention to helping them develop much-needed community. It was important to assess their available and desired microsystems (the settings in which daily life is experienced), and to help the family strengthen the mesosystem between these various communities; refer to Figure 17-4, the Jamison-Jensen family ecomap. Initial health appraisal found an infant whose growth and development was on target for her prematurity-corrected age, and who was receiving appropriate primary preventive well-child care and immunizations from a local pediatrician. This provider-family microsystem was stable and just required maintenance.

Over the ensuing year, the primary care provider was glad to team up with the Children with Special Healthcare Needs nurse in making necessary arrangements for speech, vision, physical, occupational, and developmental assessments for Danni to prevent secondary developmental delays, and for tertiary prevention and rehabilitation of existing vision and respiratory compromise. In addition, the pediatrician was grateful that the community nurse could accompany Stacie to her well-child visits and therapy appointments to help provide continuity of care and family education.

During the 13 weeks of Danni's hospitalization, the NICU and special care units had become a warm, supportive, welcoming community for Stacie, and she missed this microsystem. A new microsystem was needed to provide the support that was missing. Because Stacie derived comfort from this health care community, the Children with Special Healthcare Needs nurse helped Stacie connect with other families

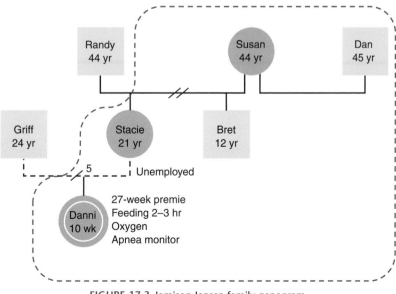

FIGURE 17-3 Jamison-Jensen family genogram.

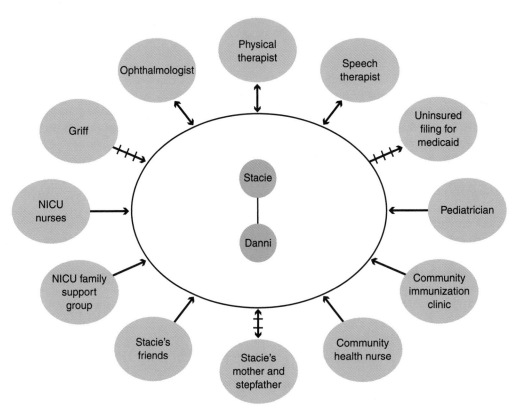

FIGURE 17-4 Jamison-Jensen family ecomap.

in her community by introducing her to a support group for parents of children with special needs. Griff had no interest in a support group but was amenable to talking to a father of an older NICU graduate who was doing well at home.

Because healthy families are the foundation of healthy communities, and because a healthy couple microsystem can be a key to a healthy family, the community/public health nurse (Children with Special Healthcare Needs nurse) needed to assess the health of the relationship between Griff and Stacie, as well as their commitment to the relationship. With Danni's health and development progressing nicely at 6 months of age (3 months corrected age), Griff felt more comfortable with supporting Stacie and caring for Danni. The relationship seemed to be a positive, nurturing one, so the nurse was able to help the parents arrange respite care so that they had some time alone as a couple without worrying too much about Danni.

Empowerment often comes through problem solving. As the family celebrated Danni's first birthday, Stacie knew that they needed to move from her parents' home and start life on their own, but having a

baby with such extensive needs, she felt hopeless about opportunities for work. The nurse answered questions about social and financial services that were available to help the family, and supported and encouraged Stacie and Griff as they completed the necessary paperwork and interviews. Helping this family move into their own home required creativity. Ultimately, they chose to move in with another family with a young infant so that child care issues could be shared. The family, with the help of the nurse, entered this new extended-family microsystem with a better understanding of the importance of communication in building stable relationships. Because Danni's grandparents had shared their home with Stacie and Danni, it was important to foster relationships among this extended family through referral to family counseling so that they could all grow in their appreciation of each other.

Empowerment also includes planning for the future. With Danni's health much improved at year's end, the Children with Special Healthcare Needs nurse and the family worked together to assess other needs before terminating the nurse-client relationship. Together, they began to probe Stacie's and Griff's desires to further their educations and improve their work situations. As they voiced these hopes, the nurse helped them find and access quality, affordable child care so that they could move forward to make a positive difference in their various communities. In addition, they discussed the impact that exosystems such as workplace or school settings might have on Danni. Working together, the Children with Special Healthcare Needs nurse helped Stacie and Griff work through the guilt that they felt when they thought of pursuing their own interests and helped them to see ways in which new experiences could have a positive impact on Danni. It was important for the nurse to be conscious of the nurse-client relationship so that the goals developed were family centered and family driven. As Stacie and Griff returned to the workplace community, macrosystemic policies were in these settings in regard to onsite child care, family leave, and medical insurance that the community nurse was able to influence both directly and by helping the family to advocate for themselves.

SUMMARY

Community/public health nursing of families is a rewarding experience for nursing students and experienced nurses alike. For the student, caring for families in a variety of community settings offers an opportunity to assess change over time, which is not possible in many other clinical settings. Community health nurses forge strong nurse-client partnerships as they maneuver through the maze of interventions and resources in providing family-centered nursing.

Community/public health nurses are concerned with the health of families and the ways in which family health influences the health of communities. The settings in which community/public health nurses work with families vary and include, but are not limited to, public and private health agencies, schools, and occupational sites. Community/public health nursing roles vary according to whether the nurse is focusing on the family as the unit of care in the context of the community, or focusing on the health of the community with families being a subunit. Students working with experienced family nurses in a variety of communities develop the skills necessary to provide family-level care and experience the satisfaction of making a difference to families

that they may come to know very well. The following case study demonstrates the highly developed skills of community health nurses.

REFERENCES

Ackerman, P. M. (1994). Competencies for the practice of effective public health nursing: Confirmation of Zerwekh's Family Caregiving Model. Unpublished Doctoral dissertation, University of Colorado, Denver.

American Public Health Association (APHA). (2008). *Public health nursing section.* Retrieved February 22, 2008, from http://www.apha.org/membergroups/sections/aphasections/phn

Ammerman, A. S., Keyserling, T. C., Atwood, J. R., Hosking, J. D., Zayed, H., & Krasny, C. (2003). A randomized controlled trial of a public health nurse directed treatment program for rural patients with high blood cholesterol. *Preventive Medicine, 36*(3), 340–351.

Anderson, D. G., Capuzzi, C., & Hatton, D. C. (2001). Families and public health nursing in the community. In S. M. Harmon Hanson (Ed.), *Family health care nursing* (2nd ed., pp. 345–361). Philadelphia: F.A. Davis.

Anderson, S. G., Halter, A. P., & Gryzlak, B. M. (2004). Difficulties after leaving TANF: Inner-city women talk about reasons for returning to welfare. *Social Work, 49*(2), 185–194.

Anonymous. (2007). Millions of Americans were uninsured for part of the year. *The Nation's Health, 37*(9), 8.

Aston, M., Meagher-Stewart, D., Vukic, A., Sheppard-LeMoine, D., Chircop, A. (2006). Family nursing and empowering relationships. *Pediatric Nursing, 32*(1), 61–67.

Bailey, K. (2007). Wrong direction: One out of three Americans are uninsured. (Families USA Publication No. 07-108) Retrieved June 2, 2009, from https://www.policyarchive.org/bitstream/handle/10207/5864/wrong-direction.pdf?sequence=1

Bender, K., Benjamin, G., Fallon, M., Jarris, P. E., & Libbey, P. M. (2007). Commentary: Exploring accreditation: Striving for a consensus model. *Journal of Public Health Management Practice, 13*(4), 334–336.

Bekemeier, B., & Butterfield, P. (2005). Unreconciled inconsistencies: A critical review of the concept of social justice in 3 national nursing documents. *Advances in Nursing Science, 28*(2), 152–162.

Berg, G. V., Hedelin, B., & Sarvimaki, A. (2005). A holistic approach to promotion of older hospital patients' health. *International Nursing Review, 522*(1), 73–80.

Bronfenbrenner, U. (2004). *Making human beings human: Bioecological perspectives on human development.* Thousand Oaks, CA: Sage.

Cassey, M. Z. (2008). Using technology to support the CLAS standards. *Nursing Economics, 26*(2), 133–135.

Clark, P. N. (1998). Nursing theory as a guide for inquiry in family and community health nursing. *Nursing Science Quarterly, 11*(2), 47–48.

Collins, A. M. & Reinke, E. (1997). Use of a family caregiving model to articulate the role of the public health nurse in infant mental health promotion. *Issues in Comprehensive Pediatric Nursing, 20*(4), 207–216.

Cunningham, M., & Henry, M. (2007). *Homelessness counts.* Research Reports on Homelessness, National Alliance to end homelessness. Retrieved April 15, 2008, from http://www.endhomelessness.org/content/article/detail/1440

Dannenberg, A. L., Jackson, R. J., Frumkin, H., Schieber, R. A., Pratt, M., Kotitzky, C., et al. (2003). The impact of community design and land-use choices on public health: A scientific research agenda. *American Journal of Public Health, 93*(9), 1500–1508.

Dewar, A. (2006). Assessment and management of chronic pain in the older person living in the community. *American Journal of Advanced Nursing, 24*(1), 33–38.

Doane, G. H., & Varcoe, C. (2007). Relational practice and nursing obligations. *Advances in Nursing Science, 30*(3), 192–205.

Doggett, C., Burrett, S., & Osborn, D. A. (2005). Home visits during pregnancy and after birth for women with an alcohol or drug problem. *Cochrane Database of Systematic Reviews, 4,* CD004456.

Doutrich, D., & Marvin, M. (2004). Education and practice: Dynamic partners in improving cultural competence in public health. *Family and Community Health, 27*(4), 298–307.

Doutrich, D. & Storey, M. (2006). Cultural competence and organizational change: Lasting results of an institutional linkage. *Home Health Care Management and Practice, 18*(8), 356–360.

Doutrich, D., Wros, P., Valdez, R., & Ruiz, M. E. (2005). Professional values of Hispanic nurses: The educational experience. *International Hispanic Health Care, 3*(3), 161–170.

Falk-Rafael, A. (2001). Empowerment as a process of evolving consciousness: A model of empowered caring. *Advances in Nursing Science, 24*(1), 1–16.

Farmer, P. (2003). *Pathologies of power: Health, human rights and the new war on the poor.* Berkeley: California University Press.

Gebbie, K., Rosenstock, L., & Hernandez, L. M. (Eds.). (2003). *Who will keep the public healthy? Educating public health professionals for the 21st century.* Washington, DC: The National Academies Press.

Glick, D. F. (1999). Advanced practice community health nursing in community nursing centers: A holistic approach to the community as client. *Holistic Nursing Practice, 13*(4), 19–27.

Hodnett, E. D., & Fredericks, S. (2003). Support during pregnancy for women at increased risk of low birth weight babies. *Cochrane Database of Systematic Reviews, 3,* CD000198.

Joint Commission: Division of Standards and Survey Methods. (2007). Office of Minority Health National Culturally and Linguistically Appropriate Services (CLAS) Standards Cross-walked to Joint Commission 2007 standards. Version 2007-1. Retrieved May 5, 2008, from http://www.jointcommission.org

Kaiser, K. L., Hays, B. J. Cho, W., & Agrawal, W. (2002). Examining health problems and intensity of need for care in family-focused community and public health nursing. *Journal of Community Health Nursing, 19*(1), 17–32.

Koniak-Griffin, D., Verzemnieks, I. L., Anderson, N. L. R., Brecht, M., Lesser, J., & Kim, S. (2003). Nurse visitation for adolescent mothers: Two year infant health and maternal outcomes. *Nursing Research, 52*(2), 127–136.

Lahr, M. B., Rosenberg, K. D., & Lapidus, J. A. (2005). Health departments do it better: Prenatal care site and prone infant sleep position. *Maternal and Child Health Journal, 9*(2), 165–172.

Lindeke, L. L., Leonard, B. J., Presler, B & Garwick, A. (2002). Family-centered care coordination for children with special needs across multiple settings. *Journal of Pediatric Health Care 16*(1), 290–297.

MacMillan, H. L., Thomas, B. H., Jamieson, E., & Walsh, C. A. (2005). Effectiveness of home visitation by public health nurses in the prevention of recurrence of child abuse and neglect: A randomized controlled trial. *The Lancet, 365*(9473), Health Module 1786.

Masters, K. R. (2005). A student home visiting program for vulnerable, community-dwelling older adults. *Journal of Nursing Education, 44*(4), 185–186.

McDaniel, S. H., Cambell, T. L., Hepworth, J., & Lorenz, A. (2005). *Family-oriented primary care* (2nd ed.). New York: Springer.

McNaughton, D. (2000). A synthesis of qualitative home visiting research. *Public Health Nursing, 17*(6), 405–414.

McNaughton, D. B. (2004). Nurse home visits to maternal-child clients: A research review. *Public Health Nursing, 21*(3), 207–219.

McNaughton, D. B. (2005). A naturalistic test of Peplau's theory in home visiting. *Public Health Nursing, 22*(5), 429–438.

Minkler, M., Frantz, S., & Wechsler, R. (2006). Social support and social action organizing in a "grey ghetto": The Tenderloin experience. *International Quarterly of Community Health Education, 25*(1–2), 49–61.

Minkler, M., & Wallenstein, N. (2003). Introduction to community-based participatory research. In M. Minkler & N. Wallenstein (Eds.), *Community-based participatory research for health.* San Francisco: Jossey-Bass.

Novick, L. F. (2003). Core public health functions: 15 year update. *Public Health Management Practice, 9*(1), 5.

Office of Minority Health (OMH); U.S. Department of Health and Human Services. (2001). *National standards for culturally and linguistically appropriate services in health care, final report.* Retrieved May 5, 2008, from http://www.omhrc.gov/assets/pdf/checked/finalreport.pdf

Office of Minority Health (OMH); U.S. Department of Health and Human Services. (2007a). *Culturally competent nursing care: A cornerstone of caring.* Retrieved May 5, 2008, from http://ccnm.thinkculturalhealth.org

Office of Minority Health (OMH); U.S. Department of Health and Human Services. (2007b). *Cultural competency CME portal.* Retrieved May 5, 2008, from http://www.thinkculturalhealth.org

Olds, D. L. (2002). Prenatal and infancy home visiting by nurses: From randomized trials to community replication. *Prevention Science, 3*(3), 153–172.

Olds, D., Eckenrode, J, Henderson, C. R., Jr., Kitzman, H., Powers, J., Cole, R., et al. (1997). Long-term effects of home visitation on maternal life course and child abuse and neglect: 15-year follow-up of a randomized trial. *Journal of the American Medical Association, 278,* 637–643.

Olds, D., Henderson, C. R., Kitzman, H., & Cole, R. (2005). The effects of prenatal and infancy nurse home visitation on surveillance of child maltreatment. *Pediatrics, 95,* 365–372.

Olds, D., Kitzman, H., Cole, R., & Robinson, J. (1997). Theoretical foundations of a program of home visitation for pregnant women and parents of young children. *Journal of Community Psychology, 25*(1), 9–25.

Olds, D. L., Kitzman, H., Cole, R., Robinson, J., Sidora, K., Luckey, D. W., et al. (2004). Effects of nurse home-visiting on maternal life course and child development: Age 6 follow-up results of a randomized trial. *Pediatrics, 114*(6), 1550–1559.

Olds, D., Pettitt, L., Robinson, J., Henderson, C., Jr., Eckenrode, J., Kitzman, H., et al. (1998). Reducing risks for antisocial behavior with a program of prenatal and early childhood home visitation. *Journal of Community Psychology, 26*(1), 65–83.

Potter, J. (2004). The importance of recognizing abuse of older people. *British Journal of Community Nursing, 10*(4), 185–187.

Sabogal, F., Marín, G., Otero-Sabogal, R., Marín, B. V., & Pérez-Stable, E. J. (1987). Hispanic familism and acculturation: What changes and what doesn't? *Hispanic Journal of Behavioral Sciences, 9,* 397–412.

Siefert, K., Heflin, C. M., Corcoran, M. E., & Williams, D. R. (2004). Food insufficiency and physical and mental health in a longitudinal survey of welfare recipients. *Journal of Health and Social Behavior, 45*(2), 171–186.

Shattuck, S. R. (2002). A domestic violence screening program in a public health department. *Journal of Community Health Nursing, 19*(3), 121–132.

Shipler, D. K. (2004). *The working poor: Invisible in America.* New York: Knopf.

Shuster, G. F., & Goeppinger, J. (2004). Community as client: Assessment and analysis. In M. Stanhope, & J. Lancaster (Eds.), *Community and public health nursing* (6th ed., pp. 342–373). St. Louis, MO: Mosby.

Smedley, B. D., Stith, A. Y., & Nelson, A. R. (Eds.). (2003). *Unequal treatment: Confronting racial and ethnic disparities in healthcare.* Washington, DC: National Academies Press.

SmithBattle, L., Diekemper, M., & Leander, S. (2004a). Getting your feel wet: Becoming a public health nurse, part 1. *Public Health Nursing, 21*(1), 3–11.

SmithBattle, L., Diekemper, M., & Leander, S. (2004b). Moving upstream: Becoming a public health nurse, part 2. *Public Health Nursing, 21*(2), 95–102.

St. John, W. (1998). Just what do we mean by community? Conceptualizations from the field. *Health and Social Care in the Community, 8*(2), 63–70.

Tuffrey, C., Finlay, F., & Lewis, M. (2007). The needs of children and their families at end of life: An analysis of community nursing practice. *International Journal of Palliative Nursing, 13*(1), 64–71.

University of Southern Mississippi School of Nursing. (2003). *Public health nursing: Pioneers of health care reform.* Retrieved August 12, 2004, from http://www.nursing.usm.edu/FacAccess/lundy/Powerpoints/chnursing_ch37.ppt

U.S. Department of Health and Human Services (DHHS). (2001). *Healthy people in healthy communities.* [Brochure]. Rockville, MD: Author.

U.S. DHHS Office of Health Promotion and Disease Prevention. (2000). Healthy People 2010. Retrieved June 1, 2009, from http://www.healthypeople.gov/

U.S. DHHS Centers for Disease Control. (2005). State and local public health agency accreditation. Retrieved June 1, 2009, from http://www.cdc.gov/od/ocphp/oseip/accred.htm

Vega, W. A. (1990). Hispanic families in the 1980's: A decade of research. *Journal of Marriage and the Family, 52,* 1015–1024.

Weman, K., & Fagerberg, I. (2006). Registered nurses working together with family members of older people. *Journal of Clinical Nursing, 15,* 281–289.

Widener, A. J. (2007/2008). Family-friendly policy: Lessons from Europe—Part ii. *The Public Manager, 36*(4), 44–49.

World Health Organization (WHO). (2000). *Community TB care in Africa.* Retrieved February 22, 2008, from http://www.afro.who.int/tb/respub/community_tb_care_in_africa.pdf

Wros, P., Doutrich, D., & Izumi, S. (2004). Ethical concerns: A comparison of values from two cultures. *Nursing and Health Science, 6,* 131–140.

Zahner, S. J., & Vandermause, R. (2003). Local health department performance: Compliance with state statutes and rules. *Public Health Management Practice, 9*(1), 25–34.

Zerwekh, J. V. (1991). A family caregiving model for public health nursing. *Nursing Outlook, 39*(5), 213–217.

Zerwekh, J. V. (1992). Laying the foundation for family self-help: Locating families, building trust, and building strength. *Public Health Nursing, 9*(1), 15–21.

Zotti, M. E., & Zahner, S. J. (1995). Evaluation of public health nursing home visits to pregnant women on WIC. *Public Health Nursing, 12*(5), 294–304.

Zurmehly, J. (2007). A qualitative case study review of role transition in community nursing. *Nursing Forum, 42*(4), 62.

CHAPTER 18

Nursing Care of Families in Disaster and War

Deborah C. Messecar, PhD, MPH, RN

Lori Chorpenning, MS, RN

CRITICAL CONCEPTS

+ Family Systems Theory can guide nursing assessment and interventions to help families dealing with the impact of disaster and war.

+ When one or more family members are traumatized by experience with war or disaster, all family members and family relationships can be affected.

+ In a disaster, all family members may be directly affected, some more than others, if the family is not all in the same location during the time of the event. War affects veterans directly, but other family members may be affected indirectly by the veteran's responses to his or her wartime experience.

+ The more severe the trauma an individual family member suffers from his or her wartime experience or disaster event, the more likely the other members of the family are to suffer secondary traumatization.

+ The family response to trauma of one or more of its members from war or disaster cannot be understood or treated by focusing on individual family members alone.

+ Trauma is the key symptom family systems experience after war and disaster. The threat or fear of death or serious injury is a salient feature of this trauma. Post-traumatic stress disorder (PTSD), which is a response to this trauma, is more likely to develop when there is a lack of social support, which is a key role of the family.

+ PTSD can be acute or chronic and can occur months, even years after a disaster or traumatic event such as war. Family members can provide key contextual information about past traumatic events and experiences that help explain current responses.

+ Family boundaries may be disrupted in wartime or during disaster situations. Family boundaries may both be protective and act as a barrier to seeking help.

+ Family systems can be divided further into subsystems, such as the spousal relationship and child-parent relationships, so that the impact of war or disaster on the functioning of these subsystems can be better understood.

*D*isasters and wars are challenging events in family life. Both are stressful for each individual in the family and disruptive to family life. Certain families, and perhaps communities, are at greater risk for traumatization, family disorganization, and post-traumatic stress disorder (PTSD). This chapter examines the similarities and the particular challenges that families face in disaster and war situations, and then describes the nursing care of families experiencing these events. This chapter begins with a summary of the demographics of families affected by disasters and wartime, and the subsequent separation and reunion. A review of the evidenced-based literature follows; it identifies major

common stressors families endure in these situations. The chapter then presents interventions by the stage of disaster for two of the most common problems encountered in both war and disaster situations: PTSD and the secondary traumatization of family members of those who have PTSD. Two case studies using Family Systems Theory illustrate the many ways that the family-focused nurse can intervene and help the family cope. Because this chapter addresses both disasters and war, it is important to know the definitions of terms that might not be common knowledge for all nurses. Box 18-1 provides a glossary of the terms used in this chapter.

BOX 18-1
Glossary of Terms

Disaster: Any event that significantly disrupts the normal functioning of a community and that overwhelms local capacity, necessitating a request to a national or international level for external assistance. Disasters can occur anytime, anyplace, and usually without warning. Disasters can be caused by natural means such as hurricanes, tornadoes, earthquakes, storms, volcanic eruptions, and even extremes of heat and cold. Disasters can also be caused by human error such as major accidents, fires, or chemical spills. Deliberate mass violence such as terrorist or wartime attacks can generate a disaster situation.

Wartime separation and reunion: These events precipitate roller-coaster patterns of family adjustment (Hill, 1949) in which the family initially goes into a state of crisis or disorganization, then reorganizes and goes into a state of recovery, and finally settles into a new level of organization. Readjustment after reunion is dependent on the emotional and social accommodations made by the family during separation.

Trauma: The person suffers or witnesses an event that involves actual or threatened death or serious injury to themselves or to others (Kessler, Sonnega, Bromet, Hughes, & Nelson, 1995). According to *Diagnostic and Statistical Manual of Mental Disorders, Fourth Edition, Test Revision (DSM-IV-TR)* criteria, to be traumatized, the person must have experienced extreme fear, helplessness, or horror.

Acute stress disorder (ASD): Individual exhibits symptoms of response to trauma; onset occurs immediately and usually resolves within 4 weeks

of the traumatic event (Kessler et al., 1995). According to the DSM IV-TR, if the symptoms persist beyond 4 weeks, then the diagnosis becomes PTSD.

Post-traumatic stress disorder (PTSD): Three symptom clusters define this condition and must be present for at least 1 month, and cause significant distress, impairment, or both (Kessler et al., 1995). Symptom clusters include re-experiencing the trauma, avoidance and emotional numbing, and increased arousal.

Substance abuse: According to the DSM-IV-TR, substance abuse is a maladaptive pattern of substance use that leads to clinically significant impairment of distress. It includes use that meets the following criteria: (1) results in failure to meet major role obligations at work, school, or home; (2) use in situations where it is physically hazardous such as driving a motor vehicle; (3) results in recurrent substance-related legal problems; and (4) use continues despite social or interpersonal problems.

Family violence: This type of abuse includes a range of physical, sexual, and emotional maltreatment by one family member against another, such as intimate partner violence and child maltreatment.

Secondary traumatization: Secondary traumatic stress is defined by the same components of PTSD, except that the person with the symptoms has not actually been exposed to the traumatic events but has developed them as a result of caring for or living with someone with PTSD (Figley & Barnes, 2005).

DEMOGRAPHICS: FAMILIES, DISASTERS, AND WAR

Because disasters and war have been considered to be isolated and infrequent events, the effects on families have been understudied. A review of the evidenced-based literature indicates that the nursing care of families experiencing stress from disasters or war needs more attention. Nurses have a crucial role in helping families cope and recover from unexpected disasters and trauma of war.

Families Affected by Disasters

Disasters are events that cause widespread destruction of property, dislocation of people, and result in immediate suffering through death or injury. A disaster produces suffering and interrupts people's ability to meet basic needs for food, shelter, or safety. It also makes recovery difficult (Veenema, 2007). Disasters can be classified as either natural or caused by humans. Natural disasters include weather and seismic events such as floods, hurricanes, and earthquakes. Human-caused disasters include events such as fires, building collapse, explosions, or acts of terrorism or war. Acts of terrorism or violence can include the use of chemical, radioactive, nuclear, biologic, or explosive weapons.

Natural disasters are the most frequent type of disasters. The International Red Cross reported that 1.1 million people across the world from 1997–2006 were killed by natural disasters (e.g., hurricanes, tornadoes, earthquakes, storms, tsunamis, and volcanic eruptions). Just during 2004 to 2005, natural disasters killed 336,540 people, and more than 300 million people were directly or indirectly affected by those disasters (International Strategy for Disaster Reduction, 2006). In the United States alone during 2007, tornadoes killed 80 people, whereas thunderstorms and the accompanying floods, lightning, winds, and hail caused another 157 deaths (National Severe Storms Laboratory, 2007). In the year 2004, the Federal Emergency Management Agency (FEMA) provided $2.25 billion in aid for families and individuals affected by disasters (U.S. Department of Homeland Security, 2004).

Human-caused disasters may include industrial accidents involving chemical spills or fires, or transportation accidents, such as airplane crashes. These types of disasters, although less frequent than natural disasters, still have a great impact on human lives. Technologic disasters killed 100,000 people from 1997 to 2006. In 2006, industrial accidents accounted for 80% of these deaths. Transportation accidents accounted for one fifth of all deaths from disasters in 2006 alone. (International Federation of Red Cross and Red Crescent Societies, 2007). Regardless of the type of event, families are affected in multiple ways when disasters strike. Some of the many stressors that occur include loss of significant others, injuries to self or family, separation from family, or extensive loss of property (Norris, 2007).

Families Affected by War

Since the turn of the century, the nature of war has changed dramatically. Warfare in the 21st century rarely involves confrontations between professional armies. Instead, wars typically are fought as conflicts involving struggles between military personnel and civilians, or groups of armed civilians in the same country in a city environment rather than in distant battlefields. As a result, innocent bystander civilian fatalities resulting from collateral injuries incurred during battles fought in towns and cities have increased to more than 90% in recent years as compared with only 5% in wars fought in the early part of the 20th century. Worldwide, the caseload of refugee children grew from 2.4 million in 1974 to 27.4 million in 1996 (Machel, 1996). In the United States, the debilitating effect of war caused by infrastructure destruction and personal injury and death, other than for refugees, is usually not part of our American experience. However, the number of families that have had to endure wartime separation and reunion during an individual's military service, the death of that military member because of their service, or both is growing.

Over time, serving in one of the branches of the U.S. military has become far less common. From 2003 to 2008, 1.6 million veterans (or less than 0.05% of the population) served in Afghanistan or Iraq, compared with the 16 million Americans, or 12% of the population, who served in World War II (Meagher, 2007). Nevertheless, the consequences for family members of military personnel are often dire and long lasting. Death, injury, and short- and long-term disability of veterans are stressors that can make life difficult for families (Cozza, Chun, & Polo, 2005). From March 2003 to March 2008,

4,124 members of the U.S. military died in Iraq (U.S. Deaths & Coalition Casualties, n.d.). Another 30,333 U.S. service members have been wounded in hostile action in Iraq (U.S. Deaths, 2008). Statistics for Afghanistan indicate that conflict has produced fewer deaths and casualties, but that the situation may be changing as Pakistan becomes less stable. In addition to these dramatic losses for the family members of the service men and women involved, much greater rates of combat stress reactions are being observed in these veterans who return home to their families (Hoge et al., 2004). Specifically, the increase in traumatic brain injury sustained during war is associated with physical health problems that include more missed work days and symptoms such as headache, chest pain, dizziness, fainting spells, and shortness of breath. All of these symptoms and problems are made worse by PTSD and depression (Hoge et al., 2008). Alarmingly, veterans represent one of every four suicides in the United States (Glauber, 2007). This is a new trend. A recent report in JAMA noted that the suicide rate among active duty Army personnel was 20.2 per 100,000 in 2008, which exceeded the suicide rate among civilians with similar demographics (19.5 per 100,000 in 2005) (Kuehn, 2009).

Veterans and their families are a population at risk. In statistics compiled by Meagher (2007), approximately 50% of the veterans who have served in the Iraq and Afghanistan conflicts are married. More than 1.9 million children have one parent or both in uniform. The telephone rang at the 24-hour help line Military OneSource, which provides counseling to veterans and their families, more than 100,000 times in the first 10 months of 2005, and the calls increased by 20% in 2006. Medical personnel wrote more than 200,000 antidepressant prescriptions for military families and service members over a 14-month period from 2005 to 2006. The report did not distinguish between prescriptions for the troops and those for their family members, and the Defense Department has not provided prescription totals for such antidepressants from before and after the United States invaded Iraq in 2003 for military populations. The lack of comparison data makes it difficult to determine if this represents an increase, but it is a trend that should be monitored.

Unidentified and untreated PTSD presents special risks for family reintegration, and may put the veterans and their families at greater danger for maladaptive responses to stress such as alcoholism, depression, and family violence (Black et al., 2004; Bremner, Southwick, Darnell, & Charney, 1996; Dansky, Byrne, & Brady, 1999; Davis & Wood, 1999). As the wars in Afghanistan and Iraq continue, military members are being deployed to combat areas multiple times. The increased risk for acute combat stress and fatigue in those serving multiple tours is more than 50%.

Familiarity with the evidenced-based literature relative to the nursing care of families experiencing stress from disasters or war is crucial for nurses. The unpredictable nature of disaster calls means that nurses need to be prepared to respond at any time.

REVIEW OF THE EVIDENCE-BASED LITERATURE

Multiple factors cause families stress during and after a disaster or war. The acute and chronic problems associated with the family effects of disaster, and wartime separation and reunion arise from key features that are part of these experiences. With both disaster and war, substance abuse can be a coping mechanism and often co-occurs with PTSD. Family violence often results from either substance abuse or PTSD, especially when PTSD is not treated. The other family stressors more specific to the family experience of either disaster or war are summarized in Table 18-1 and are explored further in this section.

Effect of Disasters on Families

Most disasters occur with little or no warning, so families have little time to prepare for the event. Some disaster events have a clear beginning point and a rapid ending, such as tornados or hurricanes, so that families know when the disaster is over. Other events, such as terrorism or flooding, have a less definitive ending, which causes more uncertainty as to when the disaster will end and recovery efforts can begin (Figley & Barnes, 2005).

Families may experience additional stress if they become separated during the disaster. Disasters have acute effects on each member of the family given their differing ages, health characteristics, and

TABLE 18-1

Comparison of Family Impact of Disaster Versus War

PROBLEMS	DISASTER	WARTIME SEPARATION AND REUNION
Acute Problems	Entire family immersed	Mostly happens out of sight of family
Timing	Usually an immediate impact	Spread out over much longer period
Direct trauma experienced	All or most family members	Only by veteran family member
Acute stress disorder	All or most family members experience it; depending on parental anxiety, child stress can be exacerbated	May have been experienced initially by veteran after combat events, then put aside; family members may have little or no knowledge about this experience
Infrastructure destruction	Widespread, witnessed by all family members and affects all equally

Difficulties presented may go on for weeks, months, or years, and interferes with family routines, getting back to normal | Only witnessed by veteran, other family members may have great difficulty picturing or understanding the veteran's experience; impact on the veteran hidden from rest of family |
Separation from other family members	May happen in immediate postimpact period after disaster; anxiety produced is immediate and profound; little or no time to prepare, and means of communicating until reunited may not exist	Some forewarning that separation will occur with at least some time to prepare; communication strategies exist to keep family members in touch during separation; requires family to form long-term strategy to manage during separation
Chronic problems	Postimpact or recovery phase	Months after reunion
Post-traumatic stress disorder (PTSD)	Multiple family members can experience acute, chronic, and or delayed PTSD; often parent stress increases child stress	Only the veteran experiences PTSD symptoms, but family members can be deeply disturbed by these symptoms
Substance abuse	One or more family members may use this as a coping mechanism to deal with trauma short and long term; often co-occurs with PTSD and can exacerbate family violence	Veteran may develop problem as coping mechanism for self-treating PTSD; often co-occurs with PTSD and can exacerbate family violence
Family violence	Can be exacerbated, especially if PTSD develops and is untreated	Can be exacerbated, especially if PTSD develops and is untreated
Secondary traumatization	More likely transmission of stress is from parent to child	Primarily occurs among spouses of veterans, but can affect children as well

needs. Disasters can also create chronic problems that can occur months after the disaster is over.

ACUTE PROBLEMS

Because trauma for family members of any age is a key feature of most disaster situations, symptoms that occur immediately after the trauma are prominent features of family response to disaster. Adult family members usually have some type of physical, psychological, cognitive, or emotional response to a trauma. Adults are more likely to report musculoskeletal pain or abdominal pain in reaction to the stress of the disaster (Gnauck et al., 2007). Adults report feelings of helplessness and hopelessness (Young, Ford, & Watson, 2007), show some difficulty concentrating and making decisions, and experience spiritual distress (Plum, 2007).

Children are more likely than adults to experience trauma symptoms as a reaction to being in a disaster. Families and nurses should use the child's developmental stage as a guide to managing their symptoms of distress in response to the disaster (American Red Cross, 2001). For example, infants sense their parents' anxiety, and demonstrate being anxious and fearful through changes in behavior such as inconsolable crying, not eating, and not sleeping. Preschool-aged children react strongly to the loss of routine and find it difficult to cope. These children often regress to an earlier developmental stage, such as sucking their thumb or wetting the bed. They may experience increased anxiety around strangers and cling to their parents. School-aged children may withdraw from friends, fear going back to school, and may regress developmentally. Adolescents may rebel at home or school, and may feel guilty for not being able to assume full adult responsibilities in helping out during the disaster response (National Mental Health Information Center, 2005; Plum, 2007).

Symptoms of acute stress responses in children after disaster are greatly influenced by the level of exposure to the disaster, the extent that children and families are affected by the disaster, and the developmental age of the children (Hagan & The Committee of Psychosocial Aspects of Child and Family Health and the Task Force on Terrorism, 2005). Children exposed to the traumas of disasters, such as seeing physical injuries to others, hearing screams of victims, or seeing dead bodies for an extended time are at greater risk for significant stress responses (Starr, 2002).

Older adults have similar stress responses to disasters and trauma as other adult family members. In addition, they may become angry, depressed, and demonstrate difficulty making decisions (Kohn, Levav, Garcia, Machuca, & Tamashiro, 2005). In some instances, older adult family members may not have the financial resources to start again after a disaster. They may find the aspects of relocation and re-establishing social contacts daunting. Older adults who have chronic medical conditions require routine medications and checkups, but after a disaster, this may be difficult for them to negotiate if their normal and routine health settings and clinicians are no longer available (Sanders, Bowie, & Bowie, 2003; Vest & Valadez, 2006).

Family separation, especially in chaotic disaster events such as 2005's Hurricane Katrina, is an acute issue. Evacuation efforts were hampered by people refusing to leave for various reasons. Some older adults had lived through previous hurricanes and felt they would be safe in their homes. Some residents had frail older or disabled family members whom they would not abandon. Many people stayed to be with their neighbors who they viewed as important parts of their extended families (Eisenman, Cordasco, Asch, Golden, & Glik, 2007). Yet, in many cases, emergency evacuation efforts could not keep communities or families together. Broughton, Allen, Hannemann, and Petrikin (2006) report that, after Hurricane Katrina, 5,000 families were fractured. Children and parents were separated by the storm, sent to different shelters, put on different transfer vehicles, and had no knowledge of their family's whereabouts. Broughton and colleagues found that, in some cases, 6 months passed before some families were reunited with their children. This delayed reunion may or may not stimulate an acute behavioral response among family members. Hurricane Katrina will be studied by emergency preparedness organizations to learn how to prevent the failures experienced in this type of disaster.

Destruction of infrastructure (the basic services, facilities, and installations needed for the functioning of the community) is a salient feature of many types of natural and human-caused disasters. Loss of infrastructure could involve loss of access to roads, destruction of buildings, including hospitals, or other essential services. Rhoads, Pearman, and Rick (2007) compared families who stayed throughout Hurricane Katrina with those families who evacuated to other parts of the country. Families who stayed throughout the hurricane were found to have more intense symptoms of stress, specifically inattentiveness, aggression, irritability, and interpersonal difficulties after the disaster. Mental health care was limited after the hurricane with only 3 of every 8 mental health clinics in operation. Access to health care was disrupted as well with hospitals damaged and entire communities destroyed. Families who relocated, however, had increased access to resources for assistance, which resulted in less severe symptoms.

CHRONIC PROBLEMS

Chronic problems may occur months after the disaster is over and include the development of PTSD, depression, substance abuse problems, family violence, and secondary traumatization. Box 18-2 lists specific symptoms and criteria for PTSD.

Depression and PTSD in both adults and children can occur months to years after the disaster (Adams & Boscarino, 2006; Kilic, Ozguven, & Sayil, 2003). Children especially are at high risk for PTSD if they are physically close to the location of the disaster (American Academy of Child and Adolescent Psychiatry, 2004; Hamblen, 2007; Vila et al., 2001) and because of their developmental vulnerability (Veenema & Schroeder-Bruce, 2002). Children are at increased risk for chronic problems if their parents, especially their fathers, demonstrate symptoms of irritability and detachment as a result of secondary traumatization (Kilic et al., 2003). Vila and colleagues have identified a correlation between mothers' stress and increased stress reactions in their children. Children react to their parents' reactions to the stresses of the disaster. The more distressed the parents, the greater the reactions to stress that their children exhibit. Norris (2007) has conducted a large meta-analysis of 121 reports from 62 natural disasters around the world and found that PTSD was identified as a stress reaction in 81% of the studies. In terms of spousal and child abuse, these problems usually existed before the disaster but were exacerbated after the disaster (Amaratunga & O'Sullivan, 2006; National Center for Children Exposed to Violence, 2006; Substance Abuse and Mental Health Services Administration, Center for Mental Health Services, National Gains Center, & the Center on Women, Violence and Trauma, 2006).

BOX 18-2
Criteria for Post-traumatic Stress Disorder

DSM-IV-TR diagnostic criteria for PTSD includes six features. Three of these features are symptom clusters associated with PTSD and include re-experiencing the traumatic event, avoidance and emotional numbing, and increased arousal. The symptoms must be present for at least 1 month, and cause significant distress, impair functioning, or both. The criteria are as follows:

Criterion A: History of trauma. The person has history of a significant stressor that involves experiencing, witnessing, or confronting an event or events that involved actual or threatened death or serious injury that produced feelings of intense fear, helplessness, or horror.

Criterion B: Intrusive recollection. The traumatic event is re-experienced by the person in one or more of the following ways:
1. Recurrent and intrusive distressing recollections and dreams of the event
2. Acting or feeling as if the trauma were reoccurring
3. Psychological distress or physiologic reactivity, or both, when exposed to cues that resemble an aspect of the traumatic event

Criterion C: Avoidant/Numbing. The person avoids stimuli associated with the trauma and has a general numbing of their responsiveness indicated by three or more of the following symptoms:
1. Avoidance of thoughts, feelings, or conversation associated with the trauma

2. Avoidance of activities that will arouse recollection of the trauma (places or people)
3. Inability to recall an important aspect of event
4. Markedly diminished interest in significant activities
5. Feelings of detachment
6. Restricted range of mood
7. Sense of foreshortened future

Criterion D: Hyperarousal. Symptoms of increased arousal as indicated by two or more of the following symptoms:
1. Difficulty falling or staying asleep
2. Irritability or outbursts of anger
3. Difficulty concentrating
4. Hypervigilance
5. Exaggerated startle response

Criterion E: Symptom duration. Symptoms in the three clusters must be present for longer than 1 month.

Criterion F: Functional impact. The distress the individual feels must interfere with social, occupational, or other important areas of life.

Source: American Psychiatric Association. (2000). Diagnostic and stastical manual of mental disorders: DSM-IV-TR (4th ed., text revision). Washington, DC: American Psychiatric Association.

Effect of Wartime Separation and Reunion on Families

Several acute and chronic problems involve wartime separation and reunion. The most difficult acute problem is the prolonged separation that veterans' families must bear. Furthermore, chronic problems, such as PTSD and substance abuse in the returning veteran, are most commonly reported. Secondary traumatization is trauma that occurs as a result of the family caring for the family member who has experienced direct trauma.

ACUTE PROBLEMS

Even though the separations endured by military families are more predictable and manageable than in the past because of better communication technologies, family members separated by wartime deployment have reported several adverse effects. Some studies of wartime separation among military families have found that temporary behavioral difficulties occurred in some children (Kelley, 1994; Nice, 1981; Rosen, Teitelbaum, & Westhuis, 1993). Yet, other studies have shown that military children are quite adaptive and are not necessarily preoccupied with the threat of war (Ryan-Wenger, 2001). High stress (Rosen, Westhuis, & Tietelbaum, 1994) and decreased psychological well-being (Knapp & Newman, 1993) have been reported by some spouses. The military personnel are also affected by the separation. A prominent theme among stress-producing factors reported by deployed personnel was concern about the well-being of their family members left behind (Mangelsdorff & Moses, 1993; Nelson & Hagedorn, 1997; Nice, Hilton, & Malone, 1994; Ryan-Wenger, 1992; Wynd & Dziedzicki, 1992).

CHRONIC PROBLEMS

Several chronic problems may develop after veterans have returned home and are reunited with their families. Classified as one of the anxiety disorders, PTSD is a syndrome of responses to extremely disturbing, often life-threatening events—for example, combat, natural disaster, torture, or rape—that fall outside of usual experience. Although not all combat veterans experience development of PTSD, a correlation does exist between PTSD and combat exposure. In fact, PTSD occurs in as many as three of five combat veterans (American Psychiatric Association, 2000). For some subgroups of veterans, the effects can be even more negative. Women, National Guard members, and reservists seem particularly vulnerable to greater rates of negative outcomes (Hotopf et al., 2006; Vogt, Samper, King, King, & Martin, 2008). U.S. studies involving personal stories of traumatic events suggest that combat exposure is among the most prevalent traumatic events that affect men (Kessler, Sonnega, Bromet, Hughes, & Nelson, 1995; U.S. Bureau of the Census, 1992). The National Vietnam Veterans Readjustment Study estimates the current prevalence of PTSD among combat-exposed Vietnam veterans to be 31% over a lifetime (Kulka et al., 1990).

It appears also that the symptoms and follow-up consequences of PTSD can be very long term and can persist or re-emerge many years after the traumatic event (Gray, Bolton, & Litz, 2004; Toomey et al., 2007). Ten years after deployment to the conflict in the Gulf in 1991, veterans had twice the prevalence of anxiety disorders and depression as nondeployed veterans (Fiedler et al., 2006). Iraq and Afghanistan combat veterans also report greater mental health difficulties (Hoge, Auchterlonie, & Milliken, 2006). Lack of follow-up resources over time appears to increase PTSD symptoms (Benotsch et al., 2000). Hobfoll (1989) has described a pattern of a loss spiral. In a loss spiral, as resource factors diminish and emotional responses to war stress increase, a reciprocal effect occurs, which exacerbates PTSD.

The costs of untreated PTSD may be high. A recent report documented a strong association of PTSD with physical health problems, even after controlling for being wounded or injured (Hoge, Terhakopian, Castro, Messer, & Engel, 2007). Moreover, the mental health consequences of PTSD include problems with family functioning, substance abuse, family violence, and secondary trauma of other family members.

Family Functioning and Post-traumatic Stress Disorder

In a study of current relationship functioning among World War II ex-prisoners of war (POW), more than 30% of those with PTSD reported relationship problems compared with only 11% of those without PTSD (Cook, Riggs, Thompson, Coyne, & Sheikh, 2004). In Vietnam veterans (which included the broader population of veterans, not just POWs), PTSD symptoms have been significantly associated with poor family functioning (Evans, McHugh, Hopwood, & Watt, 2003), and problems with marital adjustment, parenting satisfaction, and psychological abuse (Gold, Taft, Keehn, King, King, & Samper, 2007). The PTSD symptoms of avoidance and emotional numbing, in particular, have deleterious effects on parent-child relationship satisfaction (Samper, Taft, King, & King, 2004). Among Iraq and Afghanistan veterans, trauma symptoms such as sleep problems, dissociation, and severe sexual problems predicted lower marital satisfaction for both the veteran and his or her partner (Goff, Crow, Reisbig, & Hamilton, 2007).

Substance Abuse and Post-traumatic Stress Disorder

The dual diagnosis of substance abuse and PTSD is common. The rate of PTSD comorbidity among patients in substance abuse treatment is 12% to 34%; for women, it is 30% to 59% (Kessler et al., 1995; Langeland & Hartgers, 1998; Najavits, Weiss, Shaw, & Muenz, 1998; Stewart, 1996; Stewart, Conrod, Pihl, & Dongier, 1999; Triffleman, 1998). Becoming abstinent from substances does not resolve PTSD; some PTSD symptoms become worse with abstinence (Brady, Killeen, Saladin, Dansky, & Becker, 1994; Kofoed, Friedman, & Peck, 1993). Treatment outcomes for patients with PTSD and substance abuse are worse than for other dual-diagnosis patients and for patients with substance abuse alone (Ouimette, Ahrens, Moos, & Finney, 1998; Ouimette, Finney, Gima, & Moos, 1999). People with both disorders suffer greater rates of a variety of interpersonal and medical problems, including domestic violence (Dansky et al., 1999). Various subgroups have high rates of this dual diagnosis, especially combat veterans (Bremner et al., 1996, Davis & Wood,1999).

Family Violence and Post-traumatic Stress Disorder

Family violence and PTSD are clearly linked. Orcutt, King, and King (2003) have examined the effects of early-life stressors, war-zone stressors, and PTSD symptom severity on partners' reports of recent male-perpetrated intimate partner violence among 376 Vietnam veteran couples. The results indicated that several factors are directly associated with family violence, including relationship quality among the spouses, war-zone experiences of stress, and PTSD symptom severity. Experiencing PTSD symptoms as a result of previous trauma appears to increase an individual's risk for perpetrating family violence. Risk for partner violence is considerably greater among veterans with PTSD when both low marital satisfaction and alcohol abuse are present (Fonseca et al., 2006; Taft et al., 2005).

Deployment-related stress increased the rate of child maltreatment (Rentz et al., 2007). However, this study lacked the family-level deployment data that would have allowed the researchers to definitively identify if, within a family with a deployed member, the deployment was a cause of child maltreatment. In addition, for the reported statistics, nonmilitary caretakers perpetrated the largest proportion of substantiated maltreatment in military families. Therefore, although rates of child maltreatment prior to high deployment were lower than civilian counterparts, rates did increase with increased rates of deployment, but a direct causal relationship cannot be inferred. In another large study of families of enlisted Army soldiers, rates of substantiated child maltreatment were greater during combat-related deployment of the soldier parent and were primarily due to the civilian parents abuse of the child (Gibbs, Martin, Kupper, & Johnson, 2007). These two studies did not examine whether a previous pattern of child maltreatment was exacerbated by deployment. In two different studies of violence after deployment among Army soldiers, however, deployment was not a significant predictor of family violence (McCarroll et al., 2003; Newby et al., 2005). Both studies indicated that younger couples with previous history of domestic violence were at greater risk for postdeployment family violence.

Secondary Traumatization and Post-traumatic Stress Disorder

The effects of PTSD are not limited to the traumatized persons. Spouses of the injured persons seem particularly susceptible to a phenomenon called *secondary traumatization* (Dirkzwager, Bramsen, Ader, & van der Ploeg, 2005). Secondary traumatization has only recently been described and is not yet a diagnostic category in the *Diagnostic and Statistical Manual of Mental Disorders,* Fourth Edition, Text Revision (DSM-IV-TR; American Psychiatric Association, 2000). A study of Dutch Peacekeeping soldiers and their families (Dirkzwager et al., 2005), found that partners of peacekeepers with PTSD symptoms reported more sleeping and somatic problems, more negative social support, and judged the marital relationship as less favorable. Another study in Israel found that spouses of veterans with PTSD suffered from greater levels of emotional distress and a lower level of marital adjustment than the general population (Dekel, Solomon, & Bleich, 2005). In a qualitative study with wives of Israeli veterans with PTSD, Dekel, Goldblatt, Keidar, Solomon, and Polliack (2005) note that the wives were carrying a heavy burden supporting and caring for their husbands and families. In their review of the literature on secondary trauma in the United States, Galovski and Lyons (2004) identify that veterans' numbing and hyperarousal symptoms are especially predictive of family distress. Partners of veterans with combat-related PTSD experience significant levels of emotional distress (Manguno-Mire et al., 2007). The phenomenon of secondary traumatization makes using a family approach to nursing care for families experiencing wartime separation and reunion all the more critical. The effects on children need to be researched.

FAMILY NURSING PRACTICE INTERVENTIONS

The acute problems that families experience after disaster versus wartime separation and reunion are similar, yet the experience is quite different. In both situations, families are traumatized by their experiences. During disasters, most or all of the family members are at risk for experiencing trauma and injury from the widespread destruction and chaos created by the disaster. During wartime, most families in the United States are not directly traumatized

by the war experience, but rather experience the secondary trauma of living with a war veteran. In both situations, families are faced with members who have PTSD, have a tendency toward substance abuse, and are at increased risk for family violence. Because the specific trauma experience of a family living through a disaster versus a family living with a war veteran is different, however, this section presents nursing care for these families separately.

Family Nursing Care for Acute Problems After Disaster

Nurses help families and their communities prepare for and recover from disaster. How nurses help families and the community will differ depending on the phase of the disaster, which is the topic of this section.

PHASES OF A DISASTER

Disasters are unexpected events that influence families' lives. There are three phases of a disaster: (1) before the impact, (2) during the impact, and (3) after the impact. Each phase of the disaster causes different problems and requires different responses from the family. The preimpact phase is before the disaster occurs, and includes planning and preparedness. The impact phase starts when the disaster occurs and rescue efforts begin. The postimpact phase includes the recovery after the disaster (Veenema, 2007). Table 18-2 outlines the family responsibility and nursing interventions in the case of a disaster.

TABLE 18-2
Family Responsibilities and Nursing Interventions in a Disaster

PHASE OF DISASTER	RESPONSIBILITIES	NURSING INTERVENTIONS
Before impact	*Prevention and preparedness* ▪ Proactive planning ▪ Monitoring events ▪ Warnings	Emergency kits: personal, family, community Emergency plans: personal, family, workplace, community Disaster drills: personal, family, workplace, community Red Cross classes Register with county or state Disaster Volunteer List

Continued

TABLE 18-2

Family Responsibilities and Nursing Interventions in a Disaster—cont'd

PHASE OF DISASTER	RESPONSIBILITIES	NURSING INTERVENTIONS
Impact	*Response to the disaster*	Respond according to the emergency plan
	▪ Rescue	
	▪ Triage	When volunteering: arrive only when asked and assist as needed
	▪ Treat	
	▪ Shelters set up	
After impact	*Recovery*	Rebuilding
	▪ Stabilization	Repairing infrastructure
	▪ Reconstruction	Relocation efforts
	▪ Rehabilitation	Mental health interventions
	Evaluate	Future disaster planning
	▪ Review disaster action plans	Modify and practice disaster drills
	▪ Adapt plans to accommodate findings	

Source: Adapted from Veenema, T. G. (2007). Essentials of disaster planning. In T. G. Veenema (Ed.), *Disaster nursing and emergency preparedness for chemical, biological, and radiological terrorism and other hazards* (2nd ed., pp. 3–18). New York: Springer, by permission.

Before Impact Disaster Family Interventions

Events such as the September 11, 2001, terrorist attacks and Hurricane Katrina in 2005, have led to an increased awareness of the need to be prepared for disasters. Being prepared for disasters helps families to survive and cope. According to the International Council of Nurses (2006), preparedness is essential to the delivery of health care responses to the affected population. Preparedness starts with each individual and the family. Every nurse should be personally prepared with a family disaster kit and an emergency plan. This advance preparation will help the nurse be available to help other families get their disaster kits prepared before disaster occurs.

If a disaster occurs and the damage is widespread, rescue personnel and equipment will be limited. It is recommended by FEMA and the American Red Cross that everyone be prepared to "shelter in place," meaning be able to survive where they are for at least 72 hours, or 3 days, after which rescue should be able to reach all affected areas. Refer to Box 18-3 for a list of items in a family disaster kit.

One of the most important items to have available is enough water for every member of the family, both human and pets. There should be at least 1 gallon of water per person per day, and a half gallon of water for each pet per day. Water needs to be stored in clean, thick plastic containers that have

never been used for anything else. Other sources of water that could be used in emergencies are the water heater or toilet tank, but it should be purified with either water purification tablets or a water purification filter system. Other liquids such as boxed juices or canned milk should be added to the kit.

Families with children who have diabetes or other chronic illnesses need to prepare for emergencies and disasters. Children with chronic illnesses should wear or carry medical alert identification so that if the child cannot answer the rescuers' questions, information about his or her condition is available (Stallwood, 2006).

Food items in the kit need to be nonperishable items that can be eaten cold if there is no heating source. Salt content of foods should be a concern for those members of the family on salt restriction, but also because salty foods increase thirst and water intake. Peanut butter is a good source of protein.

Flashlights and lanterns are necessary light sources when no electricity is available. The batteries in items in the disaster kit should be changed every 6 months, and extra batteries should also be kept in the kit. Newer flashlights with kinetic hand-crank capabilities are helpful, so less need of batteries exists. Portable radios will be needed to obtain current information on the disaster and relief efforts, as well as weather conditions. Hand-crank

BOX 18-3

Family Disaster Kit

The family disaster kit needs to contain a 3-day supply of the following items:

WATER
- 1 gallon of water per person per day

FOOD
- Canned
  - Low-sodium foods
  - Foods that could be eaten cold
  - Foods children will eat
- Crackers
- Peanut butter
- Other fluids: juice boxes, canned milk

PETS
- Food for at least 3 days
- ½ gallon water per pet per day
- Litter box supplies for cats
- Traveling cage or box
- Copy of latest vaccinations, ID numbers
- Leash or chain

PERSONAL PAPERS: KEEP IN A WATERTIGHT CONTAINER
- Insurance: health, homeowners, car
- Copies of car or professional licenses

- Health information for each family member, including a list of medication names and daily dose for each family member
- Contact list: phone numbers and e-mail addresses for family contacts
- Out-of-state contact number for the family

NONFOOD ITEMS
- Medications: 2-week supply of all essential medications for each family member
- Money
- Light source: crank or battery operated
- Radio: crank or battery operated
- Batteries for battery-operated items
- Games and activities for all members of family
- Set of clothes, shoes for each member of family, including hats and gloves
- Nonelectric can opener
- Blankets
- Toilet paper
- First-aid kit

Source: Adapted from the American Red Cross (2007a), Federal Emergency Management Administration (2007b), and Ready America (2007), by permission.

---

radios are available, including ones that can recharge cell phones.

It is useful to have access to personal information that is kept in a central place such as a disaster kit. Copies of insurance policies or policy numbers of homeowner's, health, and car insurance policies are important. Copies of driver's or nursing licenses could be helpful when purse or wallets are lost or inaccessible. Contact information including phone numbers and e-mail addresses may help, especially if phone information is lost. All papers should be in watertight containers. External memory devices, such as thumb drives with password capabilities, could be used to store electronic information when security concerns exist.

Pets should be considered when building a disaster kit. Food and water, as well as vessels to allow pets to eat and drink, are essential. Carrying cages for smaller animals need to be accessible. Vaccination records are important, especially if the family is being evacuated to a shelter that allows animals.

Keep a leash or chain in the kit to keep the pet safe and with the family.

In addition to disaster kits, emergency plans are important for families to develop and practice. All members of the family must be involved in planning and carrying out the plan. Fire drills should be rehearsed two or three times a year so that all members of the family are comfortable knowing the escape routes and their roles. Box 18-4 provides the steps for making a family emergency plan.

Emergency contacts are essential to have during times of disaster. Families need to designate an emergency contact person who is in near proximity to the family so they can assist in times when the family phone service is not working. An out-of-state contact is necessary when local phone service might be damaged and only long-distance service is available. Designating one person to be the out-of-state contact allows information from multiple family members to be shared with other family members who will be concerned.

BOX 18-4
Family Emergency Plan

1. Develop an emergency plan. Answer the following questions:
   - What natural disasters could occur where you live?
   - What will you do for each type of disaster?
     - Fire
     - Earthquake
     - Tornado
     - Hurricane
   - What emergency exits might you need to use to evacuate the house?
   - Where will you meet if you have to evacuate the house?
   - How will you make sure each family member is safe? Know how to shut off the water and utilities to the house.
2. Practice your plan with your family.
   - Does each member of the family know the plan?
   - Plan drills with the family.
   - Walk through the drills and evacuation routes.
3. Have a map of the surrounding area.
   - Mark the closest fire stations and hospitals.
   - Mark areas where you will meet if you need to leave the immediate area.
   - Identify other safe places to go, such as shelters.
4. Arrange for someone to be an emergency contact.
   - Make sure all family members know the emergency contact person and phone number.
   - Have an in-the-area contact and an out-of-state contact.
5. Obtain an information sticker to go at the front of the house that shows how many people and how many pets reside in the house.

Source: Adapted from the American Red Cross (2007a), Federal Emergency Management Administration (2007b), and Ready America (2009), by permission.

It is important for nurses to be as prepared as possible for all types of disasters, whether it is a terrorist attack or a natural disaster. The victims will be adults, children, and infants of all ages and sizes. A national survey showed that first responders and emergency departments (EDs) were not as prepared for child and infant victims. Disaster drills rarely use children as mock victims (Timm & Reeves, 2007). EDs have minimal child-sized personal protective equipment on stock (Martin, Bush, & Lynch, 2006). Responders must be prepared for both adult and pediatric emergencies that occur in disasters.

Impact Disaster Interventions

Impact is the moment the disaster strikes. The most important aspect of impact interventions is safety for everyone involved. During the initial impact phase, damage may occur to buildings and property, making them unsafe to stay in or to enter to rescue others. Often, the initial impulse of the lay rescuer is to rescue as many people as possible, but it is important to take time to evaluate the situation and determine that the area is safe to enter. Professional rescuers will be arriving who are trained in safe rescue techniques. Classes are available at the city and state levels that teach rescue techniques.

Postimpact Disaster Interventions

Most interventions will take place during the postimpact phase of the disaster. The Red Cross offers courses to prepare individuals to manage shelter operations. Nursing students can take these courses to prepare them to volunteer in shelters and hospitals after a disaster. In shelters, the first priority is to follow the chain of command established in the rescue shelter. Families in the shelter will be looking to the nurses to provide guidance on how the shelter is set up, and how they may get situated to become more comfortable. Nurses must use the therapeutic communication skills of active listening and validation of feelings to provide necessary emotional and spiritual support. It is not appropriate to offer advice to family survivors; the goal is to ask what you can do to help or to guide families through problem solving. Of utmost importance is to provide basic physical needs such as shelter, first aid, food, and water. Once these basic needs are met, the psychosocial and spiritual needs of disaster victims must be the focus of nursing care. Self-disclosure is not an appropriate nursing intervention at this time. Assess for risk factors, such as increased family or individual stress, PTSD, or other health problems.

When working with children in a disaster situation, remember that the coping strategies for children vary by age and developmental stage (Starr, 2002). Teach parents how to provide reassurance for children infant to 3 years of age. Children of this age will mirror their parents' emotions. Coach parents and adults to use phrases such as, "I will keep you safe." Encourage parents to be factual with school-aged and adolescent children, but not to be brutally factual or tell all they know. Encourage parents to give children a role in helping the family to reestablish routines and rituals.

Getting families back to normal roles and routines is essential for family coping (Wells, 2006). Normal family routines, such as bedtime routines, add familiarity to new situations or surroundings, especially if the family or child is in a shelter. Routines, such as returning to school, help reinforce that the situation is returning to normal, as well as increase social support for older children (Gaffney, 2008; National Child Traumatic Stress Network, 2005). Because disaster coverage is usually conducted 24 hours per day 7 days per week and is inundated with repeated images that may frighten or cause the child to relive the traumatic experience, it is important to limit children's television viewing (Jordan, Hersey, McDivitt, & Heitzler, 2006). Children who watch television for long periods after a disaster have demonstrated increased stress (Kennedy, Charlesworth, & Chen, 2004).

Families who have a child with a disability are especially vulnerable because rescuers may not have the resources to handle the child's medical equipment or even remember to gather their specialized equipment. During the postimpact phase of the disaster, a family member with a disability needs to be taken into consideration when placing the family in a shelter or temporary housing.

Nurses can use their knowledge of growth and development to encourage children to express their feelings about the disaster in drawings or play. When children experience stress, they may need to repeat the details of the disaster over and over in their drawings or simulate the disaster again and again as they try to process their feelings about the disaster. Adolescents, especially teenagers, feel better if they are allowed to help in some way because this provides them control. The American Academy of Child and Adolescent Psychiatry (2003) suggests that honesty and listening to children are important interventions. Allowing children to express their feelings helps them to start coping with their disaster experience. False reassurances, not allowing the child to talk about the disaster, or allowing the child to focus only on the positives disrupt the healing process.

Adults benefit from talking about their disaster story. Providing the adult with a list of available resources has been known to help decrease stress. Working to decrease stresses starting during the impact phase of the disaster has been shown to decrease the possibilities of acute stress responses and PTSD (Hoffpauir & Woodruff, 2008).

The following section presents a case study of the Green family that illustrates nursing interventions in response to acute problems caused by a natural disaster.

Family Case Study: The Impact of Disaster

This case study addresses family nursing care after a disaster, focusing primarily on the acute problems the family will experience during and immediately after a natural disaster.

SETTING: The Greens live in the suburbs of a large metropolitan area. It is the middle of winter, with an average temperature of 39 degrees Fahrenheit. It is often windy with a wind chill factor of 32 degrees Fahrenheit. Figure 18-1 illustrates the Green family genogram.

FAMILY MEMBERS: The Green family is a multigenerational nuclear family with the maternal grandmother living with the family. The Green family genogram provides a pictorial representation of the family (see Figure 18-1).

+ Sam, 47 years, husband and father, is a long-distance trucker who has just been laid off. He is worried about the family finances, because his 18-wheeler truck payment stretches the Green's budget and is due next week. He has been drinking more and more as a result of this stress. He is often short tempered with his kids and his wife. He has been out interviewing for a new job and is considering the possibility of a menial labor job just to make ends meet.

+ Anne, 43 years old, a wife and mother, is an ED registered nurse at a trauma-designated hospital in the downtown area. She travels 15 miles to

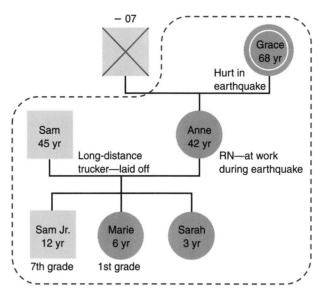

FIGURE 18-1 Green family genogram.

work and has to cross the large river that bisects the city. She works 7 a.m. to 7 p.m. three days a week.

✦ Grace, 68 years old, Anne's mother, is a widow of one year. She came to live with the Greens after her husband died. She cares all day for the youngest child and for the older children after school, which allows Sam and Anne to work.

✦ Sam Jr., the oldest child, is 12 years old. He is in the seventh grade at a school 3 miles away from the house. He rides the school bus every day.

✦ Marie, the middle child, is 6 years old. She normally goes to first grade in the elementary school, which is two blocks from the house, but she is home sick with a cold.

✦ Sarah, the youngest child, is 3 years old and stays at home with her grandmother Grace.

FAMILY STORY

At 10:20 a.m., a 6.0 earthquake hits the outer edge of the metropolitan area. There is massive destruction of buildings at the epicenter, with moderate damage to property in the area where the Greens live. Power lines are down, trees are blocking all roads in the area, the trauma center hospital has suffered moderate damage in some of the clinics, but the generators are functioning and the ED has only minor damage, mostly to the supply rooms. There is minor-to-moderate damage

to the bridges crossing over the river, all of which are older than 20 years.

Anne is not hurt, and is trying to call home on her cell phone to see if everyone is safe. She cannot leave the hospital because casualties are starting to arrive and word is passed through the ED that the bridges have been damaged and are unsafe for travel. Sam was four blocks from home after an interview when the earthquake started. The road to the house is blocked by multiple downed trees. He starts walking home. Grace's back is strained when a large bookcase falls and knocks her to the ground. She is experiencing increased pain and struggles to get to the girls. The girls were napping in their room and are not injured, just scared. Sam Jr. is at school. The school has only minor damage, and the staff immediately initiates emergency procedures for the disaster. Emergency policy announces on the radio emergency broadcast that children will not be released from school until it is safe; then they can go home by school bus or leave if a parent picks the child up.

Sam returns home with some difficulty, aftershocks are occurring frequently, and he has to dodge falling tree limbs and telephone poles. Grace has the girls with her in the hallway where there are no windows. Shortly after Sam arrives home, firemen pound on the door and tell Sam they have to evacuate the house and area immediately because of a gas main break.

They have no time to gather anything and are directed by the firemen to go to the elementary school a half mile away where a temporary shelter is being set up. Sam shows up at the shelter with Grace, who is in extreme pain, and the two girls, Marie and Sarah, who has wet herself. Sam Jr. is still at the middle school, and Anne is across town at the hospital. Cell phones are not working because the cell phone towers collapsed.

The nursing assessment and interventions for the Green family are presented using the concepts of Family Systems Theory. For more information on Family Systems Theory, see Chapter 3. Figure 18-2 depicts the ecomap developed by the nurse working with the Green family.

NURSING GOAL: The nursing goals are to work with the Green family in the shelter, and to meet the family's immediate needs and assist with obtaining resources for the family to use when they are finally allowed to go home.

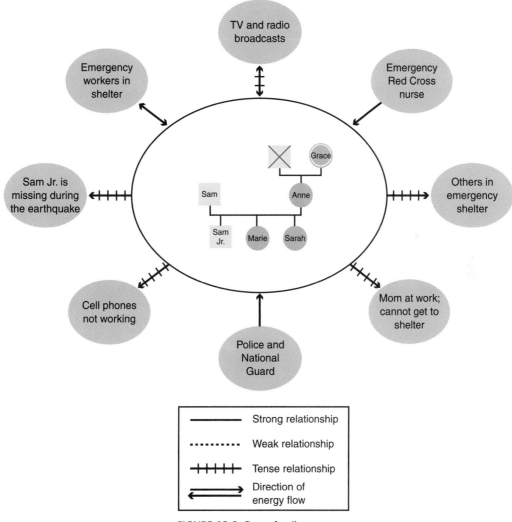

FIGURE 18-2 Green family ecomap.

FAMILY SYSTEMS THEORETICAL PERSPECTIVE

Concept 1: All Parts of the Family System are Interconnected

In a disaster, all family members may be directly affected, some more than others, if the family is not all in the same location during the time of the event. The more severe the trauma an individual family member suffers from the disaster event, the more likely the other members of the family are to suffer secondary traumatization. The children, Marie and Sarah, in addition to being frightened, have witnessed Grace being severely injured. The family is separated because Anne cannot get back to the family, and this puts more stress on Sam as the only available parent. Sam Jr. is at the middle school and can not be released until a parent can pick him up.

Concept 2: The Whole is More than the Sum of its Parts

The family response to trauma of one or more of its members from war or disaster cannot be understood or treated by focusing on individual family members alone. Trauma is the key experience that affects the family system in a disaster. The threat or fear of death or serious injury is a salient feature of this trauma. Grace's injury is producing additional stress in the family. Treating her pain and stabilizing her condition will do more than just assist her, it should also calm and allay Marie's and Sarah's fears, and decrease the stress on Sam.

Concept 3: All Systems have Boundaries Between the System and its Environment

The Green family has boundaries or borders between itself and the environment that are now disrupted. Because these boundaries or borders may both be protective and act as a barrier to seeking help, they need to be considered when planning interventions. For example, Anne is not with the family in the shelter, so there may be things the children look to her for that they now need from their father. Sam may be feeling overwhelmed, yet may view others' attempts to help as intrusive. At the same time, Grace is hurt and would ordinarily turn to Anne for help but cannot.

Other boundaries will affect the family. Their home is damaged; their city is destroyed. These losses will be overwhelming. However, disaster preparedness strategies enacted by the community before the event will help decrease stress on the family. For example, prepositioned medical supplies in the shelter can be used to treat Grace's injury. Sam may be able to obtain a change of clothes for his daughter who has wet herself. Food and water will be available to provide further comfort.

Concept 4: Systems can be Further Organized into Subsystems

The child-parent relationship for this family includes the child-grandparent relationship as well. Understood in this context, it makes it all the more imperative that Grace's roles and responsibilities be taken over for the children's sake. They will want to ensure that Grace is comfortable and will be taken care of; this might need to be addressed before Sam, Marie, and Sarah can deal with their own needs.

ASSESSMENT AND INTERVENTION CONSIDERATIONS

Assessment

Drawing on Family Systems Theory, the nurse should explore the family structure, roles, and relationships. Initially, this could be done casually in conversation, while also determining the Greens' physical and emotional needs. Grace has known medical needs, and Marie's cold will need to be monitored. Sarah has immediate hygiene requirements that necessitate clean clothes. Sam has not been able to call Anne on her cell phone and is getting increasingly worried about Sam Jr. All are tired and hungry.

Intervention

After meeting immediate needs, perform other assessments to determine future requirements. Anne will not be coming home until transportation is restored over the river, possibly weeks. Sam Jr. is reunited with the family at the shelter, and Sam, Grace, and the kids are allowed to return home after 3 days. Information obtained while in the shelter will assist Sam in determining which organizations he might go to for help.

Family Care for Chronic Problems: Disaster and War

This section covers how to assess and intervene when PTSD or secondary traumatization are complicating the recovery of a family from a disaster or wartime separation and reunion experience.

POST-TRAUMATIC STRESS DISORDER ASSESSMENT AND INTERVENTION

PTSD can develop after a traumatic event such as war or disaster. A PTSD diagnosis requires certain conditions to exist. The person must have been exposed to a traumatic event. They must experience intense feelings of fear, helplessness, or horror. They must re-experience the event through flashbacks, dreams, or disturbing memories. They will avoid any stimuli associated with the event, avoiding any reminders, thoughts, or feelings about the event. The person may be hypervigilant, having difficulties falling or staying asleep, or have an exaggerated startle response. The symptoms must have lasted longer than 1 month and must cause significant distress or impairment in functioning (National Center for PTSD, 2000). Nurses need to assess for the following risk factors and provide families with strategies for coping (Friedman, 2006).

- Suicide risk: because of positive association between numbing from trauma events and a possible suicide attempt
- Danger to others: ask about firearms or weapons, aggressive intentions, feelings of persecution
- Ongoing stressors: such as changes that have occurred at home in their absence, marital discord, problems at work
- Risky behaviors: such as risky sexual adventures, nonadherence to medical treatment, substance use and misuse
- Personal characteristics: trauma history, coping skills, relationship attachment
- Social support: can be limited by the individual's willingness to accept help and inclination to isolate
- Comorbidity: coexisting psychiatric or medical problems such as depression and chronic widespread pain (CWP)

The best evidence-based nursing treatments for the individual with PTSD include both psychotherapeutic interventions, such as cognitive behavioral therapy, and medications, such as selective serotonin inhibitors (Friedman, 2006). Partner and family engagement in PTSD treatment has been shown to improve the treatment outcomes. Predictors of partner engagement include higher income, patient-partner involvement, and lower partner caregiver burden (Sautter et al., 2006). Attention to child family members is also important.

SECONDARY FAMILY TRAUMATIZATION ASSESSMENT AND INTERVENTION

To help the traumatized family, the nurse should first realize that traumatized families rarely seek family-focused intervention. Instead, they often present with problems that are not immediately related to the traumatic events they have experienced (Figley & Barnes, 2005). Nurses should learn the parallel processes of individual and systemic stress reactions that follow a traumatic event. Figley and Barnes (2005), in their book *Families and Change: Coping with Stressful Events,* present a guide to help clinicians recognize family responses to traumatic events and what they can do to help patients and families affected by these events. The following guidelines are taken from this work.

Recognizing Secondary Trauma

For every PTSD criterion, the family members have corresponding symptoms. See the DSM-IV-TR list of symptoms (see Box 18-2). Under Criterion A: History of Trauma, families are affected by the soldier's symptoms of PTSD. They know the story of the trauma, witnessed the symptoms, and want to help in some way. As a result, the family spends more and more time caring for the traumatized member. For Criterion B: Intrusive Recollection, while the traumatic event is being persistently re-experienced by the exposed family member, the other family members are responding to the individual's increased demands for support as they struggle with recurring recollections, bad dreams, or responses to cues that resemble an aspect of the event. With Criterion C: Avoidant/Numbing, as the primary affected family member tries to avoid stimuli that remind him or her of the trauma, the other family members must devote increased time, energy, and problem solving to avoiding conversations, people, places, and things that might stimulate memories. They must tolerate the withdrawal and numbing that goes along with the primary affected family member's diminished interest in their usual activities, refusals to see old friends, and inability to express love and caring. As they help their family member with PTSD try to avoid triggers, and they put up with an unwillingness to go places and do former activities, the family becomes increasingly more isolated. Criterion D: Hyperarousal results in the other family members having to manage problems with sleep, outbursts of anger, exaggerated startle responses, and hypervigilance about safety. The family must now take on the unpleasant task of managing outbursts of anger. The secondary traumatization is considered acute if the duration is less than 3 months, chronic if the duration is 3 months or longer, and delayed if the onset is at least 6 months after the stressor.

Systems Theory Approach to Secondary Trauma

The nurse working with a traumatized family needs to explore each family member's perception of what happened both before and after the event (Figley & Barnes, 2005). The nurse needs to recognize that the family's worldview will have been altered by the traumatizing event, and that the family's attitudes and beliefs will shift to a focus on safety that may result in suspicious, distrustful attribution regarding the motivations of others. Hypervigilance and control behaviors may actually interfere with the family getting the help it needs. In addition, if the stressors impinging on the family go unattended, a pattern of triangulation and blaming may become the central family dynamic. Also, the roles in the family may shift, with some members becoming more enmeshed with the traumatized member, whereas others withdraw from the family system. One of the children may have to take on the role of emotional caretaker for the parents, and thus be compelled to hide his or her own feelings and fears, whereas other siblings act out to express anger and get parental attention. Most emerging trauma treatment has as its main shortcoming the focus on the individual rather than the family system. The following case study is used to illustrate how the broader view can help the nurse plan more effective care for traumatized families.

Family Case Study: Effect of War

This case study addresses family nursing care with the Caldwell family after surgery on a male veteran experiencing profound PTSD symptoms. This case study focuses primarily on the chronic problems that follow from his wartime exposure to trauma, and the family's struggle to deal with his PTSD and their own symptoms of secondary trauma.

SETTING: Inpatient acute care hospital surgical unit in a large metropolitan area.

FAMILY MEMBERS:
- Mr. Caldwell, father, 47 years old, fireman, Iraqi war veteran
- Mrs. Caldwell, mother, 46 years old, stay-at-home mother
- Kira, daughter, 16 years old, high-school student
- John, son, 14 years old, middle-school student

FAMILY STORY

Mr. Caldwell, a 47-year-old National Guard soldier, is in the hospital for a hernia repair. About 2 years ago he returned home from a 12-month deployment to Iraq, where he had his first exposure to combat in his 18 years of National Guard duty. Before deployment, he worked successfully as a fireman paramedic and was a happily married father with two children. He and his wife were socially outgoing with a large circle of friends from the same rural area in which they both grew up. They have been married since high school. A genogram and ecomap for the Caldwell family is provided in Figures 18-3 and 18-4, respectively.

While in Iraq recently, Mr. Caldwell has had extensive exposure to other soldiers' combat injuries as the noncommissioned officer in charge of the battlefield medical aide station in Baghdad. His unit treated the severe, crippling injuries of soldiers en route to the trauma hospital. The aide station was often overrun with multiple casualties, often resulting in death or injury to those brought to them for care. He treated soldiers from patrols and convoys in which improvised exploding devices destroyed vehicles and wounded or killed people with whom he had become close. Although he did not have to kill enemy combatants, he agonized that he may also have been responsible for the deaths of some soldiers because he simply did not have enough men or resources to treat all of the casualties

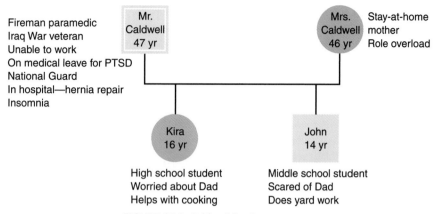

Fireman paramedic
Iraq War veteran
Unable to work
On medical leave for PTSD
National Guard
In hospital—hernia repair
Insomnia

Mr. Caldwell 47 yr

Mrs. Caldwell 46 yr

Stay-at-home mother
Role overload

Kira 16 yr

High school student
Worried about Dad
Helps with cooking

John 14 yr

Middle school student
Scared of Dad
Does yard work

FIGURE 18-3 Caldwell family genogram.

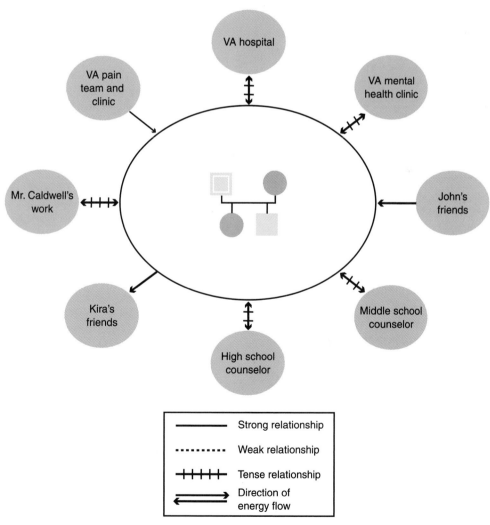

FIGURE 18-4 Caldwell family ecomap.

adequately. When asked about the worst moment during his deployment, he readily stated that it was when he was unable to intercede when a Humvee with a bleeding soldier draped over the hood and several wounded soldiers in the back drove by the aide station; the driver's view was blocked by blood gushing on the windshield and the driver could not see him waving the Humvee to safety. Mr. Caldwell never found out what happened to the soldiers, and this vision haunted him.

When he first returned home, things seemed to return to normal. But more than 2 years after coming home, he has had more and more difficulty relating to his wife. He reports feeling angry all the time, and that no one will listen to him. Sleep has become difficult. He has to sleep on the recliner in the living room because his back hurts so badly that he cannot lay flat. When he does sleep, he has a recurring, vivid nightmare about turning a corner outside of a building in Baghdad where he encounters an insurgent with a rifle who shoots him. His daughter complains that he has become so overprotective that he will not let her go out with any friends, much less any boys. His wife reports that he has been emotionally distant since his return.

His employer, who initially supported him, has reported that his work at the fire department has suffered dramatically. During a recent burning motor vehicle extradition drill, one of the car's tires exploded. The unexpected explosion rattled him so much that he became unable to go to work anymore. Mr. Caldwell says that since his deployment he no longer has an identity; he cannot work, and he no longer feels like he can fulfill his obligations as a husband and a father. He reports that he sometimes experiences strong surges of anger, panic, guilt, and despair, and that at other times he has felt emotionally dead, unable to return the love and warmth of family and friends. He does not want to get a divorce, but fears this will happen. Although he has not been actively suicidal, he reports that he sometimes thinks everyone would be better off if he had not survived his tour in Iraq. He is currently on a number of medications for back pain from his on-the-job injury at the fire department. He is reporting a lot of postoperative pain.

This composite case illustrates several kinds of war-zone stressors. Mr. Caldwell felt helpless to prevent several deaths. In addition to that feeling of helplessness, he had to witness the horror of many people dying and had to respond to emergencies on an unpredictable basis. Nurses who are taking care of patients who have had a difficult return to civilian life need to be aware of the complicated nature of readjustment. As this case illustrates, the prevalence of PTSD may increase considerably during the 2 years after veterans have returned from combat duty (Wolfe, Erickson, Sharkansky, King, & King, 1999).

The care for this family, when delivered from a Family Systems Theory perspective, will need to address Mr. Caldwell's PTSD, as well as the family's ever increasing secondary traumatization from his stress responses.

NURSING GOAL: Using a family systems theoretical approach, plan care for Mr. Caldwell that includes referral for his PTSD, and provides the family with education and resources about what they can do to address their own secondary trauma, as well as support his recovery.

THEORETICAL PERSPECTIVE

Concept 1: All Parts of the Family System are Interconnected

Because Mr. Caldwell has been traumatized by his experience with war, ultimately all of his family members and family relationships are affected. Mr. Caldwell's war experience was his alone, but his wife is being affected by the symptoms he is experiencing, symptoms that will get worse as she takes on even more of a caregiving role after his surgery. The children are baffled by the changes in their father and do not quite know what to do. Because their mom is so involved with caring for him, they do not feel like they can go to her with their problems. In addition to their parents not being available to them emotionally, both children have had to take on family roles that their parents used to manage. For example, Kira now must do more of the family meal preparation and house cleaning. The son, John, has to do all of the yard work, which has made it harder to spend time with his friends. Both teenagers are not doing as well in school because of the constant tension in the home and their fears that their parents may divorce. Because Mr. Caldwell's trauma is so severe, it is highly likely the other members of the family will suffer secondary traumatization.

Concept 2: The Whole is More than the Sum of its Parts

This family's response to the trauma of Mr. Caldwell from war cannot be understood or treated by focusing on just his care. PTSD can occur months or even years after a disaster or traumatic event such as war. In this case, Mr. Caldwell's PTSD is getting worse, not better, over time. His family members can provide key contextual information about past traumatic events and experiences that can explain current responses. In fact, they are a central and key reason why Mr. Caldwell wants to get better and resume more of his leadership roles within the family. As he has been spiraling downward, the rest of the family has followed, and all now report deteriorating mental health.

Concept 3: All Systems have Boundaries Between the System and its Environment

Boundaries or borders between the system and its environment may be protective and may act as a barrier to seeking help. It could be that Mrs. Caldwell feels it is disloyal to talk about her husband's problems with an outsider. Mr. Caldwell has many fears about admitting his difficulties and feels ashamed about how his problems have affected his wife. Mrs. Caldwell is afraid to ask for help because she does not want her husband to feel any more embarrassment than he does already. They are both suffering in silence, reluctant to talk to each other, or to anyone else. The nurse will have to create a trust relationship to overcome this natural reluctance to share family secrets. One of the things that may help is to explain how providing this information may enhance the medical team's ability to provide quality care.

Concept 4: Systems can be Further Organized into Subsystems

In this case, the spousal relationship has suffered because of Mr. Caldwell's trauma. Wartime separation and reunion, and then later problems with PTSD from combat, have created some marital dysfunction that was not there before. In this situation, the marital relationship as a subset within this family is the most problematic area. By helping the family improve this one area of family functioning through appropriate referral, the nurse could create a beneficial effect on the rest of the family subsystems. Because this is a new experience for Mr. and Mrs. Caldwell, they are not quite sure how to deal with it, plus they are reluctant to seek outside help at this time.

POST TRAUMATIC STRESS DISORDER AND SECONDARY TRAUMA: ASSESSMENT AND INTERVENTION

Why is it important for the nurse to be aware of trauma and PTSD in the health care setting? As clearly seen from this case, although Mr. Caldwell's traumatic exposure occurred some time ago, undiagnosed or inadequately treated PTSD could complicate his surgical recovery. PTSD is associated with more physical health problems and somatic symptom severity (Hoge et al., 2007). Although CWP, defined as pain in various parts of the body and fatigue that lasts for 3 months or longer, has thus far been documented only in veterans from the first Gulf war, the potential for this phenomenon to emerge in current combat veterans is high. CWP is associated with greater health care utilization and a lower quality of life (Forman-Hoffman et al., 2007). Recently, researchers working for the Veterans Administration documented that a substantial percentage of Iraqi and Afghanistan war veterans experience ongoing or new pain, of which 28% report is severe (Gironda, Clark, Massengale, & Walker, 2006).

In this instance, after surgery, Mr. Caldwell may be having more problems with pain perception, pain tolerance, and other kinds of untreated chronic pain. In addition, PTSD symptoms may make it difficult for the nurse to communicate with the patient, reduce the patient's active collaboration in evaluation and treatment, and reduce patient adherence to medical regimens.

Assessment

Recognize PTSD and secondary trauma. Because traumatization is under-recognized, patients with PTSD are not properly identified and are not offered education, counseling, or referrals for mental-health evaluation. Identify a simple screening method to screen your patients who may have undetected PTSD. One easy-to-use tool is the Primary Care PTSD Screen (Prins et al., 2004), which is posted on the National Center for Posttruamatic Stress DisorderWeb site (http://www.ncptsd.va.gov/ncmain/ncdocs/fact_shts/fs_screen_disaster.html). The tool consists of four questions proceeded by the following introduction: "In your life, have you ever had any experience that was so frightening, horrible, or upsetting that, in the past month, you... (1) Have had nightmares about it or thought about it when you did not want to? (2) Tried hard not to think about it or went out of your way to avoid situations that reminded you of it? (3) Were constantly on guard, watchful, or easily startled? (4) Felt numb or detached from others, activities, or your surroundings?" (p. 11). The screen is positive if the patient answers yes to any three items.

Next, assess the family for possible symptoms of secondary traumatization. How are Mr. Caldwell's wife and children responding to his symptoms? What symptoms are they experiencing as a result of his difficulties? Identify how roles might have shifted for this family given Mr. Caldwell's current circumstances. Is the family still functioning as a strong cohesive unit? How have things changed? How open is this family to working with the nurse? What might help facilitate this?

Intervention

Provide education about PTSD and secondary trauma. Because the family's participation is essential in identifying symptoms of PTSD and planning treatment, the nurse must create an environment that is supportive and inclusive of family members to work in partnership with the family. Several sites on the Internet can help the nurse develop educational fact sheets that can be shared with patients and families. The Veterans Affairs National Center for PTSD and the Defense Department's Walter Reed Army Medical Center collaborated to develop the Iraq War Clinician Guide (available online at: http://www.ncptsd.va.gov/ncmain/ncdocs/manuals/nc_manual_iwcguide.html). The guide provides several tools such as practice guides for treatment of PTSD, as well as background information about substance abuse, grief, and the effect of deployment on the family.

The next step that the nurse should take in intervening with the Caldwell family is referring them for further care. Set up a plan for referring to a PTSD specialist those patients who show signs of potential PTSD and who are amenable to receiving additional evaluation or counseling. In this instance, the nurse could provide the family with a list of possible options. Many local areas have lists of returning veteran's counseling services that do include counseling for couples and families. Involve the family in the plan of follow-up care.

SUMMARY

A Family Systems Theory perspective is useful for nurses when assessing and intervening with individuals and families during times of disaster and war. This particular theoretical lens to view family reactions to disasters and war suggests solutions and options for care and intervention that differ from what the nurse might do if focused on only the individual patient. For example, planning and personal preparedness were identified as important factors in reducing the stress of disasters, though we might not necessarily think of this kind of intervention if we were concerned with providing only individual emergency care.

One major family response to both disasters and wartime separation and reunion is PTSD. PTSD was identified as a risk factor in both children and adults that could occur months, even years after an event. PTSD has been associated with a host of other potential medical and psychological comorbidities such as chronic pain, substance abuse, and depression. For veterans suffering from PTSD, the importance of treating the family, rather than focusing only on the veteran, was illustrated through the Caldwell case study.

Both case studies illustrate how the family response to trauma of one or more of its members from war or disaster cannot be understood or treated by focusing on individual family members alone. For example, in the Green family case study if the nurse only focused on the grandmother or only on the father, the recovery of the family as a unit would have been delayed or not been achieved at the same level as when the family is the client of care. Secondary traumatization, though a common family response to a member with PTSD, is rarely recognized by health professionals. Because families suffering from secondary traumatization rarely seek help for this condition, this chapter highlights how important it is to use a family lens when treating individuals for PTSD. Partnering with families is key to helping the individual with PTSD, because family boundaries may otherwise act as a barrier to seeking help.

Further research is needed to develop good assessment tools for identifying secondary trauma. This phenomenon has only recently been identified in the PTSD body of literature. It is not yet part of the DSM-IV-TR, and screening tools for its identification have not yet been developed. Until the screening and assessment work is further refined, nurses can use what they know about PTSD to help them identify this phenomenon in families. This chapter provides some suggested guidelines on how the symptoms of secondary trauma might manifest in family members of those suffering from PTSD.

Natural disasters and wars have been a part of human history on Earth from the beginning of recorded history. It is important that nurses who work with people during these events, understand what happens to individuals and families during wartime and natural disasters, and be prepared to support and intervene wherever they may be.

REFERENCES

Adams, R. E., & Boscarino, J. A. (2006). Predictors of PTSD and delayed PTSD after disaster: The impact of exposure and psychosocial resources. *The Journal of Nervous and Mental Disease, 194*(7), 485–493.

Amaratunga, C. A., & O'Sullivan, T. L. (2006). In the path of disasters: Psychosocial issues for preparedness, response, and recovery. *Prehospital and Disaster Medicine, 21*(3), 149–153.

American Academy of Child and Adolescent Psychiatry. (2003, February). *Talking to children about terrorism and war.* Retrieved January 23, 2008, from http://aacap.org/cs/root/facts_for_families/talking_to_children_about_terrorism_and_war

American Academy of Child and Adolescent Psychiatry. (2004, July). *Helping children after a disaster.* Retrieved January 23, 2008, from http://aacap.org/page.ww?name=Helping+Children+After+a+Disaster&section=Facts+for+Families

American Psychiatric Association. (2000). *Diagnostic and statistical manual of mental disorders: DSM-IV-TR* (4th ed., text revision). Washington, DC: American Psychiatric Association.

American Red Cross. (2001). *Helping young children cope with trauma.* Retrieved January 23, 2008, from http://www.redcross.org/services/disaster/keepsafe/childtrauma.html

American Red Cross. (2007a). *Disaster supplies kit.* Retrieved June 24, 2008, from http://www.redcross.org/services/disaster/0,1082,0_3_,00.html

American Red Cross. (2007b). *Your family disaster plan.* Retrieved June 24, 2008, from http://www.redcross.org/services/disaster/beprepared/fdpall.pdf

Benotsch, E. G., Brailey, K., Vasterling, J. J., Uddo, M., Constans, J. I., & Sutker, P. B. (2000). War zone stress, personal and environmental resources, and PTSD symptoms in Gulf War veterans: A longitudinal perspective. *Journal of Abnormal Psychology, 109*, 205–213.

Black, D. W., Carney, C. P., Forman-Hoffman, V. L., Letuchy, E., Peloso, P., Woolson, R. F., et al. (2004). Depression in veterans of the first Gulf War and comparable military controls. *Annals of Clinical Psychiatry, 16*(2), 53–56.

Brady, K. T., Killeen, T., Saladin, M. E., Dansky, B., & Becker, S. (1994). Comorbid substance abuse and posttraumatic stress disorder: Characteristics of women in treatment. *American Journal of Addictions, 3*, 160–164.

Bremner, J. D., Southwick, S. M., Darnell, A., & Charney, D. S. (1996). Chronic PTSD in Vietnam combat veterans: Course of illness and substance abuse. *American Journal of Psychiatry, 153*, 369–375.

Broughton, D. D., Allen, E. E., Hannemann, R. E., & Petrikin, J. E. (2006). Getting 5000 families back together: reuniting fractured families after a disaster: The role of the National Center of Missing & Exploited Children. *Pediatrics, 117*(5), S442–S445.

Cook, J. M., Riggs, D. S., Thompson, R., Coyne, J. C., & Sheikh, J. I. (2004). Posttraumatic stress disorder and current relationship functioning among World War II Ex-Prisoners of War. *Journal of Family Psychology, 18*(1), 36–45.

Cozza, S. J., Chun, R. S., & Polo, J. A. (2005). Military families and children during operation Iraqi Freedom. *Psychiatric Quarterly, 76*(4), 371–378.

Dansky, B. S., Byrne, C. A., & Brady, K. T. (1999). Intimate violence and post-traumatic stress disorder among individuals with cocaine dependence. *American Journal of Drug and Alcohol Abuse, 25*, 257–268.

Davis, T. M., & Wood, P. S. (1999). Substance abuse and sexual trauma in a female veteran population. *Journal of Substance Abuse Treatment, 16*, 123–127.

Dekel, R., Goldblatt, H., Keidar, M., Solomon, Z., & Polliack, M. (2005). Being a wife of a veteran with posttraumatic stress disorder. *Family Relations, 54*(1), 24–36.

Dekel, R., Solomon, Z., & Bleich, A. (2005). "Emotional distress and marital adjustment of caregivers: Contribution of level of impairment and appraised burden": Erratum. *Anxiety, Stress & Coping: An International Journal, 18*(2), 157–159.

Dirkzwager, A. J., Bramsen, I., Ader, H., & van der Ploeg, H. M. (2005). Secondary traumatization in partners and parents of Dutch peacekeeping soldiers. *Journal of Family Psychology, 19*(2), 217–226.

Eisenman, D. P., Cordasco, K. M., Asch, S., Golden, J. F., & Glik, D. (2007). Disaster planning and risk communication with vulnerable communities: Lessons from hurricane Katrina. *American Journal of Public Health, 97*(S1), s109–s115.

Evans, L., McHugh, T., Hopwood, M., & Watt, C. (2003). Chronic posttraumatic stress disorder and family functioning of Vietnam veterans and their partners. *Australian and New Zealand Journal of Psychiatry, 37*(6), 765–772.

Federal Emergency Management Administration. (2007a). *Basic disaster supplies.* Retrieved June 23, 2008, from http://www.fema.gov/plan/prepare/basickit.shtm

Federal Emergency Management Administration. (2007b). *Plan for emergencies.* Retrieved June 23, 2008, from http://www.fema.gov/plan/prepare/plan.shtm

Fiedler, N., Ozakinci, G., Hallman, W., Wartenberg, D., Brewer, N. T., Barrett, D. H., et al. (2006). Military deployment to the Gulf War as a risk factor for psychiatric illness among US troops. *British Journal of Psychiatry, 188*(5), 453–459.

Figley, C. R., & Barnes, M. (2005). External trauma and families. In P. C. McKenry & S. J. Price (Eds.), *Families and change: Coping with stressful events and transitions* (3rd ed., pp. 379–399). Thousand Oaks, CA: Sage Publications.

Fonseca, C. A., Schmaling, K. B., Stoever, C., Gutierrez, C., Blume, A. W., & Russell, M. L. (2006). Variables associated with intimate partner violence in a deploying military sample. *Military Medicine, 171*(7), 627–631.

Forman-Hoffman, V. L., Peloso, P. M., Black, D. W., Woolson, R. F., Letuchy, E. M., & Doebbeling, B. N. (2007). Chronic widespread pain in veterans of the first Gulf War: Impact of deployment status and associated health effects. *Journal of Pain, 8*(12), 954–961.

Friedman, M. J. (2006). Posttraumatic stress disorder among military returnees from Afghanistan and Iraq. *Am J Psychiatry, 163*, 586–593.

Gaffney, D. A. (2008). Families, schools, and disaster: The mental health consequences of catastrophic events. *Family and Community Health, 31*(1), 44–53.

Galovski, T., & Lyons, J. A. (2004). Psychological sequelae of combat violence: A review of the impact of PTSD on the veteran's family and possible interventions. *Aggression and Violent Behavior, 9*(5), 477–501.

Gibbs, D. A., Martin, S. L., Kupper, L. L., & Johnson, R. E. (2007). Child maltreatment in enlisted soldiers' families during combat-related deployments. *JAMA: Journal of the American Medical Association, 298*(5), 528–535.

Gironda, R. J., Clark, M. E., Massengale, J. P., & Walker, R. L. (2006). Pain among veterans of operations enduring freedom and Iraqi freedom. *Pain Medicine, 7*(4), 339–343.

Glauber, B. (2007, March 2). Experts tackle suicide prevention among combat veterans: Doctors, social workers here join VA's drive for awareness. *JSOnline.* Retrieved from http://www.jsonline.com/story/index.aspx?id=572352

Gnauck, K. A., Nufer, K. E., Lavalley, J. M., Crandall, C. S., Craig, F. W., & Wilson-Ramirez, G. B. (2007). Do pediatric and adult disaster victims differ? A descriptive analysis of clinical encounters from four natural disaster DMAT deployments. *Prehospital and Disaster Medicine, 22*(1), 67–73.

Goff, B. S., Crow, J. R., Reisbig, A. M., & Hamilton, S. (2007). The impact of individual trauma symptoms of deployed soldiers on relationship satisfaction. *Journal of Family Psychology, 21*(3), 344–353.

Gold, J. I., Taft, C. T., Keehn, M. G., King, D. W., King, L. A., & Samper, R. E. (2007). PTSD symptom severity and family adjustment among female Vietnam veterans. *Military Psychology, 19*(2), 71–81.

Gray, M. J., Bolton, E. E., & Litz, B. T. (2004). A longitudinal analysis of PTSD symptom course: Delayed-onset PTSD in Somalia peacekeepers. *Journal of Consulting and Clinical Psychology, 72*(5), 909–913.

Hagan, J. F., & The Committee of Psychosocial Aspects of Child and Family Health and the Task Force on Terrorism. (2005). Psychosocial implications of disaster or terrorism on children: A guide for the pediatrician [Electronic version]. *Pediatrics, 116*(3), 787–795.

Hamblen, J. (2007, May 22). *PTSD in children and adolescents.* Retrieved March 14, 2008, from National Center for Posttraumatic Stress Disorder Web site: http://www.ncptsd.va.gov/ncmain/ncdocs/fact_shts/fs_children.html

Hill, R. (1949). *Families under stress: Adjustment to the crisis of war separation and reunion.* New York: Harper and Brothers.

Hobfoll, S. E. (1989). Conservation of resources: A new attempt at conceptualizing stress. *American Psychologist, 44,* 513–524.

Hoffpauir, S. A., & Woodruff, L. A. (2008). Effective mental health response to catastrophic events: Lessons learned from hurricane Katrina. *Family and Community Health, 31*(1), 17–22.

Hoge, C. W., Auchterlonie, J. L., & Milliken, C. S. (2006). Mental health problems, use of mental health services, and attrition from military service after returning from deployment to Iraq or Afghanistan. *JAMA: Journal of the American Medical Association, 295*(9), 1023–1032.

Hoge, C. W., Castro, C. A., Messer, S. C., McGurk, D., Cotting, D. I., & Koffman, R. L. (2004). Combat duty in Iraq and Afghanistan, mental health problems, and barriers to care. *New England Journal of Medicine, 351,* 13–22.

Hoge, C. W., McGurk, D., Thomas, J., Cox, A. L., Engel, C. C., & Castro, C. A. (2008). Mild traumatic brain injury in U.S. soldiers returning from Iraq. *New England Journal of Medicine, 358*(5), 453–463.

Hoge, C. W., Terhakopian, A., Castro, C. A., Messer, S. C., & Engel, C. C. (2007). Association of posttraumatic stress disorder with somatic symptoms, health care visits, and absenteeism among Iraq War veterans. *American Journal of Psychiatry, 164*(1), 150–153.

Hotopf, M., Hull, L., Fear, N. T., Browne, T., Horn, O., Iversen, A., et al. (2006). The health of UK military personnel who deployed to the 2003 Iraq war: A cohort study. *Lancet, 367*(9524), 1731–1741.

International Council of Nurses. (2006). *Nurses and disaster preparedness position statement.* Retrieved January 15, 2008, from http://www.icn.ch/psdisasterprep01.htm

International Federation of Red Cross and Red Crescent Societies. (2007). World disasters report 2007: Disaster data. *World Disasters Report.* Retrieved February 28, 2008, from http://www.ifrc.org/Docs/pubs/disasters/wdr2007/WDR2007-English.pdf

International Strategy for Disaster Reduction. (2006, July). *Disaster statistics.* Retrieved January 23, 2008, from United Nations International Strategy for Disaster Reduction Web site: http://www.unisdr.org/disaster-statistics/introduction.htm

Jordan, A. B., Hersey, J. C., McDivitt, J. A., & Heitzler, C. D. (2006). Reducing children's television-viewing time: A qualitative study of parents and their children. *Pediatrics, 118*(5), 1303–1310.

Kelley, M. L. (1994). The effects of military-induced separation on family factors and child behavior. *American Journal of Orthopsychiatry, 64*(1), 103–111.

Kennedy, C., Charlesworth, A., & Chen, J. (2004). Disaster at a distance: Impact of 9.11.01 televised news coverage on mothers' and children's health. *Journal of Pediatric Nursing, 19*(5), 329–339.

Kessler, R. C., Sonnega, A., Bromet, E., Hughes, M., & Nelson, C. B. (1995). Posttraumatic stress disorder in the National Comorbidity Survey. *Archives of General Psychiatry, 52,* 1048–1060.

Kilic, E. Z., Ozguven, H. D., & Sayil, I. (2003). The psychological effects of parental mental health on children experiencing disaster: The experience of Bolu earthquake in Turkey. *Family Process, 42*(4), 485–495.

Knapp, T. S., & Newman, S. J. (1993). Variables related to the psychological well-being of Army wives during the stress of an extended military separation. *Military Medicine, 158,* 77–80.

Kofoed, L. Friedman, M. J., & Peck, R. (1993). Alcoholism and drug abuse in inpatients with PTSD. *Psychiatric Quarterly, 64,* 151–171.

Kohn, R., Levav, I., Garcia, I. D., Machuca, M. E., & Tamashiro, R. (2005). Prevalence, risk factors and aging vulnerability for psychopathology following a natural disaster in a developing country. *International Journal of Geriatric Psychiatry, 20,* 835–841.

Kuehn. B. M. (2009). Soldier suicide rates continue to rise: Military, scientists work to stem the tide. *JAMA. 301*(11), 1111–1113.

Kulka, R. A., Schlenger, W. E., Fairbank, J. A., Hough, R. L., Jordan, B. K., Marmar, C. R., et al. (1990). *Trauma and the Vietnam War generation: Report of findings from the National Vietnam Veterans Readjustment Study.* New York: Brunner/Mazel.

Langeland, W., & Hartgers, C. (1998). Child sexual and physical abuse and alcoholism: A review. *Journal of Studies on Alcohol, 59,* 336–348.

Machel, G. (1996). Impact of armed conflict on children. Report of the expert of the Secretary-General, Ms. Graça Machel, submitted pursuant to General Assembly resolution 48/157. Retrieved June 18, 2008, from UNICEF Web site: http://www.unicef.org/graca

Mangelsdorff, D. A., & Moses, G. R. (1993). A survey of Army medical department reserve personnel mobilized in support of Operation Desert Strom. *Military Medicine, 158,* 254–258.

Manguno-Mire, G., Sautter, F., Lyons, J., Myers, L., Perry, D., Sherman, M., et al. (2007). Psychological distress and burden among female partners of combat veterans with PTSD. *Journal of Nervous and Mental Disease, 195*(2), 144–151.

Martin, S. D., Bush, A. C., & Lynch, J. A. (2006). A national survey of terrorism preparedness training among pediatric, family practice, and emergency medicine programs [Electronic version]. *Pediatrics, 118*(3), e620–e626.

McCarroll, J. E., Ursano, R. J., Newby, J. H., Liu, X., Fullerton, C. S., Norwood, A. E., et al. (2003). Domestic violence and deployment in US Army soldiers. *Journal of Nervous and Mental Disease, 191*(1), 3–9.

Meagher, I. (2007, March 11). *The war list: OEF/OIF statistics.* Retrieved July 23, 2008, from http://scoop.epluribusmedia.org/story/2007/3/12/03718/4139

Najavits, L. M., Weiss, R. D., Shaw, S. R., & Muenz, L. R. (1998). "Seeking safety": Outcome of a new cognitive-behavioral psychotherapy for women with posttraumatic stress disorder and substance dependence. *Journal of Traumatic Stress, 11*(3), 437–456.

National Center for Children Exposed to Violence. (2006, April). *Statistics.* Retrieved January 23, 2008, from http://www.nccev.org/resources/statistics.html

National Center for PTSD. (2000). *Effects of traumatic stress after mass violence, terror or disaster.* Retrieved March 14, 2008, from http://www.ncptsd.va.gov/ncmain/ncdocs/fact_shts/fs_effects_disaster.html

National Child Traumatic Stress Network. (2005). *The effects of trauma on schools and learning.* Retrieved March 4, 2008, from http://www.nctsnet.org/nccts/nav.do?pid=ctr_aud_schl_effects

National Mental Health Information Center. (2005, September). *Tips for talking to children after a disaster: A guide for parents and teachers.* Retrieved February 18, 2008, from Substance Abuse and Mental Health Services Administration Web site: http://mentalhealth.samhsa.gov/cmhs/katrina/parent_teach.asp

National Severe Storms Laboratory. (2007). *Annual Disaster/Death Statistics for United States Storms.* Retrieved June 9, 2008, from http://www.wind.ttu.edu

Nelson, J., & Hagedorn, M. E. (1997). Federal Nursing Service Award. Rhythms of war: Activation experiences during the Persian Gulf War. *Military Medicine, 162*(4), 233–239.

Newby, J. H., Ursano, R. J., McCarroll, J. E., Liu, X., Fullerton, C. S., & Norwood, A. E. (2005). Postdeployment domestic violence by U.S. Army soldiers. *Military Medicine, 170*(8), 643–647.

Nice, D. S. (1981). The course of depressive affect in Navy wives during family separation. *Military Medicine, 148,* 341–343.

Nice, D. S., Hilton, S., & Malone, T. A. (1994). Perceptions of U. S. Navy Medical Reservists recalled for Operation Desert Storm. *Military Medicine, 159,* 64–67.

Norris, F. H. (2007, May 22). Psychosocial consequences of natural disasters in developing countries: What does past research tell us about the potential effects of the 2004 tsunami? Retrieved January 27, 2008, from National Center for Posttraumatic Stress Disorders Web site: http://www.ncptsd.va.gov/ncmain/ncdocs/fact_shts/fs_tsunami_research.html

Orcutt, H. K., King, L. A., & King, D. W. (2003). Male-perpetrated violence among Vietnam veteran couples: Relationships with veteran's early life characteristics, trauma history, and PTSD symptomatology. *Journal of Traumatic Stress, 16*(4), 381–390.

Ouimette, P. C., & Ahrens, C., Moos, R. H., & Finney, J. W. (1998, November/December). During treatment changes in substance abuse patients with posttraumatic stress disorder. The influence of specific interventions and program environments. *Journal of Substance Abuse Treatment, 15*(6), 555–564.

Ouimette, P. C., Finney, J. W., Gima, K., & Moos, R. H. (1999). A comparative evaluation of substance abuse treatment III. Examining mechanisms underlying patient-treatment matching hypotheses for 12-step and cognitive-behavioral treatments for substance abuse. *Alcoholism: Clinical & Experimental Research, 23*(3), 545–551.

Plum, K. C. (2007). Understanding the psychosocial impact of disasters. In T. Veenema (Ed.), *Disaster nursing and emergency preparedness* (2nd ed., pp. 81–94). New York: Springer.

Prins, A., Ouimette, P., Kimerling, R., Cameron, R. P., Hugelshofer, D. S., Shaw-Hegwer, J., Thrailkill, A., Gusman, F.D., Sheikh, J. I. (2004). The primary care PTSD screen (PC–PTSD): Development and operating characteristics. *Primary Care Psychiatry, 9,* 9–14.

Ready America. (2007). *Get a kit.* Retrieved April 16, 2008, from http://www.ready.gov/america/getakit/index.html

Ready America. (2009). *Make a plan.* Retrieved April 16, 2008, from http://www.ready.gov/america/makeaplan

Rentz, E. D., Marshall, S. W., Loomis, D., Casteel, C., Martin, S. L., & Gibbs, D. A. (2007). Effect of deployment on the occurrence of child maltreatment in military and nonmilitary families. *American Journal of Epidemiology, 165*(10), 1199–1206.

Rhoads, J., Pearman, T., & Rick, S. (2007). Clinical presentation and therapeutic interventions for posttraumatic stress disorder post-Katrina. *Archives of Psychiatric Nursing, 21*(5), 249–256.

Rosen, L. N., Teitelbaum, J. M., & Westhuis, D. J. (1993). Children's reactions to the Desert Storm deployment: Initial findings from a survey of Army families. *Military Medicine, 158,* 465–469.

Rosen, L. N., Westhuis, D. J., & Teitelbaum, J. M. (1994). Patterns of adaptation among Army wives during Operation Desert Shield and Desert Storm. *Military Medicine, 159,* 43–47.

Ryan-Wenger, N. A. (2001). Impact of the threat of war on children in military families. *American Journal of Orthopsychiatry, 71*(2), 236–244.

Ryan-Wenger, N. M. (1992). Physical and psychosocial impact of activation and deactivation of Army reserve nurses. *Military Medicine, 157,* 447–452.

Samper, R. E., Taft, C. T., King, D. W., & King, L. A. (2004). Posttraumatic stress disorder symptoms and parenting satisfaction among a national sample of male Vietnam veterans. *Journal of Traumatic Stress, 17*(4), 311–315.

Sanders, S., Bowie, S. L., & Bowie, Y. D. (2003). Lessons learned on forced relocation of older adults: The impact of hurricane Andrew on health, mental health, and social support of public housing residents. *Journal of Gerontological Social Work, 40*(4), 23–35.

Sautter, F., Lyons, J. A., Manguno-Mire, G., Perry, D., Han, X., Sherman, M., et al. (2006). Predictors of partner engagement in

PTSD treatment. *Journal of Psychopathology and Behavioral Assessment, 28*(2), 123–130.

Stallwood, L. G. (2006). Assessing emergency preparedness of families caring for young children with diabetes and other chronic illnesses. *Journal for Specialists in Pediatric Nursing, 11*(4), 227–233.

Starr, N. B. (2002). Helping children and families deal with the psychological aspects of disaster. *Journal of Pediatric Health Care, 16*(1), 36–39.

Stewart, S. H. (1996). Alcohol abuse in individuals exposed to trauma: A critical review. *Psychological Bulletin, 120,* 83–112.

Stewart, S. H., Conrod, P. J., Pihl, R. O., & Dongier, M. (1999). Relations between posttraumatic stress symptom dimensions and substance dependence in a community-recruited sample of substance abusing women. *Psychology of Addictive Behaviors, 13,* 78–88.

Substance Abuse and Mental Health Services Administration, Center for Mental Health Services, National Gains Center, & the Center on Women, Violence and Trauma. (2006). After the crisis: Healing from trauma after disaster. *Expert Panel Meeting,* 1–10. Retrieved January 23, 2008, from http://mentalhealth.samhsa.gov/nctic/trauma.asp

Taft, C. T., Pless, A. P., Stalans, L. J., Koenen, K. C., King, L. A., & King, D. W. (2005). Risk factors for partner violence among a national sample of combat veterans. *Journal of Consulting and Clinical Psychology, 73*(1), 151–159.

Timm, N., & Reeves, S. (2007). A mass casualty incident involving children and chemical decontamination. *Disaster Management and Response, 5,* 49–55.

Toomey, R., Kang, H. K., Karlinsky, J., Baker, D. G., Vasterling, J. J., Alpern, R., et al. (2007). Mental health of US Gulf War veterans 10 years after the war. *British Journal of Psychiatry, 190,* 385–393.

Triffleman, E. (1998). An overview of trauma exposure, posttraumatic stress disorder, and addictions. In H. R. Kranzler & B. J. Rounsaville (Eds.), *Dual diagnosis and treatment: Substance abuse and comorbid medical and psychiatric disorders* (pp. 263–316). New York: Marcel Dekker.

U.S. Bureau of the Census. (1992). *Statistical abstract of the United States: 1992* (112th ed.). Washington, DC: Author.

U.S. Deaths. (2008, April 9). *The Oregonian,* p. A9.

U.S. deaths and coalition casualties. (n.d.). Retrieved July 23, 2008, from http://www.cnn.com/SPECIALS/2003/iraq/forces/casualties

U.S. Department of Homeland Security. (2004, December). *Fact sheet: U.S. Department of Homeland Security 2004 year end review.* Retrieved January 21, 2008, from http://www.dhs.gov/xnews/releases/press_release_0578.shtm

Veenema, T. G. (2007). Essentials of disaster planning. In T. G. Veenema (Ed.), *Disaster nursing and emergency preparedness for chemical, biological, and radiological terrorism and other hazards* (2nd ed., pp. 3–18). New York: Springer.

Veenema, T. G., & Schroeder-Bruce, K. (2002). The aftermath of violence: Children, disaster, and posttraumatic stress disorder. *Journal of Pediatric Health Care, 16*(5), 235–244.

Vest, J. R., & Valadez, A. M. (2006). Health conditions and risk factors of sheltered persons displaced by hurricane Katrina. *Prehospital and Disaster Medicine, 21*(2), 55–58.

Vila, G., Witkowski, P., Tondini, M. C., Perez-Diaz, F., Mouren-Simeoni, M. C., & Jouvent, R. (2001). A study of posttraumatic disorders in children who experienced an industrial disaster in the Briey region. *European Child and Adolescent Psychiatry, 10*(1), 10–18.

Vogt, D. S., Samper, R. E., King, D. W., King, L. A., & Martin, J. A. (2008). Deployment stressors and posttraumatic stress symptomatology: Comparing active duty and national guard/reserve personnel from Gulf war I. *Journal of Traumatic Stress, 21*(1), 66–74.

Wells, M. E. (2006). Psychotherapy for families in the aftermath of a disaster. *Journal of Clinical Psychology: In Session, 62*(8), 1017–1027.

Wolfe, J., Erickson, D. J., Sharkansky, E. J., King, D. W., & King, L. A. (1999). Course and predictors of posttraumatic stress disorder among Gulf War veterans: A prospective analysis. *Journal of Consulting Clinical Psychology, 67,* 520–528.

Wynd, C. A., & Dziedzicki, R. E. (1992). Heightened anxiety in Army reserve nurses anticipating mobilization during Operation Desert Strom. *Military Medicine, 157,* 630–634.

Young, B. H., Ford, J. D., & Watson, P. J. (2007). *Helping survivors in the wake of disaster.* Retrieved March 14, 2008, from National Center for Posttraumatic Stress Disorder Web site: http://www.ncptsd.va.gov/ncmain/ncdocs/fact_shts/fs_helping_survivors.html

CHAPTER WEB SITES

- *American Red Cross:* http://www.redcross.org
- *Helping young children cope with trauma:* http://Alaksa.redcross.org/media/1303en.pdf
- *American Association of Pediatricians*—offers advice on communicating with children about disasters: http://www.aap.org/disasters/pdf/youngest-victims-final.pdf
- *American Academy of Child and Adolescent Psychiatry*—helps children after a disaster plus links to facts for families: http://www.aacap.org/publications/factsfam/disaster.htm
- *National Center for Posttraumatic Stress Disorder*—lists resources for disasters and war: http://www.ncptsd.va.gov/ncmain/index.jsp
- *National Mental Health of America*—Coping with Disaster: Tips for Adults: http://www.nmha.org/reassurance/adulttips.cfm
- *Mental Health America*—Helping Children Handle Disaster-Related Anxiety: http://www.nmha.org/reassurance/children.cfm
- *Green Cross the Academy of Traumatology*—is an international, nonprofit humanitarian assistance organization comprised of trained traumatologists and compassion fatigue service providers: http://www.figleyinstitute.com/documents/gcatflyer.pdf

4

Looking to the Future

CHAPTER 19

Advancing Family Nursing

Joanna Rowe Kaakinen, PhD, RN

CRITICAL CONCEPTS

✦ In today's world, family nursing is without borders.

✦ Family nurses cannot be complacent with the current status of family health and family nursing; they need to be politically and actively involved in bringing about changes.

✦ Without health care reform, family-centered care will continue to be lost in systems that were built to address individual, acute care health needs.

✦ Nursing must step to the forefront and become actively involved in shaping health care reform locally, nationally, and globally.

✦ For family nursing practice to advance, it needs to move beyond patient-centered care to family-centered practice.

✦ It is imperative that nursing education require competency in family nursing.

✦ Family nursing practice should be theory-practice and practice-theory evidence based.

✦ Family nursing will continue to be influenced by the ability of nurses to maintain their commitment to family care.

Throughout the previous 18 chapters of this text, 37 family scholars have provided the current state of the science and practice of family nursing. These chapters are grounded in theory and evidence-based practice (EBP), illustrating the best practices of family nursing. Dr. Shirley Hanson's Foreword calls attention to the critical point that family nursing is a dynamic specialty in the discipline of nursing. Dr. Hanson notes that family nursing peaked in the United States and Canada in the 1980s and 1990s as it was valued and recognized as an important discipline area of nursing. Family nurses from other countries around the world are now contributing significantly to the science and practice of family nursing. Dr. Hanson eloquently states, "Today, it could be said that family nursing is without borders." Family nurses have much of which to be proud.

The earlier chapters in this book prove that family nursing is being practiced at a high level today. This does not mean, however, that family nurses can be complacent about the current status of family health care and family nursing. Serious worldwide problems threaten the health of families. The prime example is availability and access to health care by all people. This chapter is a call at both the national and the local levels for nurses in Canada and the United States to become more politically informed and active in health care issues. Family nurse educators are challenged to keep family nursing a central thread in curriculums and programs of study. This chapter seeks to stimulate thoughtful debate, discussion, and ideas about the future direction for family nursing. Despite these troubled times for family health care, family nurses are leading the practice arena through nurse-managed family health care initiatives, several of which are described in this chapter.

FUTURE NEEDS OF FAMILIES

Families remain the basic unit of society and have been that basic unit as long as families have been studied (Hanson, 2005a). One of the questions family scholars debate is the current status of families. One side of the argument takes the position that families are in "trouble," whereas the other side holds the position that families have always been "resilient." Clearly, the evidence offered in this book supports the view that families are resilient and are able to change their function, structure, and process to protect, care for, and buffer their family members from outside influences. Based on the family and health demographics presented in Chapter 2, families are becoming increasingly culturally diverse, and the gap between the wealth and poverty in the United States is ever widening. Webb (2005, pp. 110–102) predicts that, in the future, many families will immigrate to the United States, so these families and second-generation families will have the following characteristics:

- Experience severely limited economic growth and growth opportunities
- Be characterized by a semiextended family form made up of nonbiological kin
- More than likely live in households that speak two primary languages and have two generations
- Consist of people of color as a majority group
- Have social customs, beliefs, attitudes, and communication forms from cultures that researchers have not thoroughly studied
- Have some form of major involvement with governmental institutions (e.g., immigration, homeland security, criminal justice, public, welfare, and social services)

- Be stigmatized and misunderstood in part because the scientific community will fail to adapt their research and theories to understand these families

HEALTH CARE SYSTEM REFORM

Most of the focus for health care system reform has been on the access and financial burden for both individuals and the nation as a whole. This chapter examines the health care reform debate in the United States and in Canada, and outlines some of the challenges being faced.

Both Canada and the United States are in serious discussions about health care reform. Some suggest that Canada delivers better health care with its publically funded, single-payer health care system. Others believe that the U.S. multipayer system (private and public pay) offers more choice and availability of health care. Regardless of this debate, residents of both countries have not been satisfied with their health care system (Blendon et al., 2001).

Both countries have health disparities relative to race, income, and immigrant status (Lasser, Himmelstein, & Woolhandler, 2006). U.S. residents, on average, have higher incomes and greater relative poverty rates but are less healthy, with greater rates of obesity, physical inactivity, diabetes, hypertension, arthritis, and chronic pulmonary disease than Canadian residents (Lasser et al., 2006). However, the United States has higher 5-year survival rates for some cancers and greater low-birth-weight infant survival rates (O'Neill & O'Neill, 2008).

In the United States, unmet health needs arise primarily from financial barriers and limited access to care. The unmet Canadian health needs are from long wait times (O'Neill & O'Neill, 2008). Some studies have shown that U.S. residents have slightly higher unmet health care needs than the residents in Canada (Blendon et al., 2001; Donelan, Blendon, Schoen, Davis, & Binns, 1999; Lasser et al., 2006). In both countries, health care reform has become a priority. An unstated assumption is that if individuals can afford and access health care, families will benefit. Yet the increase in chronic, complex health care and costly institutional care has shifted more health care to families themselves. Without addressing reform in health care services, family-centered care will continue to be lost in health care systems that were built to address individual and acute care health needs.

United States Health Care System

The American health care system is "perennially in crisis yet seemingly impervious to comprehensive reform" (Oberlander, 2006, p. 245). Throughout the 20th century, the United States repeatedly failed to enact national health insurance. Of all the industrialized democracies, only Switzerland and the United States have health care systems that are primarily funded via personal out-of-pocket pay, employer-based health care, and private insurance (Oberlander, 2006). In the United States, the costs of health care continue to increase, as do the number of underinsured and uninsured. Most of the uninsured are working families who fall below the poverty line and are working in smaller businesses (Oberlander, 2006). Medical care is one of the major causes of personal bankruptcy in the United States (Oberlander, 2006). The United States has the highest paid providers (physicians) and the highest proportion of population without access to health insurance (Cutler, 2002).

It is important to understand that being insured does not mean that individuals are fairing well in the health care system (Havinghurst & Richman, 2006). Employers pass the cost of health insurance to the workers by having them pay more for their health insurance and increasing their copayments. Hourly earnings for employees have been stagnant in the last three decades because they have been forced to use their cost of living increases to cover their out-of-pocket medical copayments (Herman, 1999). Another cost to the financial health of the nation is the loss of workers who cut back on work to be an unpaid caregiver for a family member.

Increasingly, professional and national leaders are taking the political position that without government intervention toward a national tax-financed health insurance system, the numbers of uninsured and underinsured will continue to increase. Some sources predict that employer-based health insurance is ending (Brookings Institution, 2006), because health benefits continue to be one of the main issues in labor management disputes with employers transferring more of the health care costs on to the workers (Gottschalk, 2007). Fewer employees are providing health care insurance for family members. Fewer employers offer health plans to their workers, and an

increase is occurring in employers who are decreasing health care benefits to retired employees (Dixon, 2006). The Equal Employment Opportunities Commission (EEOC) supports the decrease in benefits to retired workers once they qualify for Medicare (Pear, 2004). Many large industries, such as United Airlines and General Motors, declared bankruptcy and dropped health benefits to their retired workers as a strategy to stabilize their financial status (Biddle, 2005). The fate of Medicare is largely unknown but is assumed to be tenuous.

What is the answer to these health care system problems? Many believe that the system is broken and needs to be changed entirely to a national health care system similar to the Canadian system. Problems with the Canadian system are presented next. Others believe that policy issues at the state level will provide solutions for access and availability of health care. The challenges are many. The American Hospital Association advanced the following framework to consider when designing a health care system that will improve the health of families (O'Donnell, Cox, Sharp, & Carroll, 2006).

- No child should be without health care.
- No American should become impoverished because of a major illness or injury.
- Every American deserves access to emergency medical services regardless of ability to pay.
- Poor and older Americans must be ensured continued access to high-quality hospital care. The United States must commit to adequate Medicare and Medicaid reimbursement for hospitals, physicians, and other providers (nurse practitioners). Congress must not reduce Medicare or Medicaid spending to reduce the federal deficit.
- Remove barriers to coordinating health care for all Americans, especially the chronically ill. America must commit to providing coverage for case management and other chronic care management services under all forms of insurance, not just managed care, and in doing so reduce the duplication and inefficiencies in care delivery.
- All Americans deserve high-quality health care. The United States must commit to supporting public and private partnerships for performance improvement and investing in information technologies that improve quality of care.

■ Every American should have access to important preventitive care services. The United States must commit to ensuring that critical preventitive services are available for every child and every adult through public and private sector initiatives.

■ The health care system needs to recognize mental health issues as valid and include full coverage for these health concerns.

Families will benefit from these recommendations for several reasons: (1) the cost of health care will limit using family assets to provide health care; (2) they meet the needs of individual family members throughout the health care continuum (promotion, prevention, emergency, acute, and chronic/end of life); and (3) families would be supported in accessing and coordinating services, and management of a complex health care system. The American Hospital Association recommendations reflect both public and private sector initiatives, whereas the Canadian health care system models a public sector approach.

Canadian Health Care System Reform

The Canadian health care system provides publicly funded, tax-supported coverage for almost all doctor, nurse, and hospital health care costs, which covers approximately 70% of the total cost of health care (Kenny & Chafe, 2007). The other 30% of care not covered publically is dealt with in the private sector, for example, podiatry, dentistry, and nonsurgical vision care (Kenny & Chafe, 2007). Similar to the United States, much of the delivery of care has shifted to outpatient clinics, homes, and communities. Recently, Canada has been involved in several initiatives to reform its health care system (Canadian Medical Association Task Force on the Public-Private Interface, 2006; Commission on the Future of Health Care in Canada, 2002). Some of the suggestions for reform include:

> [I]mproved information systems for patients and practitioners, development of a national human health resource plan, renewal and reform of primary care, expansion of public coverage to home care, and development of a national pharmaceutical strategy that includes public coverage for catastrophic out-of-hospital drug costs (Kenny & Chafe, 2007, p. 25).

Although the Canadian system started with a more publicly funded approach, it has expanded the discussion to include a combined funding approach: public and private. This debate has been based on the assumption that individuals have the right to some level of health and health care services. The debate of how to finance and provide these services is ongoing. Family nursing advocates need to examine initiatives from the family perspective.

Nursing Leadership in Health Care Reform

The American Nurses Association (ANA) issued a Health Policy Agenda (2005) that states that "health care is a right of all people." The ANA calls for health reform that focuses on primary preventitive care in the community and is not focused on just high-technology, hospital-based care.

Nursing and other health professionals must step to the forefront from a social justice perspective and become actively engaged in shaping health care reform locally, nationally, and globally (Feetham, 2005). Nurses are practicing in a more global health care arena given the number of families who are refugees, living in poverty, have diverse cultural and spiritual needs, and have been exposed to pandemics. One nurse has the power to influence hospital policy; several nurses have the power to influence local health policy. Many collective nursing voices can provide the power and guidance to help reform national health policy. A similar appeal to family nurses around the world was made by Suzanne Feetham during the 2005 International Family Nursing Conference (IFNC) in Victoria, Canada, and was echoed by several nurses during the 2007 IFNC in Bangkok, Thailand. Clearly, nurses have a role in health policy development and reform (Bogenschneider, 2000; Wakefield, 2004). Nurses can influence civic, religious, business, and legislative leaders across the world (Edlund, Lufkin, & Franklin, 2003).

The American Academy of Nursing (AAN) formulated a *Raise the Voice* campaign, which is a platform for nurses to make their new thinking in the health care debate heard in the public and political arenas (Bolton, 2006). The goals of this Raise the Voice campaign, as described by Bolton, (2006, p. 4) are as follows:

- Increase the visibility of nursing solutions that can fix a broken health care system.
- Provide policymakers and clinicians with nurse-developed models of care.
- Raise the level of nurse participation in discussions and deliberations focused on fixing the health care system.
- Address the nursing shortage.
- Close health disparities.
- Improve the quality of patient care.
- Address the health care needs of our aging population.

The AAN is showcasing the practice, research, and intervention programs that nurses have designed, implemented, and evaluated for improving health outcomes. The next section of this chapter presents several nurse-managed, family-centered care models.

Similarly, the Canadian Nurse Association (2008) has issued a call to all nurses to increase their own involvement in policy reform and to focus their policy work on the following three practical solutions to three critical issues that influence the quality of health care available in Canada:

- Sustaining Canada's publicly funded health system
- Reducing threats to health, particularly from environmental risks
- Recruiting and effectively deploying health professionals

It is clear that both U.S. and Canadian nursing organizations are encouraging nurses to become politically involved in health policy and system reform. Nurses have a place in policy development and need to heed this call.

FAMILY NURSING PRACTICE: FAMILY-CENTERED CARE

Family nursing practice needs to move beyond patient-centered care to family-centered practice if it is to advance as an art and science. Health is a family event. Health care is a function of the family. Health is learned in the family. Health is promoted in the family. When illness occurs in one member, it affects the whole family. When illness occurs, it is the family who provides the majority of care to the

ill family member across time. Health care providers serve as consultants to families by guiding their decision-making and treatment choices. Professionals cannot continue to use old paradigms that view health as individual autonomous decisions. Nurse and other health care professionals must practice family-centered care.

Nurses with advanced practice education have the leadership skills to design, implement, and evaluate multidisciplinary, community-centered models of care (Saxe, Janson, Dennehy, Stringari-Murray, Hirsch, & Waters, 2007). The nursing managed practice models in the following subsections have been found to improve health outcomes for patients and families. The three models presented in this section include Chronic Care Model (CCM), the Nurse-Partnership Program, and the Medical Home Model.

Chronic Care Model

The CCM was designed by Wagner, Bennett, Austin, Greene, Schaefer, and Vonkorff (2005). In the CCM, the patient and family self-manage their daily care with the health care providers as expert coaches. Shared decision making is one of the central tenets of the care approach. This model emphasizes interdisciplinary collaboration and communication with the patient and family as part of the team, with the goal of fostering continuity of care. The University of California San Francisco (UCSF) School of Nursing has been instrumental in establishing CCM pilot projects, which have demonstrated sustained positive changes for patients and families with diabetes type 2 (Janson, Kroon, & Baron, 2006), asthma, HIV, and cardiovascular disease (Dennehy et al., 2006; Landon et al., 2007; Piatt et al., 2006; Saxe, Jansen, Dennehy, Stringari-Murray, Hirsch & Waters, 2007). The goals of these CCM projects are to improve health, enhance access to care, positively influence self-management skills, decrease hospitalizations and emergency department visits, and increase satisfaction with health care. By working with families as client, these nurse-driven programs have improved patient health outcomes.

The Canadian British Columbia Ministry of Health (2006) proposes a chronic condition management model entitled the *Transitions Model of Palliative Care*. Because people are living longer with multiple comorbidities that require complex care needs, expanding pharmaceutical and treatment options that provide continuity of care is critical. Rather than using traditional models of palliative care in which referral occurs when death is expected, this newer Transition Model of Palliative Care can be applied when the patient's response to illness and needs are such that concepts involved in palliative care would help with this transition of trajectory of care. The goals would be to offer support for self-care, episodic disease management, and case management. Most people live an average of 4 years with the end-stage aspect of their disability before death; therefore, these individuals could benefit from the type of care offered in a transition model of palliative care (Lynn, Schuster, & Kabcenell, 2000), which makes this model a viable option. The family focus of this model is to extend palliative care to families and individuals sooner to enhance their quality of life. This approach works with families who are managing chronic illness.

Nurse-Family Partnerships

The Nurse-Family Partnerships (NFPs) are evidence-based programs aimed at improving the lives of at-risk, first-time mothers and their infants. NFP programs are in 23 states with 800 nurses serving 13,000 families (Dawly, Loch, & Bindrich, 2007). Nurses receive training in this program at program headquarters in Colorado. Nurses visit the families every 2 weeks from the 29th week of pregnancy until the child turns 2 years of age, except during the first month of the intervention and the first postpartum month when the nurses visit weekly. Each nurse has a caseload of about 25 families. Nurses work with the first-time mothers to encourage prenatal care, healthy nutrition, smoking and drug cessation, early infant development education, parenting skills, and development of a plan for self-sufficiency for the mother. The outcomes have shown a decrease in the rate of child abuse, child neglect, and injury in children, whereas increasing intervals between pregnancies, school readiness for the children, and maternal employment. The program has been shown to be cost-effective (Aos et al., 2004; Dawley, Lock, & Bindrich, 2007; Hill, Uris, & Bauer, 2007). It has been estimated that there is a $5.70 return for every dollar invested in the NFP (Karoly, Kilbum, & Cannon, 2005).

Medical Home Model

One of the Healthy People 2010 recommendations was the development of a *Medical Home Model of family-centered care* that offers continuous, coordinated care for children and families managing special health needs (Kelly, Kratz, Bielski, & Rinehart, 2002). These centers offer comprehensive integrative family services focused on preventitive care, early intervention, and developmental perspectives. The services help families coordinate care between home and school, access family counseling services, and handle insurance coverage issues for mental health services. A handful of these sites were developed, but few have been systematically evaluated (McMenamy & Perrin, 2004).

This brief synopsis of nurse-managed, family-centered practice models demonstrates that nursing is at the forefront of providing family health care. These practice models have proved that family-centered health care is cost-effective and can have long-term positive effects on health outcomes for all members of the family. These models offer evidence that nurses are leaders in family-centered practice.

FAMILY NURSING EDUCATION

Given the number of diverse and at-risk families, it is absolutely necessary that nursing education require competency in family nursing. Hanson (2005b) raises this issue during the IFNC in 2005 in Victoria, British Columbia, Canada. In the Foreword of this book, Hanson also calls attention to the pervasive dilution of family content within nursing curricula. With the documented increase in the number of families providing care for their members, it is a travesty that family nursing is relegated to a minimal focus in nursing curricula. As discussed in Chapter 1, the American Nurses Association Social Policy Statement (2003a) and the American Nurses Association Scope and Standards of Practice (2003b) call for family nursing to be a focus of care. Nonetheless, nursing education continues to dilute family content by integrating it throughout the curriculum of study instead of making family nursing a central aspect and foundation of nursing education. If nurse educators continue to focus competencies on individual patient care and community/public health systems of care, they are perpetuating the patient-centered care approach to health care instead of the much needed theory-guided, evidence-based, family-centered paradigm of nursing practice.

FAMILY NURSING EVIDENCE-BASED PRACTICE AND RESEARCH

In recent years, there has been a proliferation of family nursing literature and research. As such, many would posit that this research supports and validates EBP. In addition, nursing practice flows from theory. Therefore, nursing practice should be theory guided and evidence based. The reality, however, is that an inadequate transfer of family nursing theory to clinical practice occurs (Segaric & Hall, 2005).

The current movement of EBP is dominated by the Institute of Medicine, which has used the randomized clinic trial as the gold standard of science and emphasized the individual patient and not the family. The science of nursing uses descriptive studies as well, testing interventions for applicability across different situations. Nursing recognizes other ways of knowing than EBP. These ways of knowing include aesthetic knowing, symbolic knowing, personal or experiential knowing, and ethical knowing (Parker, 2006). Aesthetics involves synthesis and creativity of putting things together as a satisfying whole. A nurse's empathy is a part of the aesthetics of personal practice. Symbolic and interpretive knowing are understanding meanings expressed in rituals and the values indicated in gestures. Often this knowledge comes from immersion into situations to learn the meaning of the symbols. Knowing by experience, Patricia Benner's novice-to-expert concept (Benner, 1983), is knowledge learned as one practices. The knowing comes from having experienced a number of situations so that nurses' thinking progresses from thinking about each step of their actions to anticipating and acting intuitively based on the whole situation. Ethical knowing focuses on the "oughts" and "shoulds," that is, the moral obligations that as a discipline are perceived as a social mandate of serving families. In nursing practice, the ethical way of knowing requires an understanding of varying philosophical and ethical frameworks for evaluating what is right or good, or what ought to be done. Not all families, nor in fact

all nurses, use the same frameworks for deciding what is right or good. The current debate, interpretation, and ethic of EBP in nursing brings forward many of the following issues:

- Concern exists that EBP is widely considered to *be the truth*, thus dismissing or eliminating philosophical possibilities of other ways of knowing (Milton, 2007).
- The EBP approach to nursing is perceived by many as dehumanizing, marginalizing, and discounting the innumerable ways of knowing in nursing (Milton, 2007).
- From Parse's human becoming perspective, "Evidence in nursing practice is the humanly lived experiences and descriptions of value priorities of health and quality of life as seen through the eyes and lens of understanding of the person, family and community who are living it from moment to moment" (Milton, 2007, p. 125).
- The medical model of EBP leads one to believe that more science means nursing will automatically improve. Nursing is more than science, it is about relationships, and how the RN and patient view the condition and derive actions or interventions (Norberg, 2006).
- Nursing has such diverse ways of knowing, so adopting a medical model gives an illusion of credibility; therefore, nursing should consider a mixed methods approach (Flemming, 2007).
- Nursing should value priorities of health and quality of life as seen through the eyes and lens of understanding the person, family, and community who are living it from moment to moment (Milton, 2007, p. 125).

Medical EBP is dominating all health professions and nursing EBP, which is being developed all of the time through research, has more application to nursing with its many ways of knowing and focus on the whole patient and family.

A review of the nursing family literature revealed a paucity of EBP family nursing studies, and that few of these systematic reviews directly addressed family nursing. Box 19-1 lists these studies. Many of these studies were completed on small sample sizes, which makes it difficult to determine the strength of the summaries. The sources of EBP and national practice guidelines are listed in Box 19-2.

Using EBP in nursing will increase the likelihood of best outcomes. A systematic review of evidence

---

BOX 19-1

Evidence-Based Family Nursing Studies

1. Alverez, G., & Kirby, A. (2006). The perspective of families of the critically ill patient: Their needs. *Critical Care, 12*(6), 614–618.
2. *Breastfeeding and maternal and infant health outcomes in developed countries* [structured abstract, April 2007]. Rockville, MD: Agency for Healthcare Research and Quality. Abstract retrieved May 4, 2007, from http://www.ahrq.gov/clini/tp/brfoulttip.htm
3. Chambers, H. M., & Chan, F. Y. U. (1998). Support for women/families after perinatal death. *Cochrane Database of Systematic Reviews, 2,* CD000452.
4. Gage, J., Everett, K., & Bullock, L. (2006). Integrative review of parenting in nursing research. *Journal of Nursing Scholarship, 38*(1), 56–62.
5. Nibert, L., & Ondrejka, D. (2005). Family presence during pediatric resuscitation: An integrative review for evidenced-based practice. *Journal of Pediatric Nursing, 20*(2), 145–147.
6. *Perinatal depression: Prevalence, screening accuracy, and screening outcomes* [structured abstract, February 2005]. Rockville, MD: Agency for

Healthcare Research and Quality. Abstract retrieved May 4, 2007, from http://www.ahrq.gov/clinic.tp/perideptp.htm
7. Scott, J., Prictor, M. J., Harmsen, M., Broom, A., Entwistle, V., Sowden, A., et al. (2003). Interventions for improving communication with children and adolescents about a family member's cancer. *Cochrane Database of Systematic Reviews, 4,* CD004511.
8. Shields, L, Pratt, J., & Hunter, J. (2006). Family centered care: A review of qualitative studies. *Journal of Clinical Nursing, 17*(15), 1317-1323.
9. Stolz, P., Uden, G., & Willman, A. (2004). Support for family carers who care for an elderly person at home: A systematic literature review. *Scandinavian Journal of Caring Sciences, 18*(2), 111–119.
10. Van Horn, E., Fleury, J., & Moore, S. (2002). Family interventions during the trajectory of recovery from cardiac event: An integrative literature review. *Heart and Lung: Journal of Acute and Critical Care, 31*(3), 186–198.

---

demonstrates that there is a greater causal strength derived from using a body of research than a single study: The conclusions are more stable than results from a single research study (Stevens, 2004). The volume and complexity of science and technology is huge, and no one person can stay on top of it, so systematic reviews and other forms of meta-analysis reduce the complexity and volume into a single meaningful whole. EBP replaces research utilization because it is a complete paradigm, connecting research findings to practice, health care policy, and patient outcomes (Stevens, 2004). EBP was addressed

---

BOX 19-2

Sources of Evidence-Based Nursing Practice and National Practice Guidelines

- Cochrane Database of Systematic Reviews Web site has more than 1,500 topics; need subscription to access full-text reports: www.cochrane.org
- Agency for Healthcare Research and Quality (AHQR) Web site currently has 70 evidence reports or evidence summaries: www.ahrq.gov
- National Guideline Clearinghouse Web site has 1,500 clinical practice guidelines: www.guideline.gov
- Other guidelines can be found on the U.S. Preventative Services Task Forces segment of the AHQR
- U.K. National Institute for Clinical Excellence and National Collaborating Centre for Nursing and Supportive Care: London, England

- Registered Nurses Association of Ontario, Toronto, Canada
- New Zealand Guidelines Group: www.nzgg.org.nz
- Scottish Intercollegiate Guidelines Network, 28 Thistle Street, Edinburgh EH2 1EN, United Kingdom. Phone: 0131 718 5090. Fax: 0131 718 5114. E-mail: duncan.service@nhs.net. Web site: www.sign.ac.uk/guidelines/index.html
- National Institute for Clinical Excellence Web site: www.nice.org.uk
- Guidelines International Network Web site: www.g-i-n.net

as a Core Competency for Health Professionals in the U.S. Institute of Medicine 2003 report Priority Areas for National Action: Transforming Health Care Quality.

Given the clear benefits of EBP and the fact that nursing is a scientific discipline, the question remains why so much of nursing practice is not evidenced based in nature. The many obstacles to EBP in nursing include:

- The form of knowledge available in the literature often does not fit neatly into ways of knowing.
- Many nurses have a perceived lack of knowledge about research processes, hence they are intimidated by research (Cooke et al., 2004; Gerrish & Clayton, 2004).
- Nurses have a perception that they lack power or have limited authority to make changes in their practice settings (Cooke et al., 2004; Gerrish & Clayton, 2004).
- Nurses' access to research resources is inadequate and time consuming (Hockenberry, Wilson, & Barrera, 2006).
- Work environments provide little or no access to online search engines and online journals within the work setting (Hockenberry et al., 2006).
- A persistent belief that quantitative research is better than well-designed qualitative research eliminates many important nursing studies on newly defined concepts difficult to measure in a traditional quantitative design.
- Some EBP findings show that no particular approach to practice is better; thus, each approach studied has an equal effect. Therefore, nurses do not know which finding to incorporate into their practice (Pearson, Wiechula, Court, & Lockwood, 2007).
- The research question does not lend itself to cause-and-effect evidence; therefore, EBP research is the wrong approach to the question.

The next question is, What are the obstacles to family nursing EBP? Scholars of family nursing do not even agree on the definition of who is family, which creates difficulty when trying to conduct meta-analysis of practice. Research on family nursing is complex, because to understand family, it must be interpreted within context, culture, and process. If we use the classic definition—family is

who the patient says it is—then we are in conflict with the individual perspective and legal definitions that currently guide access, payment, and visiting privileges found in practice. Many studies investigate family, but few look across studies or build on other studies. Few of the integrative or systematic reviews that have been done have the level of rigor that is necessary for EBP. Most of the family nursing research studies are descriptive in nature. Few family nursing studies are intervention strategies or measure effectiveness of the intervention in a way that can be replicated. Limited family nursing theory that is relevant is transferred into clinical nursing practice (Segaric & Hall, 2005). All of these obstacles reveal a huge gap between the ideal and the real health care practice settings.

It is suggested that the definition of EBP in nursing and family nursing be revised to address the concerns identified earlier in this section. It must give consideration to the best evidence available and be a pluralistic approach to what constitutes legitimate evidence in family nursing. Family nursing practice should be theory-practice and practice-theory evidence based. Like others in the family nursing arena (e.g., Chesla, 2005; Loveland-Cherry, 2006), family nursing needs to accomplish the following tasks:

- Facilitate professional networking to encourage practice development internationally.
- Form an international family nursing professional nursing organization (Curry, 2007).
- Organize another family nursing "think tank" that would provide guidance and direction for family nursing and create a practice, theory, and research agenda.
- Use action research and teams to collaborate internationally via Internet technologies (Booth, Tolson, Hotchkiss & Schofield, 2007).
- Close the gap between family nursing theory and practice by internationally developing conceptual clarity about family, family health, family stressors, and coping strategies and interventions (Segaric & Hall, 2005).
- Figure out how to make family nursing theory applicable to practice settings for the nurse on the front lines, especially in ritualistic traditional medical model acute care settings (Segaric & Hall, 2005).

SUMMARY

The issues raised in this chapter are meant to bring about discussion, raise awareness, and provide ideas for future action in family nursing. Clearly, the solutions to these volatile issues are not simple; thus, debate and discussion are necessary to assure that family-centered health care remains a priority. What is known is that family nursing will continue to be influenced by the ability of nurses to maintain their commitment to family care. Nurses are and will be important health providers to lead health care reform in decreasing health disparities, encouraging universal health care for families, providing models that encourage healthy family lifestyles, supporting and guiding families during caregiving of ill members, and developing models of family-centered health care. Nurses must move beyond local work settings to enhance family nursing by becoming actively involved in policy design, adoption, and implementation. Nursing education must continue to embrace family nursing as an integral part of the curriculum. Nursing research will generate knowledge generalizable to families, as well as critical use of evidence-based guidelines to demonstrate the effectiveness of family care to enhance family health across settings, time, family structures, and cultures. Family nursing research should have a gold standard of theory guided by EBP.

REFERENCES

American Nurses Association (ANA). (2003a). *Nursing's social policy statement*. Washington, DC: American Nurses Association.

American Nurses Association (ANA). (2003b). *Nursing: Scope and standards of practice*. Washington, DC: American Nurses Association.

American Nurses Association (ANA). (2005). *Health care agenda*. Retrieved May 28, 2009, from http://www.nursingworld.org/FunctionalMenuCategories/MediaResources/PressReleases/2005/pr0613850.aspx

Aos, S., Lieb, R., Mayfield, J., Miller, M., & Pennucci, A. (2004). *Benefits and costs of prevention and early intervention programs for youth*. Olympia, WA: Washington State Institute for Public Policy. Retrieved May 28, 2009, from http://www.wsipp.wa.gov/rptfiles/04-07-3901.pdf

Benner, P. (1983). Uncovering the knowledge embedded in clinical practice. *Image: The Journal of Nursing Scholarship, 15*(2), 36–41.

Biddle, J. (2005, June 1). United air workers face biggest pension default in U.S. history. *Labor Notes, Article 315*. Retrieved May 28, 2009, from http://labornotes.org/node/824

Blendon, R. J., Schoen, C., DesRoches, C. M., Osborn, R., Scoles, K. L., & Zapert, K. (2001). Inequities in health care: A five country survey. *Health Affairs (Milwood), 23*, 182–191.

Bogenschneider, K. (2000). Has family policy come of age? A decade review of the state of U.S. family policy in the 1990s. *Journal of Marriage and the Family, 62*, 1136–1159.

Bolton, L. B. (2006). Raise the voice! Transforming America's health care system through nursing solutions. *Nursing Outlook, 16*(2), 3–4.

Booth, J., Tolson, D., Hotchkiss, R., & Schofield, I. (2007). Using action research to construct national evidence-based nursing care guidance for gerontological nursing. *Journal of Clinical Nursing, 16*, 945–953.

British Columbia Ministry of Health. (2006). *The challenge of chronic condition management in British Columbia*. Retrieved May 28, 2009, from www.health.gov.bc.ca/cdm/practitioners/challenge.pdf

Brookings Institution. (2006). *Employment-based health insurance: A prominent past, but does it have a future?* Washington, DC: Brookings Institution – New America Foundation Forum. Retrieved May 28, 2009, from www.brookings.edu/comm/events/200616.pdf

Canadian Medical Association Task Force on the Public-Private Interface. (2006). *It's about access! Informing the debate on public and private health care*. Ottawa, Ontario, Canada: Commission on the Future of Health Care in Canada.

Canadian Nurse Association. (2008). *Nursing and the political agenda*. Retrieved August 9, 2008, from http://www.cna-nurses.ca/CNA/issues/matters/default_e.aspx

Chesla, C. A. (2005). Family nursing: Challenges and opportunities: The hand that feeds us: Strings and restrictions on funding for family nursing research. *Journal of Family Nursing, 11*, 340–343.

Commission on the Future of Health Care in Canada. (2002). *Building on values, the future of health care in Canada—final report*. Ottawa, Ontario, Canada: Commission on the Future of Health Care in Canada.

Cooke, L., Smith-Idell, C., Dean, G., Gemmill, R., Steingass, S., Sunn, V., et al. (2004). Research to practice: A practical program to enhance the use of evidence based practice at the unit level. *Oncology Nursing Forum, 31*(4), 825–832.

Cutler, D. M. (2002). Equality, efficiency, and market fundamentals: The dynamics of international medical-care reform. *Journal of Economics, 40*, 881–891.

Dawley, K., Loch, J., & Bindrich I. (2007). The nurse-family partnership. *American Journal of Nursing, 107*(11), 60–67.

Dennehy, P., Saxe, J. M., Sweet, J., Budd, D., Niemen, J, Greenwald, J., & Waters, C. (2006). Service demands that have influenced nursing education and training chronic care for a homeless population. Paper presented at the Dimensions of the NP Kaleidoscope: Education Practice, Research & Advocacy, Orlando, FL. Retrieved August 11, 2008, from http://nurseweb.ucsf.edu/public/targeting.htm

Dixon, K. (2006, June 29). Most employers cutting retiree health care. *Reuters*. Retrieved May 28, 2009, from http://www.worldproutassembly.org/archives/2006/06/most_employers.html

Donelan, K., Blendon, R. J., Schoen, C., Davis, K., & Binns, K. (1999). The cost of health system change: Public discontent in five nations. *Health Affiliations (Millwood), 18*, 206–216.

Edlund, B. J., Lufkin, S. R., & Franklin, B. (2003). Long-term care planning for baby boomers: Addressing an uncertain future [Manuscript 2]. *Online Journal of Issues in Nursing, 8*(2). Retrieved May 28, 2009, from www.nursingworld.org/ojin

Feetham, S. L. (2005). Family nursing: Challenges and opportunities: Providing leadership in family nursing from local to global health. *Journal of Family Nursing, 11,* 327–331.

Flemming, K. (2007). The knowledge base for evidence-based nursing: A role for mixed methods research? *Advances in Nursing Science, 30*(1), 41–51.

Gerrish, K., & Clayton, J. (2004). Promoting evidence-based practice: An organizational approach. *Journal of Nursing Management, 12*(2), 114–123.

Gottschalk, M. (2007). Back to the future? Health benefits, organized labor, and universal health care. *Journal of Health Politics, Policy and Law, 32*(6), 923–970.

Hanson, S. M. H. (2005a). The futures of families, health, and family nursing. *Family health care nursing: Theory, practice & research* (3rd ed., pp. 479–506). Philadelphia: F.A. Davis.

Hanson, S. M. H. (2005b). Family nursing: Challenges and opportunities: Whither thou goeth family nursing. *Journal of Family Nursing, 11,* 336–339.

Havinghurst, C. C., & Richman, B. D. (2006). Distributive injustice(s) in American health care. *Law and Contemporary Problems, 69*(1), 1–6.

Herman, A. M. (1999). Futurework: Trends and challenges for work in the 21st century. Retrieved May 28, 2009, from www.dol.gov/asp/ programs/history/herman/reports/futurework/report.htm

Hill, P., Uris, P., & Bauer, T. (2007). The Nurse-Family Partnership: A policy priority: In home nurse visits are cost effective and evidence-based. *American Journal of Nursing, 107*(11), 73-75.

Hockenberry, M., Wilson, D., & Barrera, P. (2006). Implementing evidence-based nursing practice in a pediatric hospital. *Pediatric Nursing, 32*(4), 371–377.

Institute of Medicine. (2003). *Priority areas for national action: Transforming health care quality.* Washington, DC: National Academy Press.

Janson, S., Kroon, L., & Baron, R. (2006, April). Development of interdisciplinary professional education and training: Outcomes and lessons learned. Paper presented at the National Organization for Nurse Practitioner Faculties, Orlando, FL.

Karoly, L. A., Kilbum, R., & Cannon, J. (2005). *Early childhood interventions: Proven results, future promise.* Retrieved August 11, 2008, from the RAND Corporation Web site: http://www.rand.org/pubs/monographis/MG341

Kelly, M. M., Kratz, B., Bielski, M., & Rinehart, P. M. (2002). Implementing transitions for youth with complex chronic conditions using the medical home model. *Pediatrics, 110*(6), 1322–1327.

Kenny, N., & Chafe, R. (2007). Pushing right against the evidence: Turbulent times for Canadian health care. *Hastings Center Report, 37*(5), 24–26.

Landon, B. E., Hicks, L. S., O'Malley, A. J., Lieu, T. A., Keegan, T., McNeil, B. J., et al. (2007). Improving the management of chronic disease at community health centers. *New England Journal of Medicine, 356,* 921–934.

Lasser, K. E., Himmelstein, D. U., & Woolhandler, S. (2006). Access to care, health status, and health disparities in the United States and Canada: Results of a cross-national population-based survey. *American Journal of Public Health, 96*(7), 1300–1307.

Loveland-Cherry, C. J. (2006). Where is the family in family interventions? *Journal of Family Nursing, 12,* 4–6.

Lynn, Schuster, J. L., & Kabcenell, A. (2000). *Improving care for the end-of-life: A sourcebook for health care managers and clinicians,* Arlington, VA: Oxford University Press.

McMenamy, J. M., & Perrin, E. C. (2004). Filling the GAPS: Description and evaluation of a primary care intervention for children with chronic health conditions. *Ambulatory Pediatrics, 4*(3), 249–256.

Milton, C. (2007). Evidence-based practice: Ethical questions for nursing. *Nursing Science Quarterly, 20*(2), 123–126.

Norberg, A. (2006). The meaning of evidence-based nursing. *Nursing Ethics, 13*(5), 453–454.

Oberlander, J. (2006). The political economy of unfairness in U.S. health policy. *Law and Contemporary Problems, 69*(4), 245–264.

O'Donnell, R. O., Cox, K. S., Sharp, G., & Carroll, C. A. (2006). Redesigning the health care system of the future. *Missouri Medicine, 103*(1), 48–50.

O'Neill, J. E., & O'Neill, D. M. (2008). Health status, health care and inequality: Canada versus the U.S. *Forum for Health Economics and Policy: The Berkeley Electronic Press, 10*(1), Article 3.

Parker, M. E. (2006). *Nursing theories & nursing practice* (2nd ed., pp. 29–30). Philadelphia: F.A. Davis.

Pear, R. (2004, April 23). Agency to allow insurance cuts of the retired. *New York Times.* Retrieved May 28, 2009, from http://www.nytimes.com/2004/04/23/us/agency-to-allow-insurance-cuts-for-the-retired.html

Pearson, A., Wiechula, R., Court, A., & Lockwood, C. (2007). A re-consideration of what constitutes "evidence" in healthcare professions. *Nursing Science Quarterly, 20*(1), 85–88.

Piatt, G. A., Orchard, T. J., Emerson, S., Simmons, D., Songer, T. J., Brooks, M. M., et al. (2006). Translating the CCM into the community: Results from a randomized controlled trial of a multifaceted diabetes care intervention. *Diabetes Care, 29,* 811–817.

Saxe, J. M., Janson, S. L., Dennehy, P. M., Stringari-Murray, S., Hirsch, J. E., & Waters, C. M. (2007). Meeting a primary care challenge in the United States: Chronic illness care. *Contemporary Nursing: A Journal For The Australian Nursing Profession, 26*(1), 94-103.

Segaric, C., & Hall, W. (2005). The family theory-practice gap: A matter of clarity? *Nursing Inquiry, 12*(3), 210–218.

Stevens, K. (2004). *ACE star model of knowledge transformation.* Retrieved August 11, 2008, from www.acestar.uthscsa.edu

Wagner, E. H., Bennett, S. M., Austin, B. T., Greene, S. M., Schaefer, J. K., & Vondorff, M. (2005). Finding common ground: Patient-centeredness and evidence-based chronic illness care. *Journal of Alternative and Complimentary Medicine, 11*(Supp. 1), S7-S15.

Wakefield, M. (2004). Linking health policy to nursing and health care scholarship: Points to consider. *Nursing Outlook, 52*(2), 111–113.

Webb, F. J. (2005). Spotlight on theory: The new demographics of families. In V. I. Bengstons, A. C. Acock, K. R. Allen, & P. Dilworth-Anderson (Eds.), *Sourcebook of family theory and research.* Thousand Oaks, CA: Sage.

Family Systems Stressor-Strength Inventory (FS³I)

Shirley May Harmon Hanson

Karen B. Mischke

INSTRUCTIONS FOR ADMINISTRATION

The Family Systems Stressor-Strength Inventory (FS³I) is an assessment and measurement instrument intended for use with families (see Chapter 8). It focuses on identifying stressful situations occurring in families and the strengths families use to maintain healthy family functioning. Each family member is asked to complete the instrument on an individual form before an interview with the clinician. Questions can be read to members unable to read.

After completion of the instrument, the clinician evaluates the family on each of the stressful situations (general and specific) and the strengths they possess. This evaluation is recorded on the family member form.

The clinician records the individual family member's score and the clinician perception score on the Quantitative Summary. A different color code is used for each family member. The clinician also completes the Qualitative Summary, synthesizing the information gleaned from all participants. Clinicians can use the Family Care Plan to prioritize diagnoses, set goals, develop prevention and intervention activities, and evaluate outcomes.

Family Name _____ Date _____

Family Member(s) Completing Assessment _____

Ethnic Background(s) _____

Religious Background(s) _____

Referral Source _____

Interviewer _____

Source: Hanson, S. M. H. (2001). *Family health care nursing: Theory, practice, and research* (2nd ed., pp. 425–437). Philadelphia: F.A. Davis.

Family Members	Relationship in Family	Age	Marital Status	Education (highest degree)	Occupation
1. _____	_____	_____	_____	_____	_____
2. _____	_____	_____	_____	_____	_____
3. _____	_____	_____	_____	_____	_____
4. _____	_____	_____	_____	_____	_____
5. _____	_____	_____	_____	_____	_____
6. _____	_____	_____	_____	_____	_____

Family's current reasons for seeking assistance:

_____

_____

_____

Part I: Family Systems Stressors (General)

DIRECTIONS: Each of 25 situations/stressors listed here deals with some aspect of normal family life. They have the potential for creating stress within families or between families and the world in which they live. We are interested in your overall impression of how these situations affect your family life. Please circle a number (0 through 5) that best describes the amount of stress or tension they create for you.

STRESSORS	DOES NOT APPLY	LITTLE STRESS		MEDIUM STRESS		HIGH STRESS	CLINICIAN PERCEPTION SCORE
1. Family member(s) feel unappreciated	0	1	2	3	4	5	_____
2. Guilt for not accomplishing more	0	1	2	3	4	5	_____
3. Insufficient "me" time	0	1	2	3	4	5	_____
4. Self-Image/self-esteem/ feelings of unattractiveness	0	1	2	3	4	5	_____
5. Perfectionism	0	1	2	3	4	5	_____
6. Dieting	0	1	2	3	4	5	_____
7. Health/Illness	0	1	2	3	4	5	_____
8. Communication with children	0	1	2	3	4	5	_____
							_____
9. Housekeeping standards	0	1	2	3	4	5	_____
10. Insufficient couple time	0	1	2	3	4	5	_____
11. Insufficient family playtime	0	1	2	3	4	5	_____
12. Children's behavior/ discipline/sibling fighting	0	1	2	3	4	5	_____
13. Television	0	1	2	3	4	5	_____
14. Overscheduled family calendar	0	1	2	3	4	5	_____
15. Lack of shared responsibility in the family	0	1	2	3	4	5	_____

The FAMILY PERCEPTION SCORE column spans LITTLE STRESS, MEDIUM STRESS, and HIGH STRESS headings.

| | FAMILY PERCEPTION SCORE | | | | CLINICIAN PERCEPTION |
| | | | | | |

STRESSORS	DOES NOT APPLY	LITTLE STRESS		MEDIUM STRESS		HIGH STRESS		SCORE
16. Moving	0	1	2	3	4	5		_____
17. Spousal relationship (communication, friendship, sex)	0	1	2	3	4	5		_____
18. Holidays	0	1	2	3	4	5		_____
19. In-laws	0	1	2	3	4	5		_____
20. Teen behaviors (communication, music, friends, school)	0	1	2	3	4	5		_____
21. New baby	0	1	2	3	4	5		_____
22. Economics/finances/budgets	0	1	2	3	4	5		_____
23. Unhappiness with work situation	0	1	2	3	4	5		_____
24. Overvolunteerism	0	1	2	3	4	5		_____
25. Neighbors	0	1	2	3	4	5		_____

Additional Stressors: _____

_____

Family Remarks: _____

_____

Clinician: Clarification of stressful situations/concerns with family members.

Prioritize in order of importance to family members: _____

_____

Part II: Family Systems Stressors (Specific)

DIRECTIONS: The following 12 questions are designed to provide information about your specific stress-producing situation/problem or area of concern influencing your family's health. Please circle a number (1 through 5) that best describes the influence this situation has on your family's life and how well you perceive your family's overall functioning.

The specific stress-producing situation/problem or area of concern at this time is: _____

_____

_____

STRESSORS	FAMILY PERCEPTION SCORE					CLINICIAN PERCEPTION
	LITTLE		MEDIUM		HIGH	SCORE
1. To what extent is your family bothered by this problem or stressful situation? (e.g., effects on family interactions, communication among members, emotional and social relationships)	1	2	3	4	5	_____

Family Remarks: _____

Clinician Remarks: _____

| 2. How much of an effect does this stresssful situation have on your family's usual pattern of living? (e.g., effects on lifestyle patterns and family developmental task) | 1 | 2 | 3 | 4 | 5 | _____ |

Family Remarks: _____

Clinician Remarks: _____

| 3. How much has this situation affected your family's ability to work together as a family unit? (e.g., alteration in family roles, completion of family tasks, following through with responsibilities) | 1 | 2 | 3 | 4 | 5 | _____ |

Family Remarks: _____

Clinician Remarks: _____

Has your family ever experienced a similar concern in the past?
1. YES   If YES, complete question 4
2. NO   If NO, complete question 5

| 4. How successful was your family in dealing with this situation/problem/concern in the past? (e.g., workable coping strategies developed, adaptive measures useful, situation improved) | 1 | 2 | 3 | 4 | 5 | _____ |

Family Remarks: _____

Clinician Remarks: _____

STRESSORS	FAMILY PERCEPTION SCORE			CLINICIAN PERCEPTION
	LITTLE	MEDIUM	HIGH	SCORE
5. How strongly do you feel this current situation/problem/concern will affect your family's future? (e.g., anticipated consequences)	1　2	3　4	5	_____

Family Remarks: _____

_____

Clinician Remarks: _____

_____

STRESSORS	LITTLE	MEDIUM	HIGH	SCORE
6. To what extent are family members able to help themselves in this present situation/problem/concern? (e.g., self-assistive efforts, family expectations, spiritual influence, family resources)	1　2	3　4	5	_____

Family Remarks: _____

_____

Clinician Remarks: _____

_____

STRESSORS	LITTLE	MEDIUM	HIGH	SCORE
7. To what extent do you expect others to help your family with this situation/problem/concern? (e.g., what roles would helpers play; how available are extra-family resources)	1　2	3　4	5	_____

Family Remarks: _____

_____

Clinician Remarks: _____

_____

STRESSORS	POOR	SATISFACTORY	EXCELLENT	SCORE
8. How would you rate the way your family functions overall? (e.g., how your family members relate to each other and to larger family and community)	1　2	3　4	5	_____

Family Remarks: _____

_____

Clinician Remarks: _____

_____

STRESSORS		FAMILY PERCEPTION SCORE				CLINICIAN PERCEPTION
	POOR	SATISFACTORY		EXCELLENT		SCORE

9. How would you rate the overall physical health status of each family member by name? (Include yourself as a family member; record additional names on back.)

	POOR		SATISFACTORY		EXCELLENT	SCORE
a. _____	1	2	3	4	5	_____
b. _____	1	2	3	4	5	_____
c. _____	1	2	3	4	5	_____
d. _____	1	2	3	4	5	_____
e. _____	1	2	3	4	5	_____

10. How would you rate the overall physical health status of your family as a whole?   1   2   3   4   5   _____

Family Remarks: _____

_____

Clinician Remarks: _____

_____

11. How would you rate the overall mental health status of each family member by name? (Include yourself as a family member; record additional names on back.)

	POOR		SATISFACTORY		EXCELLENT	SCORE
a. _____	1	2	3	4	5	_____
b. _____	1	2	3	4	5	_____
c. _____	1	2	3	4	5	_____
d. _____	1	2	3	4	5	_____
e. _____	1	2	3	4	5	_____

12. How would you rate the overall mental health status of your family as a whole?   1   2   3   4   5   _____

Family Remarks: _____

_____

Clinician Remarks: _____

_____

Part III: Family Systems Strengths

DIRECTIONS: Each of the 16 traits/attributes listed below deals with some aspect of family life and its overall functioning. Each one contributes to the health and well-being of family members as individuals and to the family as a whole. Please circle a number (0 through 5) that best describes the extent to which the trait applies to your family.

	DOES NOT APPLY	SELDOM	FAMILY PERCEPTION SCORE USUALLY	ALWAYS		CLINICIAN PERCEPTION SCORE
MY FAMILY						
1. Communicates and listens to one another	0	1 2	3	4	5	_____

Family Remarks: _____

_____

Clinician Remarks: _____

_____

| 2. Affirms and supports one another | 0 | 1   2 | 3 | 4 | 5 | _____ |

Family Remarks: _____

_____

Clinician Remarks: _____

_____

| 3. Teaches respect for others | 0 | 1   2 | 3 | 4 | 5 | _____ |

Family Remarks: _____

_____

Clinician Remarks: _____

_____

| 4. Develops a sense of trust in members | 0 | 1   2 | 3 | 4 | 5 | _____ |

Family Remarks: _____

_____

Clinician Remarks: _____

_____

| 5. Displays a sense of play and humor | 0 | 1   2 | 3 | 4 | 5 | _____ |

Family Remarks: _____

_____

Clinician Remarks: _____

_____

| 6. Exhibits a sense of shared responsibility | 0 | 1   2 | 3 | 4 | 5 | _____ |

Family Remarks: _____

_____

Clinician Remarks: _____

_____

MY FAMILY	DOES NOT APPLY		SELDOM	FAMILY PERCEPTION SCORE				CLINICIAN PERCEPTION
				USUALLY		ALWAYS		SCORE
7. Teaches a sense of right and wrong	0	1		2	3	4	5	_____

Family Remarks: _____

_____

Clinician Remarks: _____

_____

8. Has a strong sense of family in which rituals and traditions abound	0	1		2	3	4	5	_____

Family Remarks: _____

_____

Clinician Remarks: _____

_____

9. Has a balance of interaction among members	0	1		2	3	4	5	_____

Family Remarks: _____

_____

Clinician Remarks: _____

_____

10. Has a shared religious core	0	1		2	3	4	5	_____

Family Remarks: _____

_____

Clinician Remarks: _____

_____

11. Respects the privacy of one another	0	1		2	3	4	5	_____

Family Remarks: _____

_____

Clinician Remarks: _____

_____

12. Values service to others	0	1		2	3	4	5	_____

Family Remarks: _____

_____

Clinician Remarks: _____

_____

MY FAMILY	DOES NOT APPLY	SELDOM	FAMILY PERCEPTION SCORE USUALLY	ALWAYS	CLINICIAN PERCEPTION SCORE

13. Fosters family table
    time and conversation   0   1   2   3   4   5   _____

Family Remarks: _____

Clinician Remarks: _____

14. Shares leisure time   0   1   2   3   4   5   _____

Family Remarks: _____

Clinician Remarks: _____

15. Admits to and seeks
    help with problems   0   1   2   3   4   5   _____

Family Remarks: _____

Clinician Remarks: _____

16a. How would you rate
     the overall strengths that
     exist in your family?   0   1   2   3   4   5   _____

Family Remarks: _____

Clinician Remarks: _____

16b. Additional Family Strengths: _____
_____
_____

16c. Clinician: Clarification of family strengths with individual members: _____
_____
_____
_____

Family Systems Stressor-Strength Inventory (FS³I) Scoring Summary
Section 1: Family Perception Scores

INSTRUCTIONS FOR ADMINISTRATION

The Family Systems Stressor-Strength Inventory (FS³I) Scoring Summary is divided into two sections: Section 1, Family Perception Scores, and Section 2, Clinician Perception Scores. These two sections are further divided into three parts: Part I, Family Systems Stressors (General); Part II, Family Systems Stressors (Specific); and Part III, Family Systems Strengths. Each part contains a Quantitative Summary and a Qualitative Summary.

Quantifiable family and clinician perception scores are both graphed on the Quantitative Summary. Each family member has a designated color code. Family and clinician remarks are both recorded on the Quantitative Summary. Quantitative Summary scores, when graphed, suggest a level for initiation of prevention/intervention modes: Primary, Secondary, and Tertiary. Qualitative Summary information, when synthesized, contributes to the development and channeling of the Family Care Plan.

Part 1 Family Systems Stressors (General)

Add scores from questions 1 to 25 and calculate an overall numerical score for Family Systems Stressors (General). Ratings are from 1 (most positive) to 5 (most negative). The Does Not Apply (0) responses are omitted from the calculations. Total scores range from 25 to 125.
Family Systems Stressor Score (General)

$(_{25}) \times 1 =$

Graph score on Quantitative Summary, Family Systems Stressors (General), Family Member Perception Score. Color-code to differentiate family members. Record additional stressors and family remarks in Part I, Qualitative Summary: Family and Clinician Remarks.

Part II Family Systems Stressors (Specific)

Add scores from questions 1 through 8, 10, and 12 and calculate a numerical score for Family Systems Stressors (Specific). Ratings are from 1 (most positive) to 5 (most negative). Questions 4, 6, 7, 8, 10 and 12

are reverse scored.* Total scores range from 10 through 50.
Family Systems Stressor Score (Specific)

$(_{10}) \times 1 =$

Graph score on Quantitative Summary, Family Systems Stressors (Specific) Family Member Perception Score. Color-code to differentiate family members. Summarize data from questions 9 and 11 (reverse scored) and record family remarks in Part II, Qualitative Summary: Family and Clinician Remarks.

Part III Family Systems Strengths

Add scores from questions 1 through 16 and calculate a numerical score for Family Systems Strengths. Ratings are from 1 (seldom) to 5 (always). The Does Not Apply (0) responses are omitted from the calculations. Total Scores range from 16 to 80.

$(_{16}) \times 1 =$

Graph score on Quantitative Summary: Family Systems Strengths, Family Member Perception Score. Record additional family strengths and family remarks in Part III, Qualitative Summary: Family and Clinician Remarks.

Source: Mischke-Berkey, K., & Hanson, S. M. H. (1991). *Pocket guide to family assessment and intervention.* St. Louis, MO: Mosby.
*Reverse scoring:
Question answered as (1) is scored 5 points.
Question answered as (2) is scored 4 points.
Question answered as (3) is scored 3 points.
Question answered as (4) is scored 2 points.
Question answered as (5) is scored 1 point.

Section 2: Clinician Perception Scores

Part I Family Systems Stressors (General)*

Add scores from questions 1 through 25 and calculate an overall numerical score for Family Systems Stressors (General). Ratings are from 1 (most positive) to 5 (most negative). The Does Not Apply (0) responses are omitted from the calculations. Total scores range from 25 to 125.

Family systems Stressor Score (General)

$(_{25}) \times 1 =$

Graph score on Quantitative Summary, Family Systems Stressors (General) Clinician Perception Score. Record clinicians' clarification of general stressors in Part I, Qualitative Summary: Family and Clinician Remarks.

Part II Family Systems Stressors (Specific)

Add scores from questions 1 through 8, 10, 12 and calculate a numerical score for Family Systems Stressors (Specific). Ratings are from 1 (most positive) to 5 (most negative). Questions 4, 6, 7, 8, 10, 12 are reverse scored.* Total scores range from 10 to 50.

Family Systems Stressor Score (Specific)

$(_{10}) \times 1 =$

Graph score on Quantitative Summary, Family Systems Stressors (Specific), Clinician Perception Score. Summarized data from questions 9 and 11 (reverse order) and record clinician remarks in Part II, Qualitative Summary: Family and Clinician Remarks.

Part III Family Systems Strengths

Add scores from questions 1 through 16 and calculate a numerical score for Family Systems Strengths. Ratings are from 1 (seldom) to 5 (always). The Does Not Apply (0) responses are omitted from the calculations. Total scores range from 16 to 80.

$(_{16}) \times 1 =$

Graph score on Quantitative Summary, Family Systems Strengths, Clinician Perception Score. Record clinicians' clarification of family strengths in Part III, Qualitative Summary: Family and Clinician Remarks.

---

*Reverse scoring:
Question answered as (1) is scored 5 points.
Question answered as (2) is scored 4 points.
Question answered as (3) is scored 3 points.
Question answered as (4) is scored 2 points.
Question answered as (5) is scored 1 point.

QUANTITATIVE SUMMARY OF FAMILY SYSTEMS STRESSORS: GENERAL AND SPECIFIC FAMILY AND CLINICIAN PERCEPTION SCORES

DIRECTIONS: Graph the scores from each family member inventory by placing an "X" at the appropriate location. (Use first name initial for each different entry and different color code for each family member.)

	FAMILY SYSTEMS STRESSORS (GENERAL)			FAMILY SYSTEMS STRESSORS (SPECIFIC)	
SCORES FOR WELLNESS AND STABILITY	FAMILY MEMBER PERCEPTION SCORE	CLINICIAN PERCEPTION SCORE	SCORES FOR WELLNESS AND STABILITY	FAMILY MEMBER PERCEPTION SCORE	CLINICIAN PERCEPTION SCORE
5.0			5.0		
4.8			4.8		
4.6			4.6		
4.4			4.4		
4.2			4.2		
4.0			4.0		
3.8			3.8		
3.6			3.6		
3.4			3.4		
3.2			3.2		
3.0			3.0		
2.8			2.8		
2.6			2.6		
2.4			2.4		
2.2			2.2		
2.0			2.0		
1.8			1.8		
1.6			1.6		
1.4			1.4		
1.2			1.2		
1.0			1.0		

*PRIMARY Prevention/Intervention Mode: Flexible Line   1.0–2.3
*SECONDARY Prevention/Intervention Mode: Normal Line   2.4–3.6
*TERTIARY Prevention/Intervention Mode: Resistance Lines   3.7–5.0
*Breakdowns of numerical scores for stressor penetration are suggested values.

Family Systems Strengths
Family and Clinician Perception Scores

DIRECTIONS: Graph the scores from the inventory by placing an "X" at the appropriate location and connect with a line. (Use first name initial for each different entry and different color code for each family member.)

SUM OF STRENGTHS AVAILABLE FOR PREVENTION/ INTERVENTION MODE	FAMILY SYSTEMS STRENGTHS	
	FAMILY MEMBER PERCEPTION SCORE	CLINICIAN PERCEPTION SCORE
5.0		
4.8		
4.6		
4.4		
4.2		
4.0		
3.8		
3.6		
3.4		
3.2		
3.0		
2.8		
2.6		
2.4		
2.2		
2.0		
1.8		
1.6		
1.4		
1.2		
1.0		

*PRIMARY Prevention/Intervention Mode: Flexible Line   1.0–2.3
*SECONDARY Prevention/Intervention Mode: Normal Line   2.4–3.6
*TERTIARY Prevention/Intervention Mode: Resistance Lines   3.7–5.0
*Breakdowns of numerical scores for stressor penetration are suggested values.

QUALITATIVE SUMMARY FAMILY AND CLINICIAN REMARKS

Part I: Family Systems Stressors (General)

Summarize general stressors and remarks of family and clinician. Prioritize stressors according to importance to family members.

_____
_____
_____

Part II: Family Systems Stressors (Specific)

A. Summarize specific stressors and remarks of family and clinician.

_____
_____
_____

B. Summarize differences (if discrepancies exist) between how family members and clinicians view effects of stressful situation on family.

_____
_____
_____

C. Summarize overall family functioning.

_____
_____
_____

D. Summarize overall significant physical health status for family members.

_____
_____
_____

E. Summarize overall significant mental health status for family members.

_____
_____
_____

Part III: Family Systems Strengths

Summarize family systems strengths and family and clinician remarks that facilitate family health and stability.

_____
_____
_____

Family Care Plan*

DIAGNOSIS GENERAL AND SPECIFIC FAMILY SYSTEM STRESSORS	FAMILY SYSTEMS STRENGTHS SUPPORTING FAMILY CARE PLAN	GOALS FOR FAMILY AND CLINICIAN	PREVENTION/INTERVENTION MODE		
			PRIMARY, SECONDARY, OR TERTIARY	PREVENTION/ INTERVENTION ACTIVITIES	OUTCOMES EVALUATION AND REPLANNING

*Prioritize the three most significant diagnoses.

The Friedman Family Assessment Model (Short Form)

The following Friedman Family Assessment Short Form is useful as a quick instrument to help highlight areas of family function that will need more exploration. Before using the following guidelines in completing family assessments, two words of caution are noted: First, not all areas included below will be germane for each of the families visited. The guidelines are comprehensive and allow depth when probing is necessary. The student should not feel that every subarea needs be covered when the broad area of inquiry poses no problems to the family or concern to the health worker. Second, by virtue of the interdependence of the family system, one will find unavoidable redundancy. For the sake of efficiency, the assessor should try not to repeat data, but to refer the reader back to sections where this information has already been described.

Identifying Data

1. Family Name
2. Address and Phone
3. Family Composition: The Family Genogram
4. Type of Family Form
5. Cultural (Ethnic) Background
6. Religious Identification
7. Social Class Status
8. Social Class Mobility

Developmental Stage and History of Family

9. Family's Present Developmental Stage
10. Extent of Family Developmental Tasks Fulfillment
11. Nuclear Family History
12. History of Family of Origin of Both Parents

Environmental Data

13. Characteristics of Home
14. Characteristics of Neighborhood and Larger Community
15. Family's Geographical Mobility
16. Family's Associations and Transactions with Community

Family Structure

17. Communication Patterns
    Extent of Functional and Dysfunctional Communication (types of recurring patterns)
    Extent of Emotional (Affective) Messages and How Expressed
    Characteristics of Communication Within Family Subsystems
    Extent of Congruent and Incongruent Messages

Types of Dysfunctional Communication Processes Seen in Family
Areas of Closed Communication
Familial and Contextual Variables Affecting Communication

18. **Power Structure**
    Power Outcomes
    Decision-making Process
    Power Bases
    Variables Affecting Family Power
    Overall Family System and Subsystem Power (Family Power Continuum Placement)

19. **Role Structure**
    Formal Role Structure
    Informal Role Structure
    Analysis of Role Models (optional)
    Variables Affecting Role Structure

20. **Family Values**
    Compare the family to American core values or family's reference group values and/or identify important family values and their importance (priority) in family.
    Congruence Between the Family's Values and the Family's Reference Group or Wider Community
    Disparity in Value Systems
    Presence of Value Conflicts in Family
    Effect of the Above Values and Value Conflicts on Health Status of Family

Family Functions

21. **Affective Function**
    Mutual Nurturance, Closeness, and Identification
    Family attachment diagram, Figure 14-2, is helpful here.
    Separateness and Connectedness
    Family's Need-Response Patterns

22. **Socialization Function**
    Family Child-rearing Practices
    Adaptability of Child-rearing Practices for Family Form and Family's Situation
    Who Is (Are) Socializing Agent(s) for Child(ren)?
    Value of Children in Family
    Cultural Beliefs that Influence Family's Child-rearing Patterns

Social Class Influence on Child-rearing Patterns
Estimation About Whether Family Is at Risk for Child-rearing Problems and if So, Indication of High-Risk Factors
Adequacy of Home Environment for Children's Needs to Play

23. **Health Care Function**
    Family's Health Beliefs, Values, and Behavior
    Family's Definitions of Health-Illness and Its Level of Knowledge
    Family's Perceived Health Status and Illness Susceptibility
    Family's Dietary Practices
    Adequacy of family diet (recommended 3-day food history record)
    Function of mealtimes and attitudes toward food and mealtimes
    Shopping (and its planning) practices
    Person(s) responsible for planning, shopping, and preparation of meals
    Sleep and Rest Habits
    Physical Activity and Recreation Practices
    Family's Therapeutic and Recreational Drug, Alcohol, and Tobacco Practices
    Family's Role in Self-care Practice
    Medically Based Preventive Measures (physicals, eye and hearing tests, immunizations, dental care)
    Complementary and Alternative Therapies
    Family Health History (both general and specific diseases—environmentally and genetically related)
    Health Care Services Received
    Feelings and Perceptions Regarding Health Services
    Emergency Health Services
    Source of Payments for Health and Other Services
    Logistics of Receiving Care

Family Stress, Coping, and Adaptation

24. **Family Stressors, Strengths, and Perceptions**
    Stressors Family Is Experiencing
    Strengths That Counterbalance Stressors
    Family's Definition of the Situation

25. **Family Coping Strategies**
    How the Family Is Reacting to the Stressors
    Extent of Family's Use of Internal Coping Strategies (past/present)
    Extent of Family's Use of External Coping Strategies (past/present)
    Dysfunctional Coping Strategies Utilized (past/present; extent of use)

26. **Family Adaptation**
    Overall Family Adaptation
    Estimation of Whether Family Is in Crisis

27. **Tracking Stressors, Coping, and Adaptation Over Time**

Source: Friedman, M. M., Bowden, V. R., Jones, E. G. (2003). *Family nursing: Research, theory, and practice* (5th ed). pp. 593–594. Upper Saddle River, NJ: Prentice Hall.

INDEX